Health Informatics Research Methods

Principles and Practice

Second Edition

Volume Editors

Valerie J. Watzlaf, PhD, MPH, RHIA, FAHIMA

Elizabeth J. Forrestal, PhD, RHIA, CCS, FAHIMA

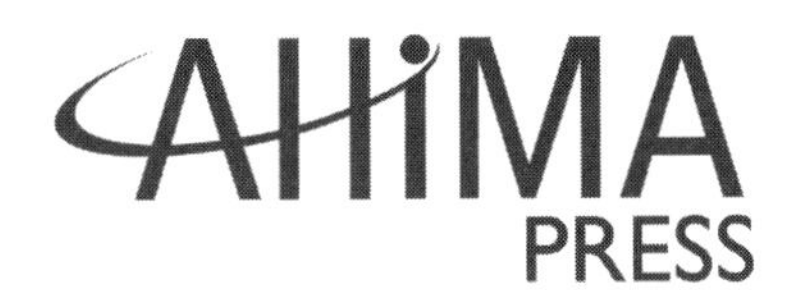

ISBN: 978-1-58426-532-0

AHIMA Product No.: AB120916

AHIMA Staff:

Jessica Block, MA, Project Editor
Chelsea Brotherton, MA, Assistant Editor
Elizabeth Ranno, Vice President of Product and Planning
Pamela Woolf, Director of Publications

Cover image: © Blueberries, iStock

For more information, including updates, about AHIMA Press publications, visit **http://www.ahima.org/education/press**.

American Health Information Management Association
233 North Michigan Avenue, 21st Floor
Chicago, Illinois 60601-5809
ahima.org

Brief Table of Contents

Table of Contents iv
About the Authors xi
Foreword xiii
Preface xv
Acknowledgments xviii
Online Resources xix

Part I Research Designs and Methods

1 Research Frame and Designs 3
Elizabeth J. Forrestal, PhD, RHIA, CCS, FAHIMA

2 Survey Research 35
Valerie J. Watzlaf, PhD, MPH, RHIA, FAHIMA

3 Observational Research 53
Valerie J. Watzlaf, PhD, MPH, RHIA, FAHIMA

4 Experimental and Quasi-Experimental Research 71
Valerie J. Watzlaf, PhD, MPH, RHIA, FAHIMA

5 Epidemiological Research 85
Valerie J. Watzlaf, PhD, MPH, RHIA, FAHIMA

6 Evaluation Methods 109
Jennifer Hornung Garvin, PhD, MBA, RHIA, CPHQ, CCS, CTR, FAHIMA

7 Data Science and Data Mining 123
Ryan H. Sandefer, PhD

8 Systematic Reviews and Meta-Analyses 141
Leming Zhou, PhD, DSc, Dilhari DeAlmeida, PhD, RHIA, and Valerie Watzlaf, PhD, MPH, RHIA, FAHIMA

Part II Research Process

9 Applied Statistics 163
Elizabeth J. Forrestal, PhD, RHIA, CCS, FAHIMA

10 Defining the Research Question and Performing a Literature Review 191
Elizabeth J. Forrestal, PhD, RHIA, CCS, FAHIMA

11 Selecting the Research Design and Method and Collecting Data 213
Elizabeth J. Forrestal, PhD, RHIA, CCS, FAHIMA

12 Analyzing Data and Presenting Results 241
Elizabeth J. Forrestal, PhD, RHIA, CCS, FAHIMA

Part III Information to Knowledge

13 The Grant Process and Proposal Writing 273
Valerie Watzlaf, PhD, MPH, RHIA, FAHIMA

14 Research and Ethics 289
Laurinda B. Harman, PhD, RHIA, FAHIMA

15 Disseminating Information 315
Elizabeth J. Forrestal, PhD, RHIA, CCS, FAHIMA

Glossary 333
Index 349

Table of Contents

Brief Table of Contents iii
About the Authors xi
Foreword xiii
Preface xv
Acknowledgments xviii
Online Resources xix

Part I Research Designs and Methods

1 Research Frame and Designs . . . 3

What Are Health Informatics Research and HIM Research? . . . 4

Purposes of Health Informatics Research and HIM Research . . . 4

Research Frame . . . 5

Scientific Inquiry . . . 9

Research Designs . . . 10

Historical Research . . . 12

Descriptive Research . . . 13

Correlational Research . . . 14

Observational Research . . . 16

Evaluation Research . . . 20

Experimental Research . . . 23

Quasi-experimental Research . . . 25

Time Frame as an Element of Research Design . . . 26

2 Survey Research . . . 35

Survey Creation . . . 37

Use of Existing Surveys . . . 37

New Survey Development . . . 37

Inclusion and Exclusion Criteria . . . 39

Types of Questions . . . 39

Scales . . . 40

Pilot Test Survey . . . 42

Validity and Reliability . . . 42

Audience . . . 43

Framing of Questions . . . 43

Incentives . . . 44

Confidential Responses . . . 44

Limitations, Bias, and Error . . . 44

Type or Medium . . . 44

Distribution of Survey . . . 45

Sample and Sample Size . . . 46

Sampling Methods . . . 46

Part I

Example of Sample Size Calculation Used for the EHR Study . . . 46
Response Rate . . . 48
Statistical Analysis of the Survey Study Data . . . 49
3 Observational Research . . . 53
Nonparticipant Observation . . . 55
Naturalistic Observation . . . 55
Simulation Observation . . . 56
Case Study . . . 56
Focused Interview . . . 58
Participant Observation . . . 62
Ethnography . . . 63
Content Analysis . . . 65
Constant Comparative Method . . . 67
Software for Content Analysis . . . 68
4 Experimental and Quasi-Experimental Research . . . 71
Elements of Experimental Research Study Design . . . 72
Randomization . . . 72
Crossover Design . . . 73
Observation . . . 73
Control Group . . . 74
Treatment . . . 74
Types of Experimental Study Designs . . . 74
Pretest-Posttest Control Group Method . . . 75
Solomon Four-Group Method . . . 76
Posttest-Only Control Group Method . . . 76
Types of Quasi-Experimental Study Designs . . . 77
One-Shot Case Study . . . 78
One-Group Pretest-Posttest Method . . . 78
Static Group Comparison . . . 79
Internal and External Validity . . . 79
Factors Affecting Internal Validity . . . 80
Factors Affecting External Validity . . . 81
Additional Concerns Affecting Validity . . . 81
5 Epidemiological Research . . . 85
Types of Epidemiology and its Effectiveness in Eradicating Disease . . . 86
Epidemiology and Health Informatics . . . 86
Epidemiological Study Designs . . . 87
Descriptive Study Design . . . 87
Analytic Study Designs . . . 90
Experimental Research Study Designs . . . 99
Epidemiological Models of Causation . . . 102
Infectious Disease Model . . . 102

Chronic Disease Model . . . 102
Using Epidemiological Models of Causation in Health Informatics . . . 103
Rules of Evidence for Causality . . . 104
6 Evaluation Methods . . . 109
Evaluations in Health Informatics and Health Information Management . . . 110
Formative Evaluation . . . 111
Summative Evaluation . . . 111
Stakeholders . . . 111
Evaluation Projects versus Evaluation Research . . . 111
Evaluation Research . . . 112
Identifying Scientific Gaps . . . 112
Identifying a Theoretic Framework . . . 112
Healthcare Organizations as Complex Adaptive Systems . . . 113
Using Design Principles for Health Information Technology . . . 114
The Five Rights of Clinical Decision Support . . . 114
User-Centered Design . . . 114
Development of an Evaluation Plan . . . 116
Theory of Change . . . 116
Evaluation Questions . . . 117
Evaluation Data Collection and Activities . . . 117
Examples of Evaluation Research Studies from the Scientific Literature . . . 118
Process Evaluation . . . 118
Goal-Based and Impact Evaluation . . . 118
Outcome Evaluation . . . 119
Additional Evaluation Resources in Health Informatics . . . 119
7 Data Science and Data Mining . . . 123
Data Science . . . 125
Business Understanding . . . 127
Data Understanding . . . 127
Data Preparation . . . 133
Modeling . . . 133
Evaluation . . . 136
Deployment . . . 137
8 Systematic Reviews and Meta-Analyses . . . 141
Steps in Conducting a Systematic Review . . . 143
Step 1: Defining the Research Question(s) . . . 144
Step 2: Creating the Systematic Review Protocol . . . 145
Step 3: Identifying the Terms of the Project . . . 146
Step 4: Defining Inclusion and Exclusion Criteria . . . 146
Step 5: Performing Searches in Databases . . . 147
Step 6: Selecting Articles According to Inclusion and Exclusion Criteria . . . 149
Step 7: Reviewing and Extracting Data from Articles . . . 151
Step 8: Conducting Quality Appraisal and Data Analysis (Meta-Analysis) . . . 152
Step 9: Writing a Final Report . . . 157

Part II Research Process

9 Applied Statistics 163

Goals of Quantitative Researchers 164

Probability 164

Random Sampling 165

Level of Data 165

Nominal, Ordinal, Interval, and Ratio Data 165

Other Terms Associated with Level of Data 166

Parametric Data Versus Nonparametric Data 166

Associations among Variables 166

Factors in Selecting a Statistical Test 167

Purpose of the Research 169

Type of Variable 169

Number of Variables 169

Nature of the Target Population 170

Number, Size, and Independence of Groups 170

Descriptive Statistics 171

Purposes of Descriptive Statistics 171

Frequency Distributions 171

Ratios and Proportions 177

Measures of Central Tendency 177

Measures of Dispersion 178

Correlation 178

Inferential Statistics 178

Independent One-Sample t-Test 179

Independent-Measures t-Test 179

Mann-Whitney U Test 179

Chi-Square Test 179

Fisher Exact Test 180

Paired t-Test 180

Wilcoxon Signed-Rank Test 180

Analysis of Variance 181

Pearson Product-Moment Correlation Coefficient 182

Spearman Rank Order Correlation 182

Simple Regression 183

Multiple Regression 183

Other Tests and Terms 184

Misuse of Statistics 184

Invalid Statistics for Ordinal Data 185

Lying with Statistics 185

Unit of Analysis Error 185

Confusing Correlation with Causation 185

Part II 10 Defining the Research Question and Performing a Literature Review . . . 191
Development and Refinement of a Research Topic . . . 192
Development of a Research Question . . . 193
Problem Statement . . . 196
Hypothesis . . . 197
Purpose Statement . . . 199
Literature Review . . . 200
Purposes of the Literature Review . . . 201
Process of the Literature Review . . . 202
Development of the Literature Review . . . 208
11 Selecting the Research Design and Method and Collecting Data . . . 213
Selecting a Research Design and Method . . . 214
Purpose of the Research . . . 214
Internal Validity and External Validity . . . 214
Other Factors in Selecting a Research Design and Method . . . 215
Planning to Collect Data . . . 215
Quantitative Plan for Data Collection . . . 215
Qualitative Plan for Data Collection . . . 216
Selection of an Instrument . . . 216
Sources of Instruments . . . 216
Validity of Instruments . . . 216
Reliability of Instruments . . . 220
Factors in Selecting an Instrument . . . 222
Examples of Instruments Used in Health Informatics and HIM . . . 227
Techniques and Tools of Data Collection . . . 227
Surveys . . . 228
Observations . . . 228
Elicitation . . . 228
Data Mining . . . 229
Sampling and Samples . . . 230
Target Population and Sample . . . 230
Data Sampling Methods and Types of Samples . . . 230
Sample Size . . . 232
Sample Size Calculation . . . 232
Response Rate . . . 233
Data Collection Procedures . . . 234
Approvals of Oversight Committees . . . 234
Training and Testing . . . 234
Pilot Study . . . 234
Assembling and Storing Data . . . 234
12 Analyzing Data and Presenting Results . . . 241
Quantitative Data Analysis . . . 243
Statistical Analysis Plan . . . 243

Part II

Statistical Significance Versus Practical Significance 244
Null Hypothesis Significance Testing and Significance Level 244
Power 245
Type I Error and Type II Error 245
Preparation of Data 245
Descriptive Statistics 247
Inferential Statistics 253
Data Analysis in Data Mining 254
Statistical Conclusion Validity 257
Quantitative Analytic Software Programs 258

Qualitative Data Analysis 258
Grounded Theory 259
Content Analysis 261
Conclusion Validity 261
Qualitative Analytic Software Programs 262

Presentation of Results and Discussion 263
Tabular and Graphical Display 263
Narrative 263

Part III **Information to Knowledge**

13 The Grant Process and Proposal Writing 273

Preparing to Write a Grant 274
Monitor Research Trends and Problems in Areas of Expertise 275
Build Credibility in Area of Expertise Through Publication 275

Sources of Grants 275
Internal Sources and Foundations 275
Local and State Entities 276
Federal Entities 276

Writing the Grant Proposal 276
Basic Application Criteria 277
Minimum Performance Requirements as Specified in Applications 278

Grant Proposal Review Criteria 282
Peer Review 282
Programmatic Requirements for Grant Recipients 282
Financial Requirements 283
Administrative Requirements 283

Key Individuals in the Granting Agency Process 283
Program Officer 283
Proposal Reviewers 284

Grant Proposal Review Process 284
Role of Proposal Reviewers 284
Panel Assessment and Ranking 286
Funding Entity's Decision 286
Reasons Why a Proposal May Not Get Funded 287

Revising Grant Proposals 287

Part III

14 **Research and Ethics** . . . 289

Biomedical Research and Ethics . . . 290

What Is Ethics in Research and Why Is It Important? . . . 290

Two Approaches to Ethics in Research . . . 290

Ethical Principles and Examples of Breaches of Ethical Principles . . . 292

Codes of Ethics for Researchers . . . 296

International Protection of Human Research Subjects . . . 297

The Nuremburg Code . . . 297

Declaration of Helsinki . . . 297

Federal Laws and Regulations . . . 298

Policy and Procedure Order 129 . . . 298

National Research Act of 1974 . . . 298

Belmont Report . . . 298

Federal Policy for the Protection of Human Subjects and the "Common Rule" . . . 299

HIPAA and HITECH Act . . . 304

Health Research Extension Act of 1985 . . . 306

Support and Training for Researchers . . . 306

Local-Level Ethical Research Guidelines and Procedures . . . 306

Bioethics Committees . . . 307

Ethical Climate for Research . . . 307

15 **Disseminating Information** . . . 315

Formats for Disseminating Research . . . 316

Presentation . . . 316

Journal Publication . . . 319

Alternative Dissemination Formats: White Paper and Research Project Website . . . 328

White Paper . . . 328

Research Project Website . . . 328

Glossary . . . 333

Index . . . 349

Online Ancillaries

Appendix 2A: EHR Survey

Appendix 2B: Excerpts from Web-based EHR Survey

Appendix 2C: Cover Letter for EHR Survey

Appendix 2D: Sample Follow-Up Cover Letter

Appendix 5A: Research Instrument for Case Control Study

Appendix 13A: Example Timeline for a Research Proposal

About the Authors

Volume Editors

Valerie J. Watzlaf, PhD, MPH, RHIA, FAHIMA, is an associate professor within the Department of Health Information Management in the School of Health and Rehabilitation Sciences (SHRS) at the University of Pittsburgh. She also holds a secondary appointment in the Graduate School of Public Health. In those capacities, Dr. Watzlaf teaches and performs research in the areas of health information management (HIM) and epidemiology. She has worked and consulted in several healthcare organizations in HIM, long-term care, and epidemiology. Dr. Watzlaf is very active in professional and scientific societies, having served on several AHIMA committees, as a board member of AHIMA and the AHIMA Foundation, and as the chair of the Council for Excellence in Education (CEE) of the AHIMA Foundation. She is currently serving on the task force for the development of health informatics curriculum competencies. She is also on the Editorial Advisory Board for the *Journal of AHIMA* and for *Perspectives in Health Information Management.* Dr. Watzlaf has published extensively in the field of HIM and is the recipient of numerous awards and professional accolades including AHIMA's Research Award and the Pennsylvania Health Information Management Association's Distinguished Member Award. She worked as a partner with CIOX Health (formerly Care Communications) as part of the CareInnoLab conducting research in HIM applications. Dr. Watzlaf received her bachelor of science degree in health records administration from the School of Health Related Professions, and her master of public health and doctorate degrees in epidemiology from the Graduate School of Public Health, all from the University of Pittsburgh.

Elizabeth J. Forrestal, PhD, RHIA, CCS, FAHIMA, is a professor emerita in the Department of Health Services and Information Management at East Carolina University, Greenville, NC. In 2001, she was awarded the designation of Fellow of the American Health Information Management Association, one of the first two individuals in the country to receive this award. She is the coauthor of *Principles of Healthcare Reimbursement,* first published by AHIMA in 2006 and currently in its fifth edition, for which she and her coauthor were recipients of AHIMA's Legacy Award in 2007. She was the first editor of *Perspectives in Health Information Management* and has delivered presentations at numerous AHIMA events. She earned her baccalaureate degree from the University of Minnesota. While working, she returned to school to earn her associate's degree in medical record technology. She completed St. Scholastica's progression program to earn her postbaccalaureate certificate in health information administration. She earned her master's degree in organizational leadership from the College of St. Catherine's and her doctorate in higher education from Georgia State University.

Contributing Authors

Dilhari R. DeAlmeida, PhD, RHIA, is an assistant professor in the Department of Health Information Management at the University of Pittsburgh. She received her bachelor of science degree in cell and molecular biology from the University of Toronto. Prior to joining the HIM department, she has more than 12 years of experience working in government, academics, and the private sector in the field of molecular biology. She received her master of science (HIS/RHIA option) and doctorate degrees from the University of Pittsburgh. Her dissertation research involved evaluating the ICD-10-CM coding system for documentation specificity and reimbursement. DeAlmeida has great interest in documentation specificity in the ICD-10 coding system and the electronic health record, and she is an AHIMA-approved ICD-10-CM/PCS trainer. In addition to research, she teaches both undergraduate and graduate courses in HIM.

Jennifer Hornung Garvin, PhD, MBA, RHIA, CPHQ, CCS, CTR, FAHIMA, is an associate professor in the University of Utah's Department of Biomedical Informatics with a secondary appointment in the Division of Epidemiology, a Core Research Investigator at the VA Salt Lake City Health Care System (SLCVAHCS) Informatics Decision Enhancement and Surveillance (IDEAS) 2.0 Research Center, and an affiliated faculty member of the SLCVAHCS Geriatric Research Education and Clinical Center. Dr. Garvin's research interests include developing and studying applied informatics to advance clinical and public health practice. She was awarded a National Library of Medicine fellowship in Woods Hole, MA for bioinformatics. Dr. Garvin's professional HIM work includes such positions as professor and program director of HIM, director of HIM, director of quality management, and consultant. She received her doctorate from the Department of Public Health at Temple University, a master of business administration from St. Joseph's University, a postbaccalaureate certificate and associate degree from the HIM Program at Gwynedd-Mercy College, and completed the Clinical Research Certificate Program at the Center for Clinical Epidemiology and Biostatistics at the University of Pennsylvania School of Medicine.

Laurinda B. Harman, PhD, RHIA, FAHIMA, is an associate professor emeritus in the Department of Health Information Management at the College of Public Health at Temple University in Philadelphia. She has been an HIM professional and educator for more than 47 years and has directed HIM baccalaureate programs at George Washington University in Washington, DC, Ohio State University in Columbus, and Temple University in Philadelphia. She was also a faculty member in the health information technology program at Northern Virginia Community College. Dr. Harman has authored 16 book chapters, 12 juried articles, and 6 AHIMA-published articles. She has made 96 presentations at local, state, national, and international professional meetings; participated in grants; and served on several AHIMA committees, including the Professional Ethics Committee. She has also served on multiple task forces and AHIMA editorial boards, including *Perspectives in Health Information Management* and *In Confidence*. She was the editor for the textbook *Ethical Challenges in the Management of Health Information* in 2001 and 2006 and received the AHIMA 2001 Triumph Legacy Award for this publication. She was the co-editor for the third edition of the book *Ethical Health Informatics: Challenges and Opportunities*, published in 2016. She received the 2011 Dorland Health Ethicist Award and the 2011 AHIMA Educator Triumph Award. She was awarded a bachelor of science degree in biology with a concentration in medical record administration from Daemen College in Buffalo, NY, a master of science degree in education at Virginia Polytechnic and State University in Blacksburg, and a doctorate in human and organizational systems at Fielding Graduate University in Santa Barbara, CA.

Ryan H. Sandefer, PhD, is chair and assistant professor in the Health Informatics and Information Management Department at the College of St. Scholastica. He teaches research methods, program evaluation, technology applications, and consumer informatics. He coedited the textbook *Data Analytics in Healthcare Research: Tools and Strategies* and is currently engaged in multiple research projects on topics including electronic clinical quality measure reporting in rural hospitals, usability of mobile technologies, and consumer personal health information. Mr. Sandefer regularly presents at national and local meetings of HIM and HIT professionals and has published articles in the areas of health policy, health workforce, and health informatics. He is a member of the American Health Information Management Association, the American Medical Informatics Association, and the Health Information Management Systems Society. He received both his undergraduate and graduate degrees in political science from the University of Wyoming and his doctorate in health informatics from the University of Minnesota–Twin Cities.

Leming Zhou, PhD, DSc, is an assistant professor of the Department of Health Information Management at the School of Health and Rehabilitation Sciences at the University of Pittsburgh. He also holds secondary appointments in the Department of Bioengineering at the School of Engineering and McGowan Institute for Regenerative Medicine at the University of Pittsburgh. Dr. Zhou's current research focus is in the areas of mathematical modeling on health related topics, information integration, data analytics, health IT system development, and comparative genomics. Dr. Zhou's research goal is to provide computational methods and tools to facilitate high quality and low cost healthcare services. His research has been supported by the National Science Foundation (NSF); the Department of Veterans Affairs (VA); the National Institute on Disability, Independent Living, and Rehabilitation Research (NIDILRR); and private companies. Dr. Zhou received a bachelor of science degree in physics from Nankai University, China, a master of science degree in computer science, a doctorate in physics, and a doctor of science degree in computer science from the George Washington University.

Foreword

It is an honor and a pleasure to write the Foreword for this second edition of *Health Informatics Research Methods* by Dr. Watzlaf and Dr. Forrestal. Research and research-like activities are more essential to the future than ever. It is estimated that there will be 25,000 petabytes, or 25 billion gigabytes, of healthcare data by 2020 (Gandhi and Wang 2016). Healthcare will be drowning in a sea of naturally collected data from electronic health records (EHRs); Internet of Things devices, such as home control devices and personal trackers; genomic data from care delivery and third-party companies; the natural and built environment; and social media. This excess of data, however, makes it ever more important to understand the health informatics and health information management (HIM) frames and designs, threats to internal and external validity, tools and techniques, and how to secure funding and effectively disseminate research results.

The collection of primary research data will remain necessary for a variety of reasons, including incomplete natural data sources and control of the research to eliminate threats to validity. Chapters 2, 3, and 4 are especially helpful. Chapter 2, on surveys, is applicable to almost all health informatics and HIM professionals. Almost all of us seek to survey someone for some reason regardless of our position or responsibilities. Creating a reliable survey is difficult. Observational research, as well as experimental and quasi-experimental research, also presents challenges. A poor survey design can lead to misleading conclusions. There are many examples of spurious correlations; that is, two concepts that may have a statistically significant correlation that means absolutely nothing. As an example, the enrollment in my school is correlated at greater than 0.8 with the stock price of a company named for a fruit. Needless to say, correlation does *not* equal causation.

Chapters 6, 7, 8, and 9 are focused on the tools and technologies mentioned previously. Evaluation methods can be used for practitioners seeking to document value for their initiatives, as well as researchers seeking to improve the application of health information technology. The large amounts of data referenced earlier will require utilization of data science techniques to some extent in our research and operations initiatives. Systematic reviews and meta-analyses are very specific types of research that have been used more frequently to combine the results from multiple studies in a bid to develop best practices in healthcare. In figure 8.1, you will see that the systematic review is considered to be the most clinically relevant evidence. Chapter 9 presents basic statistical methods that can be employed. Table 9.1, the decision table for selecting a statistical test, is helpful for all researchers. All of these chapter topics can support their own entire books. Tools and methods must be thoroughly explored to be used correctly.

Chapters 10 through 12 cover important fundamentals of research. Perhaps most challenging to many researchers is selecting a reasonable research question. Many researchers, including many students, want to choose the research question that promises to answer very broad questions; that is, they want to fix the world. A literature review can often help to narrow the research question. The ultimate result of a good literature review is the identification of gaps in the knowledge, also known as opportunities for future research. Of course, the research design is vital. The design, as well as the population selection and sampling, often impact the validity of the research. Interestingly, the move into using big data sets now means that the sample is sometimes the entire population. For example, in the past when we needed to abstract data from hard copy medical records, choosing a representative sample for quality and other measures was of vital importance. In an era of EHRs, it is possible to use the entire population for quality measure calculation. Of course, this all leads to the effective analysis of the data and presenting the results. My experience is that preparing the data for analysis as described in the chapter, the hard work of data preparation and cleaning, is 80 percent of the work, with the actual running and interpretation of the analysis the remaining 20 percent. Presenting the data so it can be understood is also known as data visualization. The rule of thumb is that figures and graphics need to be able to be understood as they stand alone.

The final chapters, 13, 14, and 15, cover overarching topics. Securing funding either via the government or foundations often requires the development of a valid, feasible research plan with preliminary data already in hand. Most funded grant applications "tell a story." Research is generally a highly regulated enterprise. All human subjects research, including that using most data, must be approved by an Institutional Review Board. However, ethical challenges remain. As described in the case of Vioxx, valid research and its findings can be used in ethically questionable ways. Finally, disseminating the research often depends on the type of research, as well as the ultimate intended audience. The decision where and how to disseminate findings should be carefully considered.

Research is hard, and fun, and exhausting, and very necessary to increasing our knowledge of our world. My experience has taught me that the "perfect" research study does not exist, nor does research ever occur exactly as planned. Research is definitely a team sport due to its complexity. I invite you and your research colleagues to use this book to learn how to produce wondrous findings that help health informaticians and health information managers improve the human condition.

—Susan H. Fenton, PhD, RHIA, FAHIMA

Gandhi, M. and T. Wang. 2016. *The Future of Personalized Healthcare: Predictive Analytics*. Rock Health. https://rockhealth.com/reports/predictive-analytics/.

Preface

Research in health informatics and health information management (HIM) is critically necessary. Now more than ever, applicable research methods and appropriate analyses are needed to support the development and the evolution of the electronic health record, the personal health record, computerized physician order entry, decision support systems, protocols for privacy and security of electronic health information, and other health information technologies and applications. Research can demonstrate why and where certain applications are most vital to improve the quality of healthcare. The authors have written this textbook to support the development of health information technologies and applications and to advance the bodies of knowledge of health informatics and HIM.

Health informatics and HIM professionals can be the leaders in the advancement of health information technologies and applications by conducting effective research. These professionals provide a myriad of services to the health sector. They work throughout the healthcare delivery system in healthcare facilities, insurance companies, vendor settings, consulting companies, government agencies, and research and development firms. Health informatics and HIM professionals also teach and conduct research in university and college settings. To conduct effective research in the applied disciplines of health informatics and HIM, practitioners and educators often collaborate.

This second edition of *Health Informatics Research Methods: Principles and Practice* supports baccalaureate- and graduate-level students, researchers, and educators. The textbook focuses on the practical applications of research in health informatics and HIM. It provides real-life examples of research studies, step-by-step research methods, and explanations of analytic procedures. The textbook's organization guides students through the process of conducting research specific to health informatics and HIM. This organization also assists faculty members in the teaching of health informatics and HIM research methods. Every chapter consists of the following features:

- Learning objectives
- Key terms with definitions included in the body of the chapter
- A real-world case
- Practical examples of research studies
- Review questions
- Application exercises

In writing this textbook, the authors have two aims: (1) that students and practitioners can read research articles and determine the appropriateness of the articles' results and conclusions for their own work environments and (2) that students and practitioners can conduct a research study that results in credible and defendable conclusions. The textbook is written to support students and practitioners as they work through the chapters' content. The authors present information in a direct and straightforward style and provide many real-world examples from health informatics and HIM.

This textbook has three parts. Part I, Research Designs and Methods, introduces research designs and research methods commonly used in health informatics and HIM research. Part II, Research Process, begins with an overview of common statistical tests used in health informatics and HIM research and then presents the processes of conducting research. Part III, Information to Knowledge, describes grant and proposal writing, ethical issues encountered in research, and the ways that researchers disseminate the information from their research investigations.

Part I, Research Designs and Methods, includes eight chapters that describe research designs and methods that are frequently used in health informatics and HIM research. The chapters include samples of current health informatics and HIM research studies.

Chapter 1 introduces research frames and seven research designs. The chapter explains that research is conducted within research frames, which have associated theories and models. The chapter also discusses the quantitative, qualitative, and mixed methods approaches and describes the differences between inductive and deductive reasoning. The research designs discussed in the chapter are historical research, descriptive research, correlational research, observational research, evaluation research, experimental research, and quasi-experimental research. The chapter includes examples of these research designs being used in health informatics and HIM research projects.

Chapter 2 centers on survey research. Steps taken to create surveys are explained and discussed, including the types of questions to use, pilot testing of the survey, testing for validity and reliability, choosing the sample, methods for improving the response rate, and statistical analysis of data.

Chapter 3 explains the purpose of observational research and how it is used in health informatics and HIM research. It describes the different types of observational research: nonparticipant observation, participant observation, and ethnography as well as steps to use to conduct content analysis.

Chapter 4 contains information on the differences and similarities between experimental and quasi-experimental research. It walks readers through the experimental designs: pretest-posttest control group method, Solomon four-group method, and posttest-only control group method. Then, it describes the quasi-experimental designs: one-shot case study, one group pretest-posttest method, and static group comparison method.

Chapter 5 explains epidemiological research and how it can be used in health informatics and HIM. It describes the models of causation (infectious and chronic disease model) and how these models can be used when assessing health informatics applications. It then describes the types of epidemiological study designs: cross-sectional or prevalence, case-control, prospective, and clinical trials.

Chapter 6 provides a rationale for the practical applications of evaluation methods in health informatics and HIM. The scope, definition, and types of evaluation research methods are explained and discussed. Examples from the published literature and a clinical practice scenario are used to illustrate the various types of health informatics and HIM evaluation methods.

Chapter 7 defines data science and provides a model to approach problems using data science. The chapter covers the steps of business understanding, data understanding, data preparation, modeling, evaluation, and deployment.

Chapter 8 describes, step-by-step, how a systematic review is conducted. The research question, research protocol, the review's terms, inclusion and exclusion criteria, database searches, article selection, data extraction, quality appraisal and data analysis, and the final report are explained and an example is provided for each step.

Part II, Research Process, includes four chapters that guide readers through the components of the research process. The second part begins with chapter 9, Applied Statistics, because the choice of statistical technique can influence other choices in the research process. The part's three remaining chapters walk the reader through the research process, which consists of defining the research question, performing the literature review, selecting the research design and method, collecting data, and analyzing and presenting results.

Chapter 9 discusses descriptive and inferential statistics and introduces readers to commonly encountered statistical terms. Factors in selecting statistical tests are explained. The emphasis of the chapter is on matching the appropriate statistical test to the researcher's goal rather than on mathematical proofs and computations.

Chapter 10 addresses how to develop the research question, formulate hypotheses, and conduct the literature review. Examples are provided throughout the chapter, which concludes with the characteristics of a well-developed literature review.

Chapter 11 focuses on choosing an appropriate research design and method and collecting data. In this chapter, the role of validity and reliability in the selection of an instrument is explained, and factors that affect the selection of instruments are discussed. The chapter also covers data sampling methods and types of samples and data collection procedures common to both quantitative and qualitative research are discussed.

Chapter 12 explains how researchers transform their quantitative and qualitative data into results. Statistical significance and practical significance are differentiated, techniques used to prepare quantitative data for analysis are presented, and the qualitative analytical techniques of grounded theory and content analysis are described. The chapter includes discussions of presenting results in tables, graphs, and narrative.

Part III, Information to Knowledge, concludes the book with three chapters.

Chapter 13 describes the grant and proposal writing process. The chapter provides information about granting agencies and the requirements of their applications. It also explains why some grants are not funded.

Chapter 14 introduces ethical principles as they relate to research. It also describes research codes of conduct, the protection of human research subjects, the role and responsibility of institutional review boards and the Department of

Health and Human Services, and the impact of federal regulations on the conduct of research. Ethical research problems are discussed and examples are provided that relate to issues such as informed consent, publication of accurate results, and integrity.

Chapter 15, the final chapter, defines dissemination and provides a practical explanation of how to effectively present research results through poster presentations, oral paper presentations, journal publications, white papers, and research project websites.

Acknowledgments

The editors and AHIMA Press staff would like to thank the authors who contributed chapters to this textbook. They shared their knowledge and helped expand the bodies of knowledge in health informatics and HIM. Writing a chapter is a labor-intensive task, and we appreciate the care and time that the authors took with their contributions.

We would like to acknowledge the authors who contributed to the previous edition of this textbook:

- C. Andrew Brown, MD, MPH
- Susan Hart-Hester, PhD, RHIA
- Carol S. Nielsen, MLS
- William J. Rudman, PhD, RHIA

We would also like to thank the technical reviewers, Shannon Houser, PhD, MPH, RHIA, FAHIMA, and Nathan Taylor, MS, MPH, CHDA, who improved the quality of this book by sharing their expertise and providing constructive criticism.

Finally, the volume editors want to acknowledge Jessica Block, MA, for her guidance throughout this project.

Online Resources

For Students

Several online appendices are provided for student use. To access these appendices, go to http://www.ahimapress.org/Watzlaf5320 and download the Online Appendices zip file. The first time you access the zip file, enter the case-sensitive password AH5320IMA_WvFe.

For Instructors

AHIMA provides supplementary materials for educators who use this book in their classes. Materials include an instructor's manual and PowerPoint slides for lectures. Visit http://www.ahimapress.org/Watzlaf5320 and click the link to download the files. Please do not enter the scratch-off code from the interior front cover, as this will invalidate your access to the instructor materials. If you have any questions regarding the instructor materials, contact AHIMA Customer Relations at (800) 335-5535 or submit a customer support request at https://my.ahima.org/messages.

PART I

Research Designs and Methods

1 Research Frame and Designs

2 Survey Research

3 Observational Research

4 Experimental and Quasi-Experimental Research

5 Epidemiological Research

6 Evaluation Methods

7 Data Science and Data Mining

8 Systematic Reviews and Meta-Analyses

1 Research Frame and Designs

Elizabeth J. Forrestal, PhD, RHIA, CCS, FAHIMA

Learning Objectives

- Use and explain the terms *research, research frame, theory, model*, and *research methodology.*
- Designate the appropriate placement of a research project on the continuum of research from basic to applied.
- Differentiate among research designs.
- Provide appropriate rationales that support the selection of a research design.
- Use key terms associated with research frames and designs appropriately.

Key Terms

Applied research
Artifact
Basic research
Case study
Causal-comparative research
Causal relationship
Comparative effectiveness research (CER)
Confounding (extraneous, secondary) variable
Context
Control group
Correlational research
Cross-sectional
Deductive reasoning
Dependent variable
Descriptive research
Empiricism
Ethnography
Evaluation research
Experimental (study) group
Experimental research
Generalizability
Health informatics research
Health information management (HIM) research
Health services research
Health technology assessment (HTA)
Historical research
Independent variable
Inductive reasoning
Longitudinal
Mixed-methods research
Model
Naturalistic observation
Negative (inverse) linear relationship (association)
Nonparticipant observation
Observational research
Parsimony
Participant observation
Positive (direct) linear relationship (association)
Positivism
Primary source
Prospective
Qualitative approach
Quantitative approach
Quasi-experimental research
Random sampling
Randomization
Randomized controlled trial (RCT)
Research
Research design
Research frame
Research method
Research methodology
Retrospective
Rich data
Rigor
Scientific inquiry
Secondary source
Simulation observation
Theory
Translational research
Triangulation
Usability testing
Variable

Research is a systematic process of inquiry aimed at discovering or creating new knowledge about a topic, confirming or evaluating existing knowledge, or revising outdated knowledge. This chapter explains the purpose of research and defines terms associated with it, such as *research frame, theory, model,* and *scientific inquiry,* and describes several research designs that are used in health informatics and health information management (HIM). Examples of these research designs being used by health informatics and HIM researchers are provided throughout the chapter.

Research answers questions and provides solutions to everyday problems. It also provides clear, step-by-step processes that result in a comprehensive approach to questions and problems. These processes allow people to collect reliable and accurate facts they can analyze and interpret. Research information is relevant to health professionals and others because research provides evidence they can use not only in fulfilling their responsibilities but also in conducting operations and improving practice. This analysis and interpretation becomes valuable information that can be used to draft policies, respond to administrative and legislative queries, and make decisions. The following real-world case illustrates how healthcare leaders can use information from research to create contingency plans and estimate risk.

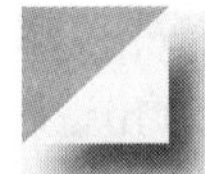

Real-World Case

According to analysts at the Health Research Institute of PricewaterhouseCoopers (PWC), nearly 40 percent of consumers "would abandon or hesitate using a health organization if it is hacked" (PWC 2015, 1). The analysts obtained this information through research. In an online survey, 1,000 US adults provided their perspectives of the healthcare environment and their preferences related to the use of healthcare services. These adults represent a cross-section of the US population in terms of their insurance status, age, gender, income, and geography. Moreover, more than 50 percent of the respondents would avoid or be wary of using Internet-connected healthcare devices, such as pacemakers and drug infusion pumps, if a security breach were reported. Healthcare leaders can factor this information into the cost projections for breaches and cyber attacks of information systems as they create contingency plans and estimate risk.

What Are Health Informatics Research and HIM Research?

Health informatics research is the investigation of the process, application, and impact of computer science, information systems, and communication technologies to health services. **Health information management (HIM) research** involves investigations into the practice of acquiring, analyzing, storing, disclosing, retaining, and protecting information vital to the delivery, provision, and management of health services. HIM research has a narrower scope than health informatics research. Both health informatics research and HIM research are at the intersection of research from several disciplines, including medicine, computer science, information systems, biostatistics, and business, to name just a few. Consequently, researchers and practitioners have conducted research in multiple ways, which reflect the investigators' range of experiences. Because health informatics and HIM researchers ask research questions covering a wide range of topics, their research projects are stimulating, dynamic, and varied.

Health informatics research and HIM research are often influenced by current events, new technologies, and scientific advancements. Recent research studies include how activity trackers and mobile phone apps can improve users' health. For example, researchers at Harvard University are using a smartphone app to collect data to assess the health and well-being of former professional football players (Harvard University 2016). While adults of all ages, genders, and cultures may participate in the research study, the research focuses on the everyday experiences of former professional football players—their memory, balance, heart health, pain, and mobility.

The sections that follow address the purposes of health informatics and HIM research, research frames, and scientific inquiry.

Purposes of Health Informatics Research and HIM Research

The purposes of health informatics research and HIM research are directly related to the definition of research—creating knowledge, confirming and evaluating existing knowledge, and revising outdated knowledge. Thus, the purposes of health informatics research and HIM research are as follows:

- To formulate theories and principles of health informatics and HIM
- To test existing theories, models, and assumptions about the principles of health informatics and HIM

- To build a set of theories about what works, when, how, and for whom
- To advance practice by contributing evidence that decision makers can use
- To train future practitioners and researchers
- To develop tools and methods for the process of health informatics research and HIM research (Wyatt 2010, 436)

Generally, the overarching purpose of health informatics research is to determine whether the application of health information technologies and the assistance of health informaticians have helped users improve health (Friedman 2013, 225). Similarly, the overarching purpose of HIM research is to determine whether the health information has the integrity and quality necessary to support its clinical, financial, and legal uses (AHIMA 2016).

Research Frame

A field's body of knowledge is built on research, and research is conducted within research frames. A **research frame**, or *research paradigm,* is the overarching structure of a research project. A research frame comprises the theory or theories underpinning the study, the models illustrating the factors and relationships of the study, the assumptions of the field and the researcher, the methods, and the analytical tools. The research frame is a view of reality for the researcher and his or her discipline. Each field has its own theories, models, assumptions, methods, and analytic tools. Fields also have preferred means of disseminating knowledge; some fields prefer books, whereas others prefer journal articles.

Theories and Models

Many theories and models are potentially applicable to health informatics research and HIM research. These theories and models come not only from healthcare but also from computer science, business, and many other fields. Researchers select the theory or model that best suits their purpose and addresses their question or problem. Table 1.1 lists many of these theories and models along with representative examples of related publications by leading theorists or developers.

Table 1.1 Selected theories and models used in health informatics and HIM research

Theories or Models	Related Publications by Noted Theorists or Developers
Adult learning theories (e.g. experiential learning theories)	Rogers, C.R. 1969. *Freedom to Learn*. Columbus, OH: Merrill Publishing.
AHIMA data quality management model	Davoudi, S., J.A. Dooling, B. Glondys, T.D. Jones, L. Kadlec, S.M. Overgaard, K. Ruben, and A. Wendicke. 2015. Data quality management model (2015 update). *Journal of AHIMA* 86(10):62–65.
Change theories	Lewin, K. 1951. *Field Theory in Social Science*. New York: Harper and Brothers Publishers.
Cybernetics theory	Wiener, N. 1948. *Cybernetics; or Control and Communications in the Animal and Machine*. New York: John Wiley.
Diffusion of innovations theory	Rogers, E.M. 2003. *Diffusion of Innovations,* 5th ed. New York: Free Press. (1st ed. 1962)
Dominant design—a dynamic model of process and product development (A-U model)	Abernathy, W.J. and J.M. Utterback. 1978. Patterns of industrial innovation. *Technology Review* 80(7):40–47. Utterback, J.M. 1996. *Mastering the Dynamics of Innovation,* 2nd ed. Boston: Harvard Business School Press.
Fuzzy set theory	Zadeh, L.A. 1965. Fuzzy sets. *Information and Control* 8(3):338–353.
General systems theory (GST; evolved into open systems theory and closed systems theory)	Von Bertalanffy, L. 1950. An outline of general system theory. *British Journal for the Philosophy of Science* 1(2):134–165.
Information behavior theories	Wilson, T.D. 1999. Models in information behavior research. *Journal of Documentation* 55(3):249–270.
Information processing and cognitive learning theories (e.g. chunking)	Miller, G.A. 1956. The magical number seven, plus or minus two: Some limits on our capacity for processing information. *Psychological Review* 63(2):81–97. Sweller, J. 1988. Cognitive load during problem solving: Effects on learning. *Cognitive Science* 12(2):257–285.

(*Continued*)

Table 1.1 (*Continued*)

Theories or Models	Related Publications by Noted Theorists or Developers
Information systems success (D&M IS success) model	DeLone, W.H. and E.R. McLean. 1992. Information systems success: The quest for the dependent variable. *Information Systems Research* 3(1):60–95.
Knowledge engineering theories	Gruber, T.R. 1993. A translation approach to portable ontology specifications. *Knowledge Acquisition* 5(2):199–221. Newell, A. 1982. The knowledge level. *Artificial Intelligence* 18(1):87–127.
Learning styles theories	Kolb, D.A. 1984. *Experiential Learning: Experience as the Source of Learning and Development*. Englewood Cliffs, NJ: Prentice-Hall.
Open systems theory	*See* General systems theory
Rough set theory	Pawlak, Z. 1982. Rough sets. *International Journal of Computer and Information Sciences* 11(2):341–356.
Seven-stage model of action	Norman, D.A. and S.W. Draper. 1986. *User Centered System Design: New Perspectives on Human-Computer Interaction*. Hillsdale, NJ: Lawrence Erlbaum Associates.
Social learning theories	Bandura, A. 1982. Self-efficacy mechanism in human agency. *American Psychologist* 37(2):122–147.
Sociotechnical theories (e.g. sociotechnical systems [STS] and sociotechnical model)	Cherns, A. 1987 (March). Principles of sociotechnical design revisited. *Human Relations* 40(3):153–161. Sittig, D.F. and H. Singh. 2010. A new sociotechnical model for studying health information technology in complex adaptive healthcare systems. *Quality and Safety in Health Care* 19 (Suppl3):i68–i74.
Swiss cheese model	Reason, J. 2000. Human error: Models and management. *BMJ* 320(7237):768–770.
System of systems (SoS) theory (e.g. chaos theory and complex systems theory)	Jackson, M.C. and P. Keys. 1984. Towards a system of systems methodologies. *Journal of the Operational Research Society* 35(6):473–486.
Systems development life cycle (SDLC) model	Benington, H.D. 1983 (reprint of 1956). Production of large computer programs. *Annals of the History of Computing–IEEE* 5(4):350–361.
Technology acceptance model (TAM)	Davis, F.D., R.P. Bagozzi, and P.R. Warshaw. 1992. Extrinsic and intrinsic motivation to use computers in the workplace. *Journal of Applied Social Psychology* 22(14):1111–1132.
User acceptance theories (e.g. unified theory of acceptance and use of technology [UTAUT])	Thompson, R.L., C.A. Higgins, and J.M. Howell. 1994. Influence of experience on personal computer utilization: Testing a conceptual model. *Journal of Management Information Systems* 11(1):167–187. Venkatesh, V., M.G. Morris, G.B. Davis, and F.D. Davis. 2003. User acceptance of information technology: Toward a unified view. *MIS Quarterly* 27(3):425–478.

Source: Adapted from Nelson and Staggers 2014, Venkatesh et al. 2003, Dillon and Morris 1996, and Gorod et al. 2008.

A **theory** is the systematic organization of knowledge that explains or predicts phenomena, such as behavior or events, "by interrelating concepts in a logical, testable way" (Karnick 2013, 29). They provide definitions, relationships, and boundaries. For example, the theory of diffusion of innovations is commonly used in studies related to health information technology (HIT). The theory explains how new ideas and products—innovations—spread, and it includes definitions of innovation and communication and elements (concepts) of the process of diffusion (Rogers 2003, xvii–xviii, 11). Using the theory of diffusion of innovations, health informatics researchers investigated what key strategic leaders knew about various information technology (IT) innovations and how those innovations were implemented. The researchers found that the strategic leaders—that is, chief information officers (CIOs), and directors of nursing—significantly disagreed on the number of IT functions available in their hospital and on the implementation status of several functions (Liebe et al. 2016, 8). The researchers concluded that leaders' agreement can initiate adoption, but disagreements among leaders could be a barrier to successful IT adoption (Liebe et al. 2016, 3).

Using theories to examine phenomena and complex relationships optimally and systematically advances scientific knowledge (Fox et al. 2015, 71; Shapira 2011, 1312). Researchers begin with informed predictions or raw theories of what they believe will happen. As they collect observations and data, they refine their theories. Researchers strive for parsimony or elegance in their theories. **Parsimony** means that explanations of phenomena should include the fewest assumptions, conditions, and extraneous complications. The best theories simplify the situation, explain the most facts in the broadest range of circumstances, and most accurately predict behavior (Singleton and Straits 2010, 25).

A **model** is an idealized representation that abstracts and simplifies a real-world situation so the situation can be studied, analyzed, or both (Gass and Fu 2013, 982). Models visually depict theories by using objects, graphic representations, or smaller-scaled versions of the situation being studied. A model includes all known properties of a theory. Health informatics and HIM researchers often select models associated with sociotechnical theories and user acceptance theories, such as Sittig's and Singh's sociotechnical model (2010) and the technology acceptance model (TAM) (Davis et al. 1992). Readers may also encounter other models applicable to health informatics and HIM research, such as the seven-stage model of action (Norman and Draper 1986), the Swiss cheese model (Reason 2000), and DeLone's and McLean's information systems (IS) success model (2003).

Sittig's and Singh's sociotechnical model, shown in figure 1.1, presents the dimensions (factors) critical to the success of HIT implementations in adaptive, complex environments (2010, 3–8). This model includes dimensions from social systems (the "socio" part of "sociotechnical"), such as workflow and communication, and technical systems, such as hardware and software infrastructure. In the sociotechnical perspective, both systems are important and complementary (Whetton and Georgiou 2010, 222). The comprehensive model illustrates eight dimensions:

- Hardware and software computing infrastructure
- Clinical content
- Human computer interface
- People
- Workflow and communication
- Internal organizational policies, procedures, and culture
- External rules, regulations, and pressures
- System measurement and monitoring (Sittig and Singh 2010)

The theorists specifically emphasize that the dimensions are not independent, sequential, hierarchical steps; instead, the dimensions are interactive and interrelated.

Figure 1.1 Illustration of the complex interrelationships between the dimensions of Sittig's and Singh's sociotechnical model

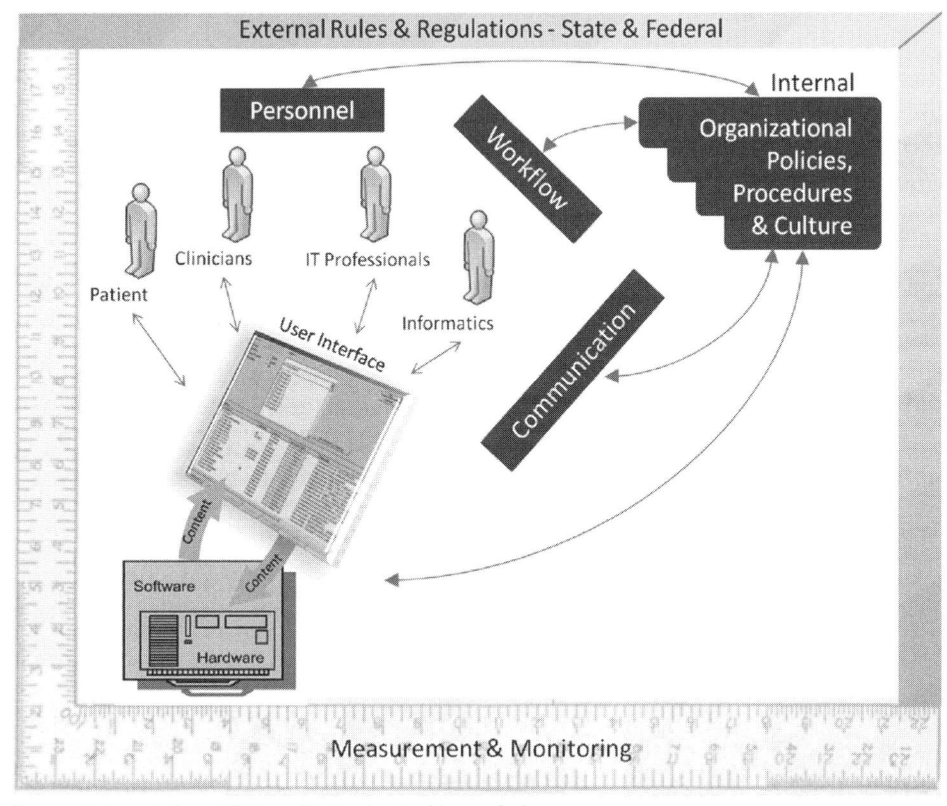

Source: Sittig and Singh 2010, p. i69. Reprinted with permission.

Sittig and Singh's model has been used to analyze a large health system's investigative reports of safety incidents related to electronic health records (EHRs) (Meeks et al. 2014, 1053). The health informatics researchers' analysis identified emerging and commonly recurring safety issues related to EHRs. Another set of health informatics researchers used the model to describe the environment in the emergency department so that a pediatric clinical decision support system would be designed with appropriate decision rules for children with minor blunt head traumas (Sheehan et al. 2013, 905).

Research Methodology

Research methodology is the study and analysis of research methods and theories. A **research method** is a set of specific procedures used to gather and analyze data. Research methodologists tackle questions such as "What is research?" or "Which method of data collection results in the greatest, unbiased response rate?" For example, researchers evaluated blogging as a way to collect data from young adults age 11 to 19 who had juvenile rheumatoid arthritis (a chronic autoimmune disorder) (Prescott et al. 2015, 1). Although the data collection method was promising, the researchers concluded that blogging probably should be combined with other collection methods.

Continuum of Basic and Applied Research Research is often categorized as basic or applied, but these two types of research are actually the ends of a continuum, not separate entities. In practice, the distinction between basic and applied research is sometimes unclear; however, research methodologists generally differentiate them as follows:

- **Basic research** answers the question "Why" and focuses on the development of theories and their refinement. Basic research is sometimes called *bench science* because it often occurs in laboratories. In health informatics and HIM, basic research comprises the development and evaluation of new methods and theories for the acquisition, storage, maintenance, retrieval, and use of information.
- **Applied research** answers the questions "What?", "How?", "When?", or "For whom?" Most health informatics and HIM researchers who conduct applied research focus on the implementation of theories and models into practice. Applied research, particularly clinical applied research, is often done in healthcare settings, such as at the bedside or in the clinic. The following are examples of clinical applied research questions:
  - What systems work best to support health professionals in making decisions?
  - What types of HIT and which methods of HIT implementation will improve the exchange of health data across the continuum of care?
  - What is the impact of accurately coded data on the financial status of healthcare organizations?
  - What features of HIT increase the safety of the administering medications?
  - When does HIT reduce the costs of the delivery of health services?
  - How can health informatics practice improve workflows in various healthcare settings and between settings?
  - How do leaders' ways of implementing health information systems affect users' satisfaction and utilization?
  - What features of HIT help people improve their health and for whom do these features work best?
  - When should training be provided to best support health professionals' use of new features of EHRs?

Most of the examples of research studies provided in this chapter and the rest of the book are applied research.

The translation of the discoveries of basic science into practice in the community has been slow, even though these discoveries have the potential to benefit individuals and populations (NCATS 2015). To spur that translation, the federal government has supported translational research, a form of applied research that health analysts and policymakers describe as "bench-to-bedside." **Translational research** has two aspects: applying discoveries generated during basic research to the development of research studies with human subjects, and enhancing the sector's adoption of best practices and cost-effective strategies to prevent, diagnose, and treat health conditions (NIH 2016). For example, translational research may take knowledge from basic science, such as a newly discovered property of a chemical, and convert that knowledge into a practical application, such as a new drug. Generally, translational research makes the benefits of scientific discoveries available to the practitioners in the community and to the public.

Quantitative, Qualitative, and Mixed-Methods Approaches to Research Research methodologists describe three overarching approaches to research: the quantitative approach, the qualitative approach, and mixed-methods research approach. The **quantitative approach** explains phenomena by making predictions, collecting and analyzing evidence, testing alternative theories, and choosing the best theory. The **qualitative approach** involves investigations to describe, interpret, and understand processes, events, and relationships as perceived by individuals or groups (Holloway and Wheeler 2010, 3). **Mixed-methods research**, also known as *mixed research,* combines (mixes) quantitative and qualitative theoretical perspectives, methods, sampling strategies, data collection techniques, data sets, analytic procedures, representational modes, or any combination of these aspects of research (Sandelowski 2014, 3). The purpose of the research question determines the approach.

In the quantitative approach, the desired end result of research is objective knowledge that has generalizability. **Generalizability** means capable of being applied to other similar situations and people. As the word *quantitative* implies, researchers using the quantitative approach collect data that can be numerically measured and lead to statistical results. The quantitative approach is informed by the philosophy of positivism (Ingham-Broomfield 2014, 33). **Positivism**, which dates back to the mid–19th century, proposes that knowledge should be based on universal laws, objectivity, and observed facts (Hasan 2016, 318–319; Comte 1853, 2). In health informatics and HIM research, an example of quantitative research would be a study that calculates the percentage of patients that use a healthcare organization's patient portal.

In the qualitative approach, the desired end result is specific knowledge that is particular to the situation. Qualitative researchers study nonnumerical observations, such as words, gestures, activities, time, space, images, and perceptions. For example, researchers using the qualitative approach explore reasons for people's decisions or attempt to interpret their actions. Qualitative researchers are careful to place these observations in **context**, which means the specific conditions of the situation, including time, space, emotional attitude, social situation, and culture. The researchers attempt to understand phenomena through their subjects' perspective and in their subjects' terms. Additionally, in the qualitative approach, research often takes place in the natural setting of the issue rather than in a researcher-created scenario or laboratory (Abma and Stake 2014, 1150). As a result, the qualitative approach is sometimes called the *naturalistic approach* (Ekeland et al. 2012, 3). In health informatics and HIM research, an example of research using the qualitative approach would be an exploration of the reasons why patients are uncomfortable using a healthcare organization's patient portal.

Mixed-methods research seeks to combine the strengths of the quantitative and qualitative approaches to answering research questions. The combination of methods may occur concurrently and simultaneously within a single study, or mixed methods might be applied sequentially across chronological phases of an investigation or across a series of related studies. Reasons to conduct mixed-methods research include corroborating the results of other studies, clarifying and expanding the results of other studies, and resolving or explaining discrepancies in other studies.

Mixed-methods research is suited to investigations of large topics or complex phenomena, such as in health informatics, HIM, and health-related issues. Consequently, many research methodologists have noted the importance of using mixed-methods research in studying HIT and health information systems (Lee and Smith 2012, 251). In health informatics and HIM research, an example of mixed-methods research would be an initial physician survey asking physicians to estimate the number of minutes that they or their extenders (nurses and physician's assistants) spend responding to patients' queries from the patient portal. In a follow-up face-to-face interview, researchers could ask the physicians to explain how they feel about the portal's effect on the patient-physician relationship.

Scientific Inquiry

Scientific inquiry is "a way of generating knowledge" (Salazar et al. 2015, 25). In scientific inquiry, people use diverse ways to systematically gather data about phenomena, critically analyze the data, propose explanations based on their evidence, and develop understanding and knowledge. One component of scientific inquiry is **empiricism**, the theory that true knowledge is based on observations and direct experiences that can be perceived through the physical senses, such as eyesight or hearing (Salazar et al. 2015, 32). Research is based on empirical data rather than other sources of knowledge, such as authority or tradition. Scientific inquiry includes the considerations of types of reasoning and rigor, concepts that will be discussed in the next sections.

Reasoning

In scientific inquiry, researchers use two types of reasoning, inductive and deductive, to justify their decisions and conclusions. **Inductive reasoning**, or *induction,* involves drawing conclusions based on a limited number of observations. Inductive reasoning is "bottom up," meaning that it goes from the specific to the general. Researchers who use inductive reasoning begin with observations, detect patterns or clusters of relationships, form and explore tentative hypotheses, and generate provisional conclusions or theories. For example, during a student's field work experience, he or she might observe that all coding professionals in the coding department at XYZ hospital had the credential of certified coding specialist (CCS). From this observation, the student might conclude that all coding professionals have the CCS credential. A potential flaw in inductive reasoning is that the observations could be abnormal or could be limited in number, omitting some possible observations. In our example, the student's conclusion would be incorrect if he or she did not observe that one coding professional had the registered health information technician (RHIT) credential instead of the CCS credential. Inductive reasoning is associated with the qualitative approach because qualitative researchers begin at the bottom with their observations (Kisely and Kendall 2011, 364).

Deductive reasoning, or *deduction*, involves drawing conclusions based on generalizations, rules, or principles. Deductive reason is "top down," meaning that deductive reasoning goes from the general to the specific. Researchers using a deductive reasoning begin with a theory, develop hypotheses to test the theory, observe phenomena related to the hypotheses, and validate or invalidate the theory. For example, the same student might use the generalization that all coding professionals have the CCS credential. Based on this assumption, the student may conclude that because Jane Doe is a coding professional in the department, she must have the CCS credential. Similar to inductive reasoning, deductive reasoning can also be flawed. A flaw in deductive reasoning can occur when the generalization or rule is wrong. As we just noted, a coding professional may have the RHIT credential. Therefore, in this example, the student's initial assumption was incorrect. Deductive reasoning is associated with the quantitative approach because quantitative researchers test hypotheses (Wilkinson 2013, 919).

Scientific inquiries can use inductive and deductive reasoning in a cyclical process. Early, exploratory research often takes an inductive approach. Researchers record observations to induce (generate) empirical generalizations. These empirical generalizations, describing and explaining the observations, are developed into theories. Researchers then use the theories to deduce (infer) hypotheses (tentative predictions). Once researchers have generated a theory, they use the deductive approach to test or validate the theory by comparing their predictions to empirical observations. The cycle can start at any point in the process and continues to loop as the researchers refine the theories (Singleton and Straits 2010, 28).

Rigor

The integrity and quality of a research study is measured by its rigor. The definition of **rigor** varies for qualitative and quantitative researchers. For quantitative researchers, rigor is the "strict application of the scientific method to ensure unbiased and well-controlled experimental design, methodology, analysis, interpretation and report of results … and includes transparency in reporting full experimental details so that others may reproduce and extend the findings" (NIH/AHRQ 2015). As a result, rigor improves objectivity and minimizes bias (Eden et al. 2011, 30). For qualitative researchers, rigor is the trustworthiness of the interpretation of the study's findings (Morse 2015, 1212; Guba and Lincoln 1989, 233). For both sets of researchers, rigor establishes the validity and reliability of the study's results and conclusions.

Research Designs

A **research design** is a plan to achieve the researchers' purpose: answering a question, solving a problem, or generating new information. The research design is the infrastructure of the study. There are seven common research designs (see table 1.2). Each of these designs has a role in health informatics and HIM research.

Table 1.2 Types of research designs and the application in health informatics and HIM studies

Type of Design	Purpose	Selected Methods	Example of Health Informatics or HIM Study
Historical	Understand past events	Case study Biography	Study of the factors that led to the creation and development of clinical decision support systems in the 1960s and 1970s
Descriptive	Describe current status	Survey Observation	Survey of clinicians to determine how and to what degree they use clinical decision support systems
Correlational	Determine existence and degree of a relationship	Survey Data mining	Study to determine the relationship among individual clinicians' attributes, the health team's characteristics, the setting, and use of clinical decision support systems

(*Continued*)

Table 1.2 (*Continued*)

Type of Design	Purpose	Selected Methods	Example of Health Informatics or HIM Study
Observational	Describe and detect patterns and regularities in existing situations or natural surroundings	Case study Ethnography Nonparticipant observation Participant observations	Study to observe clinicians' use of clinical decision support systems in the examination rooms in an academic health center's specialty clinic
Evaluation	Assess efficiency, effectiveness, acceptability, or other attribute	Survey Case study Observation Usability study Double-blind randomized controlled trial	Study to evaluate the efficacy of the implementation of a clinical decision support system in an academic health center's specialty clinic
Experimental	Establish cause and effect	Double-blind randomized controlled trial Pretest-posttest control group method Solomon four-group method Posttest-only control group	Study to evaluate the influence of a clinical decision support system on clinicians' prescribing of antibiotics for acute respiratory infections, with clinicians randomly assigned to an intervention group and a control group
Quasi-experimental (causal-comparative)	Detect causal relationship	One-shot case study One-group pretest-posttest Static group comparison	Study to investigate the antibiotic prescribing practices for acute respiratory infections of primary care clinician teams using a clinical decision support system before and after an educational intervention on the system

Source: Adapted from Forrestal 2016, 576.

Researchers choose a research design for a particular study. Many research topics are suited to any one of the designs described in table 1.2, whereas other research topics are better suited to one research design than another. Which design is appropriate depends on the study's objectives and the researcher's statement of the problem in the problem statement, which is explained in detail in chapter 10.

Researchers can choose among a variety of research designs to investigate the same broad question or problem. For example, researchers can use different designs for different aspects of the question or problem. They can extend the breadth and scope of their question or problem by exploring related issues, but they may need to adopt different research designs for those issues. Preliminary, exploratory, investigations are typically descriptive, correlational, or observational. As researchers refine these investigations, they conduct causal-comparative and experimental studies. Other possible refinements include using the results of a preliminary study to identify or test techniques for sampling or for collecting and analyzing data in subsequent studies. Researchers also combine designs to address their particular research questions or problems. For instance, studies may include both descriptive and correlational findings.

The examples of studies in the fourth column of table 1.2 represent a progression of research studies on one topic, clinical decision support systems. The progression shows how a research team might sequentially use the results from one study to guide the design of its next study. The descriptive study merely looks at the extent of clinicians' use of a clinical decision support system; in contrast, the correlational study expands the study to examine attributes, characteristics, and other factors associated with the system's use. Eventually, the research team might conduct a double-blind, randomized controlled trial on a specific aspect of the clinical decision support system that compares an intervention (experimental) group and a control (nonexperimental) group.

The following subsections describe each of the research designs listed in table 1.2: historical research, descriptive research, correlational research, observational research, evaluation research, experimental research, and quasi-experimental (causal-comparative) research. For each research design, a relevant health informatics or HIM example is discussed. Table 1.2 also lists examples of research methods typically associated with each design. Several of these research methods are explained in chapters 2 through 8. Appropriate choices of research designs and research methods increase the likelihood that the data (evidence) collected are relevant, high quality, and directly related to the research question or problem.

Historical Research

Historical research examines historical materials to explain, interpret, and provide a factual account of events (Atkinson 2012, 20). The purposes of historical research include discovering new knowledge, identifying trends that could provide insights into current questions or problems, relating the past to contemporary events or conditions, and creating official records. In historical research, the investigator systematically collects, critically evaluates, and analyzes and interprets evidence from historical materials (Polit and Beck 2012, 500). These historical materials are known as primary and secondary sources.

Primary sources, also sometimes called *primary data,* are firsthand sources. In historical research, these firsthand sources include original documents, artifacts (objects, such as computers or paper records), and oral histories (first-person, spoken accounts). Generally, these firsthand sources are created or collected for a specific purpose. For example, original data obtained by researchers in a research study to answer a specific question and the article in which they published their data might be used as a primary source. **Secondary sources**, also called *secondary data,* are secondhand sources. In historical research, these secondhand sources are created by people uninvolved with the event. Generally, secondary sources aggregate, summarize, critique, analyze, or manipulate the primary sources, and, as such, they are derived from primary sources. Clinical data warehouses are secondary sources because they aggregate many individual patient health records and because the data are used for strategic planning or trend analysis rather than treating the individual patient. This chapter is another example of a secondary source because it describes and summarizes the original reports of others. Some methodologists categorize encyclopedias, textbooks, and other references as *tertiary sources* because they summarize information from secondary sources. (See figure 1.2 for examples of primary and secondary sources.)

Figure 1.2 Primary and secondary sources

Primary Sources	Secondary Sources
Agency regulations	Administrative data
Annual reports	Annual reviews of research
Audio recordings	Census data
Catalogs	Clinical data warehouses
Charters	Encyclopedias and other reference works
Contracts	Registries
Cost reports	Textbooks
Curricular documents	Publicly available data sets:
E-mail records	✧ Basic Stand Alone (BSA) Medicare Claims Public Use Files (PUFs)
Eyewitness accounts	✧ Healthcare Cost and Utilization Project (HCUP)
Executive orders	✧ Health Services Research Information Central (HSRIC)
Films	✧ Medical Expenditure Panel Survey (MEPS)
Handbooks	✧ Medicare Provider Analysis and Review (MEDPAR) File
Health records	✧ National Health Care Surveys
Journal articles	✧ National Vital Statistics System (NVSS)
Legal decisions	✧ National Survey of Family Growth (NSFG)
Legislative bills, laws, or statutes	✧ National Health Interview Survey (NHIS)
Letters	✧ National Immunization Survey (NIS)
Logs	✧ *See also* data.gov and the CDC website
Oral histories	
Organizational charts	
Patient blogs	
Patient diaries	
Photographs	
Physician accounting ledgers	
Reports	
Video recordings	
Websites	

As noted earlier, historical researchers begin by systematically collecting sources, which means they consider all possible relevant primary and secondary sources, their location, and how to access them, and then choose the best sources for their study. Historical researchers often use records or other documents. For example, historical researchers might investigate the increasing importance of IT departments in healthcare organizations by examining organizational charts over time. Possible questions that these historical researchers could ask include the following:

- When did IT departments first begin to appear on the charts?

- What were these departments called?
- Which types of healthcare organizations first established these departments?
- Where were the departments' leaders in the organization's chain of command? Were they midlevel managers or upper administration?

In addition to using documents as a source of data, historians also use oral histories, particularly to obtain eyewitness accounts. "Oral history is a method for documenting history in a vivid way by recording the voices of those who have experienced it" (Ash and Sittig 2015, 2). Historians might record interviews with early leaders in a field, such as Dr. Lawrence Weed, who was the first in medicine to propose problem-oriented medical records as a way of recording and organizing the content of health records and advocated for EHRs (Jacobs 2009, 85). The researchers also could record interviews with staff members of a healthcare organization about how the organization's information systems functioned during a time when the facility was flooded or a natural disaster led to unusually high numbers of injuries and patient admissions. Historical research must be open to the scrutiny and critical assessment of other researchers. Therefore, historical researchers must ensure the preservation of their source documents, such as tapes and transcripts of interviews, and make them available to other researchers (American Historical Association 2011, 7).

The following are examples of hypothetical historical research investigations in health informatics and HIM:

- While detailing the history of health informatics from 1950 to 1975, health informatics researchers find previously undetected communications between hardware developers.
- While identifying trends in patients' use of social media, health informatics or HIM researchers suggest ways to increase patients' engagement with patient portals.
- While identifying trends in the development of standards organizations, health informatics or HIM researchers account for the organizations' impact on the establishment of standards.
- While relating the views of early adopters of big data to current practice, health informatics researchers predict views of clinicians in small or solo practices.
- While tracing the history of clinical vocabularies, medical terminologies, nomenclatures, and coding and classification systems, especially those that no longer exist (such as the Standard Nomenclature of Diseases and Operations), HIM researchers hypothesize about their influence on current clinical vocabularies, medical terminologies, nomenclatures, and coding and classification systems.
- While tracing the history of the American Health Information Management Association (AHIMA) or of the American Medical Informatics Association (AMIA), HIM researchers or health informatics researchers establish the official records of these organizations' development.

An example of historical research related to health informatics is the US National Library of Medicine's oral history project called *Conversations with Medical Informatics Pioneers,* which is published online (NLM 2015).

A field's history is one aspect of its body of knowledge. Therefore, historical research, while focused on the past, can inform current and future practice of health informatics and HIM.

Descriptive Research

Descriptive research determines and reports on the current status of topics and subjects. Descriptive research studies seek to accurately capture or portray dimensions or characteristics of people, organizations, situations, technology, or other phenomena. Descriptive research is useful when researchers want to answer the questions "what is," "what was," or "how much" (Bickman and Rog 2009, 16). Some descriptive research studies are also correlational, which means they detect relationships. "Descriptive studies are usually the best methods for collecting information that will demonstrate relationships and describe the world as it exists" (ORI 2015).

The data gathered in descriptive research are used to establish baselines, make policy, conduct ongoing monitoring, assess operations, or demonstrate impacts. In the practice of health informatics and HIM, descriptive research can function as a way to establish benchmarks against which outcomes of future changes can be evaluated. For example, administrators might need to establish a baseline of users' productivity on an existing health information system so that in the future the organization can compare users' productivity on a new information system to their former productivity. In another example, information specialists might need to know the clinicians' levels of familiarity with a new technology before the technology is rolled out throughout the organization.

Descriptive research is *exploratory* and typically depicts the frequency of specific elements, the number of individuals, the level or quantity of factors, or the ranges of occurrences. Tools commonly used to collect descriptive data include surveys, interviews, observations, and existing data sets, such as those listed as secondary sources in figure 1.2. Obtaining a representative sample (a small group that adequately reflects relevant characteristics of the total population that might be studied) adds to the credibility of a descriptive study. Representative sampling is detailed in chapters 2 and 11. Descriptive research can collect data about a phenomenon (such as people or organizations) at one point in time, or it can follow the phenomenon over time. (Cross-sectional and longitudinal time frames are explained later in this chapter.) Familiar examples of descriptive research are the US decennial census and opinion polls. Descriptive studies allow researchers to learn details about potential factors that may affect outcomes; however, descriptive studies do *not* allow researchers to explain whether or how factors cause outcomes. As such, descriptive studies are often precursors to *explanatory* studies, such as experimental studies (explained later in the chapter) that can establish cause-and-effect relationships.

Contemporary descriptive studies have covered several health informatics and HIM topics, such as information governance, safety of HIT, education in health informatics, impact of the Health Information Technology for Economic and Clinical Health (HITECH) Act of 2009, the information literacy of health professionals, and other issues. The real-world case presented at the beginning of this chapter is an example of descriptive research in health informatics. The researchers (analysts) obtained information on the *current status* of US adults' perspectives on the healthcare environment. The study *reported* the percentage of consumers who would abandon or hesitate using a health organization if it were hacked. The researchers' tool was the online *survey*.

In another example, Fenton and colleagues, a team of health informatics and HIM researchers, investigated what the term *medical record* meant in research consent forms (Fenton et al. 2015, 466). Prior to enrolling subjects in research studies, researchers must obtain written documentation of the subjects' voluntary and informed (knowledgeable) consent in the form of a research consent form. Fenton and colleagues wondered whether everyone involved in a research study—subjects, researchers themselves, and research support staff—understood what data were included in the term *medical record* because the content of medical records has changed over the past 20 years. In the past, the medical record was the collection of documents in the paper record. However, as medical records have been computerized, their content has expanded to include other electronic data, such as data in pharmacy management systems and blood bank systems. To investigate its question, the team reviewed the language in the research consent forms of 17 academic health centers that had received Clinical and Translational Science Awards (grants) from the National Institutes of Health. In an article about the study, Fenton and colleagues provided descriptive statistics, such as tallies on the number and types of consent forms (how many and which type—long forms, short forms, adult forms, pediatric forms, and so forth) and frequencies (number of occurrences) of *medical record* and related terms (such as health record, electronic medical record, and so forth). The team concluded, based on its findings, that the term *medical record*, as it is used in informed consent documents for research studies, is ambiguous and does not support information management and governance. Fenton and colleagues noted that a limitation of its study was that the 17 academic health centers were a convenience sample (easily accessible because their research consent forms were posted on the Internet) and, as such, may not be representative of all organizations' research consent forms. Research consent (informed consent) forms are explained in detail in chapter 14.

Correlational Research

Correlational research detects the existence, direction, and strength (or degree) of associations among characteristics. These characteristics can be phenomena, factors, attitudes, organizational features, properties, traits, indicators, performance measures, or any other attribute of interest. Correlational research is quantitative and exploratory, and it indicates existing associations that can be examined and possibly explained using experimental research studies. As mentioned in the previous subsection, correlational research is *descriptive* when the researchers are detecting associations. However, this type of research can also be *predictive* when researchers suggest that a change in one characteristic (or characteristics) will or will not follow a change in another characteristic (or characteristics). The association between the items' change is nonrandom—that is, it is *not* due to pure chance.

In correlational studies, the characteristics are often called variables. **Variables** are characteristics that are measured and may take on different values. However, based on the specific type of variable or correlational study, other terms may be used instead of the term *variable*. Variables that covary—change together—may be called *covariables* or *covariates*. In some correlational studies, such as canonical and prediction studies, the variables are known as *predictor variables (predictors)* and *criterion variables* (or *outcome variables*). For example, in a prediction study, a mother's smoking (predictor variable) predicts a low birth weight (criterion variable) in her baby.

In correlational research, data are collected on at least two measured variables. These data are collected using tools similar to those used in descriptive research: surveys, standardized tests, interviews, observations, and existing data sets, such as those listed as secondary sources in figure 1.2. Readers should note that researchers often combine data from their own questionnaires and EHRs with data from large databases, such as the Centers for Medicare and Medicaid Services' (CMS's) Hospital Compare.

For example, researchers might conduct a correlational study investigating the associations among three variables: stress, anxiety, and feelings of personal accomplishment. On a scatter plot, the researchers could graph the scores (values) of the variables and find that the scores clustered around a straight line. A straight-line association is known as a *linear association,* which can be either positive or negative, as follows:

- A **positive (direct) linear relationship (association)** exists when the scores for variables proportionately move in the *same* direction (Singleton and Straits 2010, 91). For example, the researchers in the hypothetical study about stress, anxiety, and personal accomplishment might summarize their findings by stating that as participants' scores on stress increased, their scores on anxiety also proportionately increased. The researchers could also state their findings conversely, indicating that as the participants' scores on stress decreased, their scores on anxiety also proportionately decreased. In both statements of the results, the variables are proportionately moving in the *same* direction—as one increased, so did the other, *or* as one decreased, so did the other. This association is a positive relationship because the variables' scores are moving in the same direction, as demonstrated in figure 1.3a.
- A **negative (inverse) linear relationship (association)** exists when the scores of the variables proportionately move in *opposite (inverse)* directions (Singleton and Straits 2010, 91). For example, reporting on the same hypothetical study, the researchers might state that as participants' scores on stress increased, their scores on feelings of personal accomplishment proportionately decreased. Conversely, the researchers could state that as participants' scores on stress decreased, their scores on feelings of personal accomplishment proportionately increased. In both statements of the results, the variables are proportionately moving in the *opposite* directions—as one increased, the other decreased, *or* as one decreased, the other increased. This association is a negative (inverse) relationship because the variables' scores are proportionately moving in opposite directions, as demonstrated in figure 1.3b.

Figure 1.3 Examples of positive linear relationship, negative linear relationship, and curvilinear relationship

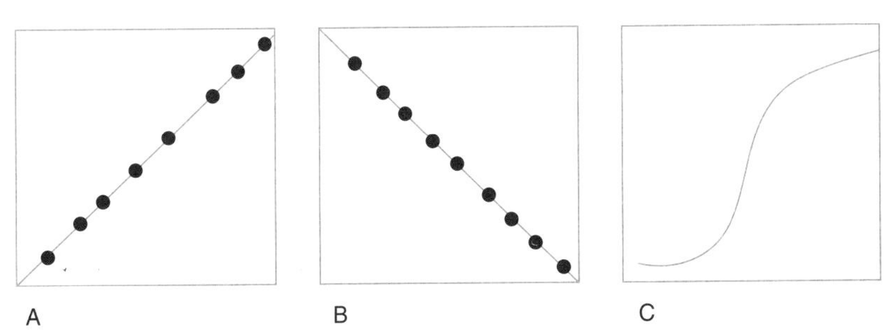

This subsection focuses primarily on linear associations because they are frequently studied in correlational research. Curvilinear associations, which are named for their shapes, such as *s*-curves, *j*-curves, and *u*-curves, are not as commonly studied. Figure 1.3c presents an *s*-curve that shows the rate of learning. In this learning curve, learning begins slowly, then rapidly increases, and then plateaus. Curvilinear and other nonlinear associations require different statistical techniques than those used to analyze linear associations.

The strength of a linear association can be understood as the accuracy of the prediction (Singleton and Straits 2010, 93). The strength of the association among variables can range from 0.00 to +1 or from 0.00 to −1, detailed as follows:

- Strength of 0.00 means absolutely no association.
- Strength between 0.00 and +1 or between 0.00 and −1 means that the variables sometimes, but not always, move together.
- Strength of 1 or −1 means a perfect association, with the variables moving exactly in tandem.

Terms and rough guidelines on cutoffs for the strength of associations are as follows:

- No or little association: 0.00 to 0.09 and 0.00 to –0.09
- Small or weak association: 0.10 to 0.29 and –0.10 to –0.29

- Medium or moderate association: 0.30 to 0.49 and –0.30 to –0.49
- Large or strong association: 0.50 to 0.10 and –0.50 to –0.10 (Ebrahim 1999, 14)

Generally, the closer the values are to +1 or −1, the stronger the linear association.

Correlational research cannot establish a causal relationship. A **causal relationship** demonstrates cause and effect, such that one variable *causes* the change in another variable. There are two reasons why researchers who conduct correlational studies cannot make causal statements:

- Correlational research is not experimental, and experimental research is one way to establish cause and effect (experimental research is covered later in this chapter).
- An unknown variable could be creating the apparent association identified in the correlational study. This unknown variable is called a **confounding (extraneous, secondary) variable** because it confounds (confuses) interpretation of the data.

In the hypothetical stress-anxiety-personal accomplishment study we have been considering, the correlational design does *not* allow the researchers to state that (1) stress *caused* anxiety to increase (or vice versa); (2) stress *caused* the feelings of personal accomplishment to decrease (or vice versa); or (3) any of the variables *caused* the other ones to change. In this case, a confounding variable, such as financial problems, poor coping skills, or low self-confidence, could explain the research's results. What the researchers who conducted the stress-anxiety-personal accomplishment study *can* state is that the variables, stress, anxiety, and personal accomplishment, are related to one another.

Finally, another shortcoming of some correlational studies is that they rely on self-reported data from the subjects. Unfortunately, retrospective self-reported data can be influenced by the subjects' biases, their selective memories, or the perceived social desirability of certain data options (study participants may tend to over report "good" behavior and under report "bad" behavior). Some descriptive studies share this shortcoming.

Researchers have conducted correlational studies on topics related to health informatics and HIM, including factors related to the adoption of HIT, patients' rates of social media usage and their ratings of providers, healthcare professionals' security practices and the personal characteristics of those professionals, use of mobile apps and maintenance of health regimens, and many more topics.

For example, researchers investigated correlations among three variables: the ability of a mobile device to monitor teens' asthma control, asthma symptoms (such as coughing), and the teens' quality of life (such as limited activities) in the short-term (Rhee et al. 2015, 1). The researchers' small convenience sample was 84 teens (42 teens with a current asthma diagnosis; 42 without asthma) between the ages of 13 and 17 years. Data came from the mobile device, the asthma teens' automated diaries, laboratory test results, and three questionnaires and were analyzed using correlational statistics (Pearson product-moment correlation coefficient and multiple regression, which are explained in chapter 9). Data from the device showed the current status of teens' asthma control and predicted the teens' asthma symptoms and quality of life. The researchers stated that the study was limited by the small convenience sample and the self-reported data on the questionnaires.

Observational Research

Observational research is exploratory research that identifies factors, contexts, and experiences through observations in natural settings. Its focus is the participants' perspective of their own feelings, behaviors, and perceptions. Observational research is highly descriptive and provides insights into what subjects do, how they do it, and why they do it. Observational researchers may use either the quantitative approach or the qualitative approach. However, most observational research is classified as qualitative research because of its emphasis on uncovering underlying beliefs and meanings.

Observational researchers observe, record, analyze, and interpret behaviors and events. They attempt to capture and record the natural, typical behavior of their participants (subjects) in their context and their natural surroundings. Observational research is intensive, and researchers amass volumes of detailed data. Common tools in observational research are case notes, check sheets, audiotapes, and videotapes. Typically, observational researchers spend prolonged periods in the setting or events being researched; however, some research topics, such as behaviors in natural disasters, prevent this type of prolonged engagement. Data collection and analysis often are concurrent with additional participant interviews, which are used to address perceived gaps or capture missing viewpoints. Observational research focuses on collecting **rich data**, thick descriptions and layers of extensive details from multiple sources. Sources of data include observations, interviews, and artifacts. **Artifacts** are objects that humans make that serve a purpose and have meaning (Malt and Paquet 2013, 354–355). Health-related examples of artifacts include administrative records, financial records, policy and procedure manuals, legal documents, government documents, flowcharts, paper-based charts, EHRs, sign-in sheets, photographs, diaries, and many more items. Through analysis, observational descriptions and details are categorized into overarching themes. The themes are then interpreted to answer the research question. Details, such as participants' narratives, are often used in the reporting of observational studies to illustrate the researchers' interpretations. Care is taken to include and to account for discrepancies, nuances, idiosyncrasies, and inconsistencies.

Observational researchers often use triangulation to support their findings. **Triangulation** is the use of multiple sources or perspectives to investigate the same phenomenon. The multiple sources or perspectives can include data (multiple times, sites, or respondents), investigators (researchers), theories, and methods (Carter et al. 2014, 545). The results or conclusions are validated if the multiple sources or perspectives arrive at the same results or conclusions. This technique lends credence to the research.

There are many types of observational research. In 1990, a research methodologist identified more than 40 types of observational studies, although many of these types overlap or are identical (Tesch 1990, 58). Three common types of observational research are nonparticipant observation, participant observation, and ethnography.

Nonparticipant Observation

In **nonparticipant observation**, researchers act as neutral observers who neither intentionally interact with nor affect the actions of the participants being observed. The researchers record and analyze observed behaviors as well as the content of modes of communication, such as documentation, speech, body language, music, television shows, commercials, and movies. Three common types of nonparticipant observation are naturalistic observation, simulation observation, and case study.

Naturalistic Observation In **naturalistic observation**, researchers record observations that are unprompted and unaffected by the investigators' actions. Researchers can conduct naturalistic studies in organizations; for example, they might study how the implementation of a type of HIT affected work flow at a hospital. Researchers conducting a naturalistic observation within an organization face the problem of remaining unobtrusive. The researchers' mere presence can affect people's behavior (known as the Hawthorne or John Henry effect). However, the strength of naturalistic studies, if researchers resolve this problem in their study's design, is that participants tend to act more naturally in their real setting than in simulated settings. Naturalistic studies are sometimes conducted after a disaster, such as a computer system breach, earthquake, hurricane, or other phenomenon. Researchers conducting natural experiments on disasters wait for the phenomenon to occur naturally. For example, researchers interested in the effectiveness of IT disaster recovery plans could establish baseline data and tools for data collection before a disaster occurred and then wait for the opportunity to record their observations of the actions and results when a disaster actually happened.

Simulation Observation In **simulation observation**, researchers stage events rather than allowing them to occur naturally. Researchers can invent their own simulations or use standardized vignettes to stage the events. For example, researchers may conduct a simulation study to evaluate an application's use, content, and format. Simulations could also develop and test the data collection tools for a naturalistic observation study of a disaster or other event. Researchers can build or use simulation laboratories to substitute for the actual setting. To allow observations of activities and behaviors, these laboratories may have one-way windows or projection screens.

Case Study A **case study** is an in-depth investigation of one or more examples of a phenomenon, such as a trend, occurrence, or incident. Case studies are intensive, and researchers gather rich data. The "case" can be a person, an event, a group, an organization, or a set of similar institutions. Depending on their research question, researchers select various types of sample cases. Types of sample cases include similar cases but with differing outcomes, differing cases but with the same outcome, diverse or contrasting cases, typical or representative cases, influential or pioneering cases, and other types. Case study researchers can also combine types of sample cases. For example, to identify general good practices researchers could select typical or representative cases that had the same successful outcome. Researchers report their case studies as detailed accounts or stories.

Participant Observation

In **participant observation**, researchers participate in the observed actions, activities, processes, or other situations. Participant observation research is used to investigate groups, processes, cultures, and other phenomena. The researchers record their observations of other people's daily lives, the contexts of people's actions, and their own experiences and thoughts. Researchers using participant observation may reflect the insiders' perspectives, which can be both an advantage and a disadvantage of this approach. As insiders, the researchers may have unique insights into the environment and context of the situation. At the same time, however, the researchers may share the biases and blind spots of insiders. Therefore, in participant observation, researchers attempt to maintain neutrality while being involved in the situation.

Researchers can participate overtly (openly) or covertly (secretly) in participant observation. Covert observation involves the deception of other participants in the study and other organizational members, and many ethicists consider it to be unethical (Spicker 2011, 118–123). Covert observation may involve breaches of the right to privacy and the principle of informed consent. Additionally, covert observation can undermine human relationships by eroding trust and disregarding honesty. On the other hand, the ethical principal of utility—the greatest good for the greatest number—and the advancement of science may override the ethical breaches of covert observation (Parker and Ashencaen Crabtree 2014, 35–36). In general, researchers who are considering covert observation as their research method should assess whether the data could be collected using another method and should seek counsel from appropriate research oversight entities.

Ethnography

Ethnography, which has its origins in anthropology, is the exhaustive examination of a culture by collecting data and making observations while being in the field (a naturalistic setting). Ethnographers amass great volumes of detailed data while living or working with the population that they are studying. This observational method includes both qualitative and quantitative approaches and both participant and nonparticipant observation. Characteristics of ethnography include immersion in the field, the accrual of volumes of data, and great attention to the environment. Ethnographers gather data with field notes (jotted observations in notebooks), interviews, diagrams, artifacts, and audio, video, and digital recordings. Ethnographers gather data about the following:

- *Environment*, such as physical spaces, participants, participants' general roles and responsibilities, and other aspects of the setting
- *Organizational characteristics*, such as strategic and tactical plans, procedures, processes, organizational charts, and division of labor
- *Flow of activities*, such as stages in a process, participants' particular roles and perspectives, and sequences of interactions and practices
- *Collaborative or cooperative actions and informal relationships,* such as conversational groups and hand-over of tasks
- *Physical, communication, and digital resources*, such as computers, audit trails, and keystroke logs (Crabtree et al. 2012, 78–84).

Ethnography can obtain insights not discoverable in other research designs. However, the design may result in quantities of data that are difficult to analyze without making large investments of money and time.

Observational research may be combined with other designs, such as descriptive research. Focused on specific contexts, observational researchers do not attempt to generalize to other situations. However, the findings of observational research may result in testable hypotheses for subsequent quantitative research studies that do seek generalizability. Characteristics of high-quality observational research are credibility, transferability, dependability, and confirmability (Guba and Lincoln 1989, 236–243). These characteristics are defined in table 1.3. However, observational research can be time-consuming, human resource–intensive, and expensive.

Table 1.3 Criteria for quality observational research

Criterion	Definition
Credibility	Procedures of the study that support the accuracy and representativeness of the thoughts, feelings, perceptions, and descriptions of the subjects under study. Examples include involvement of appropriate duration and intensity; revision of hypotheses to account for facts; and ongoing review of data, analysis, and interpretation with participants.
Transferability	Degree to which key characteristics of contexts are similar and, thus, applicable to other contexts. Transferability affects the ability to apply the results of research in one context to other similar contexts. Detailed and extensive (rich) descriptions of the context are the primary way to establish transferability.

(Continued)

Table 1.3 (*Continued*)

Criterion	Definition
Dependability	Reliability of data achieved by being able to explicitly track and account for changes in the design and methods of the study occasioned by changing conditions, identification of gaps, or other important factors. The dependability audit is the means to open decision making to public inspection.
Confirmability	Ability to trace data to original sources and ensure that another person analyzing, categorizing, and interpreting the data based on the research's documentation would confirm the logic. Confirmability is established by external reviewers conducting a confirmability audit.

Source: Guba and Lincoln 1989, 236–243.

Health informatics and HIM researchers are building a body of knowledge for evidence-based practice. Observational research supports this effort because observational research records what actually occurred in real time, rather than what subjects retrospectively recall occurred. For example, health informatics researchers can observe how users actually navigate an application, follow what really happened in an implementation, or understand other types of situations related to HIT.

The following are some reasons why health informatics and HIM researchers might choose to conduct observational research:

- **To study work flow**—Health informatics and HIM researchers can observe artifacts that support workers' use of various health information technologies and applications. Are manuals sitting by the device or are diagrams taped to the wall? Are cheat sheets and sticky tabs posted on workstations? Can these artifacts be categorized? Could the hardware or software be designed to include the necessary information; thus, eliminating the need for artifacts? Under what conditions, such as during the performance of particular tasks or at certain times of the day, do users pay attention to or ignore alerts?
- **To investigate the functioning of health information systems**—Health informatics and HIM researchers can observe the exchange and transmission of health information throughout a staged event, such as a disaster drill. In the drill, does the information system support users, both familiar and unfamiliar with the system, and provide information when and where it is needed? After an actual disaster, health informatics and HIM researchers can observe and record the actual performance of post-disaster information recovery plans.
- **To uncover why clinicians, administrators, and other personnel use (or do not use) various decision support tools**—Health informatics and HIM researchers can create scenarios of complex diagnostic or administrative problems requiring decisions for which the health information systems had embedded resources. The researchers might then ask the users to explain how they obtain the information needed to solve the problem and record the users' explanations.
- **To examine specific modules (applications) within health information systems**—How can data from health departments' syndromic surveillance systems be combined with data from health information exchange systems to support the delivery of care and services during and after disasters?
- **To investigate why healthcare organizations' online programs to engage patients work (or do not work)**—How do patients respond to targeting and how can tailoring algorithms augment engagement?

A case study of how well portals convey information to patients provides an example of an observational research study (Alpert et al. 2016, 1). The patient-participants were selected because they had used the portal at least once in the past year, were between the ages of 18 and 79 years, and had an upcoming clinic appointment. The volunteer clinician-participants (full-time physicians, residents, nurses, and an emergency medical technician) were recruited through e-mails and announcements. The researchers collected data by conducting 31 interviews with the patient-participants and by holding two focus groups of clinicians (focus groups are discussed in detail in chapter 3). In the interviews and focus groups, the researchers asked the participants to describe their best and worst experiences with the portal. The average length of the interviews was 14 minutes; the average length of the focus groups was 51 minutes. All responses were audio-recorded and transcribed. Data collection continued until the investigators identified that similar phrases and words were recurring and no new concepts were being revealed. Content analysis was used to analyze the data (content analysis is described in chapter 3). The researchers' results suggested that some simple modifications to the portals, such as increased interactivity and personalized messages, could enhance the patients' understanding of the information. The researchers noted that a limitation of the study was that the participants represented a small subset of all users in terms of ages, ethnicities, and socioeconomic classes.

Evaluation Research

Evaluation research is the systematic application of criteria to assess the value of objects (Øvretveit 2014, 6–13). *Systematic* is a key term in the definition of evaluation research. Value can be assessed in terms of merit, worth, quality, or a combination of these attributes (CDC 2012, 6). Examples of evaluated objects include policies, programs, technologies (including procedures or implementations), products, processes, events, conditions, and organizations. Criteria to assess these activities or objects can be related to many of their aspects, such as conceptualization, design, components, implementation, usability, effectiveness, efficiency, impact, scalability, and generalizability. Depending on the focus of the research, the researchers' educational background, and the research's funding source, other terms may be used for studies conducted under the large umbrella of evaluation research (see table 1.4).

Table 1.4 Terms used to describe evaluation research studies

Term	Description	Health Informatics and HIM Example
Outcomes research	Research that seeks to improve the delivery of patient care by studying the end results of health services, such as quality of life, functional status, patient satisfaction, costs, cost-effectiveness, and other specified outcomes (In and Rosen 2014, 489).	Investigation of whether a clinical decision support system that links the EHR to treatment protocols, drug information, alerts, and community resources for the care of patients with HIV infection improves patients' quality of life.
Health services research	Multidisciplinary research that studies how social factors, financing systems, organizational structures and processes, health technologies, and personal behaviors affect access to healthcare, its quality and cost, and overall health and well-being. The research is usually concerned with relationships among need, demand, supply, use, and outcome of health services (Stephens et al. 2014).	Investigation of whether the degree of an organization's adoption of health information technologies affects patient safety.
Health technology assessment (HTA)	Evaluation of the usefulness (utility) of a health technology in relation to cost, efficacy, utilization, and other factors in terms of its impact on social, ethical, and legal systems. The purpose of HTA is to provide individual patients, clinicians, funding bodies, and policymakers with high-quality information on both the direct and intended effects and the indirect and unintended consequences (INAHTA 2016). Technology, in this context, is broadly defined as the application of scientific knowledge to practical purposes and includes methods, techniques, and instrumentation. Health technologies promote or maintain health; prevent, diagnose, or treat acute or chronic conditions; or support rehabilitation. They include pharmaceuticals, medical devices, medical equipment, medical diagnostic and therapeutic procedures, organizational systems, and health information technologies.	The Technology Assessment Program of the Agency for Healthcare Research and Quality (AHRQ) conducts technology assessments based on primary research, systematic reviews of the literature, meta-analyses, and appropriate qualitative methods of synthesizing data from multiple studies (AHRQ 2016a). CMS uses AHRQ's HTAs to make national coverage decisions for the Medicare program.
Comparative effectiveness research (CER)	Research that generates and synthesizes comparative evidence about the benefits and harms of alternative methods to prevent, diagnose, treat, and monitor a clinical condition, or to improve the delivery of care. This evidence can assist consumers, clinicians, purchasers, and policymakers to make informed decisions that will improve healthcare at both the individual and population levels (AHRQ 2016b).	Investigation to determine whether a self-managed online diabetes support program or a clinician-moderated online diabetes support program is most effective or beneficial for a given patient.

(*Continued*)

Table 1.4 (*Continued*)

Term	Description	Health Informatics and HIM Example
Usability testing	Evaluation that assesses whether a product or service achieves its intended goals effectively, efficiently, and satisfactorily for representative users in a typical setting. In this evaluation, the users are the focus, not the product or service. Effectiveness is defined by whether a wide range of intended users can achieve the intended goal. Efficiency is considered in terms of the users' time, effort, and other resources. Satisfaction is defined by whether users are satisfied with the experience and also takes into account their relative opinion about this particular product or service when other alternatives are available (ISO 2013).	Investigation of whether users can schedule an appointment, obtain laboratory test results, and e-mail their provider using the healthcare organization's portal.

Common types of evaluation studies are needs assessments, process evaluations, outcome evaluations, and policy analyses (see table 1.5). Evaluation researchers conduct studies for several reasons, including the following:

- To ascertain progress in implementing key provisions of a plan, process, or program
- To assess the extent of achieving desired outcomes
- To identify effective practices for achieving desired results
- To determine opportunities to improve performance
- To evaluate the success of corrective actions (GAO 2012, 13)

Table 1.5 Common types of evaluation research studies

Type of study	Description	Health Informatics or HIM Example
Needs assessment	Collecting and analyzing data about proposed programs, projects, and other activities or objects to determine what is required, lacking, or desired by an employee, a group, an organization, or another user. Data are also collected on the extent, the severity, and the priorities of the needs (Shi 2008, 213).	Survey of patients to determine their preferences and priorities for various features in the healthcare organization's patient portal.
Process evaluation (also known as *formative evaluation*)	Monitoring programs, projects, and other activities or objects to check whether their development, implementation, or operation is proceeding as planned; may include investigation of alternative processes, procedures, or other activities or objects (GAO 2012, 15).	Assessment of the roll-out of new features in the organization's patient portal to determine whether the roll-out is achieving the project's milestones and within budget. Adjustments to the process can then be made as needed.
Outcome evaluation (also known as *summative evaluation*)	Collecting and analyzing data at the end of an implementation or operating cycle to determine whether the program, project, or other activity or object has achieved its expected or intended impact, product, or other outcome; includes investigation of whether any unintended consequences have occurred (Shi 2008, 218–219). The impact evaluation is a form of outcome evaluation that looks at long-term effects, such as what would have happened had the activity or object not been implemented or whether the impact has extended beyond the initial target population (GAO 2012, 16).	Comparison between the level of patients' interaction with the organization's patient portal and the level of interaction reported by industry peers. Organizational leaders can use the findings to help decide whether the portal vendor's contract should be renewed or revised.

(*Continued*)

Table 1.5 (*Continued*)

Type of study	Description	Health Informatics or HIM Example
Policy analysis	Identifying options to meet goals, estimating the costs and consequences of each option prior to the implementation of any option, and considering constraints of time, information, and resources (Shi 2008, 219–220).	A federal agency's identification of various ways to increase patient self-management and engagement by using health information technologies; including, for each way, an analysis of its benefits and costs; and a prediction of its consequences.

Evaluation research can involve a quantitative, qualitative, or mixed-methods approach. Moreover, evaluation research can use any of the other research designs; it is the purpose—evaluation—that classifies the design as evaluation. For example, in a descriptive evaluation study, researchers could compile data on the characteristics and numbers of people using a technology. In another example, researchers could conduct an observational evaluation study to investigate how users navigate through new features of the patient portal.

Evaluation researchers collect data by using tools such as case studies, field observations, interviews, experiments, and existing data sets, such as those identified in figure 1.2.

Evaluation research is assessed against four overarching standards, as stated below:

- **Utility:** Relevant information will be provided to people who need it at the time they need it.
- **Feasibility:** There is a realistic likelihood that the evaluation can succeed if given the necessary time, resources, and expertise.
- **Propriety:** Appropriate protections for individuals' rights and welfare are in place and the appropriate stakeholders, such as users and the surrounding community, are involved.
- **Accuracy:** The evaluation's results will be accurate, valid, and reliable for their users. (CDC 2012, 10)

Like other investigators, individuals conducting evaluation research must follow established protocols (detailed sets of rules and procedures), use defensible analytic procedures, and make their processes and results available to other researchers. Evaluation research should be capable of being replicated and reproduced by other researchers. Examples of evaluation studies include investigations of the usability, utilization, effectiveness, and impact of telehealth services, network-based registries, clinical decision support systems for various medical specialties (such as radiology, emergency medicine, and others) and conditions (such as diabetes, asthma, and others), mapping systems to capture data for decision support systems, and mobile devices. Researchers use a variety of techniques to conduct the evaluation studies.

Using a mixed-methods research approach, a contracted research agency conducted an outcome evaluation and a policy analysis of the Regional Extension Center (REC) program for the Office of the National Coordinator for Health Information Technology (ONC) (Farrar et al. 2016). As part of the HITECH Act, the REC program funded support to healthcare providers to assist them in adopting EHRs and other HIT. These providers included solo and small physician practices, federally qualified health centers and rural clinics, critical access hospitals, and other providers for underserved populations (often rural and poor).

The agency's researchers collected descriptive data through interviews and focus groups with REC representatives, an electronic survey of RECs, and surveys of Health Information Technology Research Center (HITRC) online portal users. A few examples of questions that researchers asked to evaluate the REC program included the following:

- How did RECs structure and organize their programs?
- What contextual conditions influenced the implementation and operation of the REC programs?
- Was REC participation associated with adoption of EHRs?
- Was REC participation associated with receiving incentives through the Medicare and Medicaid EHR Incentive Programs?
- Was REC participation associated with positive opinions about EHRs?

The researchers described the impact of the REC program by comparing outcomes for REC participants to outcomes for nonparticipants. The evaluation study found that 68 percent of the eligible professionals who received incentive payments under the federal meaningful use incentive program (stage 1) were assisted by an REC, compared to just 12 percent of those who did not work with an REC (Farrar et al. 2016, 5). Generally, the REC program had a "major impact" (Mason 2016). In terms of policy analysis, the evaluation study identified several points that policymakers should consider. For example, the REC model was an effective way to achieve program goals; also, tools and resources should be in place prior to the startup of a program (Farrar et al. 2016, 53–54).

Experimental Research

Experimental research is a research design in which researchers follow a strict procedure to randomly assign subjects to groups, manipulate the subjects' experience, and finally measure any resulting physical, behavioral, or other changes in the subjects. Experimental researchers create strictly controlled situations and environments in which to observe, measure, analyze, and interpret the effects of their manipulations on subjects or phenomena. Researchers conduct experimental research to establish cause-and-effect (causal) relationships. As previously noted in the subsection on correlational research, experimental research is one research design that can establish causal relationships.

Experimental research has four features, which are as follows (Campbell and Stanley 1963):

- **Randomization:** The process begins with **random sampling**, which is the unbiased selection of subjects from the population of interest. (Random sampling is discussed in detail in chapter 11.) Then, **randomization**, or the random allocation of subjects to the comparison groups, occurs. Of the comparison groups, the **experimental (study) group** comprises the research subjects who receive the study's intervention, whereas the **control group** comprises those who do not receive the study's intervention.
- **Observation:** The **dependent variable**, which is the hypothesized change, is measured *before* and *after* the intervention. Observation is used broadly and could be a pretest and a posttest. (It is acceptable to omit the *before* observation.)
- **Presence of a control group:** The experiment must compare outcomes for participants who do and do not receive the intervention.
- **Treatment (intervention):** The researcher manipulates the **independent variables**, which are the factors or actions that the researchers are proposing will cause the hypothesized change. In this context, *treatment* is defined broadly, beyond its usual meaning of therapy, to refer to any type of intervention. Treatment could mean a computer training program, an algorithm to extract medical abbreviations from bibliographic databases, a specific technology or application, or a procedure to implement health information and communication technologies.

Studies that have all four of these features are classified as *experimental*, but studies that lack any of the features are classified as *quasi-experimental*. Experimental research methods include pretest-posttest control group method, Solomon four-group method, and posttest-only group method (see chapter 4).

In experimental studies, researchers actively intervene to test a *hypothesis* (a measurable statement of the researchers' supposition). The researchers follow strict protocols, which are detailed set of rules and procedures. Protocols must be established in advance (a priori) of the study's inception. This explicit documentation of protocols assists researchers in planning their study and in consistently conducting it. Furthermore, protocols promote accountability, research integrity, and transparency (Moher et al. 2015, 8).

Experimental researchers randomly select participants (subjects) and then randomly allocate the participants into either an experimental or control group. In experimental studies, these groups are often called *arms,* with the experimental group being called the *intervention arm* and the control group known as the *control arm*. As a part of the random allocation, blinding or masking often occurs. Blinding prevents the parties involved in an experimental study—the subjects, the researchers, and the study managers or analysts—from knowing whether a participant belongs to the experimental or control group. Table 1.6 describes the various types of blinding. The purpose of blinding is to minimize the risk of subjective bias stemming from the researcher's or the subject's expectations and perceptions. These subjective biases are known as *observer-expectancy effect* and *subject-expectancy effect*. In observer-expectancy effect, the researcher (observer) expects a particular outcome and then unconsciously manipulates the experiment to achieve it. In subject-expectancy effect, a research participant (subject) expects a particular outcome and either unconsciously manipulates the experiment or reports the expected outcome.

Table 1.6 Types of blinding in research

Type of Blinding	Description
Single-blind	Only the subjects are blinded to knowing whether or not they are receiving the intervention.
Double-blind	Both researchers and subjects are blinded to knowing whether or not particular subjects are receiving the intervention.
Triple-blind	Staff members managing the study's operations and analyzing the data, researchers, and subjects are all blinded to knowing whether or not particular subjects are receiving the intervention.

According to the protocol, the researchers systematically manipulate independent variables (factors) in interventions for the experimental group. In doing so, the researchers test the variables' influences on the dependent variables (effects or outcomes). To assess the variables' influences, the researchers conduct an initial observation (measurement), such as a pretest, to establish a baseline. Then, after the manipulation—the intervention—the researchers conduct a second observation, such as a posttest (sometimes, multiple observations are made).

As they manipulate factors, experimental researchers are careful to fully control their environments and subjects. *Control* is the processes used to maintain uniform conditions during a study in order to eliminate sources of bias and variations and to remove any potential extraneous factors that might affect the research's outcome. Control is an important aspect of experimental research because the researchers' end goal is to pinpoint the cause of the intervention's effect without any possible alternative explanations related to bias, variation, or unknown factors. In a well-controlled experiment, any differences between the experimental group's measured outcomes and the control group's measured outcomes would be due to the intervention.

Given their importance in research studies, independent variables and dependent variables need more discussion. *Independent variables* are antecedent or prior factors that researchers manipulate directly; they are also called *treatments* or *interventions*. *Dependent variables* are the measured variables; they depend on the independent variables. The selection of dependent variables to measure reflects the results that the researcher has theorized. They occur subsequently or after the independent variables. See table 1.7 for a side-by-side comparison of the characteristics of independent and dependent variables. The features of experimental research—randomization, observation, control group, and treatment—and the procedures of the protocol aim to make the dependent variable—the outcome variable—the only difference between the two groups and, thereby, establish a causal relationship between the treatment and the outcome. In other words, experimental research tests whether the independent variable causes an effect in the dependent variable.

Table 1.7 Comparison of characteristics of independent variables and dependent variables

Independent Variable	Dependent Variable
Cause	Effect
Originates stimulus or is treatment	Receives Stimulus or treatment
Causes or influences change in dependent variable	Measured for effect or influence of stimulus or treatment
Manipulated	Measured for effect of manipulation of independent variable
Antecedent, prior	Successor, subsequent
Action	Consequence
Other terms: Covariable or covariate, predictor, predictor variable, treatment, treatment variable	Other terms: Covariable or covariate, criterion variable, outcome, outcome variable

Randomized controlled trials (RCTs), studies in which subjects are randomly selected and randomly assigned to an experimental group or a control group, are an important type of experimental research, particularly in medicine. *Controlled* refers to the use of a control group. Alternative terms for RCTs are *clinical trials, randomized clinical trials,* and *randomized control trials. Clinical* refers to *at the bedside,* meaning the experiment involves investigations of diagnostic and therapeutic procedures, drugs, devices and technologies, and other biomedical and health interventions.

Both health informatics and HIM researchers may conduct RCTs. RCTs related to these fields have been conducted to evaluate the effectiveness of HIT in medication safety; the impact of technologies—such as cellular phones, telehealth, the Internet, tablets, activity trackers, social media, and other technologies—on exercise and physical activity, diet, medication compliance, treatment adherence, engagement, and other outcomes; the effect of decision support systems used by various types of clinicians (nurses, surgeons, trauma physicians, and others) for various conditions (pediatric blunt head trauma, kidney disease, and other conditions) and for various functions (medication prescribing, medication reviews, diagnosing diseases, and other functions); and other studies evaluating health technologies and their use.

For example, Ford and colleagues conducted an RCT to investigate whether a single-screen display of all reports could increase the timely and accurate acknowledgement of critical and noncritical results as compared to other systems (Ford et al. 2016, 214). The researchers explained that in many current EHRs, reports—such as those providing laboratory test results—are displayed on multiple screens. The researchers obtained 100 reports each from two EHR systems and displayed them in the two systems' respective formats. Then, the researchers displayed the same 200 reports in their test single-screen display. On a single test computer, the study's participants, 12 physicians and 30 nonphysician providers, reviewed and processed the 400 reports. The study's results showed that the single-screen display was superior compared with the other two systems, both in reducing review times and improving accuracy.

Although experimental studies can lead to improvements in healthcare, health informatics and HIM researchers face barriers when conducting experimental studies. These barriers include practical constraints, such as how to blind clinicians to the fact that they are using a new technology; pressures because the timelines to implement new technologies are short; complex workflows that involve many different clinicians, professionals, and patients; and the highly regulated environments of human subjects research and healthcare delivery.

Quasi-experimental Research

Quasi-experimental studies involve nonrandomized groups, observations, and treatments. **Quasi-experimental research** searches for *plausible* causal factors or indicates that a causal relationship *could* exist. To conduct quasi-experimental investigations, researchers *approximate* the environment of true experiments. In quasi-experimental studies, researchers investigate *possible* cause-and-effect relationships by exposing one or more experimental groups to one or more treatment conditions and comparing the results to one or more control groups not receiving the treatment. However, the phenomenon or variables under study do not allow the researchers to control and manipulate all their relevant aspects. Often, a quasi-experimental study does not use randomization, a key element of a true experimental design. As the term *quasi* implies, quasi-experimental research design is "similar to" or "almost" experimental research, but quasi-experimental research lacks the ability to establish causal relationships as experimental research can. Quasi-experimental research is also called **causal-comparative research** or *ex post facto* (retrospective) *research*, when it involves a variable from the past or phenomenon that has already occurred. Types of quasi-experimental research methods include one-shot case method, one-group pretest-posttest method, and static group comparison method (see chapter 4).

In quasi-experimental studies, researchers compare the outcomes of various factors to detect differences or associations. They investigate how a particular independent variable (factor, event, situation, or other independent variable) affects a dependent variable (outcome, effect, or other dependent variable). A quasi-experimental study is the appropriate choice when any of these following situations exist:

- The independent variables cannot be manipulated (for example, gender, age, race, birth place).
- The independent variables should not be manipulated (for example, accidental death or injury, child abuse).
- The independent variables represent differing conditions that have already occurred (for example, medication error, heart catheterization performed, smoking).

These situations prevent people from being randomly assigned into experimental and control groups. To do so as a true experiment would be infeasible or unethical.

In some quasi-experimental studies, the researchers manipulate the independent variable. However, despite the manipulation, these studies are still quasi-experimental because the researchers do not randomly assign participants to groups. Data may be collected before and after an event, exposure, intervention, or other independent variable, or all the data may be collected after all the variables of interest have occurred. The researchers then identify one or more effects (dependent variables) and examine the data by going back through time, detecting differences or seeking out associations.

Quasi-experimental research studies cannot establish causal relationships because the studies may potentially have biases or confounders. First, studies that lack random assignment may be biased. Second, in other typical quasi-experimental studies, the researchers lack control over all variables. For example, the researchers observe the effect of a factor that has already occurred, such as an intervention, a diagnostic or therapeutic procedure, a risk factor, an exposure, an event, or some other factor. The investigators are not themselves manipulating the factor, and this lack of control allows the possible introduction of a confounding variable.

Quasi-experimental studies on health informatics and HIM topics have been conducted to compare physical activity and mental and cardiometabolic health between people living near a green space and people living at a distance from a green space; evaluate the effectiveness of HIT in medication safety; assess the effectiveness of decision support systems for various diseases and functions; and evaluate the impact of technologies, such as cellular phones, text messaging, delivery of telehealth services, social media, and online educational module programs on physical and health activities, knowledge and performance, treatment and medication adherence, engagement, health outcomes, and other outcomes. Study data in these quasi-experiments were often collected through questionnaires and surveys.

A quasi-experimental study conducted by Bottorff and colleagues investigated the potential of an online, man-centered smoking cessation intervention to engage men in reducing and quitting smoking (Bottorff et al. 2016, 1–2). The pretest-posttest study included one group of 117 male smokers. Data were collected through online questionnaires. The study's results revealed that the intervention's website had the potential to serve as a self-guided smoking cessation resource. Predictors of the number of times a participant attempted to quit were the number of resources he used on the website and the subject's confidence in his ability to quit. Most of the men reported they had quit smoking for 24 hours or longer since using the intervention's website. The researchers reported that limitations of their study included the sample's potential failure to represent all male smokers, the possibility that self-reported measures introduced recall and reporting bias, and smoking cessation was not verified.

Time Frame as an Element of Research Design

Time frame is an element of all seven types of research design. There are two pairs of time frames: retrospective and prospective, and cross-sectional and longitudinal.

Retrospective Time Frame Versus Prospective Time Frame

Research that uses a **retrospective** time frame looks back in time on that which has already occurred. For example, using a retrospective time frame, researchers could conduct a study about early adopters of HIT. The researchers could ask the early adopters to list factors or reconstruct events that led to their early adoption. For some types of questions, such as those related to historic events, a retrospective design is the only possible design.

Research that uses a **prospective** time frame follows subjects into the future to examine relationships between variables and later occurrences. For example, researchers could identify individuals who have successfully increased their physical activity using activity trackers. The prospective time frame would then follow these individuals or subjects into the future to see what occurs.

Cross-Sectional Time Frame Versus Longitudinal Time Frame

A **cross-sectional** time frame collects or reviews the data at one point in time. For example, researchers could conduct a study for a professional association on the characteristics of its members, such as age, gender, job titles, educational attainment, and opinions of the associations' web page. Because cross-sectional studies are snapshots, they may potentially collect data for an entirely unrepresentative time period.

A **longitudinal** time frame collects data from participants in three or more *waves* (phases) to compare changes in health, satisfaction, effectiveness, perceptions, and other variables of interest (Ployhart and Ward 2011, 414). Conducting a study using a longitudinal time frame is complex and requires more explanation than the other time frames (Ployhart and Vandenberg 2010, 95). The duration of longitudinal studies can be days, a week, months, years, or lifetimes. The study duration and the frequency and timing of the data collections (observations) depend on the topic. For example, researchers who conducted a usability study found that users' issues and problems changed as they gained experience with the technology (Rasmussen and Kushniruk 2013, 1068).

The Nurses' Health Study is an example of a longitudinal study. Since 1976, the Nurses' Health Study has followed the health of more than 275,000 nurses over their lifetimes (Nurses' Health Study 2016). Similar examples are cancer registries and other disease registries that collect data on patients from the diagnosis of their condition through their deaths.

Review Questions

1. What are the purposes of health informatics research and HIM research?
2. What is a theory, and what is the relationship between theories and research frames? What is parsimony and how does it relate to theories?
3. A health informatics researcher is designing a new storage paradigm for heterogeneous data (such as images, audio, structured data fields, and unstructured free text) and conducting research on its functioning. Is the researcher conducting basic research or applied research?
4. Provide two potential research questions for which historical research would be the appropriate research design. Suggest two primary sources for each potential research question. How do primary sources differ from secondary sources?
5. Consider the following statement: "Descriptive research studies serve no purpose in contemporary health informatics research." Why do you agree or disagree with this statement?
6. What is the difference between a positive (direct) relationship and a negative (inverse) relationship?
7. What kinds of research questions could be best answered by observational research?
8. "Control" is the managerial function in which performance is monitored in accordance with organizational policies and procedures. How are evaluation research and the managerial function of control similar? How are they different?
9. What are the four features of experimental research? Explain how experimental research is differentiated from quasi-experimental research.
10. The researchers hypothesized that active engagement with a personal health record positively affects life-long physical fitness. Why would the researchers choose to conduct a longitudinal study?

Application Exercises

1. Go to the website of the Flint Water Study organization and review its report "Chronology of MDHHS E-mails, along with Select MDHHS/MDEQ/MI State Public Statements Pertaining to Blood Lead Levels of Kids in Michigan, Primarily in Flint" (Edwards et al. 2015).

   In which type of research design(s) could the documents in the "Chronology" be used? Why are the documents categorized as primary sources? Identify additional examples of primary sources in the Final Report of the Flint Water Advisory Task Force (Flint Water Task Force 2016).
2. In health informatics, early reports of data mining of electronic records date to the 1960s (Collen 1967, 8; Collen et al. 1971, 142). As an example, read the article "Computer analyses in preventive health research" by Collen in which he reports on an automated multiphasic screening program (Collen 1967). More recently, Dr. Mona Hanna-Attisha and her colleagues mined the electronic health records of all children younger than five years who previously had a blood lead level processed through the Hurley Medical Center's laboratory (Hanna-Attisha et al. 2016, 294). The Hurley Medical Center's laboratory processes the blood lead level tests for most of children living in Genesee County, where Flint, MI, is located. Blood lead levels were obtained for both before (2013) and after (2015) the change in water source for Flint.

   What is the time frame of Collen's research? How many patients were in the program as shown in table 1, part A of the article? What data did the screenings obtain for the data acquisition center of the preventive health services research program?

   What is the time frame of the study by Hanna-Attisha and her colleagues? How many records (n) were included in the study? What data did the researchers obtain from the electronic health records?
3. Dr. Mona Hanna-Attisha and her colleagues, after obtaining the blood lead levels, assessed the percentage of elevated blood lead levels in both time periods (2013 versus 2015) and identified geographical locations through spatial analysis (analyzing locations to explain diseases or other phenomenon; geospatial analysis is discussed in chapter 7). Figure 2 in the article is the spatial analysis.

Mapping (creating a map of disease sites or other phenomenon) and spatial analysis of toxic substances and diseases are not new. In 1854, John Snow drew maps of a London district indicating the locations of cholera deaths and water pumps (Brody et al. 2000, 65). Snow was able to show that cholera mortality was related to the water source. He used the maps as visualization tools when he presented the results of his investigations (Brody et al. 2000, 68). (See figure 1.4 for Snow's map.)

Figure 1.4 Snow's map of cholera mortality and water pumps

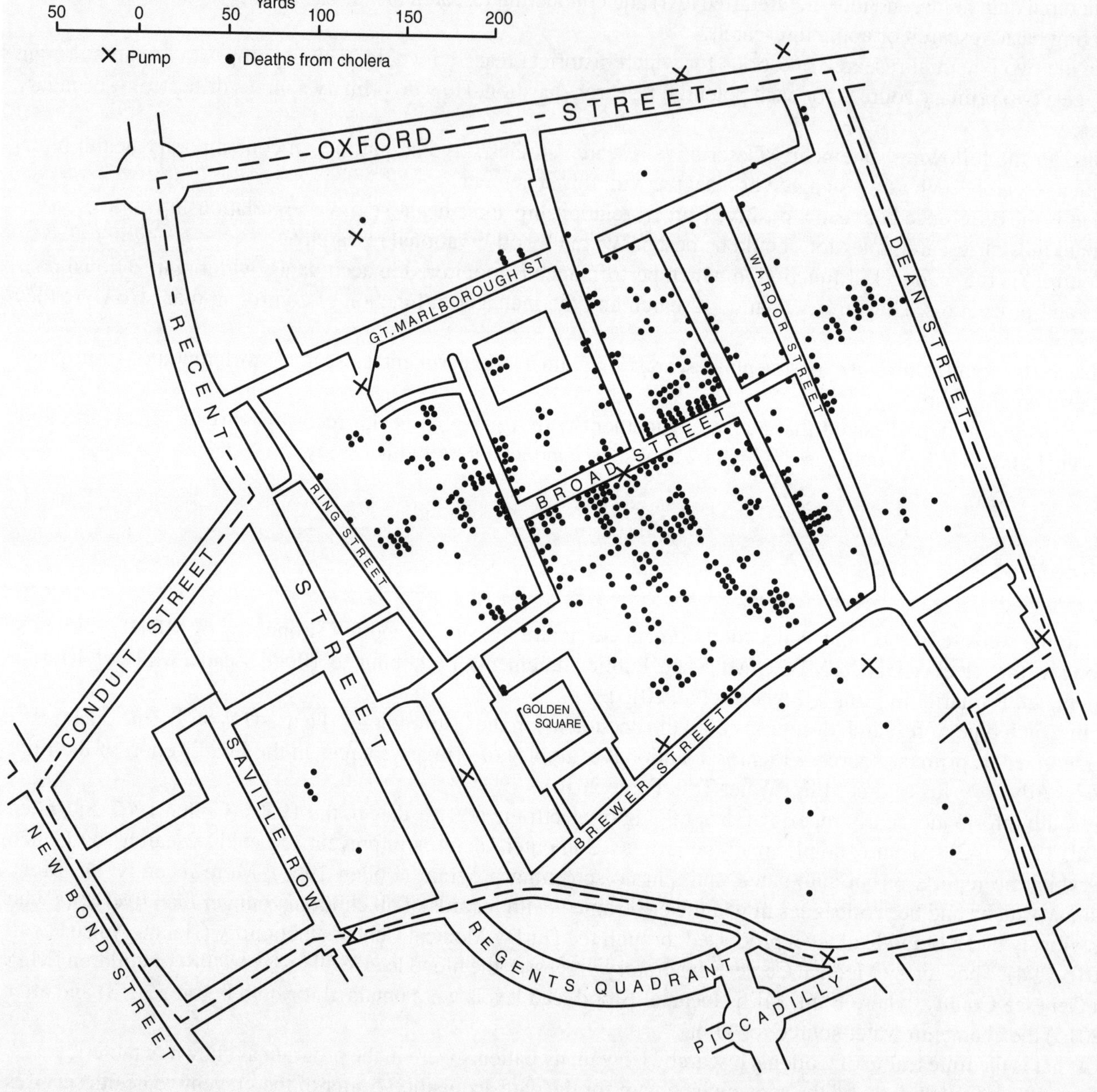

Source: Snow 1855.

The Agency for Toxic Substances and Disease Registry (ATSDR) is mandated by Congress to conduct public health assessments of waste sites, provide health consultations concerning specific hazardous substances, conduct health surveillance, maintain registries, respond to emergency releases of hazardous substances, apply research in support of public health assessments, develop and disseminate information, and provide education and training concerning hazardous substances (ATSDR 2016). As a part of these mandated functions, the ATSDR provides spatial analyses by state showing where the ATSDR has found toxic substances or diseases during its health consultations (HCs) or public health assessments (PHAs).

Go to the website of the ATSDR (2016). Click "Lead" of "Most Viewed Toxic Substances." Click on the Substances Map of the left side of the web page. Then, in "Select a Substance," select "lead" in the drop-down menu. Then, in "Select a State," select your state in the drop-down menu and click "View Map." Has the ATSDR found lead in your state? Where?

References

Abma, T.A. and R.E. Stake. 2014. Science of the particular: An advocacy of naturalistic case study in health research. *Qualitative Health Research* 24(8):1150–1161.

Agency for Healthcare Research and Quality (AHRQ). 2016a. Technology Assessment Program. http://www.ahrq.gov/research/findings/ta/index.html.

Agency for Healthcare Research and Quality. 2016b. What Is Comparative Effectiveness Research? http://effectivehealthcare.ahrq.gov/index.cfm/what-is-comparative-effectiveness-research1.

Alpert, J.M., A.H. Krist, R.A. Aycock, and G.L. Kreps. 2016. Applying multiple methods to comprehensively evaluate a patient portal's effectiveness to convey information to patients. *Journal of Medical Internet Research* 18(5):e112.

American Health Information Management Association (AHIMA). 2016. What Is Health Information? http://www.ahima.org/careers/healthinfo.

American Historical Association. 2011. Statement on Standards of Professional Conduct. https://www.historians.org/jobs-and-professional-development/statements-and-standards-of-the-profession/statement-on-standards-of-professional-conduct.

Ash, J.S. and D.F. Sittig. 2015 (January). Origins of These Conversations with Medical Informatic Pioneers. In: *Conversations with Medical Informatics Pioneers: An Oral History Project.* Edited by Ash, J.S., D.F. Sittig, and R.M. Goodwin. U.S. National Library of Medicine, Lister Hill National Center for Biomedical Communications. https://lhncbc.nlm.nih.gov/publication/pub9119.

Atkinson, M. 2012. *Key Concepts in Sport and Exercise Research Methods.* Thousand Oaks, CA: Sage Publications.

Bandura, A. 1982. Self-efficacy mechanism in human agency. *American Psychologist* 37(2):122–147.

Bickman, L. and D.J. Rog. 2009. *The Sage Handbook of Applied Social Research Methods*, 2nd ed. Thousand Oaks, CA: Sage Publications.

Bottorff, J.L., J.L. Oliffe, G. Sarbit, P. Sharp, C.M. Caperchione, L.M. Currie, J. Schmid, M.H. Mackay, and S. Stolp. 2016. Evaluation of QuitNow Men: An online, men-centered smoking cessation intervention. *Journal of Medical Internet Research* 18(4):e83.

Brody, H., M.R. Rip, P. Vinten-Johansen, N. Paneth, and S. Rachman. 2000. Map-making and myth-making in Broad Street: The cholera epidemic, 1854. *Lancet* 356(9223):64–68.

Campbell, D.T. and J.C. Stanley. 1963. *Experimental and Quasi-Experimental Designs for Research.* Chicago: Rand McNally.

Carter, N., D. Bryant-Lukosius, A. DiCenso, J. Blythe, and A.J. Neville. 2014. The use of triangulation in qualitative research. *Oncology Nursing Forum* 41(5):545–547.

Centers for Disease Control and Prevention (CDC). 2012. Introduction to Program Evaluation for Public Health Programs: A Self-Study Guide. https://www.cdc.gov/eval/guide.

Comte, A. 1853. *The Positive Philosophy of Auguste Comte*. Translated by H. Martineau. New York: D. Appleton and Co.

Crabtree, A., M. Rouncefield, and P. Tolmie. 2012. *Doing Design Ethnography*. London: Springer-Verlag.

Davoudi, S., J.A. Dooling, B. Glondys, T.D. Jones, L. Kadlec, S.M. Overgaard, K. Ruben, and A. Wendicke. 2015. Data Quality Management Model (2015 update). *Journal of AHIMA* 86(10):62–65.

DeLone, W.H. and E.R. McLean. 2003. The DeLone and McLean model of information systems success: A ten-year update. *Journal of Management Information Systems* 19(4):9–30.

Dillon, A. and M. Morris. 1996. User Acceptance of New Information Technology: Theories and Models. In *Annual Review of Information Science and Technology,* vol. 31. Edited by M. Williams. Medford, NJ: Information Today: 3–32.

Ebrahim, G.J. 1999. Simple Linear Regression. Chapter 2 in *Research Method II: Multivariate Analysis*. Oxford Journals, Journal of Tropical Pediatrics, online only area. http://www.oxfordjournals.org/our_journals/tropej/online/ma_chap2.pdf.

Eden, J., L. Levit, A. Berg, and S. Morton. 2011. *Finding What Works in Health Care: Standards for Systematic Reviews*. Washington, DC: National Academies Press.

Ekeland, A.G., A. Bowes, and S. Flottorp. 2012. Methodologies for assessing telemedicine: A systematic review of reviews. *International Journal of Medical Informatics* 81(1):1–11.

Farrar, B., G. Wang, H. Bos, D. Schneider, H. Noel, J. Guo, L. Koester, A. Desai, K. Manson, S. Garfinkel, A. Ptaszek, and M. Dalldorf. 2016. *Evaluation of the Regional Extension Center Program, Final Report*. Washington, DC: Office of the National Coordinator for Health Information Technology. https://www.healthit.gov/sites/default/files/Evaluation_of_the_Regional_Extension_Center_Program_Final_Report_4_4_16.pdf.

Fenton, S. H., F. Manion, K. Hsieh, and M. Harris. 2015. Informed consent: Does anyone really understand what is contained in the medical record? *Applied Clinical Informatics* 6(3):466–477.

Ford, J.P., L. Huang, D.S. Richards, E.P. Ambinder, and J.L. Rosenberger. 2016. R.A.P.I.D. (root aggregated prioritized information display): A single screen display for efficient digital triaging of medical reports. *Journal of Biomedical Informatics* 61:214–223.

Forrestal, E. 2016. Research Methods. Chapter 19 in *Health Information Management: Concepts, Principles, and Practice*, 5th ed. Edited by P. K. Oachs and A.L. Watters. Chicago: AHIMA Press.

Fox, A., G. Gardner, and S. Osborne. 2015. A theoretical framework to support research of health service innovation. *Australian Health Review.* 39(1):70–75.

Friedman, C.P. 2013. What informatics is and isn't. *Journal of the American Medical Informatics Association* 20(2):224–226.

Gass, S.I. and M.C. Fu, eds. 2013. *Encyclopedia of Operations Research and Management Science*, 3rd ed. New York: Springer.

Gorod, A., B. Sauser, and J. Boardman. 2008. System-of-systems engineering management: A review of modern history and a path forward. *IEEE Systems Journal* 2(4):484–499.

Guba, E. and Y. Lincoln. 1989. *Fourth Generation Evaluation*. Newbury Park, CA: Sage.

Hanna-Attisha, M., J. LaChance, R.C. Sadler, and A. Champney Schnepp. 2016. Elevated blood lead levels in children associated with the Flint drinking water crisis: A spatial analysis of risk and public health response. *American Journal of Public Health* 106(2):283–290. http://www.ncbi.nlm.nih.gov/pubmed/26691115.

Harvard University. 2016. The Football Players Health Study at Harvard University. Football Players Health Study in Motion: The New App. https://footballplayershealth.harvard.edu/join-us/teamstudy-app.

Hasan, M.N. 2016. Positivism: To what extent does it aid our understanding of the contemporary social world? *Quality and Quantity* 50(1):317–325.

Holloway, I. and S. Wheeler. 2010. *Qualitative Research in Nursing and Healthcare*, 3rd ed. Ames, IA: Wiley-Blackwell.

In, H. and J.E. Rosen. 2014. Primer on outcomes research. *Journal of Surgical Oncology* 110(5):489–493.

Ingham-Broomfield, R. 2014. A nurse's guide to quantitative research. *Australian Journal of Advanced Nursing* 32(2):32–38.

International Network of Agencies for Health Technology Assessment (INAHTA). 2016. HTA Glossary. http://htaglossary.net/HomePage.

International Organization for Standardization (ISO). 2013. Usability of Consumer Products and Products for Public Use—Part 2: Summative Test Method. https://www.iso.org/obp/ui/#iso:std:iso:ts:20282:-2:ed-2:v1:en.

Jacobs, L. 2009. Interview with Lawrence Weed, MD—the father of the problem-oriented medical record looks ahead. *Permanente Journal* 13(3): 84–89.

Karnick, P.M. 2013. The importance of defining theory in nursing: Is there a common denominator? *Nursing Science Quarterly* 26(1):29–30.

Kisely, S. and E. Kendall. 2011. Critically appraising qualitative research: A guide for clinicians more familiar with quantitative techniques. *Australasian Psychiatry* 19(4):364–367.

Lee, S., and C.A.M. Smith. 2012. Criteria for quantitative and qualitative data integration: Mixed-methods research methodology. *CIN: Computers, Informatics, Nursing* 30(5):251–256.

Liebe, J.D., J. Hüsers, and U. Hübner. 2016. Investigating the roots of successful IT adoption processes—an empirical study exploring the shared awareness-knowledge of directors of nursing and chief information officers. *BMC Medical Informatics and Decision Making* 16(10):1–13.

Malt, B.C. and M.R. Paquet. 2013. The real deal: What judgments of really reveal about how people think about artifacts. *Memory and Cognition* 41(3):354–364.

Mason, T.A. 2016 (April 12). Regional extension centers—essential on-the-ground support for EHR adoption. Health IT Buzz. https://www.healthit.gov/buzz-blog/regional-extension-centers/regional-extension-centers-essential-ground-support-ehr-adoption.

Meeks, D.W., M.W. Smith, L. Taylor, D.F. Sittig, J.M. Scott, and H. Singh. 2014. An analysis of electronic health record-related patient safety concerns. *Journal of the American Medical Informatics Association* 21(6):1053–1059.

Moher, D., L. Shamseer, M. Clarke, D. Ghersi, A. Liberati, M. Petticrew, P. Shekelle, L.A. Stewart, and the PRISMA-P Group. 2015. Preferred reporting items for systematic review and meta-analysis protocols (PRISMA-P) 2015 statement. *Systematic Reviews* 4(1):1–9.

Morse, J.M. 2015. Critical analysis of strategies for determining rigor in qualitative inquiry. *Qualitative Health Research* 25(9):1212–1222.

National Center for Advancing Translational Sciences (NCATS). 2015. Clinical and Translational Science Awards Program. https://ncats.nih.gov/files/ctsa-factsheet.pdf.

National Institutes of Health and Agency for Healthcare Research and Quality (NIH/AHRQ). 2015 (December 17). Advanced Notice of Coming Requirements for Formal Instruction in Rigorous Experimental Design and Transparency to Enhance Reproducibility: NIH and AHRQ Institutional Training Grants, Institutional Career Development Awards, and Individual Fellowships. Notice NOT-OD-16-034. http://grants.nih.gov/grants/guide/notice-files/NOT-OD-16-034.html.

National Institutes of Health (NIH) Office of Extramural Research. 2016. Grants and Funding Glossary. http://grants.nih.gov/grants/glossary.htm.

Nelson, R. and N. Staggers. 2014. *Health Informatics: An Interprofessional Approach*. St. Louis, MO: Mosby.

Norman, D.A. and S.W. Draper. 1986. *User Centered System Design: New Perspectives on Human-Computer Interaction*. Hillsdale, NJ: Lawrence Erlbaum Associates.

Nurses' Health Study. 2016. http://www.nurseshealthstudy.org.

Office of Research Integrity (ORI), US Department of Health and Human Services. 2015. Basic Research Concepts for New Research Staff, Research Design: Descriptive Studies. http://ori.hhs.gov/education/products/sdsu/res_des1.htm.

Øvretveit, J. 2014. *Evaluating Improvement and Implementation for Health*. Maidenhead, UK: McGraw-Hill Education.

Parker, J. and S. Ashencaen Crabtree. 2014. Covert research and adult protection and safeguarding: An ethical dilemma? *Journal of Adult Protection* 16(1):29–40.

Ployhart, R.E. and R.J. Vandenberg. 2010. Longitudinal research: The theory, design, and analysis of change. *Journal of Management* 36(1):94–120.

Ployhart, R.E. and A. Ward. 2011 (December). The "quick start guide" for conducting and publishing longitudinal research. *Journal of Business and Psychology* 26(4):413–422.

Prescott, J., N.J. Gray, F.J. Smith, and J.E. McDonagh. 2015. Blogging as a viable research methodology for young people with arthritis: A qualitative study. *Journal of Medical Internet Research* 17(3):e61.

PricewaterhouseCoopers (PWC) Health Research Institute. 2015. Top Health Industry Issues of 2016: Thriving in the New Health Economy. https://www.pwc.com/us/en/health-industries/top-health-industry-issues/assets/2016-us-hri-top-issues.pdf.

Rasmussen, R. and A. Kushniruk. 2013. Digital video analysis of health professionals' interactions with an electronic whiteboard: A longitudinal, naturalistic study of changes to user interactions. *Journal of Biomedical Informatics* 46(6):1068–1079.

Reason, J. 2000. Human error: Models and management. *BMJ* 320(7237):768–770.

Rhee, H., M.J. Belyea, M. Sterling, and M.F. Bocko. 2015. Evaluating the validity of an automated device for asthma monitoring for adolescents: Correlational design. *Journal of Medical Internet Research* 17(10):e234.

Rogers, E.M. 2003. *Diffusion of Innovations,* 5th ed. New York: Free Press.

Salazar, L.F., R.A. Crosby, and R.J. DiClemente. 2015. *Research Methods in Health Promotion*, 2nd ed. San Francisco, CA: Jossey-Bass.

Sandelowski, M. 2014. Unmixing mixed-methods research. *Research in Nursing and Health* 37(1):3–8.

Shapira, Z. 2011. I've got a theory paper—do you?: Conceptual, empirical, and theoretical contributions to knowledge in the organizational sciences. *Organization Science*. 22(5):1312–1321.

Sheehan, B., L.E. Nigrovic, P.S. Dayan, N. Kuppermann, D.W. Ballard, E. Alessandrini, L. Bajaj, H. Goldberg, J. Hoffman, S.R. Offerman, D.G. Mark, M. Swietlik, E. Tham, L. Tzimenatos, D.R. Vinson, G.S. Jones, and S. Bakken. 2013. Informing the design of clinical decision support services for evaluation of children with minor blunt head trauma in the emergency department: A sociotechnical analysis. *Journal of Biomedical Informatics* 46(5):905–913.

Shi, L. 2008. *Health Services Research Methods*, 2nd ed. Albany, NY: Delmar.

Singleton, R.A., Jr. and B.C. Straits. 2010. *Approaches to Social Research,* 5th ed. New York: Oxford University Press.

Sittig, D.F. and H. Singh. 2010. A new sociotechnical model for studying health information technology in complex adaptive healthcare systems. *Quality and Safety in Health Care* 19(Suppl3):i68–i74.

Snow, J. 1855. *On the Mode of Communication of Cholera,* 2nd ed. London: Churchill.

Spicker, P. 2011. Ethical covert research. *Sociology* 45(1):118–133.

Stephens, J., R. Levine, A.S. Burling, and D. Russ-Eft. 2014 (October). *An Organizational Guide to Building Health Services Research Capacity. Final Report.* AHRQ Publication No. 11(12)-0095-EF. Rockville, MD: Agency for Healthcare Research and Quality. http://www.ahrq.gov/funding/training-grants/hsrguide/hsrguide.html.

Tesch, R. 1990. *Qualitative Research: Analysis Types and Software Tools*. New York: Falmer Press.

Thompson, R.L., C.A. Higgins, and J.M. Howell. 1994. Influence of experience on personal computer utilization: Testing a conceptual model. *Journal of Management Information Systems* 11(1):167–187.

US Government Accountability Office (GAO). 2012. Designing Evaluations: 2012 Revision. http://www.gao.gov/products/GAO-12-208G.

US National Library of Medicine (NLM). 2015. Medical Informatics Pioneers. https://lhncbc.nlm.nih.gov/project/medical-informatics-pioneers.

Venkatesh, V., M.G. Morris, G.B. Davis, and F.D. Davis. 2003. User acceptance of information technology: Toward a unified view. *MIS Quarterly* 27(3):425–478.

Whetton, S. and A. Georgiou. 2010. Conceptual challenges for advancing the socio-technical underpinnings of health informatics. *Open Medical Informatics Journal* 4:221–224.

Wilkinson, M. 2013. Testing the null hypothesis: The forgotten legacy of Karl Popper? *Journal of Sports Sciences* 31(9):919–920.

Wilson, T.D. 1999. Models in information behavior research. *Journal of Documentation* 55(3):249–270.

Wyatt, J. 2010. Assessing and improving evidence based health informatics research. *Studies in Health Technology and Informatics* 151:435–445.

Resources

Altheide, D.L. and J.M. Johnson. 1994. Criteria for Assessing Interpretive Validity in Qualitative Research. Chapter 30 in *Handbook of Qualitative Research.* Edited by N.K. Denzin and Y.S. Lincoln. Thousand Oaks, CA: Sage Publications: 485–499.

Agency for Toxic Substances and Disease Registry (ATSDR). 2016. https://www.atsdr.cdc.gov/.

Barnum, C.M. 2011. *Usability Testing Essentials: Ready, Set ... Test.* Burlington, MA: Morgan Kaufman.

Cameron, R. 2011. Mixed methods research: The five Ps framework. *Electronic Journal of Business Research Methods* 9(2):96–108.

Cohen, D. and B. Crabtree. 2006. Qualitative Research Guidelines Project. Robert Wood Johnson Foundation. http://www.qualres.org.

Collen, M.F. 1967. Computer analyses in preventive health research. *Methods of Information in Medicine* 6(1):8–14. http://methods.schattauer.de/en/contents/archivepremium/issue/1311/manuscript/15365/show.html.

Collen, M.F., L.S. Davis, and E.E. Van Brunt. 1971. The computer medical record in health screening. *Methods of Information in Medicine* 10(3):138–142. http://methods.schattauer.de/en/contents/archivepremium/issue/1292/manuscript/15206.html.

Edwards, M., S. Roy, W. Rhoads, E. Garner, and R. Martin. 2015. Chronological Compilation of E-Mails from MDHHS Freedom of Information Act (FOIA) Request #2015-557. http://flintwaterstudy.org/wp-content/uploads/2015/12/MDHHS-FOIA.pdf.

Flint Water Task Force. 2016 (March). Final Report. http://www.michigan.gov/documents/snyder/FWATF_FINAL_REPORT_21March2016_517805_7.pdf.

Khong, P.C., E. Holroyd, and W. Wang. 2015. A critical review of theoretical frameworks and the conceptual factors in the adoption of clinical decision support systems. *CIN: Computers, Informatics, Nursing* 33(12):555–570.

Shortliffe, E.H. and M.S. Blois. 2014. Biomedical informatics: The science and the pragmatics. Chapter 1 in *Biomedical Informatics: Computer Applications in Health Care and Biomedicine*, 4th ed. Edited by Shortliffe, E.H. and J.J. Cimino. New York: Springer Verlag: 3–37.

US Department of Health and Human Services (HHS). 2016. What and Why of Usability. https://www.usability.gov/what-and-why/index.html.

2 Survey Research

Valerie J. Watzlaf, PhD, MPH, RHIA, FAHIMA

Learning Objectives

- Describe survey research and how it is used in health informatics.
- Display and discuss examples of structured (closed-ended) and unstructured (open-ended) questions used in health informatics research.
- Demonstrate the appropriate organization of survey questions in relation to content, flow, design, scales, audience, and appropriate medium.
- Apply appropriate statistics to measure the validity and reliability of the survey questions.
- Plan and carry out the pilot testing of the questionnaire, whether it is used as a self-survey or interview instrument.
- Calculate the appropriate sample size for the survey instrument.
- Select appropriate follow-up procedures to retrieve a good response rate.
- Depict what statistics can be generated from collecting data via a survey instrument.

Key Terms

Advisory committee
Census survey
Closed-ended (structured) questions
Cluster sampling
Convenience sample
Construct validity
Criterion-related validity
Cronbach's alpha
Face validity
Factor analysis
Health Information National Trends Survey (HINTS)
Institutional Review Board (IRB)
Interval scale
National Center for Health Statistics (NCHS)
National Health Interview Survey (NHIS)
Nominal scale
Open-ended (unstructured) questions
Ordinal scale
Pilot test
Prevarication bias
Ratio scale
Recall bias
Reliability
Response rate
Sample size
Selection bias
Simple random sampling
Stratified random sampling
Survey research
Systematic random sampling
Test-retest reliability
Validity
Web-based survey

Survey research includes a method for collecting research data by asking questions, with the responses being collected via the mail, through websites, mobile apps, or by telephone, fax, e-mail, or text message. Survey research is one of the most common types of research used in health informatics. Most of the research performed in health informatics is still new and emerging, and surveys are often used when very little is known about a particular topic. The survey method allows the researcher to explore and describe what is occurring at a particular point in time or during a specific time period.

In survey research, the researcher chooses a topic of study and begins to formulate criteria that will help develop questions he or she may have about that topic. The survey can explore, for example, a certain disease, community, organization, culture, health information system, or type of software. Often, a random sample of participants from an appropriate population is chosen to answer standardized questions. The survey questionnaire can be completed directly by the participant, with directions included within the questionnaire or cover letter, or it can be administered by mail, online, through a mobile app, by fax, or in person. Surveys also can be administered via an interview either by phone, over the Internet, or in person. The researcher needs to weigh all the variables at hand to determine the best method of administering the survey. The researcher's main goal is to collect the most appropriate and accurate data that will answer the questions most pertinent to the research topic.

Whether developing a new survey instrument or adapting an existing one, the researcher will need to address many issues, such as the content of the survey, the audience or respondents, how the survey will be administered, whether to send it to a sample of the population or the entire population, and what type of statistics will be generated.

Then, the researcher should consider whether incentives will be used to increase the response rate, how to maintain confidentiality of the responses, and how to minimize bias (error within the study design). With survey research, the study design may be limited by multiple kinds of bias, including *nonresponse bias* (the survey data are only based on responses to the survey and do not reflect what the nonrespondents might have answered), **recall bias** (respondents may not remember correctly so their answers will be inaccurate), and **prevarication bias** (respondents may exaggerate or lie in their answers to the questions, especially when answering questions related to salary or other sensitive matters). Nonresponse bias and prevarication bias are discussed later in this chapter. Recall bias is discussed in detail in chapter 5.

Once the data are collected, researchers must perform appropriate statistical analysis of the data. The results of this analysis can be displayed in tables and graphs and reported to interested audiences.

Investigators have conducted survey research studies in many health informatics areas, such as electronic health records (EHRs), coding and classification systems, population health, and so forth. Survey research in health informatics is useful and will continue to be conducted with vigor as health informatics applications advance.

The following real-world case demonstrates how the Centers for Disease Control and Prevention (CDC) and the **National Center for Health Statistics (NCHS)**, which is a part of the CDC and provides data and statistics to identify and address health issues within the United States, use survey research to compile useful statistics.

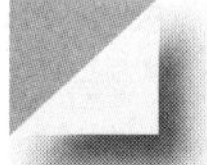

Real-World Case

The data in figure 2.1 are partially derived from the CDC's and NCHS's National Survey of Family Growth (NSFG), which collects survey data on family formation, fertility, and reproductive health. The data collected from this survey research are used to determine the pregnancy rates by age across the United States. The NSFG survey and the data derived from this survey are based on interview questions related to pregnancy history, including fetal loss. The data are collected continuously over time across all age groups and races (Curtin et al. 2015).

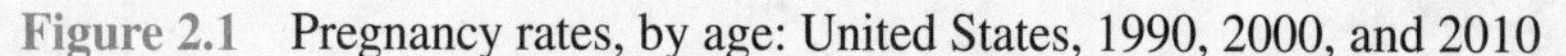

Figure 2.1 Pregnancy rates, by age: United States, 1990, 2000, and 2010

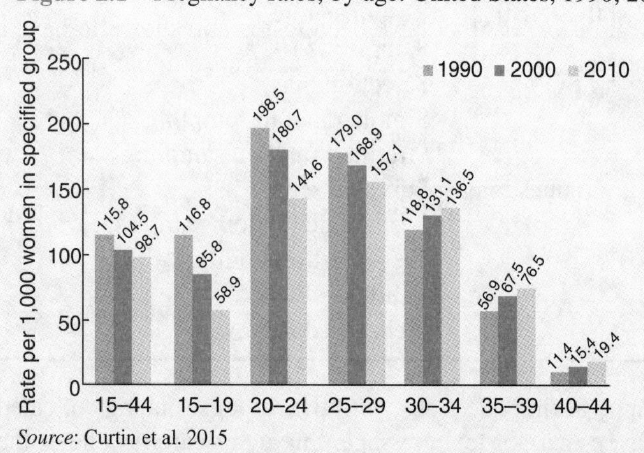

Source: Curtin et al. 2015

Survey Creation

When designing a survey research project in health informatics, one of the first questions the researcher should ask is "What should the content of the survey include to effectively answer the research questions under study?" It is also important for the researcher to determine whether a new survey needs to be created or if an existing survey can be used to answer the research questions. The health informatics researcher should decide this question by searching research journals and books, often referred to as "the literature," that is related to the topic under study to determine whether existing surveys are available that meet the needs of the new study. If no appropriate existing survey is found in the literature, the researcher should create a new survey. An advisory committee should be developed to provide feedback on the content of the survey questionnaire and help select the different types of questions and scales (nominal, ordinal, interview, and ratio) to be used. Researchers should always conduct a **pilot test**, a trial run on a small scale that enhances the likelihood of a study's successful completion because it provides an opportunity to work out the details of the research plan, on the survey questionnaire. Researchers should then review and discuss feedback with the advisory committee to determine which of the survey questions may need to be adjusted or removed as appropriate for the audience. Finally, the researcher should consider whether it is appropriate to incentivize survey response and how respondent confidentiality will be maintained.

Use of Existing Surveys

There are several areas to consider when conducting survey research in health informatics. First and foremost is the development of the survey instrument. The researcher decides whether a new survey instrument should be developed or whether an existing one can be used or adapted to fulfill the research study aim or focus. When planning a survey research project, the researcher should evaluate existing questionnaires and determine whether they could be used to answer the questions under study.

For example, the goal of the National Cancer Institute (NCI) **Health Information National Trends Survey (HINTS)** was to create a population-based survey that could be used to track trends in the use of communication technologies such as the Internet as a source of cancer information. HINTS examined several different types of existing surveys, including the **National Health Interview Survey (NHIS)**, a study from the NCHS that describes the health status of individuals and their families. However, the NCI concluded that even though existing surveys provided some of the question content, the researchers and the advisory board would need to develop several new questions and essentially a new survey (NCI 2016; Nelson et al. 2004).

Other studies have adapted existing surveys for use in different populations. For example, the eHealth Literacy Scale (eHEALS) has been widely used to examine health literacy in younger populations and has been adapted for use in older adults (Chung and Nahm 2015). The researchers examined whether the scales had reliability and validity when used with an older population. They used the **Cronbach's alpha**, which is a measure of internal consistency and determines whether all the variables within the instrument are measuring the same concept, and found that the Cronbach's alpha reliability coefficient for eHEALS was 0.94 when used with older adults. Any value close to 1, such as 0.7 and above, is considered to indicate good reliability. The Cronbach's alpha will be discussed in more detail later in this chapter. Based on this test and other psychometric tests, the authors concluded that the eHEALS survey can be used successfully with older adults.

In many cases, there are advantages to using or adapting existing surveys that have been tested and shown to have a high validity and reliability score, such as proven accuracy and consistency. However, in health informatics research, many new topics are being explored for the first time and, therefore, appropriate existing surveys are not available for use. Nevertheless, it is still important to search the literature to determine whether surveys that could be used to answer the research questions have been developed. Once the literature search has been exhausted, then the development of a new survey can begin.

New Survey Development

If the research team decides that a new survey or questionnaire is needed, they must consider the following areas when building the new questionnaire (see figure 2.2):

- The content of the questionnaire
- The audience or those individuals who will respond to the questionnaire

- The type of questionnaire and the medium in which it will be presented to the audience
- Whether a sample will be selected or the entire population will be surveyed
- The statistics to be generated

Each of these items plays a specific role in the development of the survey and is explained in more detail throughout this chapter.

Figure 2.2 Items to consider when building a survey

Content
- Consider content from existing surveys
- Use of advisory committee or SMEs to recommend survey content
- Inclusion and exclusion criteria
- Types of questions (open-ended or unstructured versus closed-ended or structured questions)
- Scales: Nominal, ordinal, interval, ratio
- Pilot testing and updating survey after pilot test

Audience
- How to frame questions to level of the audience
- Providing incentives to participants
- Confidentiality and security of responses
- Limitations, bias, or error
- Follow-up for non-responders

Type or Medium
- Electronic, web- or app-based media
- Mail
- Fax
- Phone
- In-person (individual interview or focus group)
- On-site distribution

Sample or Population?
- Sample should represent population under study
- Population or census survey for small populations
- Sample type: simple random, stratified, or systematic
- Selection bias
- Sample size calculations
- Convenience sample
- Response rate
- Collection of demographic data on non-responders to compare with the profile of responders

Statistics to Be Generated
- Frequencies
- Percentages
- Test for validity and reliability measures
- Factor analysis
- Significance testing
- Confidence intervals
- Correlation
- Regression analysis

As noted earlier in this chapter, survey researchers should, if possible, consult an **advisory committee**, a group of subject matter experts (SMEs) with experience in survey design as well as the topic of study, to assist in phrasing the questions in the appropriate manner. The advantages of forming an advisory group of SMEs are many. For example, the group can advise the research team about survey content, help develop the pilot study of the survey instrument, assist with the selection of participants in the reliability testing of the survey instrument, guide the literature review for the survey, and assess the overall quality of the survey questions. However, an advisory committee may be costly if incentives are provided to members, the amount of time to develop the survey may be more extensive when an advisory committee is used, and it may be difficult to find SMEs in the content area who can serve as advisers.

NCI used an advisory committee to develop principles and select topics and questions for the survey instrument for the HINTS, which was described previously. An advisory committee also participated extensively in the design and development of the questions for a mobile app wellness assessment survey for those living in medically underserved, trauma-affected communities in the Hill district of Pittsburgh, PA. The researchers consulted SMEs in the areas of health information technology (HIT), computer science and physics, psychiatry, psychology, internal medicine, epidemiology, and theology to help develop questions that relate to an individual's spiritual, physical, behavioral, socio-economic and relational domains. First, one member of the research team searched the literature to determine what types of questions from other surveys could be used in this new survey. Next, the research team and SMEs reviewed those existing questions and adapted them for the population under study, and they added new questions that they believed were necessary to assess the well-being of individuals affected by trauma in their community. Then, the SMEs helped the research team choose participants from the community for a pilot test of the survey. The advisory committee also assisted in the reliability and validity testing of the survey instrument. The SMEs on this advisory committee provided their expertise without being given any incentives, and the time they needed to complete this analysis was minimal. All in all, the advisory committee for this mobile app well-being survey were instrumental in its successful construction (Zhou et al. 2017).

Inclusion and Exclusion Criteria

When building a survey research study, inclusion and exclusion criteria must be set. *Inclusion criteria* identify the characteristics individuals must have to participate in the survey. Examples of inclusion criteria for a health informatics survey research study might include holding a specific job title, such as chief information governance officer (CIGO); or having certain credentials or educational backgrounds, such as having a baccalaureate degree in health informatics combined with the American Health Information Management Association (AHIMA) Certified Health Data Analyst (CHDA) credential. *Exclusion criteria* are characteristics or responses that eliminate individuals from being participants in a survey research study. In a health informatics survey research study, individuals might be excluded if they could not (or did not) use certain types of HIT, such as a mobile device and mobile app, telehealth technologies, laptops, or tablets. Another, simpler example of exclusion criteria might be age; for example, a study could exclude individuals who were not between the ages of 18 and 35 years.

Types of Questions

Survey questions can be open-ended or closed-ended. **Open-ended (unstructured) questions**, also known as *qualitative questions,* do not have a specific choice of answers, and the participant can provide their oral or written responses in their own words, similar to an essay exam. **Closed-ended (structured) questions**, also known as *quantitative questions*, require the participant to choose a particular response, similar to a multiple-choice exam. Open-ended questions are often used for phone or face-to-face interviews, whereas closed-ended questions are often used for self-assessments, web-based, mobile app or e-mail surveys, or mail and faxed surveys. Responses to closed-ended questions are easy to quantify and capture data succinctly. Open-ended questions are used when the researcher may want to collect the "why" and "why not" that closed-ended questions may not answer. Surveys can also be a mix of both closed-ended and open-ended type questions. For example, in the study entitled "Standards for the content of the electronic health record," the researchers wanted to collect data on the types of data items that are essential to have included in an EHR, and they decided to include both closed-ended and open-ended questions (Watzlaf et al. 2004a). They organized the EHR survey, which is presented in online appendix 2A, into the following parts:

- Demographic data about the facility and the individual completing the survey (closed-ended questions)
- Awareness of EHR standards (closed-ended questions)
- Type of EHR system in place or in the development stage (closed-ended questions)
- Minimum essential data set—EHR data view of all settings—which data items are in place or will be put in place if in development stage (closed-ended questions)
- Needed data elements that are not included and unnecessary data elements that should be eliminated (open-ended questions)
- Additional comments (open-ended questions)
- Definition of terms used in the questions

Scales

When deciding what types of questions to create for the survey, researchers use four measurement scales—nominal, ordinal, interval, and ratio—to categorize different types of variables and create different types of questions. As will be explained, certain types of scales are better suited to specific types of survey questions.

Nominal Scales

Nominal scales are scales that simply name, label, or categorize the response and assign a numerical value to the response for purposes of easier data analysis. This type of scale is better suited for closed-ended questions than open-ended ones. The data captured in a nominal scale do not have any units of measurement, and the ordering of the categories is completely arbitrary. For example, suppose a researcher chooses to ask survey participants, "What type of health insurance do you have?" In this survey, the following nominal scale might be used to categorize the closed-ended choices for types of insurance:

1 = Medicare
2 = Medical assistance
3 = Private insurance

As this example shows, numerical values in a nominal scale are assigned to the variables under study (here, types of insurance), but the values are only there to provide categorization; the numbers do not measure or rank the variables.

Dichotomous questions are even simpler questions than nominal ones. They provide two responses, such as "yes" and "no," "true" or "false," or "agree" or "disagree." For example, a dichotomous question might be, "In your opinion, is your computerized provider order entry (CPOE) system effective in preventing medication errors?" The two closed-end responses to this question would be 1 = Yes, and 2 = No.

Ordinal Scales

An ordinal scale is used when the answer to a question or value can be rank-ordered, such as with patient satisfaction surveys where 1 = not satisfied and 4 = very satisfied. Notably, the higher numbers indicate greater satisfaction, but the distance from 1 to 2 may not be the same as the distance from 3 to 4. The numerical value assigned to each ranked response is not a true numerical value, just a method of ranked categorization.

For example, a two-part study conducted in one long-term care facility (LTCF) interviewed residents and healthcare providers about clinical care topics related to care at this LTCF (Watzlaf et al. 1995). The interview instrument covered 25 clinical care areas, and the residents were asked to listen to a discussion of each clinical care topic and then rank the topic's importance to their lives on a scale of 1 to 5 (1 being most important and 5 being least important). The healthcare providers were given the same clinical areas to rank but were told to think about them in relation to the residents' care.

A portion of the interview instrument and the ranked scale is provided in figure 2.3.

Figure 2.3 Excerpt of an interview instrument with an ordinal scale

	Scale 1 = Most important 2 = Very important 3 = Important 4 = Somewhat important 5 = Least important	Do you want to discuss your ranking?
1. Medications	1 2 3 4 5	
2. Use of restraints	1 2 3 4 5	
3. Treatment plan (aware of treatment plan and involved in process of developing treatment plan)	1 2 3 4 5	
4. Freedom of choice (right to choose physician, participate in planning care and treatment)	1 2 3 4 5	

Source: Watzlaf et al. 1995.

This instrument enabled the researchers to determine the most important clinical care areas for residents and healthcare providers. Based on this information, researchers could make comparisons between what the residents believed was important versus the healthcare providers. To do this, the researchers computed the mean rankings for each of the clinical care topics and then rank-ordered them for residents and healthcare providers. For example, residents ranked freedom of choice as the most important topic, whereas healthcare providers ranked it number 20 out of the 25 clinical care topics (Watzlaf et al. 1995).

Interval and Ratio Scales

Interval scales and ratio scales have true numerical meaning because the distance between the variables relates to the numerical value assigned. In a **ratio scale**, continuous data have both equal intervals and an absolute zero (0) point that is clearly defined and meaningful, whereas an **interval scale**, in which the intervals between adjacent scale values are equal with respect to the attributes being measured, does not have a meaningful absolute zero. Examples of interval scales include the Fahrenheit and Celsius temperature scales and standardized test scores such as the SAT, GRE, or IQ. Examples of ratio scales include weight, age, height, blood pressure, pulse rate, and the Kelvin temperature scale. (In the Kelvin scale, zero degrees is the absolute bottom, signifying "no heat.") The following is an example of a survey question that incorporates an interval-scale response.

Students in the nursing clinical rotation program must record the temperature of each patient correctly. Therefore, after Dr. Watson takes the patient's temperature, it is recorded in the EHR. Then the nursing student is asked to take the temperature and record their response. Following is one of the questions that is asked on their practical exam.

What is the temperature of Mary Jones, a patient in Dr. Watson's office?

a. 100°F
b. 98.6°F
c. 104°F
d. 102°F

Note that the response choices have true numerical meanings because the distance between variables has a defined numerical value assigned to it, which is not the case with ordinal scales, such as those that rank a person's preferences or level of pain.

Students in nursing clinical rotation program must record the pulse rate of each patient correctly. Therefore, after Dr. Watson takes the patient's pulse rate, it is recorded in the EHR. Then, a nursing student is asked to take the patient's pulse rate and record their response. Below is one of the questions that is asked on the student nursing practical exam.

The following is an example of a survey question that incorporates a ratio response:

What is the patient's pulse rate?

a. 72
b. 55
c. 82
d. 64

In this example, the ratio scale has all the properties of the interval scale *plus* the true value of zero, which is the absence of the variable being measured. In this case, if a patient's pulse rate was "0," he or she would have no pulse (and might be dead). The next section discusses how survey data and the responses collected via certain numerical scales can be analyzed statistically.

Use of Appropriate Statistics with Different Scales

After ascertaining which types of scales will be incorporated into the questionnaire, the researcher will be able to know which types of statistics to generate. Means, standard deviations, and variance are all appropriate to use with interval and ratio scales because these scales have continuous variables. Frequencies and percentages are appropriate for nominal data, and medians, percentages, and ranges are appropriate for ordinal data. Note that, even though medians and ranges are best to use for ordinal data, many researchers (such as those who conducted the LTCF survey discussed earlier) will generate means or averages because they are easier to display in tables and graphs, and because many readers are more familiar with means or averages. When using means for ordinal data, the means do not have true numerical value but they demonstrate a method of ranked categorization in relation to the ranked scale.

Pilot Test Survey

Once the questions are framed and included into a first draft of the survey questionnaire, researchers should use the draft in a pilot test with a small group of respondents. As much as possible, these individuals should reflect the sample of respondents expected for the true survey, and the pilot test should be designed to provide an accurate simulation of how the survey questionnaire will be administered.

Researchers should review all comments from the pilot testing and discuss them with the advisory board to determine any changes to the questionnaire. It is extremely important to pilot test every questionnaire before it is distributed to respondents.

Validity and Reliability

For new surveys, it is important to test for validity and reliability and also conduct factor analysis if the sample size is large enough. **Validity** means the right thing was measured. Validity demonstrates accuracy. **Reliability** means the survey consistently produces the same results. Reliability is also referred to as *reproducibility* or *repeatability*. It is possible to have reliability without validity, but validity cannot be achieved without reliability. Validity and reliability testing of the survey instrument is essential and may involve determining face validity, criterion validity, construct validity, and content validity, as well as reliability coefficients. A more sophisticated assessment of the survey questionnaire may use factor analysis to determine which questions conform to a particular factor or area of interest.

Validity

Several types of validity can be examined for each survey developed. The four major types are face, criterion-related, construct, and content validity. Refer to table 2.1 for definitions and examples of these types.

Table 2.1 Validity for survey research

Validity	Definition	Example
Face validity	Confirmation at the surface level ("face value") that the survey seems to measure what it set out to measure.	Researchers arrange survey questions in a certain order to study the respondents' understanding of health informatics concepts. The first section may include demographics of the respondents, and the second section may include questions related to health informatics concepts such as artificial intelligence, audit trail, and so forth.
Criterion-related validity	Measurement of the accuracy of the intended survey instrument through comparison to another method that has been shown to be valid.	Researchers evaluate computer skills of employees in a healthcare facility by providing a hands-on computer skills test that has been shown to be accurate as well as a written test on computer concepts.
Construct validity	Agreement between a theoretical concept and the survey instrument. Can be separated into two parts: *convergent validity* (agreement among ratings collected independently on issues that should be agreed on theoretically) and *discriminant validity* (disagreement on issues measured that should be disagreed on theoretically).	When seeking to study the concepts of what constitutes quality of healthcare, researchers first establish, in theory, the concepts of quality healthcare. Then, the practical relationships of these theoretical concepts can be measured. Next, the results from the practical data can be used to determine how well the survey instrument will collect quality of care data.
Content validity	The survey instrument captures the information the researchers intended to measure.	If researchers aim to study physicians' documentation practices in the EHR, but only examine practices related to the history and physical examination section of the EHR, the study would not demonstrate content validity because it excludes other areas in which physicians conduct documentation practices.

Source: Adapted from Howell et al. 1993–2017.

In the 2004 EHR study survey by Watzlaf and colleagues, discussed earlier in this chapter, both face validity and content validity were achieved. The survey had face validity because it was used in a pilot study in which it was found to be understandable and to flow well; additionally, most comments from the pilot study were incorporated into the final version of the survey. The survey had content validity because an advisory committee of EHR experts ensured that the survey instrument included all the appropriate topic content. Face validity is a weak measure of validity whereas content validity is a much stronger measure of validity. Further information on both content and face validity is available in chapter 11.

Reliability

In a study that developed and tested a survey instrument that measured the benefits of a nursing information system, the survey's reliability was established by using the Cronbach's alpha to determine internal consistency of the items included in the survey. A Cronbach's alpha of 0.97 was found (Abdrbo et al. 2011). Reliability coefficients close to 1 have very high internal consistency and those close to 0 have very low internal consistency. Therefore, the Cronbach's alpha for this study shows that the survey had high internal consistency and all items in the instrument were measuring the same concept (Cronk 2016).

Test-retest reliability determines whether the survey instrument is consistent over time or when given multiple times. The test-retest reliability coefficient is a correlation coefficient for the relationship between the two total scores given on two different times to the same group of individuals. In the well-being assessment scale developed by Zhou and colleagues, test-retest reliability was conducted for each of the domains within the survey, and the correlation coefficient for reliability was 0.834 (Zhou et al. 2017). The assumptions for test-retest are the same as the Cronbach's alpha. Values close to 1 indicate strong reliability and those values close to 0 indicate poor reliability. The correlation coefficient of 0.834 indicates that the survey instrument used in Pittsburgh was very reliable when administered multiple times (Cronk 2016).

Factor Analysis in Refining Survey Questionnaires

Sometimes, researchers need to refine the number of questions that are used in a survey questionnaire. One way to do this is by using factor analysis. **Factor analysis** is a statistical technique in which a large number of variables are summarized and reduced to a smaller number based on similar relationships among those variables. For example, researchers in the nursing information system study did a factor analysis to obtain a valid survey instrument for collecting information related to nurses using a health information system. Factor analysis was performed to reduce the number of items that were not associated with a common factor, and it revealed that items were mostly related to just four factors within the survey: saving time and efficiency, quality of care, charting, and professional practice. The researchers concluded that more research on this survey questionnaire was needed so that all items included would relate to the specific aims and factors of the study intent (Abdrbo et al. 2011).

Audience

Successful survey questions are targeted to the level of the audience. For this reason, it is extremely important to understand who the audience will be. Questions can be worded very differently depending on whether young adults or chief information officers (CIOs) will be responding. The researcher should use clear, unambiguous terms when developing the survey questions because it is easy for the intended audience to misinterpret certain questions. For example, in the original draft of the EHR survey, a "not sure" response was included. This response was determined, through the pilot testing for the survey, to be unclear and therefore was not used in the final EHR survey. This example illustrates the value of pilot testing the survey to a small sample of the intended audience before final distribution. By doing this, the researcher is better able to understand his or her intended audience and their ability to answer specific survey questions.

Framing of Questions

To obtain accurate data, researchers take care to determine the order of the questions as well as the order of the response choices. For example, in a study on the perceived effects of ICD-10 coding productivity and accuracy among coding professionals, the survey contained 13 questions, with the first one addressing the demographics of the coding professionals (level of education, years of experience). The researchers next asked about the type of facility that employed the respondent before asking about the main topic of coding productivity and accuracy (the perceived impact of ICD-10 implementation on coding productivity and accuracy) (Rudman et al. 2016). Thus, this framing of questions for this survey research followed a logical order, which made it easy for the intended audience to provide accurate information.

Incentives

Some researchers offer incentives to survey participants. Although incentives such as the chance to win a $200 gift certificate may entice the respondents to answer all the questions, the researcher should consider that incentives may influence responses and some respondents may hurriedly complete the survey to take part in the incentive. Therefore, the researcher should decide whether an incentive is necessary and whether any possible increase in response rates offsets the risk of gathering inaccurate data.

Confidential Responses

Respondents expect that their responses will be kept confidential when completing a survey questionnaire. The **institutional review board (IRB)**, which is the institutional body that provides review, oversight, guidance, and approval for research projects carried out by employees serving as researchers, regardless of the location of the research (such as a university or private research agency) and which is responsible for protecting the rights and welfare of the human subjects involved in the research, also will want to know how the researcher maintains the confidentiality of the responses generated. The level of research in which the study is approved (exempt, expedited, full-board approval, and so forth) determines how the researcher will collect and maintain the data. (See chapter 14 for additional discussion of IRB approval.)

For example, in the EHR study described in this chapter, Watzlaf and colleagues received exempt approval from the IRB, which means that no identifying information could be linked with the survey responses. An e-mail was sent to each facility with the online survey URL included. Although some other studies require the users to log in, the researchers in the EHR study believed that a log-in requirement would discourage users from proceeding in the study and would produce errors as well. Therefore, an individual, nonidentifying number and password were included in the URL. A database separate from the survey responses was developed to include the ID number and facility name and was only used to determine who responded and who did not, and therefore aid in the follow-up process. No identifying information about respondents could be linked with the survey responses, and all information that was reported in presentations and journal articles was reported in aggregate form so that no respondents could be identified. The facility was assured that survey responses would remain completely confidential and that only aggregate data was used in the reporting of the results (Watzlaf et al. 2004a).

Limitations, Bias, and Error

Every researcher must deal with error when conducting studies. Some respondents will not be able to provide an accurate response because they do not understand the question or do not have the appropriate time to respond, or because they have difficulty recalling past experiences relevant to the question. For these reasons, it is important to ask questions that are unambiguous and that do not require extensive recollection. If the respondent needs to remember an experience to answer a question, a picture, graph, table, or other type of illustration can be used to help jog the respondent's memory and increase the chances of an accurate response. Sometimes, respondents may exaggerate their responses to questions. This prevarication bias may occur when collecting salary information or other sensitive pieces of data. Therefore, it is important to phrase the questions clearly and, when possible, to give a choice of ranges to keep the respondents' answers as accurate as possible. (Refer to chapter 1 for more information on bias). It is also important to plan the type of medium the researcher will use to administer and distribute the survey. The type of medium and distribution of the survey may reduce the amount of bias or error the researcher may find when conducting survey research.

Type or Medium

Once all aspects of the survey audience have been articulated, the researcher determines the appropriate medium with which to administer the survey. This may include web- or Internet-based surveys, e-mail, mail, fax, telephone, or group administered surveys. The goal is to obtain the highest response rate while still obtaining accurate response data.

Web-Based Surveys

Web-based surveys, which are administered to participants via a website, have many advantages, including the following:

- Reduced cost in comparison with paper
- Less or no data entry (because data can be automatically downloaded to a database or spreadsheet)

- Ease of data analysis
- The use of pop-up instructions and drop-down boxes
- Ability to present questions in random order (Gunn 2002)

However, web-based surveys also have the following disadvantages:

- Exclusion of potential respondents who do not have a computer or other mobile device or access to the Internet
- Increased time in developing an effective questionnaire
- Need for a person with skills in web-based survey design and development
- Difficulty making changes to the questionnaire once on the web
- Reluctance of some respondents to provide their responses over the Internet due to lack of confidence in privacy and security

In the EHR survey study, the researchers weighed the advantages and disadvantages and decided to post the final version of the survey on a web server for easy access by recipients.

Providing the survey questionnaire in several media can help increase the number of respondents. For example, there are many things a researcher can do to make the web-based survey compatible for a mobile device. To this end, Pew Research Center recommends the following:

- Use software that automatically detects the type of device used and modifies the layout of the questions for that device type, especially screen size.
- Keep the length of the survey short.
- Use radio buttons, checkboxes, or text boxes rather than fancy features such as sliders.
- Group several questions on the same or similar topic on the same screen.
- Include a unique URL in the survey invitation, so that users are automatically brought to the survey when they click the link (McGeeney 2015)

Many researchers are required to use a specific type of software to administer their survey questions. The survey must be developed in this medium when presented in a proposal to the IRB. For example, a university may require use of specific survey software, such as Qualtrics, to build the survey questionnaires, provide summary statistics, and allow the university and IRB to keep track of all the data that are collected by their researchers.

Surveys by E-mail, Mail, Fax, and Phone

Some researchers have used both mailed survey questionnaires and phone interviews to compare responses as well as to supplement data collected or to validate the responses received from the survey questionnaire. Although the web was the primary medium for administering the EHR survey discussed in this chapter, the researchers found that several facilities preferred the survey to be mailed or faxed, or for the information to be taken over the phone. Thus, researchers had to provide the survey in each of these media. (Please see online appendix 2A for the non-web–based EHR survey and online appendix 2B for excerpts of the web-based version.)

In one study, researchers used both phone and mailed surveys to collect data from respondents regarding their weight management. The researchers did this because in their original randomized controlled trial of weight management, 85 percent of the study subjects were lost to follow-up, and the investigators wanted to find out which method of data collection was best. The response rate from the phone interview was 59 percent compared with 55 percent for the mail survey. Notably, the phone survey tended to provide more reports of weight loss than were reported from the mailed surveys (Couper et al. 2007).

Group-Administered Surveys

In some cases, surveys can be made available for a particular group at one location, such as during a meeting or conference, or at a retirement community or physician practice, so that respondents can complete the survey and immediately submit it to the researchers.

Distribution of Survey

It is important to determine how the survey will be distributed. For example, in the EHR study, researchers contacted each of the randomly selected facilities by phone or e-mail to explain the study, determine whether the facility was willing to participate in the study, and obtain the name and contact information of the individual at the facility best suited to answer questions related to the EHR standards. The participants were assured that their responses would remain completely confidential and that only aggregate data would be used in the results report. Identifying information related to the facility was stored separately from the participants' responses. No identifying information was displayed on the survey form; only a coded number was used for follow-up purposes. The facilities received a copy of the results and a complimentary copy of the *Journal of American Health Information Management Association* for participating. The cover letter described information related to research study participation (online appendix 2C).

Once the names of the individuals identified as eligible to complete the survey were obtained, they were contacted via e-mail and were provided a copy of the cover letter and survey through a corresponding URL. If the participant did not have access to a computer, the cover letter and survey were faxed or mailed, whichever was preferred by the participating facility. The deadline date to return the survey was two weeks after receipt of the survey. After two weeks, if the participants at a facility did not respond, a follow-up e-mail (with follow-up cover letter attached) or phone call was made to request that a facility representative complete the survey. The importance of the study and its results were reiterated, and any questions regarding the survey were answered. See online appendix 2D for a sample follow-up cover letter.

Sample and Sample Size

Most survey research in health informatics is performed on a sample of the population under study. A **census survey** examines an entire population. If a sample is chosen, it is extremely important to make sure that it accurately represents the relevant characteristics of the population under study. For example, for a survey of physicians about their views on patients using a personal health record, it would be best to select physicians from many different specialties. A survey of pediatricians only would not accurately represent the entire physician population. Researchers can determine the **sample size**, the number of subjects needed in a study to represent the population, to survey by using software applications such as the SPSS statistical package. Several methods of sampling are available to researchers; once a sampling method is determined, the sample size is calculated.

Sampling Methods

Because most survey research is performed by using a sample, it is imperative to apply an appropriate sampling method. The most commonly used method is **simple random sampling**, which gives every member of the population under study an equal chance of being selected. Various software programs can easily and quickly provide effective random samples, or researchers can use a table of random numbers to select a good random sample. Other methods of random sampling include the following:

- **Stratified random sampling**—Separate the population by certain characteristics, such as physician specialties, nursing units, or diagnosis-related groups (DRGs), and then choose the random sample.
- **Systematic random sampling**—Draw the sample from a list of items such as diagnoses, ICD-10-CM codes, or discharges and select every *nth* case.
- **Cluster sampling**—Separate the total population into "clusters" (smaller groups), such as neighborhoods within a city, and then randomly sample the clusters, surveying everyone within the sampled clusters.

Convenience samples are obtained by selecting units from the population based on easy availability or accessibility; they are not random, so the results are not generalizable. An example of a convenience sample would be a survey of everyone in an HIT department to determine their knowledge of Health Level 7. The survey can generate quick results, but those results cannot be generalized to everyone in HIT settings nationwide. To do that, a random sample of all HIT employees in the United States would be needed. See chapter 11 for more specific information on sampling methods.

Example of Sample Size Calculation Used for the EHR Study

When conducting survey research it is important to select a random sample that best represents the population under study. A sample size calculation can assist in this process. If the sample is not accurate, the data collected from the sample will not be accurate and could potentially damage the accuracy of the entire study. Therefore, researchers should take care to conduct this calculation accurately.

The EHR study we have been discussing in this chapter illustrates how to calculate sample size and select respondents. This study used stratified random sampling to select a sample of healthcare facilities. The population of US healthcare facilities identified in the American Hospital Association (AHA) guide (numbering approximately 15,000) was stratified by state and by type of facility, such as acute, subacute, long-term care, ambulatory care, and so forth. A subgroup was defined as all facilities of the same type within the same state (for example, acute care facilities in Pennsylvania and LTCFs in Virginia), and a random number-generating procedure was used to draw a random sample from each subgroup.

The healthcare facilities selected by this method comprised one of three components of the total sample. To be certain that facilities with an EHR in place are included in the total sample, the second component was made up of all healthcare organizations recognized by the Nicholas E. Davies EHR Recognition Program, a program sponsored by the Healthcare Information and Management Systems Society (HIMSS).

The third component of the total sample was a sample of vendors of EHR systems, which included all information system vendors on the list published by *Health Care Informatics* magazine (approximately 100 vendors) and all 28 EHR vendors on the list of those reviewed by the American Academy of Family Physicians. Table 2.2 represents the composition of the total sample.

Table 2.2 Composition of the total sample for the EHR study

Type of Facility or Organization	Total Population	Sample Size	Sample 2 (If Applicable)
Acute, subacute, rehabilitation, and so forth	15,000	390	Approximately 3% per state and facility type
Nicholas E. Davies EHR Recognition Facilities	14 (could increase when 2001 winners are selected)	14	Not applicable
Vendors	128	128, unless there were overlap between the two lists used to calculate the total population	Not applicable

Source: Watzlaf et al. 2004b.

To determine the number of healthcare facilities to include in the first component of the sample, the following formula was used:

$$n = Npq / [(N - 1)D] + pq$$

Where: n = sample size number; N = population size number; p = 0.5, the proportion of facilities that are aware of the EHR standards, using a conservative or largest estimate; q = 1 – p; and D = B/4 where B = 0.05/4 = 0.000625

The bound for the error of estimate (B) was set at 5 percent, which is considered an acceptable margin of error for many studies. To determine the sample size for the facilities, the value for the proportion of facilities that are aware of the EHR standards (p) was set at 0.5, because this value produces the most conservative, or the largest, value for the required sample size. Substituting the appropriate values into the formula resulted in a sample size requirement of 390 facilities.

When stratified random sampling is used, the most typical way of distributing the total sample size among the subgroups (or strata) is for subgroups to be represented in the sample in the same proportion that they are represented in the population. To achieve this result, the same sampling fraction, 390/15,000 or approximately 3 percent, was applied to each subgroup. For example, if there were 300 acute care facilities in Pennsylvania, 3 percent of them (9 acute care facilities) were selected; if there were 67 LTCFs in West Virginia, 3 percent of them (2) were selected.

Thus, the total sample size for healthcare facilities was computed as follows:

$$n = Npq / [(N - 1)D] + pq$$

$$n = (15{,}000)(0.5)(0.5) / [(15{,}000 - 1)0.000625] + [(0.0.5)(0.05)]$$

$$= 3{,}750/9.624375$$

$$= 389.636 \text{ (rounded up to 390)}$$

When the other two samples (14 for Nicholas Davies Winners and 128 for Vendors) were included, the grand total sample size equaled 532 (390 + 14 + 128).

Each of the sample size estimates for the healthcare facilities was oversampled to allow for facility refusal, nonresponse, and so forth. There are limitations to the sample. It does not include all types of healthcare facilities in the United States, only those listed in the *AHA Guide to the Health Care Field: United States Hospitals, Health Care Systems, Networks, Alliances, Health Organizations, Agencies, Providers*, which also includes a convenience sample of "elite" facilities with EHR systems and the top 100 vendors.

Response Rate

Achieving an adequate **response rate**, the percentage of subjects answering the survey, is extremely important in survey research. Sometimes, however, even a low response rate in an area that has not been researched in depth before may provide useful data.

In one study on health information management (HIM) practices, 1,000 surveys were sent out to AHIMA members and only 200 were returned (Osborn 2000). Even though the 20 percent response rate may seem low, the study was one of the first of its kind to examine practices and productivity of HIM functions in acute care hospitals. Therefore, the study provided preliminary information about HIM practices that had never before been examined, such as average completion times for chart assembly, chart analysis, coding, and billing, as well as mean turnaround time for release of information activities and other additional HIM functions.

One method used to increase the response rate is to follow up with parties who have not responded to ask them if they would complete the survey. Follow-up can be performed by mailing a postcard, through e-mail, or by phone or fax. Follow-up should include the title of the research study, when the survey questionnaire was sent, the importance of the study and how important the respondent's reply is to the research study, as well as the maintenance of confidential responses and any incentives (if stated in the initial cover letter of the survey). The survey should be attached again so the respondent does not need to look for it in a previous e-mail or letter.

Follow-up should never be overly annoying or intrusive. As part of the protection of research subjects, IRBs have guidelines about follow-up methods, and some IRBs will specifically ask the researcher to state the number of times respondents will be contacted to respond to the survey questionnaire.

In the EHR study, the researchers sought to obtain a response rate from the facilities of greater than 50 percent of the surveys sent, and they believed that using different types of survey media as well as follow-up e-mails or phone calls was essential in obtaining this rate. (See online appendix 2D for a sample of the follow-up cover letter for the EHR study.) The researchers reported two response rates for facilities in the EHR study. A total of 1,129 surveys were sent out to facilities. Respondents completed 192 surveys, and 271 surveys with at least one page completed were received. Thus, the response rate based on the desired sample size of facilities (390) was between 49 percent for all pages completed to 69 percent for at least one page completed. Response rates based on the total number of surveys sent was much lower (17 percent to 24 percent).

Factors limiting the success of the response and completion rates included the length of the paper and web-based survey, respondents not having an EHR on site and therefore not understanding that they could complete the survey, and respondents not having the ability to answer the survey online.

If a response rate is very low, researchers may seek to determine whether the nonresponders are similar to the responders in relation to relevant demographic characteristics (such as age, gender, geographic region, and so forth). If they are, the researchers may conclude that the responders are similar to the general population under study. However, to reach this conclusion, the researchers would need to collect demographic information about the nonresponders and compare it with the demographics of the responders, and researchers often do not have this data on the nonresponders. However, if demographic data are available, a comparison can be made, and researchers may conclude that the response rate was low but representative.

Selection bias may be a factor in the response rate when participants choose to answer the survey questionnaire or be part of the survey research study because, for example, they have an EHR in their facility. **Selection bias** is the ability of some participants to choose to answer the survey questionnaire or be part of the survey research study. It can bias survey results when responders take part in the research study for specific reasons. For example, in the EHR study, some of the respondents may have decided to respond to the survey because they had an EHR in place in their facility, but some other potential participants may not have responded because their facilities did not have an EHR. The researchers may have missed getting input from this latter group of participants.

Statistical Analysis of the Survey Study Data

Statistical analysis of survey data is usually quite simple and includes calculating frequencies, percentages, correlation coefficients, tests of significance, or confidence intervals. (These topics are covered in more detail in chapters 9 and 12.) It may also involve the creation of graphs and tables that reflect these statistics. In the analysis, each section of the open-ended or unstructured questions should be reviewed and summarized into specific categories. Specific or additional comments can be reproduced in a separate section of the report so that no important information is missed.

Examples of statistical tables for analysis of closed-ended and open-ended question responses for the EHR study are shown in table 2.3 and figure 2.4. Respondents were asked to review each data element and then state whether they believed it should be a standard part of the provider data for the EHR. Table 2.3 shows simple frequencies and percentages for closed-ended, or quantitative, data. Figure 2.4 shows open-ended, qualitative, data.

Table 2.3 Example of a closed-ended response summary for data elements for provider

Data Element	Yes		No		N/A		Total
	#	%	#	%	#	%	#
Provider agency ID code	97	51%	70	36%	25	13%	192
Admission surgeon role	121	62%	33	17%	41	21%	195
Practitioner current role	131	68%	47	24%	14	7%	192
Anesthesiologist	132	69%	24	13%	36	19%	192
Practitioner address	134	69%	47	24%	12	6%	193
Practitioner universal ID #	141	73%	39	20%	12	6%	192
Therapy performance practitioner	140	74%	26	14%	24	13%	190
Provider address	145	74%	40	21%	10	5%	195
Admission surgeon	151	76%	10	5%	37	19%	198
Practitioner profession	152	77%	37	19%	9	5%	198
Practitioner authentication	163	84%	23	12%	8	4%	194
Provider ID number	168	86%	16	8%	12	6%	196
Provider type	170	86%	19	10%	9	5%	198
Practitioner name	184	92%	7	4%	8	4%	199
Provider/practitioner name	196	97%	0	0%	7	3%	203

Source: Watzlaf et al. 2004a.

Figure 2.4 Example of open-ended responses for provider data

Provider Data Elements Added

- All practitioners and appropriate information
- Practitioner's status—active vs. inactive
- Practitioner's title—MD, FNP, MSW, PA, and so forth
- Other contact information-specifically, provider e-mail, phone number, fax number, beeper number (2)
- Provider should always be identified with specialty and by role such as ordering or prescribing, attending, admitting, primary, interpreting, treating (3)
- Name of consultant and specialty consultants during an episode of care. Type, date of order, date consultation completed, consultant's report (2)
- Admission/encounter consultant; admission/encounter referring
- DEA and state license numbers
- Primary RN
- Pharmacy provider information
- Social service provider information
- Insurance plans providers participate with
- Admission/encounter surgeon role

(*Continued*)

Figure 2.4 (*Continued*)

- Include space for resident staff
- Name of any laboratory or radiology services used

Provider Data Elements Removed

- Provider agency ID code...goal should be to strive for a universal standard number for physicians and other providers

Additional Comments

- Would provider type be better served by provider taxonomy code? How/who will define provider type?

Source: Watzlaf et al. 2004a.

Review Questions

1. Why is survey research one of the most common types of research performed in health informatics?
2. Why is it important for the researcher to determine whether an existing survey can be used to answer the research questions?
3. Why should an advisory committee be formed when developing the survey?
4. What is the major purpose of the 2004 EHR study by Watzlaf and colleagues?
5. What are examples of open-ended questions relevant to health informatics?
6. What are examples of closed-ended questions relevant to health informatics?
7. Why is it important to pilot test the survey before it is administered?
8. What does a Cronbach's alpha of 0.345 tell the researcher about the survey?
9. What should a researcher do if the response rate is low?
10. What are some examples of statistics that should be generated from survey research?

Application Exercises

1. You have chosen to research the use of computer-assisted coding in healthcare organizations, and you have decided to survey coders in their healthcare organizations. Construct examples of closed-ended and open-ended questions.
2. Review the National Ambulatory Medical Care Survey (NAMCS) (NCHS 2008) and the National Electronic Health Record Survey (NCHS 2014). Do they contain face validity and content validity? Refer to table 2.1 for definitions and examples of face and content validity.
3. Referring back to the real-world case, read the article "2010 Pregnancy Rates Among U.S. Women" (Curtin et al. 2015) and answer the questions that follow.
   a. Why would the NCHS want to continue examining birth rates when their decline has been well documented?
   b. What else declined other than birth rates? How much of a decline was found?
   c. What would you do if you wanted to collect more current data on pregnancy rates from 2016? How would you go about collecting this data?

References

Abdrbo, A.A., J.A. Zauszniewski, C.A. Hudak, and M.K. Anthony. 2011 (Summer). Development and testing of nurses information system benefits instrument. *Perspectives in Health Information Management*. http://perspectives.ahima.org/development-and-testing-of-a-survey-instrument-to-measure-benefits-of-a-nursing-information-system/.

Chung, S. and E. Nahm. 2015. Testing reliability and validity of the eHealth Literacy Scale (eHEALS) for older adults recruited online. *Computers, Informatics, Nursing: CIN*. 33(4): 150–156. doi: 10.1097/CIN.0000000000000146.

Couper, M.P., A. Peytchev, V.J. Strecher, K. Rothert, and J. Anderson. 2007. Following up non-respondents to an online weight management intervention: Randomized trial comparing mail versus telephone. *Journal of Medical Internet Research* 9(2):e16.

Cronk, B.C. 2016. *How to Use SPSS,* 9th ed. Glendale, CA: Pyrczak Publishing.

Curtin, S.C., J.C. Abma, and K. Kost. 2015. 2010 pregnancy rates among U.S. women. NCHS Health e-Stat. http://www.cdc.gov/nchs/data/hestat/pregnancy/2010_pregnancy_rates.htm.

Gunn, H. 2002. Web-based surveys: Changing the survey process. *First Monday* 7(12). http://firstmonday.org/issues/issue7_12/gunn/index.html.

Howell, J., P. Miller, H. Park, D. Sattler, T. Schack, E. Spery, S. Widhalm, M. Palmquist. 1993–2017. Reliability and validity. Writing@CSU Guide. Colorado State University. http://writing.colostate.edu/guides/guide.cfm?guideid=66.

McGeeney, K. 2015. Tips for creating web surveys for completion on a mobile device. PewResearchCenter. http://www.pewresearch.org/2015/06/11/tips-for-creating-web-surveys-for-completion-on-a-mobile-device.

National Cancer Institute (NCI). 2016. Health Information National Trends Survey (HINTS). Accessed 26 June 2016. http://hints.cancer.gov/about.aspx.

Nelson, D.E., G.L. Kreps, B.W. Hesse, R.T. Croyle, G. Willis, N.K. Arora, B.K. Rimer, K.V. Viswanath, N. Weinstein, and S. Alden. 2004. The Health Information National Trends Survey (HINTS): Development, design, dissemination. *Journal of Health Communication* 9:443–460.

Osborn, C.E. 2000. Practices and productivity in acute care facilities. *Journal of the American Health Information Management Association* 2:61–66.

Rudman, W., K. Jackson, P. Shank, D. Zuccarelli. 2016. Perceived effects of ICD-10 coding productivity and accuracy among coding professionals. *Perspectives in Health Information Management.* http://perspectives.ahima.org/perceived-effects-of-icd-10-coding-productivity-and-accuracy-among-coding-professionals.

Watzlaf, V.J., J. Mazzoni, and A. Pandolph. 1995. Quality assessment in a long-term care facility using the medical record as principal data source. *Journal of Health Information Management Research* 3(2):24–36.

Watzlaf, V.J., X. Zeng, C. Jarymowycz, and P. Firouzan. 2004a (Winter). Standards for the content of the electronic health record. *Perspectives in Health Information Management*: 1.

Watzlaf, V.J., X. Zeng, C. Jarymowycz, and P. Firouzan. 2004b. Composition of the total sample for the EHR study. Unpublished developmental material.

Zhou, L., V. Watzlaf, P. Abernathy, M. Abdelhak. 2017 (Summer). The adoption of enabling technologies for personalized interventions of the medically underserved: A multidisciplinary team solution. *Perspectives in Health Information Management.* Forthcoming.

Resources

National Center for Health Statistics (NCHS). 2014. National Electronic Health Records Survey. https://www.cdc.gov/nchs/data/ahcd/2014_NEHRS_Long_Form.pdf.

National Center for Health Statistics (NCHS). 2008. National Ambulatory Medical Care Survey. https://www.cdc.gov/nchs/data/ahcd/NAMCS_1_2008.pdf.

3 Observational Research

Valerie J. Watzlaf, PhD, MPH, RHIA, FAHIMA

Learning Objectives

- Explain the purpose of observational research and how it is used in health informatics.
- Describe the following types of observational research: nonparticipant observation, participant observation, and ethnography.
- Determine how to record and collect data for each type of observational research.
- Conduct the constant comparative method of analysis for observational research.
- Discuss which types of observational research are most appropriate for health informatics.

Key Terms

Case study
Constant comparative method
Content analysis
Direct observation
Field notes
Focus group
Focused interview
General interview guide
Grounded theory
Group case study
Indirect observation
Individual case study
Informal conversational interview
Institutional case study
Standardized open-ended interview

Observational research is research that explores a particular topic and can include both quantitative or qualitative approaches. However, most observational research is categorized as qualitative because it allows an investigator to get to know the nuts and bolts of a study subject, program, or facility. This type of research strives to examine perceptions, interactions, feelings, and attitudes in an uncontrolled study setting. By collecting these types of data, observational research adds depth, substance, and meaning to the results of the research study that may be lacking when performing the quantitative approach.

Researchers conduct observational research for many reasons. Observational research is usually conducted when little is known about the study subject, when the researcher is studying relationships between the research participants and the setting, or when the researcher is studying a transitional program and the change or impact it may have on research study participants' attitudes, feelings, and behaviors. It can be used to prepare for larger, quantitative studies, or it can stand alone, especially when a topic is studied for the first time.

Observational researchers use various methods to obtain robust and meaningful data (see table 3.1). Some observational research studies use a combination of observation, field interviews, health record reviews, and ethnographic

Table 3.1 Observational research methods

Method	Definition	Example in Health Informatics
I. Nonparticipant Observation	The observation of actions of study participants in which the researcher limits his or her interference with their actions.	Researcher observes how employees react to a new documentation software system.
a. Naturalistic	A type of nonparticipant observation in which the researcher observes behaviors and events as they occur naturally in the normal environment.	Researcher observes employee behavior at a healthcare facility to determine whether the cancer registry is being properly utilized.
b. Simulation	Observation of participants in an environment that has been created for them, rather than in their normal environment.	Researcher selects websites and observes how well individuals with visual disabilities use them.
c. Case Study	Nonparticipant observational study to thoroughly assess an individual, group, or institution.	See examples for individual case study, group case study, and institutional case study, below.
i. Individual Case Study	Detailed observation of an individual as he or she progresses through a certain disease, procedure, treatment, cultural, or system change.	Researcher follows and evaluates a patient to determine how he or she uses an assistive technology device.
ii. Group Case Study	Detailed observation of a group of individuals as it progresses through a certain disease, procedure, treatment, cultural, or system change.	Researcher observes the moral reasoning skills of medical students when dealing with ethical issues.
iii. Institutional Case Study	Detailed observation of a institution or facility to determine how it conducts a particular process, system, or procedure.	Department of Veterans Affairs healthcare system used the institutional case study method to describe how their electronic health record system is used in home-based primary care programs (Shea 2007).
d. Focused Interview	An interview method used when the researcher wants to collect in-depth, rich, robust information to open-ended questions. Four types of focused interviews include: focus group, informal conversation, general interview guide, and standardized open-ended interview.	Examples of each type of focused interview are provided below.
i. Informal Conversation	A discussion that moves forward based on what the study participant would like to discuss, without preset questions.	Researcher and participants discuss living with dementia while in a nursing facility.
ii. Standardized Open Ended Interview	An interview using specific open-ended questions.	Researcher interviews participants about automated coding software and the potential to decrease fraud and abuse.
iii. General Interview Guide	An informal interview based on an outline of issues.	Medical schools use the general interview guide to reassess team-based learning.
iv. Focus Group	Observation of a group of subjects, usually experts in the particular area of study, who are brought together to discuss a specific topic.	Researcher convenes a focus group of experts to evaluate ICD-10-CM and its effectiveness in capturing public health-related diseases.
II. Participant	The observation of actions of study participants in which the researcher is an actor in the environment he or she is observing.	Researcher observes how well employees in healthcare facilities abide by Health Insurance Portability and Accountability Act (HIPAA) privacy rules.
III. Ethnography	An in-depth investigation of a culture or organization to learn everything there is to know about it and to develop new hypotheses.	Researcher closely observes and assesses interactions between physicians and patients when the EHR is used.

methods. When designing an observational study, it is important to pay particular attention to the observation site, time period, what will be observed, how it will be recorded, who will conduct the observation, how the data will be analyzed, and how the results will be disseminated.

Health informatics researchers can use observational research methods when they want to obtain a qualitative perspective on a problem. For example, observational researchers in healthcare facilities can gather data from in-depth observations, interviews, or ethnographic accounts of what occurs in interactions between patients and physicians, as well as information about the feelings of patients diagnosed, for example, with dementia or colon cancer. Observational research provides extensive amounts of data that need to be evaluated using content analysis, the analysis of observational data using patterns, themes, and other more complex methods, but it can provide the researcher with information about the feelings, perceptions, attitudes, and thoughts that experimental research methods (discussed in chapter 4) will not provide.

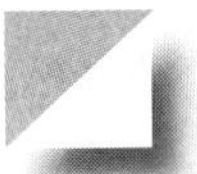

Real-World Case

In a leadership study, researchers used multiple observational and qualitative techniques to study health information management (HIM) professionals. The investigators began by conducting individual interviews with colleagues and bosses of HIM directors. Next, the researchers interviewed HIM directors and managers and held focus groups with management and staff. They also conducted separate focus groups with HIM staff as well as observations of enterprise-wide and department meetings, with the observations recorded on an informational data sheet. All data were analyzed for similar patterns and themes across the different leaders to determine what constitutes a leader in HIM (Sheridan, Watzlaf, and Fox 2016).

Nonparticipant Observation

Field observation may include direct or indirect observation. During a **direct observation**, researchers are present in the environment they are observing so they can personally conduct the observation. For example, researchers might personally observe someone using a tablet to collect wellness assessment information. During a direct observation, researchers may record observations by taking extensive and meticulous notes about the phenomena they observe. During an **indirect observation**, researchers use audio or video recording so that the environment is not changed in any way from the norm; this practice reduces the effect the researcher may have on the behavior of those they are observing. For example, the investigators might video record someone using a tablet to collect wellness information and analyze the recording later.

As the comparison between direct and indirect observations suggests, the observational researcher may influence the actions of the individuals being observed. Therefore, the researcher should determine whether a nonparticipant or participant observational method is best for a specific research topic (Giacomini and Cook 2000). In a nonparticipant observation, the investigator observes the actions of the study subjects while trying not to interfere in their activities. In participant observation (which will be discussed in more detail later in this chapter), the researcher is also a part of the environment he or she is observing.

Researchers can use nonparticipant observation to examine, for example, how employees react to a new documentation software system. In such a study, the researchers might observe how employees are educated about and trained in the system, their collection or use of data with the new system, and their use of the results that the system provides. Acting as neutral observers of the discussions, actions, or issues of the study subjects, the investigators record the feelings, behaviors, attitudes, and perceptions of the employees regarding the new documentation software system. By using nonparticipant observation, the investigators can determine potential problems in the software system and begin to correct them. Nonparticipant observation may include four different types: naturalistic observation, simulation observation, case study, and focused interviews.

Naturalistic Observation

Researchers use naturalistic observation to study behaviors or events that occur naturally in the normal environment, as noted in chapter 1. The study subjects normally should not know what researchers are observing or when observations are made. This approach ensures that the study participants or events that are being observed are as similar as possible to the real or natural environment, and it allows the study participants to display behaviors that tend to occur in their normal environment. Researchers may choose this type of observation when they want to know, for example, whether individuals are following a specific procedure, rule, law, or policy.

A research study incorporated naturalistic observation to determine the age, gender, and ethnicity of the customers of vape shops (stores that sell e-cigarettes) and the activities that may take place when customers enter the shop. The investigators used observation forms to record demographic characteristics (age, gender, ethnicity) as well as purchases made, activities, and conversations. To be sure that the age estimations were valid, the observer performed age estimations in a pilot study on a university campus and then asked the people being observed their exact ages. Correlation between the estimated age and actual age indicated high accuracy of the estimates ($r = 0.95$). Nonparticipant observations were conducted during the workday of customers staying in the vape shop for over 20 minutes. The observer stayed at least 15 feet away from all customers and observed what products were purchased, the conversations that took place, the amount of time the customers stayed in the shop, and what they did while there. It was found that the average age of customers was 30 years, 53 percent of customers were white, and 79 percent were male. Conversations centered around vaping topics, sampling e-juices (mixtures used in vapor products), and receiving assistance on products. Customers tended to stay in the shop lounging and talking with other customers and the owner of the shop. This example shows how nonparticipant observations can assist in the understanding of the use of e-cigarettes and may provide information for future public health policies on tobacco and nicotine control (Sussman et al. 2016).

In another example of nonparticipant naturalistic observation, Swedish researchers investigated patients' experiences of care before, during, and after a hip fracture to determine their pain and nutrition needs (Hallström et al. 2000). The study used nonparticipant observation, informal field interviews, and abstraction of nursing notes and health records with patients and relatives. Nine patients were followed throughout their care for their hip fracture, including time spent in the emergency department (if applicable), hospitalization, and rehabilitation for up to four months after discharge to home. Observation periods lasted between one and four hours, and total observation time per patient was approximately 20 hours. Field notes were recorded either immediately after the observation or during short breaks between observations. The observer's role was primarily that of a listener while patients created the topics for conversation. Observers were registered nurses, did not have any personal or medical involvement with the patients, and wore street clothes during all observations. No information collected from the observers was given to hospital staff at any time, which is the normal procedure when naturalistic observation methods are used. The researchers used open coding to determine themes from the data collected in observations. A theme was found when a response appeared many times or if the response could lead to major changes in their care although it was only mentioned once. The researchers found that the most important method of data collection used in this study was nonparticipant naturalistic observation. "Observations revealed information that would not have been obtained from interviews or questionnaires" (Hallström et al. 2000, 644). The study concluded that nursing care could be improved with a focus on pain needs and nutrition protocols for hip fracture patients.

Simulation Observation

The simulation observation method is another type of nonparticipant observation used by researchers. It is usually conducted by observing study subjects in an environment created for them instead of in their natural environment. In health informatics, simulation observation can be a helpful method in usability studies in which researchers evaluate how subjects use a new health information technology. Usability outcomes can include the time to complete a specific task, number of user errors, severity of the errors, and the ability to recover from the errors, user satisfaction, the length of time it takes to complete a task (efficiency of use) and how fast a user can learn a new system (ease of learning).

A usability study observed individuals with visual disabilities using the Internet in a simulated setting by choosing which websites the study subjects would examine. The researchers had the study subjects answer questions about the websites to determine how well they navigated through each website and how accessible the sites were for persons with visual disabilities. The researchers conducted observations as subjects used a transcoding technology and again when they did not use the new technology. By identifying specific problems, the researchers have contributed to efforts to make websites fully accessible to persons with visual disabilities (Hackett 2007).

Case Study

The case study method is a type of nonparticipant observation that is used when the researcher wants to know detailed information about characteristics of an individual, a group of individuals, or a particular facility, organization, or institution. Data collection methods include field notes, photographs, and audio and video recordings. Each of these aspects is examined in great detail and includes collecting specific characteristics (demographic, disease, religious, social, cultural, technological system and software, community) about the individual, group, or institution.

Individual Case Study

The individual case study is one of the oldest methods of observational research. Historically, it has been used when physicians and other healthcare providers want to learn more about a new disease that has afflicted certain individuals. In an **individual case study**, the researcher collects as much relevant information as they can on an individual as he or she progresses through a certain disease, procedure, treatment, cultural, or health information system change.

A landmark individual case study sought to determine the feasibility of a 74-year-old man swimming the English Channel. The researchers were interested in knowing whether the man could swim for 21 hours in water as cold as the English Channel without becoming unconscious from hypothermia. They also wanted to test two thermal protective suits to determine their effectiveness and to offer advice to others who might attempt to swim long distances in cold water. Therefore, the researchers observed his long-distance training three times a week for several months. The swimmer's body temperature, water temperature, types of body covers used, length of swims, diet, and general comments about the swimmer's attitude were recorded. The researchers concluded that the man should not attempt to swim the English Channel because he could not tolerate the cold water. The study also provided some information for marathon swimmers, such as the length of time swimmers should spend training in cold water for long cold-water swims (Kanaar and Hecht 1991).

Individual case studies are occasionally performed in health informatics, although such studies are uncommon. For example, individual patients may be closely observed and their actions recorded as they use a specific assistive technology device and healthcare providers could be observed as they proceed throughout their work day to determine which technological devices may increase their work productivity. Researchers could also record how an administrator of a large healthcare facility interacted with healthcare employees, patients, and family to determine the current communication techniques used, and to evaluate whether communication could be improved with health information technology (HIT) systems. In Catalonia, researchers used a multiple case approach to determine whether an integrated healthcare network improved the quality of care for chronic obstructive pulmonary disease (COPD) patients. Individual interviews were conducted with the COPD patients and their family members. For each case, the researchers also interviewed the person who the patient believed was the most relevant health professional in their COPD care (general practitioner, pulmonologist, or case manager). Health records were also examined (Waibel et al. 2015).

Group Case Study

The **group case study** resembles the individual case study except the interviews or observations are performed on a group of individuals instead of just one individual.

The group case study method was used to evaluate the moral reasoning skills of medical students. Small groups of 8 to 10 students and 2 faculty members were used to discuss clinical cases that presented many different types of ethical issues. The faculty group leaders were asked to encourage students to take a stand on each of the ethical issues and defend their position. Moral reasoning skills were assessed by using standardized tests and tabulated results, both before and after the students participated in medical ethics education classes. It was found that teaching medical ethics can significantly increase medical students' moral reasoning skills (Self et al. 1998).

Institutional Case Study

The **institutional case study** is used to observe a healthcare institution or facility to determine how it conducts a process, system, or procedure. Individual case studies may be included within the institutional case study, but the focus is on the institution-wide system, process, or procedure.

The US Department of Veterans Affairs (VA) healthcare system used the institutional case study method in a study about how its electronic health record (EHR) system is used in home-based primary care programs (Shea 2007). The report explains how the EHR can be accessed remotely, throughout the United States, by the home and hospice care team whenever a patient referral occurs, and the efforts that are taken to keep patient information confidential. The study further examines the importance of the institution-wide EHR in relation to traumatic events such as Hurricane Katrina, which illustrated the need for a backup system to retrieve patient information should the electronic system become inoperable. It also describes the parts of the EHR and how the tabs at the bottom of the computer screen (cover sheet, problems, order, medications, notes, surgery reports, labs, discharge summary, and so forth) resemble information found in paper-based health records, and it recounts how home healthcare providers use the EHR to prepare for a home visit. For example, the study shows how the nurse can review the medication list, which includes medications currently taken as well as over-the-counter (OTC) medications that are self-reported, and the EHR will provide alerts from the pharmacy when the OTC medications are not compatible with prescribed medications. The nurse can further assess the patient's blood pressure over time through past readings as well as with graphs. At the same time, the social worker, dietician, and occupational therapist can review specific parts of the EHR, such as advance directives, diet education history, and fall history. The study includes a case report on one patient and how the use of the EHR enhanced care for this individual (Shea 2007).

Overall, this institutional case study report provides a complete overview of the institution-wide EHR system at the VA and how it is used successfully within home and hospice care. Other organizations can review the report and develop similar institutional case studies to determine the effectiveness of other HIT systems from the standpoint of ease of use. It also would be interesting to use the institutional case study method to examine whether the use of the EHR improved patient care.

Focused Interview

A **focused interview** uses open-ended questions to solicit the interviewee's opinions about a specific topic. Focused interviews are used extensively in observational research when the researcher wants to collect in-depth information that would not be obtained from the responses to close-ended questions. There are four primary types of focused interviews:

- **Informal conversational interviews**, which are loosely structured and may flow like a conversation between the person being interviewed and the researcher.
- **Standardized open-ended interviews**, in which researchers develop a set of questions ahead of time and then follow the wording and order of questions closely when conducting the interview.
- **General interview guide** interviews, which are conducted using an outline or checklist format rather than standardized questions; the interviewer can choose which areas to cover and may not cover all of them.
- **Focus groups**, which are a group of subjects, who are often experts in an area of study, who discuss a specific topic in a focused interview with a moderator.

Informal Conversational Interview

The informal conversational interview moves forward as the subject discusses certain topics of conversation. No specific topics or questions are developed ahead of time, and the researcher aims to learn about a setting, culture, system change, or person. This interview method is used most in participant observation, and its main goal is to learn as much as possible about the situation as the subject or group of subjects discuss topics of interest to them in their own words.

Farre and Cummins (2016) used the informal conversational interview method when striving to understand how a new computerized provider order entry (CPOE) system was implemented in a UK pediatric facility, how the system changed over time, the users' perspectives, and how the system may have affected healthcare outcomes. Examples of questions asked in the informal conversational interviews about using the CPOE system included the following:

- Do pediatricians and pediatric nurses feel their practice will be/is safer when CPOE is used?
- Do pediatricians feel that remote access to the system will ease/has eased their workload?
- Do pediatric nurses feel that the technology will facilitate/facilitates their interaction with pharmacists and doctors to check/amend prescriptions in a timely fashion (Farre and Cummins 2016)?

Standardized Open-Ended Interview

In a standardized open-ended interview the same specific questions written in advance by the research team are asked of all participants, and interviewers treat all respondents the same way. Standardized open-ended interviews do not always work well in observational research. Because the questions are designed by the researcher, the subject may be led to answer in a certain manner inconsistent with their own experiences instead of speaking freely.

The standardized open-ended focused interview was used extensively in a 2005 descriptive research study that examined the types of automated coding software available across healthcare settings, vendors, and users, as well as the software's ability to reduce fraudulent activities by preventing errors, increasing the accuracy of coded data, and detecting false claims (AHIMA et al. 2005). The objectives of this research project were as follows:

- To identify the characteristics of automated coding systems that have the potential to detect improper coding

- To identify the components of the coding process that have the potential to minimize improper or fraudulent coding practices when using automated coding and to determine their effectiveness with the use of the EHR
- To develop recommendations for software developers and users of coding products to maximize antifraud practices

The study had several parts, including two that involved focused interviews. In the first part, the researchers used standardized open-ended questions (figure 3.1) to interview representatives from appropriate federal agencies regarding their experiences with improper reimbursement or potential fraud involving automated coding software.

Figure 3.1 Standardized open-ended questions asked during interviews with federal employees about improper reimbursement and fraud involving automated software

1. In your view, what are the best processes to prohibit fraud and abuse?
2. What problems do you foresee in relation to fraud and abuse when the electronic health record (EHR) is used?
3. As discussed in an AHIMA practice brief, automated coding was defined as the use of computer software that automatically generates a set of medical codes for review, validation, and use based upon clinical documentation provided by healthcare practitioners. Are you aware of specific facilities or settings that use automated coding systems or automated coding? Have you found patterns of abuse with automated coding?
4. Are you aware of incorrect coding or abuse detected with Natural Language Processing (NLP)? If you are familiar with the approach of the NLP, was it a rules-based approach or data-driven approach? Please describe.
5. Have you found a pattern of abuse with any particular commercial software product that assists in the determination of codes? Examples of products include: bar codes, pick or lookup lists, coding templates or coding protocol, automated superbills, logic or rules-based encoders, groupers, imaged and remote coding applications, hard coding via charge master tables. Please describe any patterns found.
6. According to *Managed Healthcare Executive*, the most effective antifraud and recovery programs include elements of process assessment, both retrospective and prospective technology, and investigations and resolutions. Do you agree? Please discuss.
7. With the proliferation of EHRs with embedded reference terminology, such as SNOMED CT, do you envision this to affect fraud and abuse in automated coding systems? Please discuss.
8. What in your view are the weak links in antifraud software, education, and compliance practices?
9. What general patterns of abuse have you found by setting (for example, physician office, SNF [skilled nursing facilities], hospitals, and so forth) with services that:
   - Were never rendered, either by adding charges to legitimate claims, or by using actual patient names and health insurance information to fabricate claims?
   - Were upcoded?
   - Were a deliberate provision of medically unnecessary services, which include tests, surgeries, and other procedures?
10. Are you aware of programs in which consumers have been educated to alert governmental agencies of fraud? If yes, how has it worked? What is the extent of fraud found by this means and are there any patterns of reporting by setting, diagnosis, or procedure?

Source: AHIMA et al. 2005, 37.

The second part of the research study included an evaluation of automated coding software, coding optimization software, antifraud software, and coding application tools such as bar codes, pick or lookup lists, and so forth, to determine their use as well as the cost of these systems. To identify vendors that participated in the development of coding optimization, coding automation, and anti-fraud software, an extensive search of coding vendors and users was conducted via both the Internet and telephone interviews. Approximately 40 vendors were contacted and given the opportunity to complete a product information form, which is shown in figure 3.2. Once the research team received a completed form, they reviewed it and determined whether an interview with the vendor was warranted. Following the format shown in figure 3.3, researchers interviewed representatives of all vendors that had the specific coding-related software relevant to this research, and then developed three product matrices that demonstrate the extent of use and cost of these systems.

Figure 3.2 Product information form

Vendor Name:

Address:

E-mail Address:

Phone:

Contact Person:

Title of Respondent:

Place an X in the appropriate setting for each product listed that your company provides. The following definitions are from the *Coding (AHIMA Practice Brief) Glossary:* ED = Emergency Department; SDS = Same Day Surgery; HH = Home Health, LTC = Long-Term Care

	ED	SDS	Other Outpatient	X-ray	HH	LTC	Acute	Physician Office	Hospice
Coding optimization software									
Antifraud Software: Software that provides aggregate data analysis and record-specific audits									
Antifraud software									
Automated coding: Software that automatically generates a set of medical codes for review/validation and/or use based upon clinical documentation provided by healthcare practitioners									
Automated coding with NLP									
Automated coding with structured text									
Automated coding products									
Coding Tools: Tools used by coding professionals in the code assignment process									
Bar codes									
Pick lists or lookup lists									
Automated superbills									
Logic or rules-based encoders									
Groupers									
Imaged coding applications									
Remote coding applications									
Hard coding via chargemaster tables									
Automated coding-NLP system									
Automated coding-structured text									
Other automated coding systems									
Maintenance									

Source: AHIMA et al. 2005, 40–41.

Figure 3.3 Vendor interview form

As discussed in AHIMA's practice brief, automated coding is defined as the use of computer software that automatically generates a set of medical codes for review, validation, and use based upon clinical documentation provided by healthcare practitioners.

1. What type of automated coding system do you provide?
2. When was your first installation of the automated coding system? How many installations (users/clients) do you have and in what settings?
3. What is the average installation and training time?
4. Did coder quality change with the use of your automated coding system? Please describe what occurred in terms of coding quality and define how you evaluated coder quality. If coder quality was affected, by what percent was it affected?
5. Do you provide a remote coding application? Has this application improved coding productivity? Please describe what occurred in terms of productivity and by what percent the productivity changed. Please describe the number of outpatient records and inpatient records per hour before and after use of the remote coding application. What was the percent change?
6. How is the automated coding system used with the EHR? What are your thoughts regarding automated coding systems and what will transpire when the EHR is fully implemented?
7. How is the automated coding system used within the coding and billing process? Include the workflow from the coder assigning codes to billing to the payer.
8. What are the antifraud features available and how do they link to the automated coding system? Do you have future recommendations for antifraud features within automated coding systems?
9. How do you use the coded data in your analytics? Please elaborate on rules-based vs. statistics-based approach, as well as statistical modeling applications you may be using with the automated coding software.
10. Can you recommend any users of automated coding systems or vendors who are using or developing automated coding applications that we can also interview?
11. What do you believe are the weak links in fraud/abuse software, education, and compliance practices?

Source: AHIMA et al, 2005, 38.

The third part of the research study included describing the available automated coding software tools, how these tools were being used in the coding and billing process, the impact of these tools on coding and billing accuracy, and the characteristics and limitations of antifraud features that were currently available in automated coding software. Special attention was paid to "weak links" in automated coding and fraud and abuse software, user education, and compliance practices. This section of the research study will be discussed in more detail later in this chapter, in the section on content analysis.

The fourth part of the research study included an extensive search of users of automated coding systems. Focused interviews following the format presented in figure 3.4 were conducted by telephone and in person to augment the information that was found via the Internet and literature searches and to determine the effectiveness of the automated systems currently in use.

Content analysis of the interview data (discussed later in this chapter) was performed, and results were categorized into common themes related to strategies for reducing the fraud and abuse risk. Guidelines for developers and best practices for users of automated coding products were developed. Also, detailed recommendations regarding the development of automated coding tools and their use were compiled.

Figure 3.4 Standardized open-ended questions asked of users of automated coding systems

1. What type of automated coding system do you use within your facility?
2. Is the automated coding system natural language processing (NLP) or structured text?
3. What is the approximate cost of the automated coding system (including education and training)?
4. When was the automated coding system developed?
5. How long did it take to implement the automated coding system on-site, including education and training?
6. What is the level of accuracy in coding and billing?
7. How is the automated coding system used with the EHR?
8. How is the automated coding system used within the coding and billing process?
9. What are the antifraud features available and how do they link to the automated coding system?
10. What do you believe are the "weak links" in fraud/abuse software, education, and compliance practices?

Source: AHIMA et al. 2005, 39.

Use of standardized open-ended interviews for this study enabled the researchers to compile important recommendations regarding automated coding software that are now being used by system developers, users, and federal agencies. Without the use of the focused interview as a data collection technique, many of the candid remarks regarding the automated coding software may not have been recorded and used to develop recommendations.

General Interview Guide Interviews

Interviews that use a general interview guide are a bit more structured than informal conversational interviews. Here the researcher uses an outline of issues that he or she may want to explore during the interview process. The outline is used as a checklist, and as each topic is discussed during the interview, it is checked off on the outline. Sometimes, questions are listed on one side of the guide with additional prompts listed across from the questions. Interviews conducted with a general interview guide tend to be very long. Therefore, they are usually recorded so that none of the information is lost and the researcher has time to focus on the interview process while all important information is documented.

Researchers from several different medical schools across the United States used an interview guide to reassess team-based learning (TBL) among 10 medical schools since TBL's initial evaluation in 2003 (Thompson et al. 2007). Faculty members using the TBL approach were interviewed using the interview guide. Parts of the interview guide are listed in figure 3.5 to demonstrate how this method of observational research is used.

Figure 3.5 Sample questions from team-based learning interview guide

Has team learning been introduced into new courses?

Prompts:
Why? (Explore specific enablers and inhibitors)
When and how did it happen?
What elements of team learning are used?
What unexpected outcomes have occurred?

Source: Thompson et al. 2007.

Focus Group

A focus group is a group of subjects, usually experts in the area of study, who discuss a specific topic in a focused interview. A focus group typically consists of approximately 6 to 12 people and usually has a moderator who is not a member of the research team. The moderator ensures that all members of the focus group have equal time to discuss the issue and may be the person to record important information through audio or video recording. The group discusses issues as they are presented by the moderator. This allows the focus group members to hear one another's opinions and to comment on them. The focus group of subject matter experts provides an excellent way for the research team to learn more about the area of study because a group of experts is brainstorming together about it. It also enables the researcher to see how the group interacts and responds to particular study participants. Some studies may have more than one focus group (Shi 1997).

Watzlaf and colleagues examined whether the *International Classification of Diseases, Tenth Revision, Clinical Modification (ICD-10-CM)* can be effectively used to capture public health information about diseases by conducting a focus group with experts in ICD-10-CM, public health, and classification systems. For example, members of the research team developed a listing of required reportable diseases to the Centers for Disease Control and Prevention (CDC) and state departments of health. The researchers coded each of the diseases using ICD-10-CM and the *International Classification of Diseases, Ninth Revision, Clinical Modification (ICD-9-CM)*. The principal investigator and co-investigators provided rankings for each of the disease categories. The rankings ranged from 1 = "Coding system does not capture the disease" to 5 = "The coding system fully captures the disease." The focus group then came together to discuss each of the rankings and determine where changes in the ranking system needed to be made. The use of the focus group in this capacity provided the researchers with validated information that was used to clarify many of the final rankings (Watzlaf et al. 2007).

Participant Observation

As discussed previously under nonparticipant observation, participant observation is an observational method in which the observer may be a part of the observed environment. In healthcare research, the participant observer may be a researcher or a person who works in the healthcare environment. When considering participant observation, it is important to evaluate whether the openness, attitudes, feelings, and behaviors of the study's subjects can truly be observed when the observer is also a participant.

For example, healthcare facilities that are interested in how well their employees abide by Health Information Portability and Accountability Act (HIPAA) regulations may use the participant observation method. Investigators may observe employees' behavior on the elevators of the healthcare facility to determine whether patient-specific information is kept confidential. Investigators may also observe HIM employees as they process requests for health record information, observing whether they checked for completeness of the request form, including appropriate signatures, dates, and health record forms. To document the behaviors, the researchers can document the information using check sheets or audio or video recordings. Because much of the information involved in the study is confidential, researchers must take steps to maintain the confidentiality of the data collected, which includes keeping the information in secure systems, whether on paper or electronic, and abiding by any other requirements that the institutional review board (IRB) may determine necessary. The researchers, who also may be employees within the facility, may ultimately use the information collected to improve the processes and systems related to compliance with HIPAA regulations.

Hofler and colleagues used the participant method of observational research when examining HIPAA-compliance activities at the University Health Systems of Eastern Carolina (UHSEC). Their study included physical inspection or observation, staff interviews, review of the information related to privacy and security, and observation and review of automated system activity. The privacy officers conducted the physical observations or "walkabouts," which included elevator observation, cafeteria conversation observation, trash-can content review, and informal interviews with staff. Walkabouts were unannounced, and reports of results were provided to managers so that they could fix any noncompliance problems. Conversations with staff included education as the problems were found. The privacy officers, who were also the observers, used the study findings to provide education and training to staff so that compliance of HIPAA regulations could be maintained. Site visits at each of the UHSEC facilities examined the physical layout, operations, and privacy issues of each of the sites. Audits of specific practices revealed that some patients' notice of privacy practices (NPP) was not always provided on a consistent basis. A report generated from the automated patient admission system verified whether the NPP was provided to patients on admission. Further review and analysis of the data collected led the privacy officers, information technology (IT) security officers, and risk management staff to develop and implement an activity review process that identified the greatest compliance risks. A matrix was developed that outlined which activity should be monitored, who should be responsible for the review, how often it should occur, and what should be reviewed (Hofler et al. 2005). Table 3.2 shows an excerpt from the matrix using IT Infrastructure Activity as an example.

The participant observational method that UHSEC researchers used as part of their process to analyze HIPAA compliance is an excellent way to address this most complex and ongoing issue. Although the authors know that achieving compliance will be a "process in evolution," their creative methods to assess it and develop tools for ongoing evaluation and analysis will certainly aid in their ability to consistently examine this extensive requirement (Hofler et al. 2005).

Table 3.2 Excerpt from the UHSCE HIPAA activity monitoring matrix

IT Infrastructure Activity		
Responsible Party	**Frequency**	**Reviewed**
IT security	TBD	❖ Network traffic activity ❖ Firewall activity ❖ Intrusion detection system activity ❖ Wireless activity ❖ E-mail activity ❖ File transfer activity ❖ Virus management ❖ Internet activity ❖ Remote activity ❖ Software licenses

Source: Adapted from Hofler et al. 2005.

Ethnography

Ethnography, defined in chapter 1, involves the observer delving into a culture or organization to learn everything there is to know about a population and develop new hypotheses. Ethnography can be broken into two parts. The first part includes the method of cultural anthropology, in which the researcher seeks to answer questions concerning the ways of life of living human beings. Ethnographic questions include the links between culture and behavior and how cultural processes develop over time. Researchers or field workers tend to live among the people they are studying and participate in as much of the day-to-day activities as possible. Even mundane events, such as preparing meals and eating, provide pieces of information that field workers may use in their data collection process. Even though cultural research is where ethnography is most often used, it can also be necessary when examining healthcare. Reasons to use the ethnographic approach to examine the healthcare industry include the variety of healthcare facility types and the clinical culture within facilities, health policy issues, and the behaviors that take place between patients and caregivers (Goodson 2011). The second part includes the writing up and reporting of results. Ethnographic research tends to be subjective. Researchers who conduct ethnographic research may come to different conclusions about the same population studied because each ethnographer has his or her own background and ideas. No two ethnographers will examine a specific culture or organization the same way. Unlike experimental research, which is discussed in chapter 4, ethnography is not replicable. It also does not collect large numbers, rates, or percentages, or identify trends in large databases; instead, it focuses on people and provides insights into their culture and life.

Field notes, the documentation the ethnographic researcher maintains, are an important part of ethnographic research. Field notes should be written immediately after leaving the field site and should include the following four parts:

- Jottings or brief notes written at the field site immediately upon observation that will be expanded when the full field notes are written
- A more complete description—that is, full field notes—of everything the researcher can remember about the observation event, such as a meeting or encounter
- Analysis of brief notes and descriptions that link back to specific research questions, which might be about the culture, policy, or regulation

- Personal reflection on what the researcher learned and felt while doing the observation, such as how comfortable the investigator felt while collecting information in the field (Hall 2007). This is an important part of ethnography because it should include the observer's opinions as data collection from the environment under observation takes place

Ethnography can include both qualitative and quantitative approaches. Ethnographic researchers can use both participant and nonparticipant methods, although the participant approach is used more often. When the participant approach is used, researchers collect extensive field notes, conduct open-ended and unstructured interviews, and review and collect documents that are pertinent to the setting (Hall 2007; Savage 2000). Review of certain ethnographic books and articles enable the researcher to better understand how to conduct ethnographic methods.

For example, Dale and colleagues (2016) used ethnographic methods to better understand the oral care practices of healthcare professionals when administering care to patients in intensive care units (ICU) in a large teaching hospital in Canada. Researchers conducted four-hour "go-along" sessions to observe nurses as they were caring for patients and asked them questions during the observations. After one month, semi-structured interviews with the same nurses were conducted to clarify any information that was collected during the longer go-along interviews. Also, other members of the interprofessional team were interviewed to understand the overall picture of oral care in the ICU. Analysis of the data collected was performed in NVivo 9 Software (QRS International), a software program that is used for ethnographic and other qualitative studies for storage, organization, and analysis. Overall, the study identified major obstacles to providing oral care to patients while in the ICU and concluded that more research, education, and training may be needed for healthcare professionals (Dale et al. 2016).

Ethnographic research tends to move in a cycle. Figure 3.6 demonstrates how this occurs. First, the researcher begins by reviewing the literature and developing multiple tentative hypotheses, rather than one that is easily tested. Next, the researcher collects data through field notes, interviews, and documents, and then analyzes and organizes the information. As this occurs, the ethnographic researcher revises tentative hypotheses and creates new ones. Once the new hypotheses are created, the researcher sets out to collect more data to answer questions about them. This cycle continues until the entire culture or organization is known extremely well, and developing hypotheses and research questions are answered. This method of using several different approaches to collect data, answer the research questions, and support the conclusions made is called triangulation.

Figure 3.6 Cycle of ethnographic research

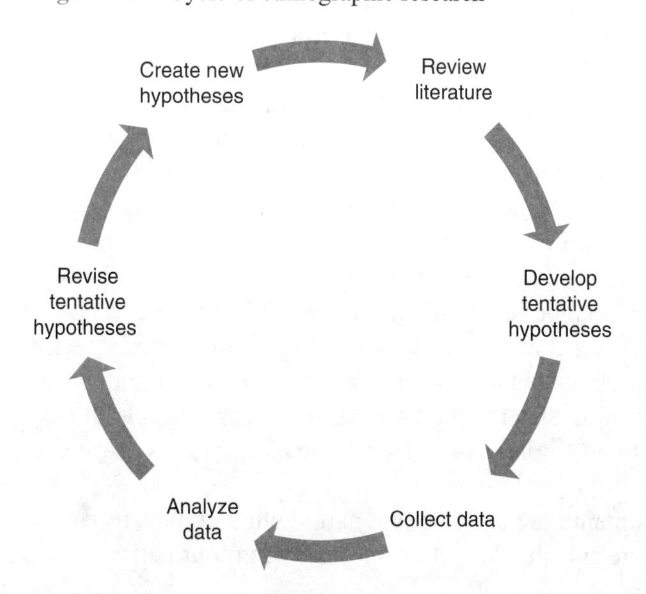

Ethnography was used as the core research method in assessing physicians, patients, and the EHR in four primary care practices in Oregon (Ventres et al. 2006). In 80 hours of participant observation, the researchers observed physicians and patients interacting with the EHR. The investigators examined the physical layout of the office, including the waiting rooms, reception areas, medical assistant stations, exam rooms, and physician work areas, and shadowed patients, medical assistants, and physicians. The researchers asked participants open-ended questions about their experiences and made extensive field notes as well as drawings showing the positions of physicians and patients in relation to the computer in the examination room. Seventy-five open-ended interviews and five focus group interviews (most of which were audiotaped) were conducted with three main groups:

- Professionals with knowledge about the use of EHRs
- Randomly selected patients
- Randomly selected physicians

The focus of the interviews centered on the participants' perspectives of their experiences with the EHR. The researchers videotaped 29 convenience sample clinical encounters to observe physician-patient interactions with EHR use. After each videotaped visit, physicians were interviewed about the impact the EHR has on physician-patient behavior. Individual physicians were also asked to review one videotaped visit that the researchers thought best reflected that physician's clinical behavior in relation to the EHR and write down their thoughts on the major aspects of the visit. Data continued to be collected until the researchers were assured that the observed patterns were valid.

The researchers used several different steps and techniques to analyze the collected data. First, the audiotaped transcripts from the individual and focus group interviews were reviewed independently from the field notes. Prominent themes were highlighted, and descriptive quotations were recorded. The researchers then discussed the themes together, and all members of the research team had to agree on the interpretations. The researchers identified data to confirm or refute the interpretations, and then themes were categorized. The investigators reviewed and discussed videotapes using similar methods used with the audiotape interviews, and all members of the team agreed upon interpretations. Field notes from observations and brief interviews were analyzed; prominent factors were listed; and themes were categorized. A medical anthropologist reviewed all results. Study results were also reviewed by four key participants, and then the researchers assessed their comments and revised the study results based on these comments. The following four themes emerged around the14 factors that were identified regarding how EHR use influenced physician-patient encounters:

- **Spatial or geographical:** How the physical presence of the EHR influenced behavior between physician and patient
- **Relational:** How patients and physicians perceived and used the EHR for each specific clinical visit
- **Educational:** How proficient the physician is in using the EHR and how well the patient understands the use of the EHR for a medical visit
- **Structural:** Institutional and technological forces that influence how the physician perceives their use of the EHR

Examples of factors for each of the themes include the following:

- **Spatial:** Many physicians positioned the monitor so the patient could see it to bring the patient into the interaction rather than the computer pulling the physician away.
- **Relational:** Benefits of use of EHR were context-dependent because some diagnoses (such as upper respiratory infection) could be documented easily using a drop-down menu whereas others (such as depression) needed extensive documentation.
- **Educational:** Patients were uninformed as to how the EHR could benefit them and how it was used in their medical care. These feelings were not expressed to their physicians.
- **Structural:** EHR notes were concise but lacked depth and tended to look similar due to menus and protocols (Ventres et al. 2006).

Content Analysis

Observational methods often result in the collection of large volumes of textual information such as notes, transcribed recordings, and existing documents. The qualitative methods used to analyze all this data to answer research questions and finalize conclusions are quite different than methods used in quantitative research. **Content analysis** is the process of examining all textual data collected and detecting the number of recurrent words or phrases to determine emerging themes and factors reflective of the culture or institution examined. Content analysis can include an array of processes and can be performed with a variety of software. One of the more well-known methods is called the **constant comparative method**, in which researchers compare and refine results as data are mined.

Content analysis was performed in the 2005 AHIMA computer-assisted coding (CAC) fraud and abuse study discussed earlier in this chapter. Table 3.3 summarizes the themes seen from interviews with the federal government, vendors, and users of CAC systems. An antifraud model, shown in table 3.4, was developed to summarize all the data collected and provide methods used to combat fraud in the coding industry.

Table 3.3 Weak links in fraud and abuse software, user education, and compliance practices

Respondent	Software	Education	Compliance
Federal government	✣ Autocoding software may facilitate incidents of fraud. ✣ Access to the data can be inhibited because of the type of software used. For example, if the coding system is proprietary, it may be difficult to obtain access to the data. ✣ Most individuals in crime detection and compliance are not technologically savvy and so they may not be able to deal with the increased technological patterns. ✣ Antifraud software is turned off, ignored, or the issues detected are not addressed—it is a disincentive, if not a deterrent.	✣ There is ignorance of automated coding and technology and fraud. ✣ More education is needed regarding EHRs and how they will work. Further, it is important to know how interoperability will come into play. ✣ It is important to teach law enforcement professionals and investigators how antifraud software will work; the more that investigators understand, the more they will be able to apply their knowledge to ongoing work in the area of concern. ✣ Educate beneficiaries about fraud. As they become more aware, they can help with antifraud activities. Provide education about how to report inaccuracies on the Medicare Summary Notices (MSN) and especially the medication report.	✣ Compliance staff will need to understand automated coding, EHR technology, and how they impact fraud. ✣ More education about EHR is needed so that compliance staff can use appropriate software within the context of interoperability of systems. ✣ There are mechanisms provided in HIPAA to allow beneficiaries to report fraud (Beneficiary Incentive Program from HIPAA, 63FR31123 published June 8, 1998, 42 CFR 420.400).
Vendor	✣ Rules may be inconsistent when audits are conducted because software edits are bypassed or software is not used. ✣ It is difficult to cross-check the accuracy of information from system to system. ✣ Prospective designs may be difficult to conduct because of prompt payment laws. ✣ All vendors require a final evaluation by an experienced or expert coding professional. Coding accuracy of automated coding alone would be problematic. ✣ Much of the software is rules-based or statistics-based; a combination of both is needed to improve accuracy. ✣ Standards are loose and data quality is poor, especially for claim elements that are not tightly linked to payment.	✣ Clinician dictation or documentation can be inaccurate, but coding professionals should be able to confirm whether information is correct. ✣ Fellows and interns lack education on how the language they use can change the code. ✣ Education is lacking for providers, government personnel, payers, and consumers regarding what constitutes fraud and how to detect it. ✣ HIM education on how the coded data interfaces with revenue cycle is also lacking. ✣ Dictation and autocoding systems lack reminders for physicians on what to include in their documentation.	✣ There is tension between the payer and provider communities. ✣ Limited administrative power leads to failure to monitor medical necessity. ✣ Facility compliance is not always done correctly or consistently even though the facility has a compliance officer. ✣ A payer may not have aggregate data evaluation capabilities they can query regarding a claim's accuracy. ✣ There may be a lack of incentives for insurance payers to pursue and eradicate fraud.

(Continued)

Table 3.3 (*Continued*)

Respondent	Software	Education	Compliance
User	❖ Automated coding systems are never 100% accurate. ❖ Users do not know the weaknesses of the automated coding system. ❖ Users do not know if automated coding software improved coding quality. ❖ Users need to have capabilities to cut and paste the documentation and need to change content to show what was documented that day.	❖ Automated coding systems are not used correctly by physicians. ❖ Education and background of coder, if lacking, can make a huge difference in the quality of coded data. ❖ Proficient coders are scarce, which can also impact cost and quality of coded data. ❖ There is reliance on physicians to code without appropriate coding education.	❖ There is an inaccuracy of codes of the automated coding product. ❖ It is difficult to determine if compliance is being performed consistently. ❖ There are no benchmarking standards. ❖ The control of whether a test is necessary, ordered appropriately, or completed as ordered is a much bigger underlying issue than whether software is effective.

Source: Adapted from AHIMA et al. 2005, 50–51.

Table 3.4 Features, processes, and staffing for the ideal antifraud system or model

Features	Processes	Staffing
Automated coding with NLP with a rules-based and statistics-based combination	Prepayment fraud detection using data profiling, advanced analytic models, and rank scoring	Advanced coder analyst to edit and check all processes for accurate code assignment IT staff for maintenance of current technology and health information systems staff to train office staff and physicians
A standardized system of data (based on a representative sample of standardized claims information) for statistical reference Private development of software for code assignment facilitated by the federal government, which may also establish criteria or certification procedures for software	Prepayment fraud detection that uses a standardized method to derive the statistical aspects of code assignment and data analysis	Payer, provider, vendor all working together to combat fraud through education and incentives
ANN (artificial neural network) and predictive modeling to determine where potential for fraud lies	Postpayment fraud detection	Consumer involvement and education
Audit trails		

Source: AHIMA et al. 2005, 52.

Constant Comparative Method

The constant comparative method is used to analyze qualitative data. It is also known as **grounded theory**, which uses both quantitative and qualitative findings (although qualitative findings are used more often) and enables researchers to develop a theory substantiated by data. The constant comparative method seeks to examine what *is* going on instead of what should go on, in the ability to analyze qualitative data. The constant comparative method is made up of four stages:

1. Comparing incidents applicable to each category
2. Integrating categories and their properties
3. Delimiting the theory
4. Writing the theory

The constant comparative method was used by researchers examining patients with colorectal cancer (Tang 2007). Researchers used a semi-structured interview guide to interview respondents about four topic areas:

- **Cancer experiences:** When and how they discovered the cancer and what treatment was received

- **Physical and emotional distress:** Emotional feelings when they were informed of the diagnosis, during treatment, and about the future after treatment
- **Coping strategies:** Ways they coped with the physical discomforts and emotional stress
- **Meaning-searching pathways:** Whether they thought cancer was attributable to possible causes and any positive implications or benefits from cancer experiences, with further probing guided by respondents' answers

The researchers used the constant comparative method and began with open coding of the interviews. All transcripts were read, and words that reflected respondents' ideas and thoughts were labeled. Codes were derived from these words, and codes sharing similar meanings were grouped into categories for further analysis. All information was then connected to the theory or to objectives, which included the following:

- To characterize the disorientation experiences
- To explore the factors that foster the process of sense-making and benefit-finding
- To examine the growth through meaning-searching

Finally, the results and their theoretical insights were organized and published.

Software for Content Analysis

Several different types of software are available to assist the researcher in conducting content analysis; the type of software to select will depend on what types of textual documents will be analyzed. These programs count word frequencies, category frequencies, concordance (each word on the document in alphabetical order), cluster analysis (groups together words used in similar contexts), and co-word citation (the occurrence of pairs of words). However, the software can be expensive and it may not be easy to use without extensive training. The researcher must weigh the risks and benefits to determine whether to use a software program for content analysis (Audience Dialogue 2007).

Review Questions

1. The text states that some observational research may use a combination of methods to fully conduct the study. What are the methods that can be used?
2. What is one health informatics example of each observational research method?
3. What are the different areas a researcher should pay attention to when conducting observational research?
4. What is the difference between direct observation and indirect observation?
5. What is one example of naturalistic observation in health informatics?
6. What is an example of simulation observation in health informatics?
7. What is an example of an individual case study in health informatics?
8. Perform a web search to find an example of an institutional case study other than the one discussed in the chapter. What type of case study is it, and how do you know?
9. Why is the informal conversational interview unique?
10. What is content analysis and how is it used in observational research?

Application Exercises

1. Read the article "Using video-based observation research methods in primary care health encounters to evaluate complex interactions" by Asan and Montague (2014).
   a. Based on the article, what may be the advantages and disadvantages of using video-based observations for research when examining different types of health encounters?
   b. Why might video data introduce more risk of breaching confidentiality than other methods?

c. How might the IRB ask you as a researcher to explain the justification for using video-based observation methods?
2. Read the article "Trust in telemedicine portals for rehabilitation care: An exploratory focus group study with patients and healthcare professionals" by VanVelsen and colleagues (2016), which illustrates the observational method of focus groups to collect data:
   a. How were the focus groups conducted? How many people were in each focus group?
   b. What types of questions were asked?
   c. Do you think this was a good method to use to determine trust in telemedicine portals for rehabilitation care? Explain.
3. Read the article about using NVIVO software for use in qualitative research by Hilal and Alabri (2013):
   a. How is this software used to analyze observational methods research?
   b. How can the software be used in health informatics when doing observational research?
   c. Is it better to use software instead of doing the analysis by hand?

References

American Health Information Management Association (AHIMA), University of Pittsburgh, HHS, and ONC. 2005 (July 11). Automated Coding Software: Development and Use to Enhance Anti-Fraud Activities. HHS Contract Number: HHSP23320054100EC. http://bok.ahima.org/PdfView?oid=65240.

Audience Dialogue. 2007. Software for Content Analysis. http://www.audiencedialogue. org/soft-cont.html.

Dale, C., J. Angus, T. Sinuff, and L. Rose. 2016. Ethnographic investigation of oral care in the intensive care unit. *American Journal of Critical Care* 25:249–256. doi: 10.4037/ajcc2016795.

Farre, A. and C. Cummins. 2016. Understanding and evaluating the effects of implementing an electronic paediatric prescribing system on care provision and hospital work in paediatric hospital ward settings: A qualitatively driven mixed-method study protocol. *BMJ* 6(2):e010444. doi: 10.1136/bmjopen-2015-010444.

Giacomini, M., and D.J. Cook. 2000. A User's Guide to Qualitative Research in Health Care. Evidence Based Medicine Informatics Project, Centre for Health Evidence. http://jamaevidence.mhmedical.com/Book.aspx?bookId=847.

Goodson, L. and M. Vassar. 2011. An overview of ethnography in healthcare and medical education research. *Journal of educational evaluation for health professions* 8(4):1–5. http://www.jeehp.org/upload/jeehp-8-4.pdf.

Hackett, S. 2007. "An Exploration into Two Solutions to Propagating Web Accessibility for Blind Computer Users." PhD diss. Pittsburgh, PA: University of Pittsburgh.

Hall, B. 2007. How to Do Ethnographic Research: A Simplified Guide. https://docs.google.com/presentation/d/1lGXCn2FStoWuCEQOTq2OU9H3aWA6JBQ45-W25J3TLhI/edit?authkey=CIW_h_0K#slide=id.i0.

Hallström, I., G. Elander, and L. Rooke. 2000. Pain and nutrition as experienced by patients with hip fracture. *Journal of Clinical Nursing* 9(4):639–646.

Hofler, L.D., J. Hardee, D. Burleson, and J. Grady. 2005. HIPAA audit and system activity review: Developing a process that focuses on the greatest risks first. *Journal of American Health Information Management Association* 76(3):34–38.

Kanaar, A.C., and M.W. Hecht. 1991. Marathon swim training in a 74-yr-old man: Personal experience. *Medicine and Science in Sports and Exercise* 24(4):490–494.

Savage, J. 2000. Ethnography and health care. *BMJ* 321:1400–1402.

Self, D.J., M. Olivarez, and C.B. DeWitt. 1998. The amount of small-group case study discussion needed to improve moral reasoning skills of medical students. *Academic Medicine* 73(5)521–523.

Shea, D. 2007. Use of the electronic record in the home-based primary care programs at the Veterans Affairs Health Care System. *Journal for the Home Care and Hospice Professional* 25 (5):323–326.

Sheridan, P.T., V. Watzlaf, and L. Fox, L. 2016 (Spring). Health information management leaders and the practice of leadership through the lens of Bowen theory. *Perspectives in Health Information Management*. 1–36. http://perspectives.ahima.org/health-information-management-leaders-and-the-practice-of-leadership-through-the-lens-of-bowen-theory.

Shi, L. 1997. Health Services Research Methods. Chapter 6 in *Qualitative Research.* Albany, NY: Delmar Publishers: 125–141.

Sussman, S., J. Allem, J. Garcia, J. Unger, T. Cruz, R. Garcia, R., and L. Baezconde-Garbanati. 2016. Who walks into vape shops in southern California? A naturalistic observation of customers. *Tobacco Induced Diseases.* 14:18. doi: 10.1186/s12971-016-0082-y.

Tang, V.Y., A. Lee, C. Chan, P. Leung, J. Sham, J. Ho, and J. Cheng. 2007. Disorientation and reconstruction: The meaning of searching pathways of patients with colorectal cancer. *Journal of Psychosocial Oncology* 25(2):77–102.

Thompson, B.M., V.F. Schneider, P. Haidet, R. Levine, K. McMahon, L. Perkowski, and B. Richards. 2007. Team-based learning at ten medical schools: Two years later. *Medical Education* 41:250–257.

Ventres, W., S. Kooienga, N. Vuckovic, R. Marlin, P. Nygren, and V. Stewart. 2006. Physicians, patients, and the electronic health record: An ethnographic analysis. *Annals of Family Medicine* 4(2):124–131.

Waibel, S., I. Vargas, M. Aller, R. Gusmao, D. Henao, and M. Vazquez. 2015. The performance of integrated health care networks in continuity of care: A qualitative multiple case study of COPD patients. *International Journal of Integrated Care.* 15:e029. https://www.ncbi.nlm.nih.gov/pmc/articles/PMC4512888.

Watzlaf, V.J., J. Garvin, S. Moeini, and P. Firouzan. 2007. The effectiveness of ICD-10-CM in capturing public health diseases. *Perspectives in Health Information Management* 4(6):1–31. http://perspectives.ahima.org/the-effectiveness-of-icd-10-cm-in-capturing-public-health-diseases/.

Resources

Asan, O. and E. Montague. 2014. Using video-based observation research methods in primary care health encounters to evaluate complex interactions. *Informatics in Primary Care.* 21(4): 161–170. doi:10.14236/jhi.v21i4.72. https://www.ncbi.nlm.nih.gov/pmc/articles/PMC4350928/pdf/nihms663130.pdf.

Glaser, B. 1965. The constant comparative method of qualitative analysis. *Social Problems* 12(4):436–445.

Hilal, A.H. and S.S. Alabri. 2013. Using NVIVO for data analysis in qualitative research. *International Interdisciplinary Journal of Education* 2(2).

Van Velsen, L., S. Wildevuur, I. Flierman, B. Van Schooten, M. Tabak, and H. Hermens. 2016. Trust in telemedicine portals for rehabilitation care: an exploratory focus group study with patients and healthcare professionals. *BMC Medical Informatics and Decision Making* 16:11. doi: 10.1186/s12911-016-0250-2.

4 Experimental and Quasi-Experimental Research

Valerie J. Watzlaf, PhD, MPH, RHIA, FAHIMA

Learning Objectives

- Differentiate between experimental and quasi-experimental research types and methodologies and decide when each should be used in health informatics.
- Distinguish between the pretest-posttest control group method and the Solomon four-group method and how they are used in health informatics.
- Explain when the posttest-only control group method should be used.
- Provide examples of when to use the one-shot case study.
- Demonstrate when to use the one-group pretest-posttest method and when to use the static group comparison method.

Key Terms

Attrition
Comparison group
Crossover design
Experimental procedures
External validity
History
Instrumentation
Interaction of factors
Internal validity
Intervention
Maturation
Midtests
Nonrandom selection
One-group pretest-posttest method
One-shot case study
Posttest-only control group method
Pretest-posttest control group method
Solomon four-group method
Static group comparison method
Statistical regression
Testing
Time-series tests

Experimental study designs, which were first discussed in chapter 1, are one of the most powerful designs to use when trying to establish cause and effect; however, in cases when conducting an experimental study would be unethical, prospective and even retrospective studies can show a causal relationship. They can be used when exploring the use of new treatment modalities, such as providing a placebo to one group of subjects and an experimental medicine to another, or when comparing two or more things, such as two different types of EHR systems and their impact on patient outcomes, or when validating a theoretical result or concept, such as testing health information exchange systems that have been described but not implemented. Experimental research study designs expose participants to different interventions to compare the result of these interventions with the outcome.

The **intervention** is the independent variable (factor you wish to measure), that is manipulated to determine its effect on the dependent variable (outcome under study). Examples of interventions are medications, diet, exercise, education, or health information systems. Examples of dependent variables include survival time for patients with cancer, frequency of pressure sores in patients using wheelchairs, and the number of adverse events in healthcare facilities that use a computerized provider order entry system (CPOE). Experimental research can involve multiple experiments to determine how much the independent variable affects the dependent variable. For example, if an experiment finds that a specific dose of medication slows the progression of cancer, the next experiment might test whether a higher dose is more effective. These types of medication experiments establish a dose-response relationship.

Internal validity is an attribute of a research study design that contributes to the accuracy of its findings and can be threatened by factors or influences outside the study, such as confounding variables. **External validity** is the extent to which a research study's findings can be generalized to the broader population, people, or groups. Researchers sometimes find that if they remove a specific variable from the environment, it decreases the incidence of certain outcomes. For example, if radon is removed from homes, or if the radon level is decreased substantially, researchers may find that the incidence of lung cancer decreases (EPA 2016). However, it is sometimes difficult for the researcher to prove that the specific independent variable caused the dependent variable without any interference from other factors or events. This is one example of problems with internal validity and there are certain things the experimental researcher can do to reduce the amount of internal validity problems.

Quasi-experimental research, defined in chapter 1, is similar to experimental research and is also effective at establishing cause and effect. Quasi-experimental research does not include randomization of participants. The independent variable may not be manipulated by the researcher, and there may be no control group (Barnes et al. 2012, 3). For example, a researcher may study the effects of an automated coding system on the quality of clinical coding to determine whether there is a difference in reimbursement to the hospital before and after the system is implemented. Health informatics researchers use quasi-experimental research designs more often than experimental research designs. The quasi-experimental design tends to be more common for many reasons, including the challenges of randomization and control groups as well as ethical concerns related to, for example, withholding a particular health information system from a specific group of patients. However, an experimental design can be used in some situations. For example, different types of educational interventions for personal health record (PHR) use can be randomly assigned to a group of subjects (in this case, one group of subjects receives an instructional video, one group of subjects receives classroom instruction, and one group of subjects receives a pamphlet) to determine if there are improvements in their use of the PHR (dependent variable). An experimental design may be appropriate because withholding a specific educational intervention is not considered to cause harm.

Several examples of experimental and quasi-experimental studies and the methodology used in the health informatics and healthcare setting demonstrate that these study designs can be viable options for health informatics research.

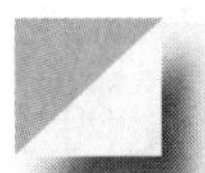

Real-World Case

The US National Institutes of Health (NIH) provides a service called ClinicalTrials.gov, a website that documents clinical trials (a type of experimental research study) that are recruiting participants, are being conducted, or have been completed. One example is the "Trial Study of an Exercise Program for Youth with Persistent Symptoms After Concussion." The purpose of this randomized controlled trial (RCT), which was recruiting participants as this book was being written, is to determine whether low-intensity exercise plus the standard level of care is better than standard care alone in reducing postconcussion symptoms such as headaches, dizziness, and memory issues and improving participation in daily activities in youth who have persistent postconcussion symptoms (Holland Bloorview Kids Rehabilitation Hospital 2016).

Elements of Experimental Research Study Design

When conducting experimental research, several important elements should be addressed and described. These elements include randomization, crossover design, observation, control group, and treatment.

Randomization

Randomization means study participants or groups of participants are randomly assigned to a type of intervention or no intervention. The intervention group is called the experimental group, and the group with no intervention is called the control group. Sometimes, **comparison groups** are used when a different intervention is used as a comparison for the intervention being investigated. For example, a researcher may be interested in determining whether individuals retain more new knowledge if they do high-intensity exercise before they learn how to use the PHR. To test this, three different groups of participants might be established. The first group (experimental group) would run for 30 minutes before sitting in front of the computer to learn to use their PHR, the second group (comparison group) would walk for 30 minutes before learning to use the PHR, and the third group (control group) would not do any type of exercise before learning to use the PHR. Randomization would need to be employed for this study. Randomization (which is *not* the same as random sampling) is when a group of participants are randomly chosen to be in the experimental, control, or comparison group using a random method, such as probability sampling, so that each participant has an equal chance of being selected for each of the groups. Randomization can be done by developing a list of all the study participants, numbering them, and putting all their numbers in a hat. Each of the numbers are picked out and allocated to a group. For example, the first number drawn will go into the experimental group, the second number to the control group, the third number to the comparison group, and so forth until all the numbers are drawn and participants allocated. The goal is for the experimental, control, and comparison groups to be as similar as possible except for the intervention being studied. Randomization techniques can also be performed using statistical software.

In studies where it may be unethical to withhold a certain intervention from one group of participants, two comparison groups may be used instead of an experimental group and a control group. In this way, the intervention under study is used, but all members of the study are receiving some type of intervention. For example, if researchers want to assess the effect of using health information exchange (HIE) to decrease the incidence of nosocomial infections in nursing facilities in a region, they could decide that some of the nursing facilities will be randomly allocated to use the HIE-based data, and some of the nursing facilities will be randomly allocated to use some other type of database to minimize the unethical consequences of not providing any type of data to some of the residents.

Crossover Design

A **crossover design** uses two groups of participants as both the experimental and control group. It also can be used to minimize some of the more difficult aspects of experimental designs, such as providing the interventions to both groups and being able to easily provide for control groups. It works as shown in figure 4.1 by having two groups of participants start out with random assignment to one of the intervention groups and receive the intervention assigned to that group for a period of time, such as six months or one year. If a study intervention involves a medication, for example, there is an intermediate "wash out" period for the intervention to leave the subjects' system before they switch with the other group and receive a different (comparison) intervention or no intervention for another six months to one year.

The crossover design may be used, for example, when studying whether certain types of telerehabilitation improve the outcomes of patients with multiple sclerosis (MS). Two groups of patients with MS may start out with one group using telerehabilitation and a mobile app for recording and collecting their functional levels (Intervention A) and another group using the traditional face-to-face in-house therapy monitoring (Intervention B). At a later point, the groups cross over so that the one using Intervention A now uses Intervention B and vice versa. The same group is used as the comparison group and the experimental group, but the researcher must be careful with this design because the use of one group for both the intervention and the comparison may bias the results, especially if the wash out period is called for but not conducted or is not long enough.

Figure 4.1 Crossover design for experimental studies

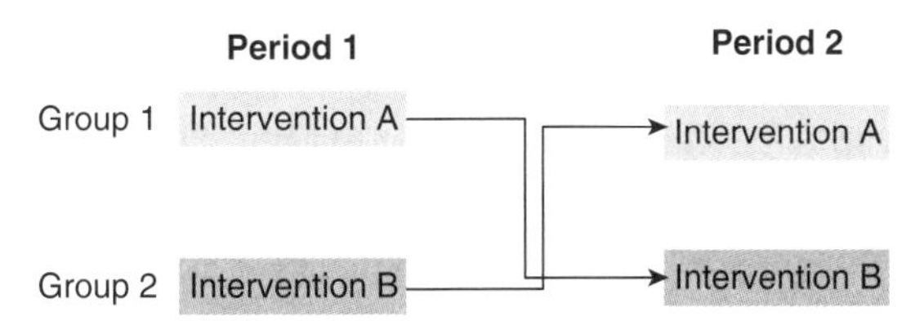

Observation

Observation, or pretest and posttest, includes monitoring the experimental and control groups before (pretest) or after (posttest) the intervention. Although the terms *pretest* and *posttest* are used to describe the observations before and after the intervention, the observations may not always include an actual test. For example, the observation could measure blood pressure before and after the administration of a certain medication, exercise, or diet, or a questionnaire might be used to determine levels of depression before and after a medication intervention.

Observations that are administered at the midpoint of a study are called **midtests**. In some studies, observations called **time-series tests** may be conducted at intervals throughout the study period. For example, a researcher might use the time-series test to examine the number of breaches of confidentiality after the implementation of the Health Insurance Portability and Accountability Act (HIPAA). These rates could be compared to each other over time and to rates before HIPAA was implemented. Other follow-up tests might be conducted several months or years after the intervention ends to determine its long-term impact.

When pretests and posttests are used in education-related intervention studies, the same pretest and posttest is usually administered so that the researcher can determine whether the study participants improved their performance after the intervention. However, using the same test may bias the results because some participants may remember the questions when responding the second time. Researchers can control for this bias by adding a group that takes just the posttest. The Solomon four-group method employs this design. Bias is addressed in more detail in the discussion of internal and external validity issues in experimental and quasi-experimental research, later in this chapter.

Control Group

The control group is the group of individuals who will not receive the intervention or who will receive an alternative intervention. Use of a control group may enable the researcher to determine whether an outcome can be attributed to the intervention and not extraneous factors or confounding variables. Sometimes, especially in clinical trials when medication is being tested as the intervention, the participants in the control group are given a placebo so that their treatment is as similar as possible to how the participants in the intervention group are treated.

Treatment

In experimental and quasi-experimental research, *treatment* and *intervention* are synonyms. Treatments or interventions are also the independent variable in these study designs. They may include a variety of different components, depending on what the researcher wants to test in the study. For example, treatments or interventions may include use of medications; changes in an individual's behavior, such as smoking or alcohol cessation; or changes in a particular assistive device, technology, software, or system. Whatever treatment is administered, it must be administered in the same way for all participants in the experimental group. For example, if physical therapists are going to be educated and trained online in using a new rehabilitation electronic health record (EHR) system, the hours of training, content of the education and training, and amount of time using the EHR system should be the same for all physical therapists in the experimental group. The control group may consist of physical therapists who will receive traditional in-class education and training. The hypothesis could be that the physical therapists trained online will demonstrate a skill level in using the EHR that is equal to or better than the skill level of those trained using the in-class method.

Types of Experimental Study Designs

The most common experimental study designs as described by Campbell and Stanley (1963) include the pretest-posttest control group method, Solomon four-group method, and posttest-only control group method. Experiments that use the **pretest-posttest control group method** (a classic experimental design) randomly assign participants to either the intervention (experimental) or a nonintervention (control) group. (Note that "nonintervention" does not necessarily mean "no intervention"; in some experiments, participants assigned to the control group may receive an intervention other than the one under study.) Pretests are given to both groups at the same time to assess the groups' similarities and differences. Posttests are given to both groups after the intervention to determine its effects. The **Solomon four-group method** is similar to the pretest-posttest design but includes two intervention or experimental groups and two control groups. Pretests are used for one of the intervention groups and one of the control groups. Posttests are used for all groups. In other words, the first experimental group receives the pretest, the intervention, and the posttest: the first control group receives the pretest, does not receive the intervention, and is given the posttest; the second experimental group receives the intervention and the posttest; and the second control group does not receive the intervention and is given the posttest. The extra groups are included to neutralize the effect of the pretest, which may influence the responses of recipients on the posttest.

The posttest-only control group method is similar to the pretest-posttest control group method except that the posttest-only method does not use a pretest (Campbell and Stanley 1963). Randomization, which is the random assignment of participants to the intervention or control group, is used in all of these experimental study designs (Shi 2009). Randomization is vital in experimental research because it is the most reliable method used to provide equality of treatment groups which lessens judgment or bias in the final study results. Each of these designs will be described in more detail in the following sections. Table 4.1 provides a brief summary of each experimental study design.

Table 4.1 Summary of experimental research designs
Key: R = randomization O = observation X = intervention

Study Design	Characteristics	Diagram
Pretest-posttest control group method	• Participants are randomly assigned to intervention or nonintervention (control) group. • Pretests given to both groups. • Posttests given to both groups after intervention.	Treatment: R---O---X---O Control: R---O--- ---O
Solomon four-group method	• Participants are randomly assigned to one of two intervention groups or one of two control groups. • One intervention group and one control group are administered the pretest. • Same intervention is used in both experimental groups. • Posttest is used in all four groups.	Treatment: R---O---X---O Control: R---O--- ---O Treatment: R--- ---X---O Control: R--- --- ---O
Posttest-only control group method	• Participants are randomly assigned to intervention or nonintervention (control) group. • No pretest is given. • Posttest is given to both groups.	Treatment: R--- ---X---O Control: R--- --- ---O

Pretest-Posttest Control Group Method

The pretest-posttest control group method is often used in the RCT or clinical trial discussed in chapter 5. The pretest-posttest control group method has excellent internal validity because participants are randomly assigned to intervention groups, and control or comparison groups are also used. The external validity or generalizability of the results may be affected somewhat by the pretesting in some instances.

An experimental pretest-posttest control group design was used to assess a smartphone mobile application that provided personalized, real-time advice about sun protection to adults ages 18 years and older who owned an Android smartphone (Buller et al. 2015). The mobile app, called Solar Cell, provided advice and visual and audible alerts about sun protection—including when to apply sunscreen or get out of the sun—hourly UV index forecasts and the amount of vitamin D produced by the skin based on the forecasted UV index, phone's time and location, and user input. The authors hypothesized that providing personalized information to adults through a mobile app when they are in the sun, based on time and location from the phone as well as user input, may help reduce sun exposure. The study included 454 non-Hispanic and Hispanic white adults recruited from a survey panel that represents the US adult population. Participants were randomly assigned to either the intervention or control group. Those in the intervention group completed a pretest survey, used the mobile app and received information when in the sun, and then completed a posttest survey. Those in the control group received no intervention but completed a pretest and posttest survey.

Results of the study indicate that the Solar Cell app provided some assistance in sun protection but not as much as the researchers anticipated. However, the researchers concluded that the Solar Cell app may help individuals with high-risk skin types and those who spend a great deal of time outdoors to make appropriate prevention decisions that reduce their exposure to the sun.

Another example of an experimental pretest-posttest control group method was conducted by researchers trying to improve the outcomes of older adults with Type 2 diabetes mellitus (Miller et al. 2002). In this study, an information processing model was used to teach older adults how to better manage their diabetes. Several theories and models of knowledge acquisition were used as a framework during the intervention to teach participants how to evaluate nutrition information on food labels when purchasing food for meal planning and preparation. Major instructional parts of the intervention included an overview of nutrition concepts that were discussed at the beginning and summarized at the end of each instructional session; having participants apply knowledge of food labels and carbohydrate counting methods; and having participants assess their current eating patterns, monitor their food intake, and write their weekly goals. All participants received an examination to assess their cognitive ability. Researchers collected data related to their medical and diet history. Participants were then randomly allocated to the intervention or control group. The intervention included 10 weekly group educational sessions lasting ninety minutes to two hours. Those in the control group did not have any further contact with the researchers until the posttest data were collected. Blood tests were given at pretest and posttest to determine cholesterol, triglyceride, glucose, and hemoglobin levels. Results showed that the fasting glucose and hemoglobin levels of the experimental group showed statistically significant improvement over those in the control group ($P = 0.005$). Also, the total cholesterol values at posttest for the experimental group were closer to their treatment goals than those in the control group ($P < 0.05$).

Solomon Four-Group Method

The Solomon four-group design may be modified to use three groups instead of four. For example, researchers used an adaptation of the Solomon four-group design to evaluate the effectiveness of a multimedia tutorial to teach dental students to recognize and respond to domestic violence (Danley et al. 2004). The tutorial was developed based on an approach that includes asking, validating, documenting, and referring (AVDR). *Asking* refers to asking the patient about abuse; *validating* refers to providing support to the patient that abuse is wrong while still verifying the patient's self-worth; *documenting* refers to including notes and photos of the potential signs and symptoms of abuse in the dental record; and *referring* includes making sure patients are properly referred to domestic violence experts. The participants were randomly assigned to one of three groups. The first experimental group of dental students took the pretest, were given the tutorial (intervention), and then took a posttest. The second experimental group were given the tutorial and then took the posttest. The third group (control group) took the pretest and the posttest. The control group received the tutorial after the posttest so they could learn its useful information, but that had no effect on the experiment's results. The researchers did not use a fourth group (posttest only with no pretest and no tutorial) because the authors believed the addition would not serve any purpose in the study. The tutorial is 15 minutes long and shows interaction between a dentist and a patient who shows signs of domestic abuse during her dental visit. The tutorial works through the four stages of AVDR in referring to the specific patient example. The pre and posttests were developed by the researchers and included 24 online questions related to the AVDR approach. For example, a question under the documentation section included: "If I identified a patient as being abused, I would document the abuse in the patient's chart. How much do you believe you know about how to document abuse in the dental chart?" Items were scored on a Likert scale.

The pretest and posttest had the same questions but in a different order. Results showed that of the 161 dental students and 13 dentists that completed the study, those in the experimental groups who used the tutorial had significantly higher mean scores than those in the control group on most of the test items.

In another example, researchers used the Solomon four-group design to assess whether an e-learning curriculum improved medical knowledge, measured by posttests and in-training exam scores, among pediatric residents and students at pediatric emergency medicine rotations (Chang et al. 2014). Here, researchers randomly assigned 458 residents and fourth year medical students from four large pediatric care centers from across the US to one of the following four groups:

- Pretest–e-learning modules–posttest (experimental group 1)
- Pretest-posttest (control group 1)
- e-Learning modules–posttest (experimental group 2)
- Posttest only (control group 2)

The pretest and posttest included 27 multiple-choice questions that were developed, tested and retested by pediatric medicine residents, fellows and attending physicians. Results showed that the e-learning modules were effective in improving the medical knowledge of pediatric residents and fourth year medical students across multiple pediatric institutions. E-learning modules raised the mean posttest scores from 18.45 to 21.30 ($P < 0.0001$) across all groups.

Posttest-Only Control Group Method

The experimental posttest only control group design randomly assigns participants to an experimental group or a control group, and posttests are the only means of observation. Pretests are not used to reduce the effect of familiarity that comes with exposure to a pretest. By eliminating the pretest, the researcher reduces the amount of recall that may influence responses on the posttest. However, not using a pretest eliminates the ability to assess an improvement in test or observation scores from before the intervention to after the intervention. Therefore, only an evaluation of current utilization of the effectiveness of the intervention can be assessed.

Researchers used the experimental posttest-only control group method to study the effect of community nursing support on patients with schizophrenia (Beebe 2001). Twenty-four participants were randomly assigned to the control group (routine follow-up care and informational telephone contact with clinical staff at 6 and 12 weeks) and 24 participants were randomly assigned to the experimental group (weekly telephone intervention plus routine follow-up care provided by clinical staff for three months). All participants were followed for three months after hospital discharge to determine the length of survival in the community setting (that is, the number of days in the community before rehospitalization or until the end of study) as well as frequency and length of stay for rehospitalizations. Fifteen participants from the experimental group and 22 from the control group fully completed the intervention and follow-up phase. The treatment intervention consisted of a 10-minute telephone call from clinical staff with questions such as "Are you having problems with your medication?" or "Did you have any follow-up appointments scheduled this week? How did that go?" Also, the researchers asked participants about specific symptoms related to their illness based on review of their medical records from previous hospitalizations. Control participants received a 1-to-3-minute phone call to collect data on any hospitalizations at any point in the past. If readmissions were found through the phone calls, medical records were reviewed for length of stay data. This phone call was provided only twice during the study, at 6 and 12 weeks. Outcome measures included the following:

- Duration of community survival, in days
- Duration of rehospitalizations, in days
- Frequency of rehospitalizations: Number of admissions to inpatient psychiatric units

Other confounding variables also were collected, such as demographic characteristics, symptoms leading to hospitalization, alternative care sought before hospitalization, and so forth. Confounding variables are discussed further in chapters 1 and 5.

Results showed that, overall, the experimental participants survived in the community longer than the control participants. When readmissions occurred, the duration of hospitalization was 27 percent shorter in the experimental group compared to the control group.

Another example of the experimental posttest only control group method was conducted in hospitals and healthcare centers in Greece (Saounatsou et al. 2001). Researchers evaluated whether hypertensive patients improve in their compliance with medication and overall self-care when given direct education from public health nurses. The study randomly assigned 20 hypertensive patients to the intervention group and 20 to a control group. The intervention group received education from a public health nurse through four to five individual visits and phone contacts twice per week, with nurse emphasizing the importance of compliance with medications and the risks of not taking medications as prescribed. The control group did not receive the educational contacts from the public health nurse, but after the study they did receive educational instructional kits regarding compliance. The dependent variable (outcome measure) was compliance and was measured on a 5-point Likert scale ranging from 1 = noncompliant to 5 = full compliance. Compliance was based on the number of medication doses taken as prescribed per month. For example, if patients took between 21 to 30 doses in one month, they would be considered in poor compliance, whereas if patients took 51 to 60 doses in one month, they would be in full compliance. The results support the hypothesis of the study in that hypertensive individuals who are educated about the importance of their medication will show improved compliance with their medication use compared to those who do not receive this education.

Types of Quasi-Experimental Study Designs

Common quasi-experimental study designs as described by Campbell and Stanley include the one-shot case study, one-group pretest-posttest method, and the static group comparison method. The **one-shot case study** is a simple design in which an intervention is provided to one group and they are followed forward in time after intervention to assess the outcome (posttest). The **one-group pretest-posttest method** is similar to the one-shot case study except that the pretest is used before the intervention. The **static group comparison method** is when two groups are examined; one with the intervention and one without, and then a posttest is given to assess the result of the intervention (Campbell and Stanley 1963) Randomization is not used in any of the quasi-experimental study designs, and most of the quasi-experimental designs are used on units or groups, so randomization can be quite difficult to execute (Shi 2009). Each of these designs will be described in more detail in the following sections. Table 4.2 provides a brief summary of each quasi-experimental study design. When reviewing study designs, it is important to recognize that, even though a researcher may categorize the study design into one of the methods discussed here, they may add certain attributes to the study design, such as an additional control group or pretest.

Table 4.2 Summary of quasi-experimental research designs
Key: O = observation X = intervention

Study Design	Characteristics	Diagram
One-shot case study	❖ Simple design ❖ One group ❖ Intervention ❖ Posttest	Treatment: ---X---O
One-group pretest-posttest method	❖ One group ❖ Pretest ❖ Intervention ❖ Posttest	Treatment: O---X---O
Static group comparison method	❖ Two groups ❖ Intervention ❖ No intervention ❖ Posttest for both groups	Treatment: ---X---O Control: --- ---O

One-Shot Case Study

In the quasi-experimental one-shot case study, researchers are able to see if a specific group responds to a specific intervention and assess the outcome. However, no randomization, no control group, and no pretest are included; therefore, there is no baseline measurement to provide a comparison to the intervention outcome. Therefore, although the results may be used to provide hypotheses that may enable research to move on to conducting experimental studies, they should not be generalizable to other populations (external validity) nor should their study methods be considered accurate (internal validity).

Researchers conducted a quasi-experimental one-shot case study to determine whether an automated two-way messaging system can help patients with human immunodeficiency virus (HIV) comply with complex medication treatments (Dunbar et al. 2003). The study followed 19 HIV-positive patients who were provided with two-way pagers that included reminders to take all medication doses (for example, “Good morning, JT, time for your indinavir”) and follow any dietary requirements. Additional messages provided information on the importance of medication compliance, adverse effects, sleeping patterns, mood, any stressful events, drug use, and any difficulties with the messaging system. Messages also include questions, such as “Any problems with your medications over the weekend?” Respondents then received various possible responses, such as “Took all but not all on time.” There was no control group in this study design, and outcome measures were the number of times participants reported missing one or more medication doses or reported medication side effects. Other outcome variables included the participants’ satisfaction level in using the messaging system. Overall results showed that participants had favorable opinions of the two-way messaging system and thought that it did help them with medication compliance (Dunbar et al. 2003).

One-Group Pretest-Posttest Method

The limitation of the one-group pretest-posttest study design is that there is no control group and no randomization. However, the quasi-experimental one-group pretest-posttest method can be used when it would be unethical or inappropriate to withhold the intervention from a group of participants.

Researchers assessed the timeliness of care and access to healthcare services using telemedicine in individuals ages 18 years and younger in state correctional facilities (Fox et al. 2007). Data were collected one year before implementation of a telemedicine program and two years after implementation. The telemedicine intervention consisted primarily of remote delivery of behavioral healthcare services as well as other types of care. Timeliness of care and use of healthcare services before and after telemedicine implementation were examined. The timeliness of care was measured by examining the time from referral to date of service at a behavioral healthcare facility. Healthcare use was measured by recording the number of outpatient, emergency, and inpatient visits per month per person. The data were collected primarily from medical records, other claims, and information assessment logs. Results showed that the average wait time from referral to date of service decreased by 50 percent after one year of implementation of telemedicine and by 59 percent after two years of implementation. Outpatient visits increased by 40 percent after implementation of telemedicine. However, some healthcare facilities did not show significant improvements in the number of outpatient visits; researchers thought that this was due to difficulty in implementing the telemedicine program (Fox et al. 2007).

In another example of a study using the quasi-experimental one-group pretest-posttest method, researchers examined clinicians' responses to computerized detection of nosocomial infections (Rocha et al. 2001). An expert reminder system, Computerized Pediatric Infection Surveillance System (COMPISS), was provided to clinicians, and a pretest and posttest observation was done before and after implementation of the system. COMPISS is a rules-based system used to generate alerts and reminders that are divided into three areas: educational, managerial, and therapeutic. An educational reminder may advise the clinician to notify infection control about a reportable disease, whereas the managerial reminder may relate to medical management of the infection (other than appropriate medication), such as use of an isolation room. Therapeutic reminders include suggestions about what medications should be prescribed to patients. COMPISS was implemented in three units within the hospital setting, and all clinicians were trained on its use. The number of suggestions to treat and manage infections before and after use of COMPISS made up the outcome measures for this study. No statistically significant findings between infection treatment recommendations before and after use of COMPISS were found. The authors noted that this finding might be attributed to a lack of documentation in the health record to show that the clinician had followed the reminders (Rocha et al. 2001).

Static Group Comparison

In the static group comparison method, subjects are not randomly assigned to groups, but a control group is used. Most static group comparison methods do not use a pretest.

An example of the static group comparison design can be found when researchers assessed the perceived use of alcohol in patients after a traumatic brain injury (TBI) based on patients' and relatives' reports (Sander et al. 1997). This study examined the validity of patients' reports of their alcohol use by comparing those reports to descriptions of the patients' post-injury alcohol use from relatives. In this design, researchers used the TBI as the intervention and then assessed, via a post-injury questionnaire, whether drinking habits as perceived by the patient with the TBI and the close relative were similar or different. Results showed that a high rate of agreement was found between the 175 patients and their relatives for each of the alcohol use measures. Lesser rates of agreement were found for those with more severe TBIs (Sander et al. 1997).

In another study, the static group comparison method was adapted to investigate whether cooperative learning (small-group learning) techniques with case studies positively affect nursing students' problem-solving and decision-making skills when compared to other learning techniques (Baumberger-Henry 2005). This study divided a convenience sample of 123 students into one experimental group and three comparison groups, with no randomization of group assignments. The experimental group was taught using cooperative learning methods and a case study. The first comparison group was taught by lecture and a large-group case study; the second comparison group was taught by lecture only; and the third comparison group was taught by lecture and a case study, and was used as the posttest only control group. In the experimental group and the first two comparison groups, two instruments were used to assess self-perception of problem-solving inventory (PSI) and clinical decision making in nursing scale (CDMNS) skills before and after the different teaching interventions, at the beginning and end of the semester. The third comparison group was tested only at the end of the semester (posttest only). Both the PSI and CDMNS instruments had Cronbach's alpha ranging from 0.82 to 0.88. Results showed that no significant differences were found across the groups, suggesting that the different teaching methods had no effect on the self-perceptions of problem-solving and decision-making skills in nursing students (Baumberger-Henry 2005).

Internal and External Validity

A research study is internally valid if it demonstrates that the dependent variable (outcome measure) is only caused by the independent variable (intervention) rather than by other confounding variables. External validity means the findings of a research study can be generalized to populations other than the participants in the study (Campbell and Stanley 1963). The factors that affect an experimental or quasi-experimental study's internal or external validity will be discussed in the sections that follow.

Factors Affecting Internal Validity

Several factors can play a part in whether a study has internal validity, including history, maturation, testing, instrumentation, statistical regression, nonrandom selection, attrition, and interaction of factors.

History

History, or the events happening in the course of the experiment, can potentially impact the results. For example, a researcher collects data about the level of functioning in hip-replacement patients before and after the use of a new physical therapy device. During the time that this device is being used, the developer becomes ill and is unable to fully train all physical therapists in its proper use. Therefore, the study may be affected by inadequate time in training rather than the device itself (Key 2002; Shi 2009).

Maturation

Maturation refers to the natural changes of research subjects that occur during the length of time that they are in the study. For example, older individuals may become very fatigued after completing a training session on using a computer to manage their finances. Their fatigue could then affect their responses on the posttest, which means that test would not accurately measure the effect of the independent variable (the training session) and therefore the study's internal validity would be compromised (Key 2002; Shi 2009).

Testing

As related to internal validity, **testing** refers to the effect created when participants are exposed in the pretest to questions that may be on the posttest. For example, researchers give a pretest and a posttest to participants of a study to assess whether a course module on the use of privacy and security within the EHR improves their knowledge of this subject. However, the students taking the posttest have already been exposed to the pretest and may recall some of the test questions; if they do, their answers on the posttest may be influenced by their experience with the pretest. Therefore, the researchers cannot tell whether the use of the pretest or the course module on privacy and security of the EHR has caused test scores to change in the posttest (Key 2002; Shi 2009).

Instrumentation

Variations in **instrumentation**, which includes how a particular survey, interview, procedure or intervention may be performed, also may affect internal validity. Changes in instruments, interviewers, or observers all may affect a study's results. For example, a study using multiple interviewers may get different sorts of answers from participants if the interviewers are not consistently trained how to ask questions and some ask more probing questions than others (Key 2002; Shi 2009).

Statistical Regression

Statistical regression (regression toward the mean) can affect the internal validity of a study when extreme values (outliers) unduly affect the calculation of the mean. For example, coding professionals who performed inadequately on an ICD-10-CM coding examination are selected to receive training. The mean of their posttest scores could be higher than their pretest scores because outliers affect the statistical regression, not necessarily because the ICD-10-CM training session had any effect (Key 2002; Shi 2009). Statistical regression is covered in more detail in chapter 9.

Nonrandom Selection

Nonrandom selection is the selection of subjects that is not random. It is also known as nonprobability sampling because each subject's probability of being selected is unknown and could be either equal or unequal; generally associated with the qualitative approach. Nonrandom selection can affect internal validity if the characteristics, such as knowledge or ability, of subjects in the experimental group are systematically different than the characteristics of the comparison group.

For example, a study might compare a group of subjects who voluntarily viewed an instructional video on how to give themselves insulin injections to another group who did not volunteer and were therefore given pamphlets on insulin injection instead. Because the groups were not randomly assigned to the different interventions, the researcher will be unable to determine that any differences in the group outcomes are caused by the video intervention (Key 2002; Shi 2009).

Attrition

Attrition (also called *mortality*) is the withdrawal of subjects from the study. Individuals who leave a study can be very different than those who remain, and these differences can affect the results. For example, researchers conduct a one-year study on how to reduce the number of incomplete health records due to incomplete nursing documentation; before the study ends, 15 nurses leave the experimental group and 2 nurses leave the control group. The 15 nurses who leave may be unlike those who remain in the experimental group in terms of critical factors such as technical aptitude, patience, or willingness to learn new processes (Key 2002; Shi 2009).

Interaction of Factors

An **interaction of factors**, a combination of the factors affecting validity, may also bias the final results. Therefore, the researcher needs to be aware of how such factors can interact and their combined impact on internal validity (Shadish and Cook 1998; Key 2002; Shi 2009). For example, if a researcher is conducting research on older individuals who have a chronic debilitating disease, such as cancer or Parkinson's disease, then they may have to deal with multiple internal validity factors at once, such as the combination of maturation, attrition, and testing.

Factors Affecting External Validity

There are several factors that affect external validity. Testing, selection bias, and other study procedures may affect external validity. The researcher must be aware of these factors and work towards limiting them as much as possible when developing the research study design. However, no research study is perfect and each will have limitations.

Testing

As noted previously, a pretest can affect internal validity. It can also have an impact on a study's generalizability because individuals who are pretested may be different from the general population. The participants may have learned information from the pretest that influences their responses in the posttest. If this effect is present in the outcome of the study, the participants could be unrepresentative of the population under study. One way to mitigate testing is to choose a study design that does not include a pretest, but then it is more difficult to see changes over time.

Selection Bias

When evaluating whether the results of a study can be generalized to an entire population, the method used to select study participants is a crucial consideration. If the chosen participants are not representative of the target population, *selection bias* affects the study's external validity. Sometimes, health informatics studies use patients as subjects; however, if the participants are frequently under medical care, they are not representative of the general population. Also, volunteers and subjects who receive compensation for participating in a study are not necessarily representative of the general population. Volunteers may be willing to participate in a study because they are interested in the study topic, are especially motivated to improve their health, or have more free time than the general population. Subjects who are compensated for being in the study may choose to be in the study for the compensation, which means they are not representative of people who would not consider the compensation to be an incentive.

Additional Concerns Affecting Validity

Still other concerns about internal and external validity include poor **experimental procedures** (how the intervention or treatment is applied in the study) that may lead to the control group being exposed to part of the intervention under study; multiple treatment interference, which is when subjects are given several different interventions at one time; the length of time of the program or treatment intervention because time may affect the study outcomes more so than the intervention itself; attrition rates or loss of subjects because subjects who then remain in the study are different than those who leave and therefore may be different than the general population; and other potential confounding variables that may influence the outcomes of the study (Shadish and Cook 1998; Key 2002; Shi 2009).

Several tools can be used to control for internal and external validity concerns in experimental studies. Randomization can help control for selection, regression to the mean, and interaction of factors. It also improves external validity because random assignment of subjects to experimental and control or comparison groups helps limit selection bias. The use of groups that are not pretested helps control for the use of pretests. Including groups that are not given an intervention helps to control for the use of experimental procedures because they provide a good control for some of the issues that arise when using an intervention. Use of a control or comparison group may help control for the effects of history, maturation, instrumentation, and interaction of factors because the control group serves as a good comparison group to much of the effects consumed by the experimental group (Key 2002; Shi 2009).

Review Questions

1. The text states that experimental research studies are considered one of the most powerful when trying to establish cause and effect. Do you agree or disagree? Why?
2. What is the independent variable? Provide examples.
3. Experimental research also tries to determine how much of an effect the independent variable will have on the dependent variable. What does this mean?
4. When deciding whether to use the experimental research design, the researcher should consider which three issues?
5. What is the difference between quasi-experimental and experimental research?
6. What are the different types of experimental study designs?
7. What is an example in health informatics of a pretest-posttest control group method?
8. What is an example in health informatics of the posttest-only control group method?
9. What is a one-shot case study?
10. What are the internal and external validity factors to be aware of when conducting experimental research study designs?

Application Exercises

1. Describe how you would study the following hypothesis and whether you would use an experimental or quasi-experimental design. Explain why you chose either type of design.

   A researcher would like to determine whether light exercise, such as walking, or listening to classical or calm music improves the overall mood of college students. The hypothesis is that light walking or classical music will improve the mood of the college students more so than doing nothing at all. The researcher would like to evaluate this hypothesis in a short time period, such as one month.
2. Describe how you would perform a quasi-experimental study in health informatics. Be sure to address the following areas:
   - Topic chosen
   - Quasi-experimental study design chosen
     - One-shot case study
     - One-group pretest-posttest method
     - Static group comparison method
   - History
   - Maturation
   - Testing
   - Instrumentation
   - Statistical regression

  - Selection
  - Attrition
  - Interaction of factors
  - Selection bias
  - Other experimental procedures
3. Visit the website for ClinicalTrials.gov and search for a clinical trial that you are interested in exploring. Once you have chosen the study, address the following:
   a. What is the purpose of the study?
   b. What makes this study an experimental study design?
   c. What are the independent and dependent variables?
   d. What is the intervention?

References

Barnes, L., J. Hauser, L. Heikes, A.J. Hernandez, P.T. Richard, K. Ross, G.H. Yang, and M. Palmquist. 1994–2012. Experimental and Quasi-Experimental Research. Writing@CSU. Colorado State University Department of English. http://writing.colostate.edu/guides/research/experiment.

Baumberger-Henry, M. 2005. Cooperative learning and case study: Does the combination improve students' perception of problem-solving and decision making skills? *Nursing Education Today* 25(3):238–246.

Beebe, L.H. 2001. Community nursing support for clients with schizophrenia. *Archives of Psychiatric Nursing* 15(5):214–222.

Buller, D., M. Berwick, K. Lantz, M.K. Buller, J. Shane, I. Kane I, and X. Liu. 2015. Smartphone mobile application delivering personalized, real-time sun protection advice: A randomized clinical trial. *JAMA Dermatology* 2015;151(5):497–504. doi: 10.1001/jamadermatol.2014.3889.

Campbell, D.T. and J.C. Stanley. 1963. *Experimental and Quasi-Experimental Designs for Research.* Chicago: Rand McNally.

Chang, T., P. Pham, B. Sobolewski, C. Doughty, N. Jamal, K. Kwan, K. Little, T. Brenkert, D. Mathison. 2014. Pediatric emergency medicine asynchronous e-learning: A multicenter randomized controlled Solomon four-group study. *Academic Emergency Medicine* 21(8):912–919. doi: 10.1111/acem.12434

Danley, D., S.A. Gansky, D. Chow, and B. Gerbert. 2004. Preparing dental students to recognize and respond to domestic violence: The impact of a brief tutorial. *Journal of the American Dental Association* 135:67–73.

Dunbar, P.J., D. Madigan, L.A. Grohskopf, D. Revere, J. Woodward, J. Minstrell, P.A. Frick, J.M. Simoni, and T.M. Hooton. 2003. A two-way messaging system to enhance antiretroviral adherence. *Journal of the American Medical Informatics Association* 10(1):11–15.

Fox, K.C., G.W. Somes, and T.M. Waters. 2007. Timeliness and access to healthcare services via telemedicine for adolescents in state correctional facilities. *Journal of Adolescent Health* 41:161–167.

Holland Bloorview Kids Rehabilitation Hospital. 2016. Trial Study of an Exercise Program for Youth with Persistent Symptoms After Concussion (clinical trial). ClinicalTrials.gov identifier: NCT02257749. https://clinicaltrials.gov/ct2/show/NCT02257749?term=concussions&rank=2.

Key, J.P. 2002. Experimental Research and Design. Module R13 in Research Design in Occupational Education. Oklahoma State University. http://www.okstate.edu/ag/agedcm4h/academic/aged5980a/5980/newpage2.htm.

Miller, C.K., L. Edwards, G. Kissling, and L. Sanville. 2002. Nutrition education improves metabolic outcomes among older adults with diabetes mellitus: Results from a randomized controlled trial. *Preventive Medicine* 34:252–259.

Rocha, B.H., J.C. Christenson, R.S. Evans, and R.M. Gardner. 2001. Clinicians' response to computerized detection of infections. *Journal of the American Medical Informatics Association* 8(2):117–125.

Sander, A.M., A.D. Witol, and J.S. Kreutzer. 1997. Alcohol use after traumatic brain injury: Concordance of patients' and relatives' reports. *American Journal of Physical Medicine and Rehabilitation* 78:138–142.

Saounatsou, M., O. Patsi, G. Fasoi, M. Stylianou, A. Kavga, O. Economou, P. Mandi, and M. Nicolaou. 2001. The influence of the hypertensive patient's education in compliance with their medication. *Public Health Nursing* 18(6):436–442.

Shadish, W.R. and T.D. Cook. 1998. Donald Campbell and evaluation theory. *American Journal of Evaluation* 19:417–422.

Shi, L. 2009. Health Services Research Methods. Chapter 7 in *Experimental Research,* 2nd ed. Albany, NY: Delmar Publishers: 164–187.

US Environmental Protection Agency (EPA). 2016. Health risk of radon: Exposure to radon causes lung cancer in non-smokers and smokers alike. https://www.epa.gov/radon/health-risk-radon#head.

5 Epidemiological Research

Valerie J. Watzlaf, PhD, MPH, RHIA, FAHIMA

Learning Objectives

- Explain the purpose of epidemiology and its importance in health informatics.
- Apply epidemiological principles and models to examine health informatics topics.
- Describe the different types of epidemiological study designs and how they can be used in health informatics research.
- Assess the impact of confounding, recall bias, and other types of bias in epidemiological studies.
- Determine which statistical tests should be used for each study design, such as the odds ratio (OR) for the retrospective study and the relative risk (RR) for the prospective study.
- List and explain the rules of evidence when considering whether an association is causal.

Key Terms

Agent
Analytic study
Case-control study design
Cases
Chronic disease model
Clinical trial
Cohen's kappa (κ) coefficient
Cohort study
Community trial
Cross-sectional (prevalence) study
Diagnostic trials
Environment
Epidemiologists
Epidemiology
Historical-prospective study
Host
Incidence cases
Incidence rate
Infectious disease model
Multivariate analysis
Odds ratio (OR)
Phase I clinical trials
Phase II clinical trials
Phase III clinical trials
Phase IV clinical trials
Prevalence rate
Prevention trials
Protocol
Quality-of-life (QOL) trials
Relative risk (RR)
Screening trials
Sensitivity rates
Specific aims
Specificity rates
Survival analysis
Treatment trials
Univariate association

Epidemiology examines the patterns of disease occurrence in human populations and the factors that influence these patterns in relation to time, place, and persons. Epidemiologists study changes in the incidence and prevalence of diseases over time, variations in the incidence of diseases among communities, and whether individuals with a disease have characteristics or risk factors that distinguish them from individuals without the disease (Lilienfeld and Stolley 1994, 3). Based on this information, epidemiologists may be able to determine ways to prevent the disease from occurring.

Although epidemiology is generally linked more to public health than healthcare informatics, it is an essential tool when developing specific research methodologies in health informatics. Applications of epidemiology can be applied to health services planning, quality monitoring, policy development, system development, and finance. The types of epidemiology and their effectiveness in eradicating disease, types of epidemiological study designs, epidemiological models of disease causation, and the rules of evidence in determining disease causality will be covered in this chapter.

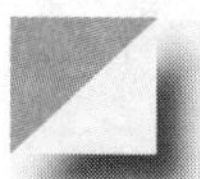

Real-World Case

Focus Pittsburgh Free Health Center (FPFHC) in Pittsburgh, PA, is working with faculty and students in the Health Information Management (HIM) Department at the University of Pittsburgh to perform epidemiological research and use health informatics to assess the health and wellness of a medically underserved community in four domains (physical, behavioral, spiritual and socio-economic). The research is using descriptive prevalence study designs. Trained behavioral health community organizers use mobile apps to deploy a new health-and-wellness survey tool throughout the community, and informatics algorithms are applied to the data collected to generate recommendations to healthcare providers about personalized interventions (healthcare, job training, housing, volunteerism, and so on) that can be used with members of the community (University of Pittsburgh School of Health and Rehabilitation Sciences 2016).

Types of Epidemiology and Its Effectiveness in Eradicating Disease

Epidemiology originated with the study of epidemics to determine what caused them and how they could be controlled and prevented. As mentioned in chapter 1, John Snow used epidemiological principles and methods to determine the source of a cholera outbreak in London in 1854. He found that several water companies supplied water to different parts of London, and he used maps to determine how the water was distributed to certain houses, discovering that some houses on the same street received their water from different sources. He then compared cholera death rates by water distributors for the initial weeks of the epidemic and found that the cholera mortality rates of the households that were supplied water by one company were eight to nine times higher than those supplied by other water companies. Snow's quantitative approach in analyzing the data revealed the source of the epidemic. His findings led to legislation to require that all water companies in London filter their water by 1857 (Lilienfeld and Stolley 1994, 28). The field of epidemiology expanded rapidly beyond the study of infectious diseases into the study of all types of illnesses. Current types of epidemiology include cancer epidemiology, pharmaco-epidemiology, environmental epidemiology, nutrition epidemiology, chronic disease epidemiology, and health services epidemiology.

Epidemiology and Health Informatics

Many health informatics systems need to be studied to determine whether they are effective in the delivery of healthcare services or if they improve patient outcomes. The basic study principles, designs, and methods of epidemiology are used to examine many of the health informatics systems and structures that currently sustain the healthcare system. The key is to know which epidemiological study design to use to inspect a problem. Many types of epidemiological study designs can be used to examine health informatics. These include the descriptive (cross-sectional or prevalence), analytic (retrospective case-control or prospective cohort), and the experimental (clinical and community trial) study designs. Most epidemiologists conduct research by beginning with the descriptive designs and then proceed to the analytic and experimental study designs. Table 5.1 summarizes the epidemiological study designs in relation to their usefulness in health informatics.

Table 5.1 Epidemiological study designs and their use in health informatics

Study Design	Uses in Health Informatics	Examples in Health Informatics
Descriptive: Cross-sectional, prevalence study	To study new ideas, concepts or systems to determine their use in a community, practice, or region	American Hospital Association study to examine the prevalence of health information technology in the United States (AHA 2016)

(Continued)

Table 5.1 *(Continued)*

Study Design	Uses in Health Informatics	Examples in Health Informatics
Analytic: Case-control (retrospective) Prospective/cohort/longitudinal Historical-prospective	To examine a system over time to determine its effectiveness when compared with another system or when comparing computer-based analysis to human analysis	Case-control study to examine nonsteroidal anti-inflammatory drug (NSAID) use and myocardial infarction (MI) rates using the QRESEARCH database (Vinogradova et al. 2014; Vindogradova et al. 2015) Prospective study to compare accuracy of physicians' diagnosis of acute myocardial infarction (AMI) to an artificial neural network diagnosis (Manson 1999) Historical-prospective study to examine breast cancer recurrence and mortality in postmenopausal women using the cancer registry, health records, and existing clinical databases (Katoh 1994)
Experimental: Clinical trial Community trial	To study an intervention or treatment over time to test its impact	Clinical or community trial using the STAR database to examine patients' ability to use computers to record symptoms and their ability to do activities of daily living (Massachusetts General Hospital 2016)

Epidemiological Study Designs

To examine disease prevalence and incidence as well as whether diseases can be prevented or kept from spreading, epidemiologists use descriptive, analytic, and experimental study designs. These epidemiological study designs can also be applied in health informatics research (refer to table 5.1). Epidemiologists often begin their research with the cross-sectional or prevalence study and then progress to the case-control, prospective, and experimental study designs. Each of these study designs is subsequently described in detail, as are their uses in health informatics.

Descriptive Study Design

A descriptive study in epidemiology explores a disease by first determining the prevalence in a community or geographic area and generates new ideas rather than proving existing hypotheses. A **cross-sectional study** (also called **prevalence study**) is a type of descriptive study performed when little is known about a disease or health characteristic. The cross-sectional study is used to describe disease or health characteristics in an environment at one point or period in time, such as one month or one year; it is not used to determine causality or explain whether specific risk factors led to a particular outcome. In other words, a prevalence study determines the **prevalence rate**, the proportion of people in a population who have a particular disease or health characteristic at a specific point in time or over a period of time. (The calculation for prevalence rate is shown in figure 5.1).

Figure 5.1 How to calculate prevalence rate

a. Equation for calculating disease prevalence:

$$\frac{\text{All new and preexisting cases during a given time period}}{\text{Population during the same time period}} \times 10^n$$

b. Equation for calculating prevalence of a personal attribute:

$$\frac{\text{Number of people with the attribute during a given time period}}{\text{Population during the same time period}} \times 10^n$$

The value of 10^n is usually 1 or 100 for common attributes. The value of 10^n might be 1,000, 100,000, or even 1 million for rare attributes and for most diseases.

Source: CDC 2012.

This design can be useful when little is known about a disease or factor because it describes the disease's or factor's prevalence in the environment at a specific time. Characteristics of the cross-sectional study design are listed in figure 5.2.

Figure 5.2 Components of the epidemiological cross-sectional study

- Describes health charasteristics at one point or one time period
- Determines whether the disease or health characteristic currently exists
- Performed when very little is known about a disease or health characteristic
- Generates hypotheses and new ideas
- Excellent design to adapt to study of new concepts in health informatics

The cross-sectional study design can be applied in health informatics as well as epidemiology. Cross-sectional studies in health informatics can provide basic but informative statistics that can be used for managing health services, administrative planning, and business intelligence. For example, a health informatics professional may be interested in determining the prevalence of digital radiology systems across acute-care hospitals in the United States. To do this, the factor to be studied (that is, digital radiology) must be defined before the study is launched.

Digital radiology systems allow the radiologist, physician, and other healthcare providers to view images immediately within the EHR. These systems have many advantages, such as decreasing the amount of effort and cost for radiology services, whether in-house or outsourced. However, many facilities will not pay the cost to implement a digital radiology system. Therefore, as part of the prevalence study, researchers may need to determine not only the expected amount of use of these systems but also the start-up and maintenance costs, including how those costs vary among several types of systems offered by multiple vendors. Then, the researchers can compare these costs to a facility's current radiology costs to determine whether a digital radiology system is a good investment.

The researchers would need to develop inclusion criteria related to the digital radiology system to be certain that data about comparable systems are collected. Criteria could include whether the system is:

- Used for at least 75 percent of all radiology reports within the healthcare facility
- Provided by a vendor or developed in-house
- Able to be used with the EHR
- Able to provide final validation checks on the quality of the image or for false-positive reports

Once the inclusion criteria are established, the prevalence rate can be calculated for a population. For example, the following equation shows how the prevalence of digital imaging systems in ambulatory care facilities is calculated:

$$\frac{\text{Number of US ambulatory healthcare facilities that use digital radiology systems}}{\text{Number of US ambulatory care facilities}} \times 10^n$$

In this example, the value of 10^n might be 1,000 to express the rate per 1,000 facilities, 10,000 to express the rate per 10,000 facilities, and so forth.

With this study design, the researchers could make statements of association—for example, the prevalence rates for various types of facilities could be compared to determine whether ambulatory care facilities use digital radiology more (or less) than other healthcare facilities. From this assessment, the researchers might generate new hypotheses that branch the research in new directions. For example, the researcher could develop a hypothesis that digital radiology systems are more prevalent than had been presumed because the images they offer are better quality than x-rays. Additional research would be needed to determine whether this hypothesis is valid.

Bell and colleagues used a cross-sectional survey study to determine whether physician offices located in high-minority and low-income neighborhoods in southern California had different levels of access to information technology than offices located in lower-minority and higher-income areas of the same region. The survey had a response rate of 46 percent and found that 94 percent of physician offices in both populations had at least one computer, 77 percent had Internet access, 29 percent had broadband Internet access, and 53 percent used a computerized practice management system to include computerized scheduling and billing systems. The researchers also found that physician offices surveyed in both categories had high levels of interest in using online clinical systems but had concerns regarding the security and confidentiality of online patient information systems (Bell et al. 2003, 487–489). This example shows that researchers continue to use epidemiological principles like those that Snow developed and expand their use beyond the study of disease.

A study by Linder and colleagues provides a real-world example of how cross-sectional studies can be helpful in new and emerging areas of health informatics (Linder et al. 2006). In this study, the investigators used a cross-sectional design to examine whether electronic billing diagnoses of acute respiratory infections (ARI) and urinary tract infections (UTI) and electronic prescribing (writing and sending a prescription to the pharmacy through the EHR) of antibiotics are accurate when compared with the full electronic clinical record. The researchers compared the electronic claims data to abstracted clinical records. The clinical records abstracted by the researchers were considered the gold standard. This study took place at nine clinics in Brigham and Women's Primary Care Practice Based Research Network in the Boston area. During the study, which took place from 2000 to 2003, a primary diagnosis of ARI or UTI was made at 65,285 visits. Initially, 1,000 were randomly selected and stratified by calendar year; however, only 827 visits were analyzed; the other cases were excluded due to the following: no clinical note found (68 visits), duplicate encounters (3 visits), or the clinic was not using an EHR (102 visits). Because the study was a descriptive, cross-sectional design, descriptive statistics about the beneficiaries in the study were generated, including the mean age (37 years); race and ethnicity (43 percent white, 29 percent Hispanic, 10 percent black, and 18 percent other); gender (79 percent women); and insurance type (26 percent HMO, 21 percent private, 15 percent Medicaid, 12 percent self-pay, 7 percent Medicare, and 19 percent other or missing) (Linder et al. 2006, 63).

Sensitivity and specificity rates were then determined for each of the electronic diagnoses collected. **Sensitivity rates** and **specificity rates**, defined in table 5.2, are measures of validity that are used when assessing whether measurement or labeling are correct. (These rates are discussed in further detail in chapter 12.) The sensitivity and specificity rates for ARI were 98 percent and 96 percent, respectively, and the sensitivity and specificity rates for UTI were 100 percent and 87 percent, respectively. When comparing electronic prescribing of antibiotics to data abstracted from the visit notes (gold standard), the sensitivity and specificity rates were 43 percent and 93 percent, respectively (Linder et al. 2006, 64).

Table 5.2 Sensitivity and specificity terms and definitions

Term	Definition	Type of Labeling
True positive (TP)	Correct labeling of a true case as a case (a *case* is an individual with the disease or outcome)	Valid
False negative (FN)	Incorrect labeling of a true case as a noncase (a *noncase* is an individual without the disease or outcome)	Invalid
True negative (TN)	Correct labeling of a noncase as a noncase	Valid
False positive (FP)	Incorrect labeling of a noncase as a case	Invalid
Sensitivity	Percentage of all true cases correctly labeled: TP/(TP + FN)	
Specificity	Percentage of all true noncases correctly labeled: TN/(TN + FP)	

Source: Adapted from Lilienfeld and Stolley 1994.

In the study by Linder and associates, the sensitivity rate of 98 percent for ARI diagnoses suggests that the electronic diagnosis system correctly identified cases of ARI 98 percent of the time, but 2 percent of the time it incorrectly identified the disease in patients who did not actually have it (Linder et al. 2006). Although 2 percent may seem like a small percentage, the undiagnosed patients would not receive proper treatment. The specificity rate of 96 percent for ARI diagnoses suggests that the electronic diagnosis correctly identified individuals without ARI 96 percent of the time, but 4 percent of the time it incorrectly indicated that patients had ARI when they actually did not have it. The sensitivity rate of 100 percent for UTI diagnoses indicates that the electronic diagnosis system correctly identified all true cases of UTI; however, the specificity rate for UTI diagnoses was much lower, at 87 percent. This means that out of all the UTI diagnoses, the electronic diagnosis system mislabeled patients with a UTI 13 percent of the time. The consequences of a false-positive diagnosis may not be as severe as missing a true diagnosis, but a false-positive could nevertheless result in inappropriate treatment, which can lengthen hospital stays, increase costs, and cause harm to patients (Linder et al. 2006).

Another example of a cross-sectional study in health informatics comes from the American Hospital Association (AHA) (2016). AHA conducted a cross-sectional study by surveying AHA-member hospitals to determine their use of HIT. Survey instruments were sent to hospital chief executive officers (CEOs) from all types of hospitals and from different geographic areas across the United States. The survey included questions related to the use of specific types of HIT, such as whether the hospital's current computerized system allows for electronic clinical documentation, results viewing, computerized provider order entry (CPOE), decision support, bar coding or radio frequency identification (RFID) for medication tracking, and other functionalities such as telehealth, and use of mobile apps. It also requested information about functionalities such as medication management, quality reporting, and public health reporting that are required under the meaningful use provisions of the Affordable Care Act. A separate section of the survey focused on health information exchange (HIE) and the EHR system and HIT vendor used by the hospital (AHA 2016). Results from the AHA survey showed that 75 percent of hospitals had at least a basic EHR in place by 2014—almost five times what was seen in 2010. Furthermore, in 2014, 64.3 percent of hospitals had provided ways for patients and consumers to access their health information, a notable change since 2013, when 10.4 percent of hospitals had done this. Also, hospitals showed a large improvement in sharing of health information outside of their healthcare system (AHA 2016).

The AHA 2016 study demonstrates how a cross-sectional study can lead to new hypotheses and suggest areas for further study. For example, the study found that even though progress has been made in HIE, the lack of compatibility of EHR systems across vendors makes the exchange of health data a problem. Ensuring privacy and security while exchanging health information across health care systems was also an issue. Based on this information, researchers may decide to conduct additional studies, to determine what the information exchange barriers are across EHR systems and to see whether such barriers are more prominent in certain types of EHR systems. Based on the results, researchers may be able to determine better systems to use to promote HIE.

Analytic Study Designs

In the **analytic study** design, the epidemiologist determines whether there is a relationship between two variables, the independent variable (the exposure or risk factor) and the dependent variable (the disease or health outcome). One method used to determine the relationship between the two variables is the retrospective **case-control study design**. Epidemiologists use the case-control study design when the disease or outcome is rare and when it is relatively easy to assess the independent variable by looking back in time. Another method is the prospective **cohort study** design. In this design, epidemiologists follow participants with the independent variable (risk factor) and those without it, over time, to determine whether the participants develop the dependent variable (disease). A more time-efficient version of the prospective design is the **historical-prospective study** (also called retrospective-prospective study), which allows the researcher to use existing information found in past records or vital statistics to establish the independent variables. Then, participants are examined in the present time and possibly forward in time to determine their health outcomes. Each of these epidemiological study designs allows researchers to support cause and effect between two variables. These topics and their epidemiological uses will be covered in the sections that follow.

Case-Control Study Design

In case-control design, researchers choose **cases** (individuals who have the disease under study) and compare them to controls (individuals without the disease) to determine whether the independent variable is historically more prominently associated with the cases than in the controls. This study design is usually performed when a researcher is trying to support cause and effect or when one variable leads to an outcome. A summary of the steps in a case-control study follows.

- **Step 1:** Determine the hypothesis and decide whether to use prevalence cases (existing cases of disease) or incidence cases (new cases of disease).
- **Step 2:** If using prevalence cases, seek out cases from the state or hospital-based cancer registry. If using incidence cases, have healthcare facilities provide new cases as they are treated.
- **Step 3:** Decide who will be part of the study by using inclusion criteria to validate the disease under study, such as ICD-10-CM codes, laboratory reports, radiology reports, and health records.
- **Step 4:** Randomly select the cases by obtaining a list of possible cases (either from the state or hospital-based cancer registry or from a list of ICD-10-CM codes, and so forth) and using a systematic sample, such as choosing every fifth case.
- **Step 5:** Choose controls from siblings or friends who are the same gender and of similar age and socioeconomic status, or from similar patients at the same hospital. Controls and cases should share all characteristics except the disease under study. For example, if studying melanoma, controls could be chosen from the same hospital-affiliated cancer registry as the cases, but the controls would have another type of cancer, such as colon cancer or lung cancer. Select these controls from a list of cancer cases identified by their ICD-10-CM code and validate the diagnosis through pathology reports and health records. Also, choose control participants from this list who are similar in age by at least five years.

- **Step 6:** Decide whether to match the cases and controls for certain variables. Matching on variables such as age, gender, race, and so forth should only be used when the researcher is certain that there is a relationship between a given variable and the dependent variable. For example, age is always related to cancer because the likelihood of developing cancer increases as people age. Therefore, age is a confounding variable in case-control studies of cancer because it may be the underlying factor that leads to the development of the cancer. Matching patients by age will reduce the chance that age confounds the study of the specific cancer risk factor being studied.
- **Step 7:** Design the instrument used to collect the exposure or risk factor data. Collect data through phone or in-person interviews, self-report questionnaires, or abstracts from existing sources such as the EHR, cancer registry, birth certificates, death certificates, and financial records. Some researchers, such as Watzlaf, design a research instrument to collect both interview-related data and health record data (Watzlaf 1989). The full research instrument is provided in online appendix 5A. It is extremely important that the researcher choose appropriate data sources so that information related to both the cases and controls can be found.
- **Step 8:** Analyze the data to include the appropriate statistics.
- **Step 9:** Summarize the results and determine if they support or refute the hypothesis.
- **Step 10:** Publish the results.

Other areas that will be covered in the case-control study design include the selection of controls, recall bias, instrument design, the odds ratio and an example of a case-control study design used in health informatics.

Recall Bias After selecting cases and controls, the researchers would interview the cases and controls to determine their health history and other health characteristics, such as the number and severity of sunburns. Because researchers would be asking subjects to think back about events that may have happened several years ago, recall bias is a weakness of this study design. Recall bias refers to the fact that memory is imperfect and therefore a respondent's answers may not completely accurate. To decrease the amount of recall bias, researchers employ various methods to improve the reliability of their memory, such as showing subjects lists of medications so that they can choose the medications they have taken or using pictures to help participants understand concepts (such as the severity of sunburns) and recall their own history.

Odds Ratio The **odds ratio (OR)** is an estimate of the relative risk that is computed from the case-control study; **relative risk (RR)** is a measure of the strength of an association between the exposure (independent variable) and the disease or outcome (dependent variable). The OR can be used in conjunction with the case-control study design to quantify the differences in exposure for the cases versus the controls. These differences can be illustrated in a 2 × 2 table, as shown in table 5.3.

Table 5.3 Example of 2 × 2 table to calculate OR

	Disease (Cases)	**No Disease (Controls)**
Exposure	A	B
No Exposure	C	D
Totals	A + C	B + D

When viewing the table, one can calculate from the first column, Disease (Cases), the proportion of cases exposed to the risk factor—A/(A + C)—and the proportion of cases not exposed to the risk factor = C/(A + C). The odds of exposure for the cases is calculated as [A/(A + C)]/[C/(A + C)], which can be simplified to A/C. Next, the odds of exposure for the controls are calculated the same way but using the values in the second column, No Disease (Controls), resulting in B/D. Finally, to determine the OR—whether the odds of exposure for the cases (A/C) are greater than the odds of exposure for the controls (B/C)—the OR of the two groups is calculated as follows (Friis and Sellers 2014):

$$OR = \frac{A/C}{B/D} = \frac{A \times D}{B \times C}$$

For example, to determine whether exposure to tanning lamps increases the risk of melanoma, the data on cases and controls can be inserted into the 2 × 2 table (table 5.4) and used to determine the OR.

Table 5.4 Example of OR in 2 × 2 table for melanoma study

	Melanoma (Cases)	**No Melanoma (Controls)**
Tanning lamp exposure	200 (A)	500 (B)
No tanning lamp exposure	10 (C)	100 (D)
Totals	210	600

$$OR = \frac{AD}{BC} = \frac{200 \times 100}{500 \times 10} = \frac{20,000}{5,000} = 4$$

The OR of 4 means that the individuals who used tanning lamps are 4 times more likely to develop melanoma than the individuals who did not use tanning lamps. If the OR for this example equaled 1, the risk for melanoma would be equal for the cases and controls, meaning that use of tanning lamps would not be a risk factor for melanoma. If an OR were less than 1, the use of tanning lamps would decrease the risk of disease, thereby providing a protective effect.

Examples of Case-Control Studies Related to Health Informatics Watzlaf conducted a case-control study to examine whether health records could be used to identify possible risk factors associated with epithelial ovarian cancer. Early diagnosis of ovarian cancer can be difficult because the initial symptoms are mild ones (such as backache, bloating, and nausea) that are common to many other less-severe illnesses. Therefore, if a specific risk factor associated with ovarian cancer can be identified in health records, early detection might be advanced (Watzlaf 1989).

In this study, researchers contacted the health record departments or cancer registries at 10 hospitals (after institutional review board [IRB] approval) to obtain the number of patients in whom epithelial ovarian cancer had been diagnosed. The study used patients newly diagnosed with ovarian cancer (patients newly diagnosed with a disease are called **incidence cases**) because the researchers thought that the health record would likely provide the most complete history of medical information when a patient is newly diagnosed. Once the patients agreed to be part of the study and signed consent forms, their health records were abstracted and they were interviewed. For each case, a control was randomly selected from the same healthcare facility as the case. Controls and cases were matched by age (within 5 years), discharge date, and hospital; controls did not have a cancer diagnosis (Watzlaf 1989).

Research assistants with backgrounds in HIM abstracted data from the health records and conducted telephone interviews. The questionnaires and abstracts used the same questionnaire format as the ovarian cancer study questionnaire presented in online appendix 5A. At the start of the study, the research assistants were trained in abstracting health records and interviewing techniques. The training sessions taught the assistants to examine the entire health record before recording a "no" answer to any of the questions used in the abstract. For example, the research assistants looked at the entire record for "no history of cervical fibroids" before indicating "no history" in the abstract. If the risk factor was simply not mentioned anywhere in the medical record, it was considered "not documented" rather than "no history" (Watzlaf 1989).

The telephone interviews were necessary in cases where the health records lacked some of the necessary information. However, many of the participants were too ill to be interviewed, which lessened the sample size and hindered the researchers' ability to examine the risk factors related to ovarian cancer and calculate ORs. Therefore, the researchers decided to focus on the health record data. Three individuals independently reviewed and abstracted which risk factors were and were not found in the health records of cases and controls. Percentages of agreement and Cohen's kappa (κ) coefficients (kappa statistics) were computed. The *percentage of agreement* is the number of occurrences in which abstractors agreed on the recording of a risk factor within the medical record. The **Cohen's kappa (κ) coefficient** provides a value that states whether the levels of agreement seen among reviews by different abstractors are real or due to chance (see chapters 8 and 11). Kappa values greater than 0.60 show a good level of agreement. The abstractors found that, in the health records of the cases, history of any cancer was documented 50 percent of the time (84 percent agreement, kappa = 0.67), whereas smoking and alcohol use was documented 94 percent of the time (80 percent agreement for alcohol, kappa = 0.68; 86 percent agreement for smoking, kappa = 0.69), and oral contraceptive use was documented 15 percent of the time (96 percent agreement, kappa = 0.71) (Watzlaf 1989). These kappa values demonstrate good agreement.

Including an epidemiological approach in assessing health status supports healthcare providers in collecting and documenting risk factors, as shown in figure 5.3. This approach improves the quality of documentation in the health record, whether it is paper-based or electronic, and in turn leads to better diagnosis, treatment, and prevention of disease.

Figure 5.3 Epidemiological approach in assessing health status

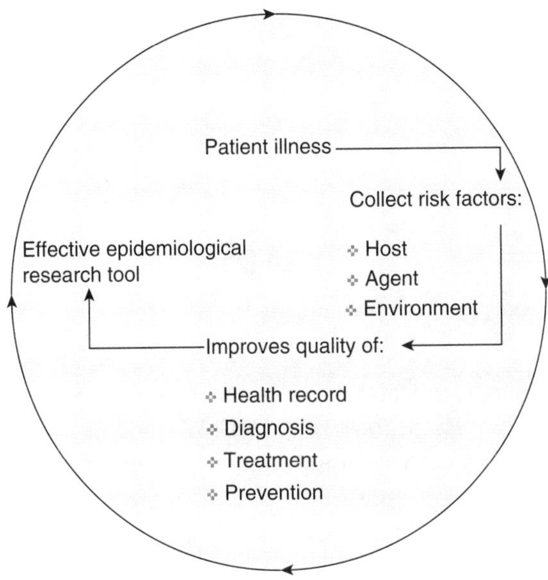

In another example of a case-control study, Vinogradova and colleagues analyzed 5,500 cases of venous thromboembolism (VTE) from QRESEARCH and 5,062 cases of VTE from Clinical Practice Research Data link (CPRD) databases, which have been tested and validated in the United Kingdom, to examine the relationship between oral contraceptives and risk of VTE. Data within these databases were tested and analyzed and found to be valid in more than 90 percent of the cases when compared with paper-based records. The information in the databases includes birth date, gender, height, weight, smoking status, diagnoses, symptoms, and prescribed medications, including the use of oral contraceptives. Diagnosis of VTE was based on the READ codes that were included in the EHR. Cases were women with VTE, and one case or woman with VTE was matched with up to five female controls of the same age and from the same physician practice but without VTE. Odds ratios were computed to examine whether the women who took oral contraceptives were more likely to have VTE. Combined oral contraceptives were associated with an increased risk of VTE (OR = 2.97). Confounding variables (other variables that can play a part in the development of VTE) were also collected and controlled for in the statistical analysis; these variables included smoking status, alcohol consumption, ethnic group, body mass index, comorbidities, and other contraceptive medications (Vinogradova et al. 2014; Vinogradova et al. 2015).

This research study demonstrates how healthcare informatics can be used effectively to examine important epidemiological relationships. Without the use of the QRESEARCH and CPRD databases, the cases, controls, and the prescribing data could not have been retrieved in such large volume with complete and consistent data content. Because electronic clinical databases are available across large geographic regions such as this one in the United Kingdom, epidemiologists and other clinical researchers can conduct effective, efficient, case-control studies.

Cohort Study Design

The analytic study design known as a cohort study (also referred to as a prospective study and incidence study) follows two groups of study participants—one with exposure to an independent variable and one without the exposure—forward in time to determine whether and when they develop the disease or outcome variable under study. For example, a prospective study about alcohol use and liver disease could start by identifying individuals with the exposure of interest, such as alcohol use, and ones without the exposure, such as those who do not drink alcohol, and then follow both groups to determine whether the alcohol users develop liver disease at a greater rate than the group that does not use alcohol.

This study design generates the **incidence rate**, the rate at which new cases of a disease or health characteristic occur, for each group. The incidence rate of the disease in the exposed group is then compared with the incidence rate of disease in the unexposed group to obtain the RR. The RR compares the risk of a disease, health attribute, or death among one group with the risk among another group (CDC 2012). (See figure 5.4 for these formulas.) The magnitude of the RR measures the strength of the association—the greater the RR value, the greater the association between the exposure and the disease (Lilienfeld and Stolley 1994). For example, an RR of 3 indicates a stronger association between the exposure and the disease than an RR of 2. In addition, RRs of less than 1 demonstrate a protective effect between the exposure and the disease.

Figure 5.4 How to calculate incidence rate and RR

a. Incidence rate $= \frac{\text{Number of new cases of a disease over a period of time}}{\text{Population at risk}} \times 10^n$

b. Relative risk (RR) $= \frac{\text{Incidence rate of the exposed group}}{\text{Incidence rate of the unexposed group}}$

Population at risk refers to the population that is free of the disease at the start of the study. The value of 10^n is usually 1 or 100 for common attributes. The value of 10^n might be 1,000, 100,000, or even 1,000,000 for rare attributes and for most diseases.

Source: CDC 2012.

RR indicated a protective effect in a landmark study by Manson and colleagues, in which the authors examined exercise and heart disease in women and found that brisk walking and vigorous exercise decreased the risk of coronary heart disease. Age-adjusted RRs in this study ranged from 0.77 in the least physically activity group (0 to 2 hours per week of brisk walking or vigorous exercise) to 0.46 in the highest physical activity group (more than 21 hours per week of brisk walking or vigorous exercise) (Manson et al. 1999, 652). When the authors controlled for other confounding variables, walking was found to be inversely related to coronary heart disease. In addition, women who walked 3 or more hours per week at a brisk pace were found to have an RR of 0.65 when compared with women who walked infrequently (Manson et al. 1999, 655).

RR can also be used to explore adverse relationships. For example, suppose researchers are interested in determining whether the risk of migraines is greater in children who play video games. These researchers could conduct a prospective study in which the exposure is playing video games and the disease is migraines. Two groups of children, one that plays video games at least three times per week, four hours per day and one group that does not play video games, could be followed forward in time to determine their incidence of developing migraines. Table 5.5 shows the 2 × 2 table framework for calculating incidence and RR. Table 5.6 shows the numbers that might be entered in such a table for this hypothetical study of video games and migraines. Using those numbers, the calculation for the RR is as follows:

$$\text{Incidence Rate of Exposed Group} = \frac{A}{(A+B)} = \frac{200}{275} = 0.727$$

$$\text{Incidence Rate of Unexposed} = \frac{C}{(C+D)} = \frac{25}{325} = 0.077$$

$$RR = \frac{[A/(A+B)]}{[C/(C+D)]} = \frac{[0.727]}{[0.077]} = 9.4$$

Table 5.5 Relative risk 2 × 2 table

Exposure	Disease	No Disease	Total
Yes	A	B	A + B
No	C	D	C + D

Table 5.6 Relative risk 2 × 2 table for hypothetical prospective study of video games and migraines

Exposure	Disease	No Disease	Total
Yes	200	75	275
No	25	300	325

In this hypothetical example, the RR of 9.4 indicates a strong association between use of video games and migraine headaches. Those children who play video games are more than nine times more likely to develop migraine headaches than those who do not play video games.

Tierney and colleagues documented what occurred when 105 patients in an urban health system were able to restrict healthcare providers' access to information in their EHR. In this cohort study, about 50 percent of patients were cases, or those choosing to restrict access to providers, and the other 50 percent were controls, or those not restricting any access to providers. Patients could choose to allow or restrict access by provider or by data type, including medications, diagnoses, results, and reports or only sensitive data such as STDs, HIV, drugs, alcohol use, behavioral health information, and so on. The EHR data shown to providers was redacted based on patient preferences, although providers had access to information in free-text entries and had the option to "break the glass" to quickly gain access to patient information when necessary to provide optimal care. The 31 providers in the study "broke the glass" over 100 times to gain access to EHR information needed to provide patient care, including 92 times for those patients in the study who did not have data redacted, 10 times for those that restricted it by data type, and 5 times for restrictions to a specific provider. Twenty-four providers completed a 5-point Likert scale questionnaire about their opinions of patients having control over access to their EHR information. Results from the questionnaire showed that although 46 percent of providers agreed that they were comfortable with patients restricting them from seeing some of the information in their EHR, 71 percent of the providers believed restricting access could lead to poor quality of care for patients (Tierney et al. 2015).

Historical-Prospective Study Design

In a historical-prospective study, study groups are identified from data about characteristics in existing data sources and the groups are followed over time, usually from the time the data were first collected to the present or into the future, to examine their outcomes. For example, Katoh and colleagues (1994) and Watzlaf and associates (2002) conducted historical-prospective studies to examine the association between body mass index (BMI) and breast cancer recurrence and survival in postmenopausal white and African-American women. Participants were divided into categories of "obese" and "not obese" based on BMI.

In the earlier study, Katoh's team examined this relationship in data from 301 postmenopausal women diagnosed with breast cancer between 1977 and 1985. Most of the women had been diagnosed at a local hospital in Pittsburgh and had estrogen receptor (ER) and progesterone receptor (PR) analyses performed on breast cancer tissue. (Testing the tumor tissue for ER and PR is a standard part of a breast cancer diagnosis. These receptors are helpful in determining the risk of breast cancer recurrence and choosing the optimal type of treatment, such as hormonal therapies like Tamoxifen.) The study did not find a significant association between obesity and breast cancer recurrence or death from breast cancer. However, most of the women in the study were white, and some interesting data were noted about the 18 postmenopausal African-American participants: 12 of them (67 percent) were obese, and 7 of the 12 obese African-American subjects (58 percent) had documented recurrences of breast cancer (Katoh et al. 1994).

Based on this finding, Watzlaf and associates (2002) decided to investigate whether the association between obesity and breast cancer recurrence and survival could be stronger in African American women than in Caucasian women. If a relationship was found in obese African American women, then diet intervention studies might be conducted for this population to evaluate whether weight loss could reduce breast cancer recurrence and mortality.

Data for both studies were collected from health records and the cancer registry (see figure 5.5). Because some of the data from the 1994 study could not be found (192 cases could not be used due to lack of documentation regarding BMI, cause of death or recurrence status, ER, PR, staging and number of positive lymph nodes, which led to a total of 301 cases used when we started with 493). Watzlaf's team could not use those cases in the 2002 study, which limited the sample size (n = 301). In the studies, postmenopausal status was assumed in patients older than 55 years and determined in patients younger than 55 years by reviewing the health record, cancer registry data, and physician office records. Obesity was defined as BMI greater than 27. (BMI is the ratio of weight in kilograms to the square of height in meters [kg/m^2]). Recurrence and survival classifications are shown in figure 5.6 (Watzlaf et al. 2002).

Figure 5.5 Data items collected for two historical-prospective studies of breast cancer recurrence and mortality

Age
Age at diagnosis
Weight
Height
Date of diagnosis
Menopausal status
Diagnosis and coding of tumor (histopathology and topography)
Number of positive nodes
Estrogen receptor (ER) and progesterone receptor (PR) analyses
Site of distant metastasis
First course of treatment
Additional treatment
Five-year recurrence and survival
Stage and size of tumor

Source: Watzlaf et al. 2002.

Figure 5.6 Classifications of recurrence and survival in two breast cancer studies

Recurrence status
Never free of disease
No recurrence
Alive with recurrence
Death due to breast cancer recurrence
Breast cancer recurrence at the time of any cause of death
Survival status
Alive
Death from other causes
Death due to breast cancer

Source: Watzlaf et al. 2002.

Tables 5.7 and 5.8 demonstrate the statistical analyses used in the 2002 study to determine whether obesity was related to mortality in African-American women with breast cancer (Watzlaf et al. 2002). In their analyses, researchers calculated the OR instead of the RR for two reasons. First, the OR should be used when performing logistic regression analyses. Second, it is best to use the OR when conducting a historical-prospective study because the exposure is an estimate of the true exposure retrieved from past data, and the outcome (death due to breast cancer) is considered rare.

Table 5.7 shows univariate associations between each variable studied by Watzlaf and colleagues and case fatality (Watzlaf et al. 2002). (The **univariate association** is the relationship between a variable and a dependent variable). For each variable in table 5.7, the specific (univariate) associations analyzed are indicated. The following variables had significant associations ($P < 0.05$):

- PR-negative versus PR-positive
- Level of treatment: Surgery and therapy versus surgery
- Stage II cancer versus stage I cancer, stage III versus I, and stage IV versus stage I (cancer stages refer to the progression of the disease, with stage I being the least advanced)
- Size of tumor (≥ 2 cm versus < 2cm)
- Nodal status (1 to 3 + nodes versus 0 nodes, and ≥ 4 nodes versus 0 nodes) (nodal status indicates whether the cancer has spread to lymph nodes, which can be a prognosticator of cancer outcomes)

The ORs were consistent for these associations. Associations that lacked significance consisted of age, ER, and obesity (Watzlaf et al. 2002).

Table 5.7 Univariate association between variables and case fatality in study of breast cancer in obese African-American women*

Variable	*P* Value	Odds Ratio (OR)	95% Confidence Interval
Age			
≥ 63.2 years vs. <63.2 years	0.475	1.16	[0.77, 1.76]
Estrogen receptor (ER)			
ER-negative vs. ER-positive	0.079	1.57	[0.95, 2.59]
Progesterone receptor (PR)			
PR-negative vs. PR-positive	0.037	1.72	[1.03, 2.88]
Level of treatment			
Surgery + therapy vs. surgery alone	0.000	8.07	[4.04, 16.11]
Obesity			
Yes vs. no	0.364	1.21	[0.80, 1.85]
Stage			
II vs. I	0.002	2.97	[1.51, 5.85]
III vs. I	0.000	12.62	[5.53, 28.8]
IV vs. I	0.000	88.31	[23.9, 326.5]
Size of tumor			
≥ 2.0 cm vs. < 2.0 cm	0.000	4.15	[2.3, 7.5]
Nodal status			
1 – 3 + vs. 0	0.016	2.21	[1.16, 4.21]
≥ 4 vs. 0	0.000	7.56	[4.02, 14.2]

*Derived using logistic regression
Source: Watzlaf et al. 2002.

Watzlaf and colleagues expanded the statistical analysis by using multiple logistic regression for predicting death from breast cancer while simultaneously controlling for the independent variables (see table 5.8). A **multivariate analysis** shows the relationship between multiple independent variables and a dependent variable. In the analysis presented in table 5.8, case fatality is the dependent variable and PR, level of treatment, obesity, cancer stage, size of tumor, and nodal status are the independent variables. These variables were chosen because they were statistically significant ($P < 0.05$) from the univariate analysis, except for obesity, which was not statistically significant from the univariate analysis. PR, level of treatment, and nodal status (4+ versus 0) emerged from this analysis as significant predictors. All other variables, including obesity, did not show significance (Watzlaf et al. 2002).

Table 5.8 Multivariate analysis for predicting case fatality in study of obese African-American women with breast cancer*

Variable	*P* Value	Odds Ratio	95% Confidence Interval
Progesterone receptor	0.036	2.23	[1.05, 4.73]
Level of treatment	0.002	8.91	[2.27, 34.9]
Obesity	0.362	1.41	[0.67, 2.94]
Stage			
II	0.345	1.85	[0.52, 6.66]
III	0.310	2.25	[0.47, 10.75]
IV	0.514	13.38	[0.98, 181.9]
Size of tumor	0.594	1.38	[0.42, 4.47]

(*Continued*)

Table 5.8 (*Continued*)

Variable	*P* Value	Odds Ratio	95% Confidence Interval
Nodal status			
1–3+ vs. 0	0.756	0.86	[0.33, 2.23]
≥ 4 + vs. 0	0.028	2.86	[1.12, 7.34]

*Derived using multiple logistic regression analysis. The appropriateness of fit of the model was evaluated using the Hosmer-Lemeshow chi-square statistic.
Source: Watzlaf et al. 2002.

The 2002 study indicated that obesity is not significantly associated with fatality because the *P* value is not less than 0.05 and, therefore, the OR of 1.21 could be due to chance (Watzlaf et al. 2002). This result may have occurred because of the small sample size. The researchers also hypothesized that the lack of significance might be because obesity was differentiated by just two categories: obese = BMI > 27 and not obese = BMI < 27. However, when the authors calculated the BMI values into quartiles and ran the analysis again, obesity was still not found to be related to case fatality or breast cancer recurrence (Watzlaf et al. 2002).

In these studies, the lack of certain data, such as height and weight, limited the total number of cases that could be used, making the study size much smaller than the investigators originally anticipated (table 5.9). Data for simple but important variables such as height or weight must be collected if the health record and cancer registry are to be considered reliable data sources for epidemiological research. Also, other important variables such as ER and PR values, stage of cancer, number of positive nodes, and so forth must be documented 100 percent of the time to improve the quality of patient care as well as the advancement of breast cancer research. Figure 5.7 lists selected ways that health informatics professionals can contribute to improving data capture methods for breast cancer research.

Table 5.9 Data items not documented in the health records and tumor registry used as sources for study of breast cancer recurrence and mortality

Item Type	# Not Documented (N = 493)	% Not Documented
Demographic data		
Birth date	0	0%
Age at diagnosis	1	0.2%
Date of diagnosis	0	0%
Marital status	27	5.5%
Occupation	68	13.8%
Diagnostic data		
Height	49	9.9%
Weight	42	8.5%
BMI	57	11.6%
ER value	181	36.7%
ER (+/–)	120	24.3%
PR value	210	42.6%
PR (+/–)	175	35.5%
Summary stage	27	5.5%
Tumor size	44	8.9%
Number of positive nodes	112	22.7%
Number of nodes examined	103	20.9%
Site of distant metastases	294	59.6%

(*Continued*)

Table 5.9 (*Continued*)

Item Type	# Not Documented (N = 493)	% Not Documented
Family history of cancer	127	25.8%
First course of surgery	5	1.0%
Surgery date	12	2.4%
Survival data		
Follow-up of cases	493	100%
Recurrence status	39	7.9%

Abbreviations: BMI, body mass index; ER, estrogen receptor; PR, progesterone receptor.
Source: Watzlaf et al. 2002.

Figure 5.7 Selected ways that health informatics professionals can improve data capture for breast cancer research

- Work closely with administration, the medical staff, and other direct healthcare providers.
- Demonstrate the importance of proper and complete documentation.
- Develop documentation policies and procedures specific to breast cancer.
- Assist in developing electronic databases specific to breast cancer risk factor data so healthcare providers know what risk factors are important and which ones should be documented.
- Assist in the development of a standardized breast cancer registry abstract.
- Move toward concurrent record analysis to capture missing, incomplete, or incorrect data quickly.
- Assist in developing methods to encourage direct data capture through mobile apps, online tools, voice recognition, and so forth.
- Encourage the use of national and state breast cancer registries and databases to enhance local data.
- Stay informed of the most effective methods of data capture for breast cancer research, which in turn leads to improvements in the quality of patient care.
- Learn the data-mining and data-warehousing capabilities in breast cancer databases that can then be linked with local cancer registry data.
- Make sure that EHR data are of good quality, can be easily accessed, and can be linked to other important databases throughout the healthcare facility.
- Encourage standard-setting organizations to include height, weight, menopausal status, and hormone receptor analysis as required data elements.
- Encourage registry software vendors to include specific risk factors related to breast cancer as required data elements.

Source: Adapted from Watzlaf et al. 2002.

Experimental Research Study Designs

Experimental research is considered one of the most powerful designs to establish cause and effect. Experimental research studies confirm causality by exposing participants to different interventions (independent variables) to compare the result of these interventions with the outcome (dependent variables). Two examples of experimental research studies in epidemiology are the clinical trial and the community trial.

Clinical trials are designed to test new approaches to the diagnosis, treatment, or prevention of specific diseases in a controlled environment. Many clinical trials enroll patients who have the disease being studied or are at high risk for developing the disease on a volunteer basis. Clinical trials are commonly used to test new medications, surgical procedures, and new treatments or combinations of treatments to prevent disease, and many trials have provided information that has advanced diagnosis, treatment, and prevention of disease. **Community trials** are like clinical trials except that, as the name suggests, community trials take place in a community and researchers therefore have less control over the intervention than they would have with the clinical trial (which is usually conducted in a controlled environment such as a clinic rather than the participant's community or home environment). The community trial's goal is to produce changes in a specific population within a community, organization, or association and its participants include all members of the community. The intervention tends to be provided throughout the population with less control than in the clinical trial (Friis and Sellers 2014, 322–323; UPMC 2015). The protocols for clinical and community trials, types and phases of clinical trials, how clinical and community trials can be applied to health informatics, and the statistical analysis that can be performed with these trials will be discussed in the next sections.

Clinical and Community Trial Protocols

Every clinical and community trial should follow a protocol—a step-by-step plan on how the trial will be conducted. It should address the following components:

- **Rationale and background:** There must be a reason for conducting the clinical or community trial, which should be related to background information about the disease under study and the intervention that will be used in the trial.
- Specific aims: The purpose or goal of the trial must be established and documented before the trial begins. Both long- and short-term goals may be provided and should explain the major aim of the study. For example, if a community trial is examining how use of a PHR by parents affects the management of their children's asthma, one aim might be to compare the number of asthma-related visits to the emergency department (ED) for children whose parents use the PHR to the number of asthma-related ED visits for children whose parents do not use the PHR.
- **Randomization:** Refer to chapter 4 for discussion of randomization.
- **Blinding:** Refer to chapter 1 for more information on blinding.
- **Types and duration of treatment:** The protocol should explain all types of interventions (treatments) used in the clinical or community trial. Types of treatments may include medications, surgery, vaccines, dietary changes, exercise intervention, smoking cessation, use of a software system, education intervention, and so forth. The dose and duration of treatment must be specified.
- **Number of subjects:** The number of subjects needed for the clinical or community trial to be valid should be explained. A sample size calculation may need to be performed to determine the best sample size necessary to see differences between the intervention group and the control group.
- **Criteria for including and excluding participants:** Researchers list the selection criteria for participants, such as age older than 50 years, familiarity with using a mobile phone app and so forth, as well as criteria that exclude individuals from entering the study, such as not having the disease being studied or having other health conditions that might confound the independent variable.
- **Outline of treatment procedures:** Treatment procedures should be specified to include the dose and duration of the treatment, how follow-up will be conducted, and any additional tests or use of interviews or questionnaires.
- **Procedures for observing and recording side effects:** The protocol should state how observations will be made, how side effects will be documented, and what will be done to treat participants who experience adverse effects. Patients are free to leave trials at any time, and this fact should be explained in the protocol and informed consent.
- **Informed consent:** Every clinical and community trial must be approved by the institutional review board (IRB). The IRB reviews all human research studies to make sure that participants are protected and that all procedures within the trial are ethical and appropriate for the subjects. (See chapter 14 for additional information about IRBs.)
- **Analysis of data:** Once data are collected, they should be analyzed by calculating the RR, survival analysis, number needed to treat (NNT), and tests of significance.
- **Dissemination of results:** Results may be provided before the study is completed if the preliminary findings establish that the medication or other intervention has substantial effects, such as improving disease outcomes or causing harm. The possibility of stopping the trial and providing the intervention to both groups must be considered if the outcomes of treatment are shown to be beneficial. After the study is completed, results should be disseminated to both the experimental and control groups, and further treatment options may be discussed as well. (Dissemination is further discussed in chapter 15.)

Types of Clinical Trials

The many different types of clinical trials include treatment, prevention, diagnostic, screening, and quality-of-life (QOL) trials.

- Treatment trials test experimental treatments, new combinations of medicines, and various types of surgery, radiation therapy, or chemotherapy. For example, researchers at the University of Washington are examining carpal tunnel syndrome and upper extremity pain in a randomized controlled trial (RCT) that compares surgical and nonsurgical treatments for patients with early, mild to moderate carpal tunnel syndrome. This study will also evaluate the ability of a new magnetic resonance imaging (MRI) technique to predict who can benefit from carpel tunnel surgery (University of Washington 2016).

- **Prevention trials** aim to prevent disease in a person who has never had the disease or to prevent it from advancing or recurring. These types of trials may use vitamins, diet, vaccines, medications, or lifestyle changes such as smoking cessation or exercise. For example, the goal of the Alzheimer's Disease Prevention trial sponsored by the National Institute on Aging (NIA) was to determine whether estrogen use can prevent memory loss and Alzheimer's disease in women with a family history of Alzheimer's disease (NIA 2010). Each clinical trial has inclusion and exclusion criteria. For example, for the Alzheimer's Disease Prevention trial, the inclusion criteria included all healthy women age 65 years or older with a family history of memory problems who were not currently on estrogen. Exclusion criteria for this study included significant neurologic impairment, current estrogen use, and history of breast cancer. History of breast cancer was excluded because estrogen use is a risk factor for breast cancer, and the researchers would not want to provide estrogen to women who have had breast cancer because it might lead to a recurrence (NIA 2010).
- **Diagnostic trials** are conducted to find better tests, procedures, or screenings to detect a disease or condition. For example, one diagnostic trial sponsored by the Rabin Medical Center in Israel plans to examine prostate cancer screening methods among men with high-risk genetic predisposition. This trial is currently recruiting participants and is looking for men between the ages of 40 and 70 years with the BRCA1 or BRCA2 gene. All candidates for the study who meet the inclusion criteria will undergo several tests including PSA, MRI of prostate, and a prostate biopsy. The goal of this diagnostic trial is to estimate the prevalence, stage and grade of prostate cancer; assess the impact the BRCA1 and BRCA2 gene mutations have on benign prostatic hypertrophy (BPH); and build a urine, serum, and tissue bank that can be used for future research (Rabin Medical Center 2016).
- **Screening trials** examine the best method to detect diseases or health conditions. A trial run by VeraLight Inc. compared screening methods for early evidence of diabetes that might be an improvement over existing screening methods, which are inconvenient and inaccurate. The researchers examined the accuracy of a new device called SCOUT which detects HbA1c in screening persons for pre-diabetes or diabetes by comparing it to the reference standard screening test (fasting plasma glucose) (VeraLight Inc. 2012).
- **Quality-of-life (QOL) trials** explore methods used to improve comfort and the QOL for individuals, such as people with a chronic disease or disability. For example, a QOL trial run by the University of Bergen tested COSMOS (COmmunication Systematic pain assessment and treatment, Medication review, Occupational therapy, and Safety), a practical intervention that aimed to improve clinical and psychiatric challenges, in nursing home patients in Norway. The goal of this study was to determine whether COSMOS improved QOL in nursing home residents while also reducing healthcare costs (University of Bergen 2014).

Phases of Clinical Trials

Most clinical trials are categorized as phase I, II, III, or IV based on the size of the population and the intervention being tested. The Food and Drug Administration (FDA) provides guidelines for the different types of clinical trials. According to the FDA, **Phase I clinical trials** usually test a new drug or treatment in a small group of people (20 to 100) for the first time to evaluate its safety, determine a safe dosage, and identify any side effects. **Phase II clinical trials** study the intervention in a larger group of people (100 to 300), and **Phase III clinical trials** study it in even larger groups of people (300 to 3,000) to confirm its effectiveness, monitor side effects, compare other treatments, and collect data to affirm that the drug or treatment can be used safely. **Phase IV clinical trials** are carried out after a drug or device has been approved by the FDA; these postmarket safety monitoring studies collect additional information after the drug has been marketed, such as the drug's risks, benefits, and optimal use (FDA 2016).

Clinical and Community Trial Applications in Health Informatics

The principles relative to clinical and community trials can be used when examining health information systems, such as mobile apps. For example, a clinical trial at Massachusetts General Hospital will study whether a mobile app with cognitive behavioral therapy (CBT) exercises could decrease anxiety levels of patients with terminal cancer when compared to an online health education program. The HAM-A (Hamilton Anxiety Rating Scale) will be used at baseline and then after the intervention to determine participants' anxiety levels before and after the intervention (Massachusetts General Hospital 2016).

Statistical Analysis

Statistical analysis used in clinical trials may include RR, survival analysis, or basic statistics such as the gain in a specific score from before the intervention to after the intervention. **Survival analysis**, also called life table analysis, examines survival of study subjects over time and compares whether the intervention group survived longer than the control group. It can be used when subjects are lost from follow-up because it accounts for those subjects who withdrew from the study before it was completed. Survival curves are developed to estimate survival over time between the two groups.

Epidemiological Models of Causation

Epidemiologists use models of potential influences that affect disease occurrence. Two models of disease occurrence have evolved from epidemiology: the infectious disease model and the chronic disease model. These models will be described in more detail as well as the epidemiological models of causation in health informatics.

Infectious Disease Model

As shown in figure 5.8, the **infectious disease model** demonstrates how infectious disease is influenced by three factors: the agent, the host and the environment.

The **agent** of the disease is the cause of the disease. Examples include the following:

- Nutritional agents (deficiencies in calcium or overabundance of saturated fat)
- Chemical agents (lead, pesticides, and medications)
- Physical agents (noise, vibration, hot or cold temperatures)
- Infectious agents (bacteria, viruses, and so forth)

When studying agents, researchers consider factors such as the severity of the disease or illness, the speed in which the disease multiplies within the host, the capability of the agent to cause disease, and antibody production within the host.

Figure 5.8 Infectious disease model

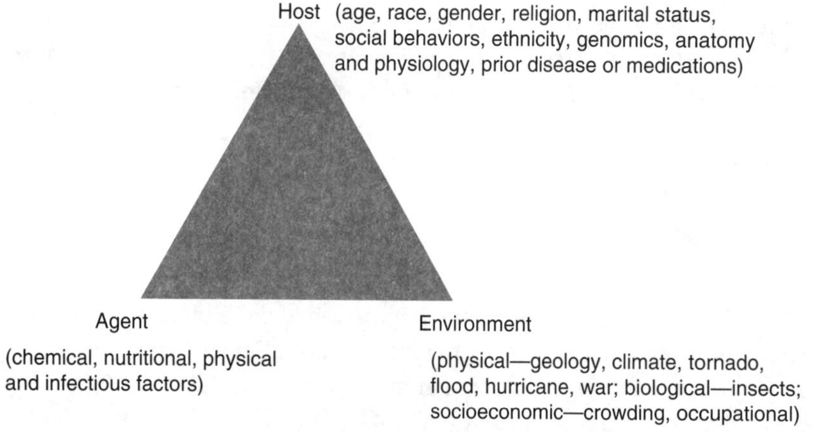

Source: Adapted from Gordis 2004; Lilienfeld and Stolley 1994; CDC 2012.

The **host** is the person who has the disease. Anything that influences disease development or immunity is considered a host factor—including age, gender, race, religion, marital status, family history or genetics, ethnicity, anatomy and physiology, social behaviors, and prior illness or chronic disease. The host is affected by its resistance to the agent and by the agent's portal of entry into the body (for example, intact skin or open wound).

The **environment** of the host and agent includes the physical environment as well as environmental influences such as disasters (tornado, flood, hurricane, war), crowding, neighborhood density, housing, and workplace conditions. Epidemiologists often seek to identify environmental factors that can expose hosts to disease agents. For example, people in areas with a large deer population may be at higher risk of contracting Lyme disease because the ticks that cause the disease are spread by deer; similarly, in certain regions of the world, people living near open water may have a greater risk of contracting West Nile virus or the Zika virus because the mosquitoes that spread these viruses breed in open water (Gordis 2004, 16; Lilienfeld and Stolley 1994, 37–38).

Chronic Disease Model

One risk factor may not lead to disease, but the combination of several may increase a person's chance of contracting a chronic disease. Therefore, the **chronic disease model** (shown in figure 5.9) demonstrates that a mix of factors may increase risk for a chronic disease, and that the presence of multiple factors over a long period of time may also increase risk of chronic disease (Schlomo and Kuh 2002, 286). For example, by applying the model to chronic lung disease (figure 5.10), it is apparent that multiple factors influence disease development (ALA 2016).

Figure 5.9 Chronic disease model

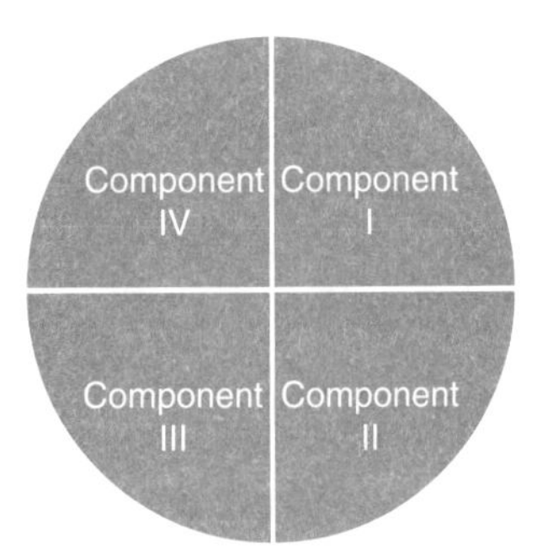

Source: Adapted from Gordis 2004 and Lilienfeld and Stolley 1994.

Figure 5.10 Application of chronic disease model to chronic lung disease

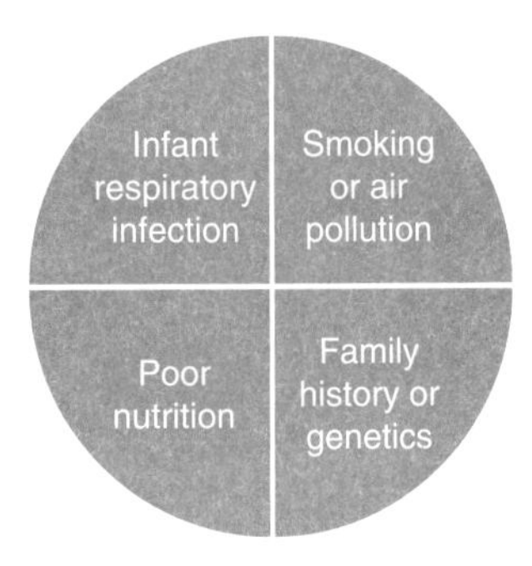

Source: Adapted from ALA 2016.

Using Epidemiological Models of Causation in Health Informatics

Epidemiological models of causation can be used as a logical framework for examining concepts within health informatics. For example, as can be seen in figure 5.11, the infectious disease model may help a researcher evaluate coding professionals' resistance to computer-assisted coding (CAC) systems. What agent is causing the resistance? Is the computer-based system capable of accurate coding? Is the system user-friendly, or is it easier for the coding professional to perform the coding manually? How is the host (the coding professional) responding to the agent, and why? Is the response related to the level of the host's experience, amount of training, and understanding of the system? Does the environment aid in the use of the CAC system, or does incomplete documentation in the electronic health record (EHR) hamper the CAC's ability to code correctly?

Figure 5.11 Application of the infectious disease model to users' resistance to computer-assisted coding (CAC)

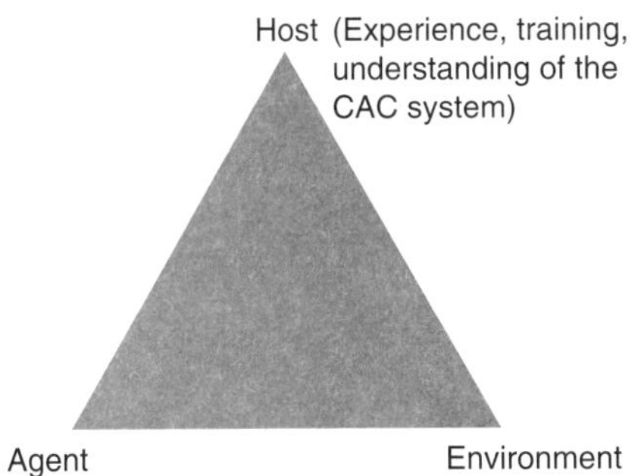

The chronic disease model can be used to evaluate what factors may be affecting outcomes associated with a health information technology (HIT) application. For example, as seen in figure 5.12, the chronic disease model could be used to examine why certain individuals do not use a personal health record (PHR). There may be a combination of reasons why the PHR is not used, and determining which combination of reasons may help advance efforts to attract more individuals to use one.

Figure 5.12 Application of the chronic disease model to patients' reluctance to use personal health records

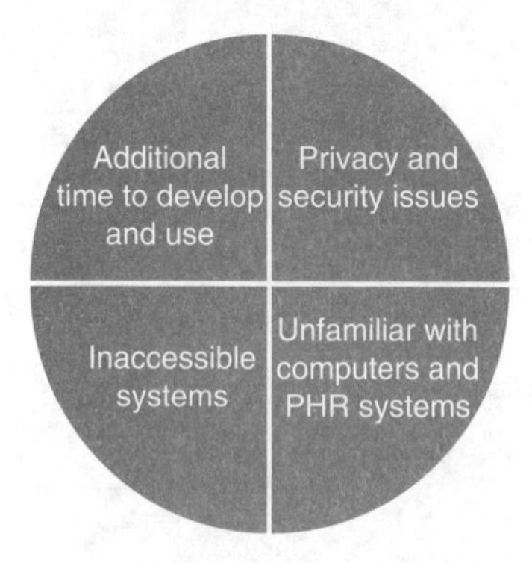

Rules of Evidence for Causality

In order to provide evidence that a causal association between a variable and an outcome is exhibited, the nine rules of evidence should be observed. The researcher does not need all nine rules to support causality, but it helps to have most of them for final results of the epidemiological study:

- **Strength of association:** The strength of the association is measured by the RR. A strong RR is important, and those greater than 2 are effective to show causality. However, repeated findings of weak RRs may be of equal importance if they are found in studies with reliable methodology.
- **Consistency of the observed association:** Consistency of the observed association includes confirmation of results in many different types of epidemiological studies in different populations and different settings.
- **Specificity:** A one-to-one relationship between an independent variable and a dependent variable, or between the exposure and the disease is necessary to add weight to claims of causality. However, because some exposures may lead to many different adverse outcomes, it may not be possible to establish specificity. In these cases, the lack of specificity does not mean an association cannot be causal.
- **Temporality:** The independent variable must precede the dependent variable, not follow it. For example, to state that clinical decision support systems decrease medical errors, the use of the decision support system must precede the development of the medical error. Sometimes, the temporal sequence is not easy to determine. A prospective study design can help support this rule.
- **Dose-response relationship:** As the dose of the independent or exposure variable changes, the response (the dependent variable such as incidence of a disease) should change in a corresponding manner. For example, epidemiological research studies have shown that dose and duration of smoking cigarettes increase risk of disease. In health informatics, to test whether clinical reminder systems for colonoscopy reduce the incidence of new cases of colon cancer, one could design a study to see whether increased use or more widespread use of the reminder system was associated with more colonoscopies and few cases of colon cancer, or whether the implementation of clinical reminders for another type of cancer screening showed similar effects to those observed when the reminders about colonoscopies were introduced.
- **Biological plausibility:** The relationship found in a study must make sense in relation to what is known about that association in the sciences, animal experiments, and so forth.
- **Experimental evidence:** A well-conducted RCT may confirm the causal relationship between an independent variable and a dependent variable.
- **Coherence:** The association should be in accordance with other factors known about the disease.

- **Analogy:** If similar associations have demonstrated causality, that makes it more likely this association is also causal. (Lilienfeld and Stolley 1994)

The rules of evidence for causality provide a guideline that health informatics professionals can use when determining whether their work or someone else's meets the rigors of proving whether a specific attribute leads to an outcome. It is very important to meet all the nine rules to say that the evidence indicates cause and effect. This was demonstrated when researchers found evidence that smoking and secondhand smoke cause lung cancer and other pulmonary diseases, and the findings were used to justify public health changes such as bans on smoking in the workplace and other environments.

Review Questions

1. What are the major goals of epidemiologists?
2. How are epidemiology and health informatics related?
3. Which model of disease causation examines how combinations of risk factors influence the severity of illnesses?
4. What are four examples of the agent of disease?
5. What is the host and its associated factors?
6. Epidemiological models of causation can be used as a logical framework when examining concepts within health informatics. What is one example of this?
7. What are two examples of cross-sectional or prevalence studies used in health informatics?
8. What is an example of the historical-prospective study design in health informatics?
9. What are the steps in a clinical trial protocol? Summarize each step.
10. What are the nine rules of evidence for causality?

Application Exercises

1. Visit the Care First website (Staywell 2016) and take the Colorectal Cancer Risk Assessment to determine your risk of colon cancer. Then, answer the following questions:
   a. How do you think this risk assessment tool works?
   b. How does the risk assessment level or score compare to the relative risk?
   c. How does it compare to the odds ratio?
   d. Do you think this is a good risk assessment tool? Why or why not?
2. Describe how you would use one of the epidemiological study designs to assess a health informatics topic. Address the following areas:
   - Topic chosen
   - Epidemiological study design chosen
     - Cross-sectional study
     - Case-control study
     - Cohort study
     - Clinical trial
     - Community trial
3. Visit the Framingham Heart Study (NHLBI 2016) website and answer the following questions:
   a. Is the Framingham Heart Study an epidemiological study?
   b. What type of study design is used?
   c. What is the purpose of the study?
   d. Is the study currently being conducted?
   e. Which groups have been studied?

References

American Hospital Association (AHA). 2016. Hospitals advance information sharing, but external barriers to increased data exchange remain. *TrendWatch.* http://www.aha.org/research/reports/tw/16feb-tw-hitadoption.pdf.

American Lung Association (ALA). 2016. What Causes COPD. http://www.lung.org/lung-health-and-diseases/lung-disease-lookup/copd/symptoms-causes-risk-factors/what-causes-copd.html.

Bell, S.B., D.M. Daly, and P. Robinson. 2003. Is there a digital divide among physicians? A geographic analysis of information technology in southern California physician offices. *Journal of the American Medical Informatics Association* 10(5):484–493.

Centers for Disease Control and Prevention (CDC). 2012. Measures of risk. Lesson 3 in *Principles of Epidemiology in Public Health Practice: An Introduction to Applied Epidemiology and Biostatistics,* 3rd ed. https://www.cdc.gov/ophss/csels/dsepd/ss1978/lesson3/section2.html.

Friis, R.H. and T.A. Sellers. 2014. *Epidemiology for Public Health Practice.* Sudbury, MA: Jones and Bartlett Publishers.

Gordis, L. 2004. *Epidemiology.* Philadelphia, PA: Saunders.

Katoh, A., V.W. Watzlaf, and F. D'Amico.1994. An examination of obesity and breast cancer survival in postmenopausal women. *British Journal of Cancer* 70:928–933.

Lilienfeld, D.E. and P.D. Stolley. 1994. *Foundations of Epidemiology.* New York: Oxford University Press.

Linder, J.A., D.W. Bates, D.H. Williams, and M.A. Connoly. 2006. Acute infections in primary care: Accuracy of electronic diagnoses and electronic antibiotic prescribing. *Journal of the American Medical Informatics Association* 13(1):61–66.

Manson, J.E., F.B. Hu, J.W. Rich-Edwards, G.A. Colditz, M.J. Stampfer, W.C. Willett, F.E. Speizer, and C.H. Hennekens. 1999. A prospective study of walking as compared with vigorous exercise in the prevention of coronary heart disease in women. *New England Journal of Medicine* 341(9):650–658.

Massachusetts General Hospital. 2016. Mobile App of CBT for Anxiety and Cancer (clinical trial). Clinicaltrials.gov identifier: NCT02238652. https://clinicaltrials.gov/ct2/show/NCT02286466?term=clinical+trials+mobile+apps&rank=8.

National Institute on Aging (NIA). 2010. Alzheimer's Disease Prevention Trial. ClinicalTrials.gov identifier: NCT00000176. https://clinicaltrials.gov/ct2/show/NCT00000176?term=prevention+trial&rank=19.

Rabin Medical Center. Prostate Cancer Screening Among Men with High Risk Genetic Predisposition (clinical trial). 2016. ClinicalTrials.gov identifier: NCT02053805. https://clinicaltrials.gov/ct2/show/NCT02053805?term=diagnostic+trial&rank=8.

Schlomo, Y.B., and D. Kuh. 2002. A life course approach to chronic disease epidemiology: Conceptual models, empirical challenges, and interdisciplinary perspectives. *International Journal of Epidemiology* 31:285–293. http://arctichealth.oulu.fi/suomi/documents/Life-course_2.pdf.

Tierney, W., S. Alpert, A. Byrket, K. Caine, J. Leventhal, E. Meslin, and P. Schwartz. 2015. Provider responses to patients controlling access to their electronic health records: A Prospective cohort study in primary care. *Journal of General Internal Medicine* 30(1):31.

University of Bergen. 2014. Improving Quality of Life in Nursing Home Residents: A Cluster Randomized Clinical Trial of Efficacy (COSMOS). ClinicalTrials.gov Identifier: NCT02238652. https://clinicaltrials.gov/ct2/show/NCT02238652?term=quality+of+life+trials&rank=9.

University of Pittsburgh Medical Center (UPMC). 2015. Frequently Asked Questions About Research and Clinical Trials. http://www.upmccancercenter.com/research/faq.cfm.

University of Pittsburgh School of Health and Rehabilitation Sciences. 2016 (Spring). Health information management: A strong partnership reaps benefits for all. *Facets*, p.30.

University of Washington. 2016. Carpal Tunnel Syndrome: Diagnosis and Treatment Trial. https://clinicaltrials.gov/ct2/show/NCT00032227.

US Food and Drug Administration (FDA). 2016. http://www.fda.gov/forpatients/clinicaltrials/types/default.htm

VeraLight Inc. 2012. Screening for early evidence of diabetes (SEED) (clinical trial). ClinicalTrials.gov identifier: NCT00614783. https://clinicaltrials.gov/ct2/show/NCT00614783?term=screening+trials&rank=50.

Vinogradova Y., C. Coupland, and J. Hippisley-Cox. 2014. Exposure to combined oral contraceptives and risk of venous thromboembolism: A protocol for nested case-control studies using the QResearch and the CPRD databases. *BMJ Open* 4: e004499. doi:10.1136/bmjopen-2013-004499.

Vinogradova, Y., C. Coupland, and J. Hippisley-Cox. 2015. Use of combined oral contraceptives and risk of venous thromboembolism: Nested case-control studies using the QResearch and CPRD databases *BMJ* 350:h2135. doi: 10.1136/bmj.h2135.

Watzlaf, V.W. 1989. Is the medical record an effective epidemiological data source? *Proceedings of the National Center for Health Statistics Public Health Conference on Records and Statistics*. Washington, DC: National Center for Health Statistics: 57–60.

Watzlaf, V., A. Katoh, and F. D'Amico. 2002. Obesity and breast cancer recurrence: Obstacles/improvements in data capture and results. Paper presented at the AHIMA National Convention and Exhibit, San Francisco, CA, Sept. 21–26. http://bok.ahima.org/PdfView?oid=30733.

Resources

National Heart, Lung and Blood Institute (NHLBI). 2016. Framingham Heart Study. https://www.framinghamheartstudy.org.

Staywell. 2016. Colorectal cancer risk assessment. http://carefirst.staywellsolutionsonline.com/InteractiveTools/RiskAssessments/42,ColorectalCancerRisk.

6 Evaluation Methods

Jennifer Hornung Garvin, PhD, MBA, RHIA, CCS, CPHQ, CTR, FAHIMA

Learning Objectives

- Demonstrate appropriate use of terms related to evaluation methods and theory.
- Explain the rationale for conducting an evaluation or evaluation research.
- Apply evaluation or evaluation research methods to a scenario.
- Outline the steps in an evaluation of health information technology.

Key Terms

Complex adaptive system (CAS)
Cost-benefit analysis (CBA)
Cost-effectiveness analysis (CEA)
Evaluation methods
Five rights of clinical decision support
Formative evaluation
Impact evaluation
Implementation evaluation
Implementation science
Logic model
Needs assessment
Outcome evaluation
Process evaluation
Semistructured interview
Sociotechnical system
Stakeholders
Summative evaluation
System Usability Scale (SUS)
Theory of change
User-centered design

Evaluation methods are used to measure program activities and determine value of the program, to undertake quality improvement, and to contribute to generalizable scientific knowledge (Alkin 2011). Such methods are needed in both professional projects and evaluation research. When undertaking evaluation research (discussed in chapter 1) researchers use social science methods and a theoretic framework or model as part of exploratory or hypothesis-driven research. Evaluation research often uses experimental or quasi-experimental design so that the findings are generalizable. Credible data are systematically collected and analyzed to assess the worth of a product, service, technology, or process. The purpose of this chapter is to provide information about evaluation and evaluation research. Evaluation and evaluation research in health informatics and health information management (HIM) professionals are undertaken when health information technology (HIT) or new processes related to HIT are developed or implemented. Evaluation of any sort is multifaceted in healthcare because healthcare organizations are complex systems within which individuals continually adapt to evolving aspects of the healthcare system. Therefore, during the development of new HIT or processes, alignment with the intended purpose should be determined so that those impacted by its implementation will have the opportunity to influence development. It is also essential to assess the final product or process. To do these important tasks we develop an evaluation plan. Examples throughout and at the end of this chapter illustrate the evaluation and evaluation research processes.

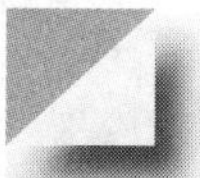

Real-World Case

Researchers have found an important gap in clinical care. Chronic systolic heart failure is a prevalent, resource-intensive condition. Patients with chronic systolic heart failure have better symptom management and improved cardiovascular outcomes when treated in accordance with the clinical guidelines (Yancy 2016). The use of evidence-based medications (in this case, beta blockers) at maximally tolerated doses can reduce morbidity and mortality. However, not all eligible patients are prescribed beta-blocker medications at guideline-recommended doses, perhaps because titration (a process of providing incrementally higher doses to the maximally tolerated dose for a given patient) is required. A clinical decision support process to titrate a patient to maximally tolerated doses is proposed using existing electronic health record (EHR) technology (Yancy 2016). It is possible to close the gap in clinical care through the use of HIT. Evaluation and evaluation research can be used to engage stakeholders in design and evaluation of HIT. Evaluation processes will measure the effectiveness of the HIT in achieving the goal of prompting the use of beta blocker medications and improving outcomes.

Evaluations in Health Informatics and Health Information Management

When health informatics and health information management (HIM) professionals develop or implement health information technology (HIT), or undertake new processes related to HIT, the system functions may require evaluation. Evaluation can be undertaken for many reasons, including quality improvement, return on investment, and research. For example, an evaluation may be needed to determine whether a given segment of the EHR is functioning as planned, evaluate the clinical stakeholders' perceived value of a new HIT component, or measure how HIT affects the efficiency of a process. In addition, health informatics and HIM professionals may conduct full-blown evaluation research to assess the effectiveness and safety of clinical decision support, clinical reminders, and other components of the EHR, or for other ends. The steps of the evaluation process are as follows:

1. **Learn about the organization, project, or HIT**—Gather information about how the process is undertaken or the purpose for the HIT.
2. **Identify stakeholders**—Determine who has funded the evaluation, who the beneficiaries are, and who will be involved in the development of the project or tool.
3. **Identify logic model elements**—Describe the outcomes and the preceding input and activities.
4. **Identify evaluation scope**—Describe what is included and what is excluded in the evaluation.
5. **Identify critical evaluation activities**—What are the evaluation questions and what activities should be undertaken in order to answer the questions?
6. **Clarify the role of the evaluator**—Determine who will undertake the evaluation activities and champion the resulting data.
7. **Clarify the evaluation plan**—Review and address the evaluation plan.
8. **Collect data**—Undertake the evaluation activities and collect the related data.
9. **Share and analyze the data**—Summarize the analysis of the evaluation results.
10. **Develop findings and final report**—Develop results with stakeholders and disseminate the final report.

Evaluation can take the several forms within two broad categories of formative and summative evaluation (Pell Institute 2016). Formative evaluation is undertaken to obtain feedback during development of projects or tools whereas summative evaluation takes place near the end of the project or after it is complete to provide information about how well the project met its goals. Stakeholders are key individuals who will be involved in the evaluation and may be the funders or the recipients of the project or tool. Evaluation projects do not involve human subjects but establish value to the stakeholders. Evaluation research involves exploration or hypothesis-driven research with the subsequent development of generalizable findings. Both evaluation projects and evaluation research can address similar topics and use similar social science methods. The most important difference between an evaluation project and evaluation research is the need in research to protect human subjects. These topics will be discussed in more detail in the sections that follow.

Formative Evaluation

Formative evaluation measures or assesses improvement in delivery methods with regard to technology used; quality of implementation of a new process or technology; information about the organizational placement of a given process; type of personnel involved in a program; or other important factors such as the procedures, source, and type of inputs. It occurs during the program cycle as the stakeholders or end-users provide feedback about how to further develop the system, software, or process. This feedback is used to adjust the process or the software to achieve the goals of the project. For example, formative evaluation could be used to determine whether a clinical decision support process using existing EHR technology works as it was expected to when it was proposed. The project team could use design principles that are known to be effective to design a clinical decision prototype using existing functionality within the EHR. The team could also develop a draft set of test patients and use the prototype with stakeholders, the primary care providers, for their review and feedback. The project team could then incorporate feedback into the design of the clinical decision support.

The types of formative evaluation include needs assessment, implementation evaluation, and process evaluation. A **needs assessment** determines organizational goals and gaps between the actual state and the desired state. It also identifies the parties that need resources and what kinds of resources are needed. Needs assessment can be undertaken to align programs, software development, and new processes with the desired goals of the organization. **Implementation evaluation** is used to examine the fidelity of the actual program delivery as compared to the planned delivery; that is, how well the planned events are actually occurring and whether the implementation is meeting the expected time frames. **Process evaluation**, which focuses on the operational aspects of the project, is used to determine how well the project was carried out.

Summative Evaluation

Summative evaluation occurs at or near the end of the project or research and is undertaken to assess effectiveness of the program. Two kinds of summative evaluation are outcome evaluation and impact evaluation. **Outcome evaluation** assesses whether the specifically defined target outcomes were demonstrated. **Impact evaluation** assesses the overall effects of the program or software implementation in terms of the larger organization, community, or system. Cost-effectiveness analysis and cost-benefit analysis (CBA), two components of summative evaluation, address questions of efficient use of resources to achieve goals within the constraints of cost (Pell Institute 2016). **Cost-effectiveness analysis (CEA)** compares the costs to the outcomes of various courses of action. According to the CDC, "CEA is best used when comparing two or more strategies or interventions that have the same health outcome in the same population—such as is vaccination more cost-effective than chemoprophylaxis in prevention of a case of influenza in people aged 65 or older?" (CDC 2013). A **cost-benefit analysis (CBA)** weighs the inputs (cost) to the outcome (benefit) of a program, showing strengths and weaknesses from an institutional or societal perspective; to conduct a CBA correctly, all costs and benefits must be placed in a common value (CDC 2013).

Stakeholders

While planning an evaluation, the researcher will identify key stakeholders and critically think through the project to identify what they value, decide how to measure this value, and communicate the value and be accountable to stakeholders (NSW Department of Environment and Conservation 2004). **Stakeholders** in evaluation projects and evaluation research include the recipients of the product, service, technology, or process being evaluated as well as participants in the evaluation. Operationally, the primary stakeholders are individuals who make decisions, have requested or commissioned the evaluation, and those who will use the evaluation results; these people will be intimately involved in the evaluation process (Alkin 2011).

Evaluation Projects versus Evaluation Research

The distinction between evaluation used for a work project, such as quality improvement or return on investment, and evaluation research that requires approval from an institutional review board (IRB) depends on the motivation and approach to the analysis as well as the intended application of the results. (Chapter 14 discusses IRBs in detail.) In some circumstances, evaluation may be considered quality improvement, or an analysis of the return on investment of a project or process, rather than research. Work projects requiring evaluation are common in health IT and health informatics. For example, the following all require evaluation of some sort:

- Implementation or redesign of EHRs
- Design or modification of software components
- Development of programs and processes that are associated with health IT
- Leading or participating in teams

If the intent of the work project is to improve care processes or demonstrate financial benefit, the evaluation generally does not constitute research. However, if the objective of the evaluation is to gain generalizable knowledge or to formally compare two processes using experimental methods, especially when the processes involve human subjects, then the study probably meets the definition of research. In these cases, the study requires IRB review to determine whether it is human subjects research (Baily et al. 2006, 11). Additionally, all proposed projects that are intended to be published should be submitted to the IRB to determine whether the project constitutes research as IRB certification of human subject or nonhuman subject research may be required by the journal. Both the institutional policy of the organization conducting the research and the source of the funding should be considered in this determination because an organization or funding agency can impose additional requirements for what needs reviewed by the IRB.

Evaluation Research

Like other forms of research, evaluation research begins with a theoretic framework and the development of a hypothesis. Using the real-world case example to improve beta-blocker medication titration, the development team could use clinical evidence from practice guidelines, essentially a form of evidence-based medicine to prompt titration. Before the researchers begin to develop scientific methods, they must formulate their questions about prompting for beta-blocker titration. Identifying scientific gaps helps researchers determine what questions they should seek to answer. Gaps in the existing research are usually found by undertaking a literature review. Once the focus of research is determined, researchers should select a theoretic framework or model suited to the variables under study.

Identifying Scientific Gaps

In the real-world case example, researchers determined there was a gap in care based on the evidence in clinical guidelines and the actual dosages of medication provided to patients. The first step in determining this gap was to search the scientific literature to learn about whether or not there was descriptive research about the beta blocker dosages patients were prescribed. The descriptive research found that the study data reflected that the average dose of beta blocker medication was lower than recommended by guidelines. Once a gap in care is identified, the researchers should review the scientific literature once again to determine if any interventions have successfully improved medication titration. The researchers should investigate whether any health information technology, for example decision support, might be helpful to improve titration. Similarly we will identify a theoretic framework or model that helps us to design our technology.

Identifying a Theoretic Framework

Once a literature review is undertaken and the gap in the scientific area of study is the process or the HIT is understood, the concepts related to the area of study can be matched to a model, framework, or scientific theory that can be used to guide the research design. The research may be exploratory or hypothesis driven. The theoretic framework assists in determining what concepts are relevant to observe, measure, describe or are predictive of outcomes.

One theoretic framework that could be used is the Promoting Action on Research Implementation in Health Services (PARIHS) framework, which is related to **implementation science**, a discipline that studies how and why implementation of evidence in clinical practice succeeds or fails (Nilsen 2015). The PARIHS framework focuses on three main domains: evidence, context, and facilitation (Kitson 2008, 1). Evidence-based medicine is the use of the best research evidence in caring for individual patients. Levels of evidence range from 1 (the best evidence) to 4 and are determined based on the type of research that generates the evidence comes from. Implementation science frameworks can be used to study how well the evidence is adopted in clinical practice. The PARIHS framework is helpful to the design of HIT because it emphasizes studying the context of use of evidence as well as barriers and facilitators of the use of the evidence. The use of clinical decision support is a facilitator of adoption and uptake of evidence (Goldstein 2008). Another framework that could be used is the Health Belief Model (HBM). This model, which explains and predicts health behaviors, consists of concepts such as perceived barriers and perceived benefits among others (University of Twente 2016). Using the real-world case as an example, a research hypothesis could be developed; for instance, more patients will receive beta-blocker titration when a clinical reminder that considers clinical context is used compared to patients whose providers use a clinical reminder without clinical context. Or, using the HBM to generate a hypothesis, when a provider perceives a benefit to beta blockers, they will prescribe them to patients.

Once the researchers find a theoretic framework or model, they begin to develop their research methods.

Healthcare Organizations as Complex Adaptive Systems

As described earlier in the chapter, evaluation in healthcare is complex and dynamic. Research shows that a healthcare organization is a **complex adaptive system (CAS)**, which is defined as an entity with many diverse and autonomous components or parts (called *agents*) that are interrelated and interdependent with many interconnections. The component parts behave as a unified whole in learning from experience and in adjusting to changes in the environment. Each agent maintains itself in an environment that it creates through its interactions with other agents (McDaniel 2009). In order to identify the relevant stakeholders, study the concepts of importance to the evaluation, and control for confounding (if applicable), knowing the characteristics of a CAS that may need to be studied is necessary. Healthcare organizations have the following characteristics of a CAS:

- **Diverse agents that learn**—For example, providers, patients, and other stakeholders
- **Nonlinear interdependencies**—The concept that if small changes are made in the system, this may or may not result in a change at the system level, which reduces predictability about system outcomes (Kannampallil 2011)
- **Self-organization**—A process by which a pattern emerges based on the interaction of the components (Prokopenko 2009)
- **Emergence**—A process in which patterns arise from the system based on the individual agents as well as the specific interactions undertaken within the system (Kaisler and Madey 2008)
- **Coevolution**—The concept that both the system and the agent evolve (McDaniel 2009)

As the real-world case suggests, HIT functions and processes, such as information governance, EHRs, computer-assisted coding, clinical decision support, and computerized patient order entry form a **sociotechnical system** within the larger CAS that is the healthcare organization. Therefore, when researchers evaluate or undertake evaluation research about how well implementation of HIT or projects work, they must evaluate the sociotechnical components of the CAS because healthcare providers, patients, and other "agents" may have different skills and interactions at one point in time compared to another because their work in a CAS causes them to be in a dynamic state of change (McDaniel 2009).

Sittig and Singh have created a sociotechnical model of HIT that provides a framework we can use to study specific aspects of the technology to determine how well it is working from a safety standpoint (2010). They describe eight dimensions that address "challenges involved in design, development, implementation, use, and evaluation of HIT within complex adaptive healthcare systems"(Sittig and Singh 2010):

- **Hardware and software**—The computing infrastructure as well as the software used in patient care and the ancillary aspects of healthcare
- **Clinical content**—The data that is contained within the application
- **Human-computer (user) interface**—What the end-users of the application can see and touch
- **People**—Anyone who interacts with the application from developer to end-user
- **Workflow and communication**—The essential processes for carrying out patient care
- **Internal organizational features**—Policies, procedures, organizational culture, and so on
- **External rules and regulations**—For example, changes in clinical guidelines or reimbursement policies
- **Measuring and monitoring**—Processes to evaluate the use of the system, including how well use of it achieves the intended goals and whether there are unintended consequences of use as well (Sittig and Singh 2013)

As depicted in figure 1.1 in chapter 1, these eight dimensions identify aspects of HIT that can be evaluated to learn what is working well and what could be improved. These evaluation findings can be used to iteratively revise software, processes, or components of the HIT to improve the safety of either the *use* of the technology or the *technology* itself.

The sociotechnical dimensions of HIT diagrammed in figure 1.1 can be used to design HIT that increases the use of optimal doses of beta blockers to treat patients with chronic heart failures. For example, a group of primary care providers (PCPs) may want to have electronic access to specific kinds of patient data, such as the ejection fraction (a measurement of the percentage of blood leaving the heart each time it contracts) and current medications with dosages. When the evaluation project team engages providers to undertake a formative evaluation of the tools, they may also request clinical guidelines and a set of steps to assess the patient for safe titration as part of the clinical content for the reminder. In this example, the project team may evaluate the hardware and software in their healthcare organization in terms of the EHR functionality to determine how this data could be captured and delivered to the PCPs through existing mechanisms. The team may also develop an evaluation of the human-computer interface to determine if the clinical reminder has embedded decision support similar to other clinical reminders, and therefore will be familiar in format to the PCPs. The team would need to identify everyone who would interface with the clinical reminder and engage them as stakeholders. The internal organizational features of the healthcare organization may require modification to allow PCPs to refer patients, via a consult order, to clinical pharmacists if titration of the beta-blocker doses proved difficult. Both the project team and the providers would likely be aware of the external clinical guidelines that described the optimal doses of beta blockers. The project team could then set up a surveillance system to monitor any emergency department visits and unexpected admissions that were related to the beta-blocker titration process in patients with heart failure. They could also developed a theory of change (as discussed in the next section) and an evaluation plan.

Using Design Principles for Health Information Technology

When evaluating HIT, it is important to determine whether good design principles are present. User-centered design relates to the human-computer interface dimension of the sociotechnical model described above. Research has identified principles to guide safe, effective and user-friendly HIT development. An overview of several key design principles is provided in this section. Additional study of these areas is encouraged, as it will further develop the reader's expertise in design. Some of the stated principles are specific to a given kind of HIT, such as clinical decision support, but they can potentially be generalized to other kinds of HIT. For example, it is always important to include the "five rights" in any design and implementation when applicable. User-centered design is also vital to evaluate. If HIT is user centered, it will align with workflow and the tasks undertaken by the person using it.

The Five Rights of Clinical Decision Support

The **five rights of clinical decision support** states that optimal design and implementation of clinical decision support will be achieved if the system provides (1) the right information (2) to the right person, (3) in the right format, (4) through the right channel, and (5) at the right time in the workflow. To determine what the right information is, who the right person is, what the right format is, what the right channel is, and what the right time is, a multidisciplinary project team will need to study the clinical process and determine how to fulfill the rights. The "five rights" are essentially a framework for formative evaluation for HIT. We can use them to examine whether we have all the information, stakeholders, and processes required to develop and implement a well-designed product, service, technology, or process that fulfills the "five rights." Following planning, design, and prototype development, it is important to test the design with those who will use it, not only to inform further development but also to determine if the design is user-centered (Sirajuddin 2009).

User-Centered Design

User-centered design is founded on an "explicit understanding of users, tasks, and environments; is driven and refined by user-centered evaluation; and addresses the whole user experience" (HHS 2017a). To help focus evaluation efforts related to HIT, this section provides an overview of general guidelines for user-centered design. Figure 6.1 depicts the iterative nature of developing HIT. First, designers have an innovative design but before it can be created, users are studied, the use case for the HIT is defined, and then a prototype is designed. This is followed by a formative evaluation and finally a validation or summative evaluation process is undertaken with end users. This cycle provides a method to develop HIT with good design principals.

Figure 6.1 User-centered design

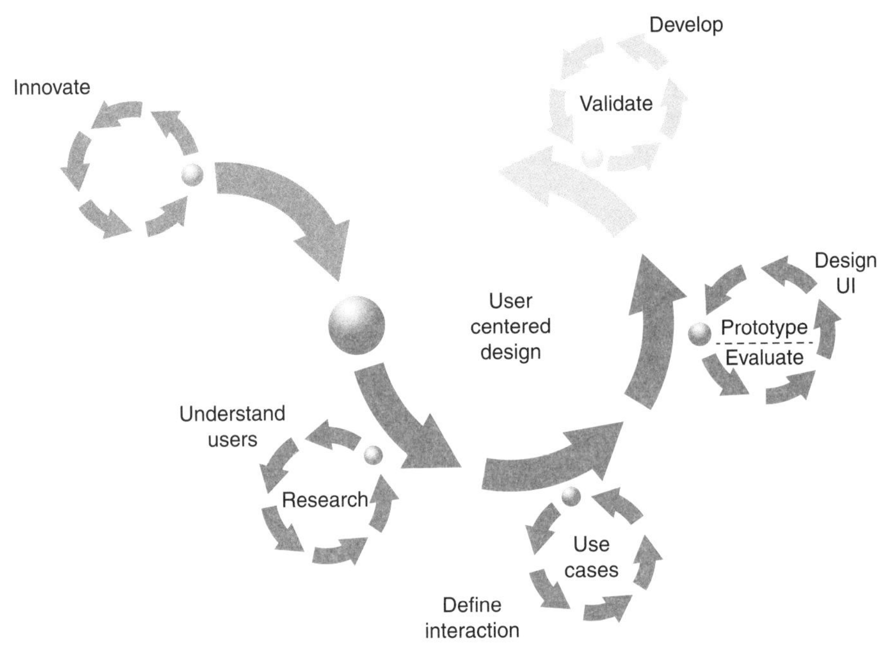

Source: Creately 2016.

Above all, the healthcare-related product, service, technology, or process should be designed for the users and their tasks. Therefore, a new or existing system should be task-oriented. Additionally, there should be consistency of the design elements among components of the system. The language and terminology should be simple and familiar to the user. The user should be able to focus on the task rather than how to interact with the computer or new system, so simplicity and transparency of use are important. The user should know whether their actions are successful, and feedback to this end should be provided. The user must have information about how to navigate the system; this aspect of user-centered design is commonly accomplished by providing familiar mechanisms, such as scroll bars and titles to windows. Similarly, it must be clear how to exit the program. As a whole, user-centered design empowers the users to easily, quickly, and accurately select the information in the sequence they need to support the task (Usabilitynet 2006).

Usability tools can measure how user-centered a system is. For example, the **System Usability Scale (SUS)** is a 10-item questionnaire that measures usability of products and services based on the respondents' Likert-scale responses indicating their level of agreement with the questions; these scores are then converted to numbers (HHS 2017b). The SUS is shown in figure 6.2. Despite its complex scoring system, the SUS is used frequently because it is simple for participants to use yet informative. In healthcare, the tool is used by having participants use a type of HIT, such as software, an EHR or personal health record, or a clinical reminder. Following the use of the technology under evaluation, the participants would complete the SUS. Once the evaluation team scores the SUSs, the findings can potentially inform a modification in the design.

Figure 6.2 The System Usability Scale

1. I think that I would like to use this system frequently.
2. I found the system unnecessarily complex.
3. I thought the system was easy to use.
4. I think that I would need the support of a technical person to be able to use this system.
5. I found the various functions in this system were well integrated.
6. I thought there was too much inconsistency in this system.
7. I would imagine that most people would learn to use this system very quickly.
8. I found the system very cumbersome to use.
9. I felt very confident using the system.
10. I needed to learn a lot of things before I could get going with this system.

Source: HHS 2017b.

Continuing with the real-world case example, the project team observed primary care clinicians to determine what information they look for in a patient's record when determining if the patient can be safely titrated with beta-blocker medication. The team made notes about the information and the location in the record. Based on discussion with the clinicians, the team determined with the clinician stakeholders that the best time in the workflow to deliver the information to the clinician was when he or she initially opened a new note for the patient visit in primary care. The team developed a prototype that it used with several primary care clinicians and tested the system to validate the accuracy of the information delivered to the providers. When a final iteration of the prototype was created, the five clinicians were identified as evaluation participant stakeholders. They were asked to use the clinical reminder during a simulated patient care visit and then were asked the SUS questions.

Development of an Evaluation Plan

When developing an evaluation plan, the complex nature of healthcare processes that are undertaken within a sociotechnical system should be considered. Further, most processes must be user centered in order for people to want to use them. At the beginning of an evaluation, it is important to develop and summarize the theory of change, evaluation questions, and data collection and evaluation activities to create an evaluation plan.

Theory of Change

The first step in developing an evaluation plan is to establish the **theory of change**, a statement that explains how activities will produce a series of results (Rogers 2014). This theory is not a scientific theory but rather a description of what the intended goal is and what needs to occur to achieve the intended goal. It is important to write a theory of change statement and develop a diagram depicting the resources and activities that will result in the output, effects, or results. The diagram can be in the form of a **logic model** (a graphic representation of the logic of how things work), or a simpler diagram of the sequence of the activities can be used. Figure 6.3 shows a sample diagram. In the figure, *inputs* and *resources* describe what will be included to obtain the overall goal as well as any barriers or constraints; *activities* describe what will be done with the resources or constraints; *outputs* are any available evidence that the activities were undertaken as intended; and *effects* are the results of the activities and resources as well as consequences, outcomes and impact of the efforts (University of Kansas Workgroup for Community Health and Development 2016).

Figure 6.3 Diagram template for theory of change

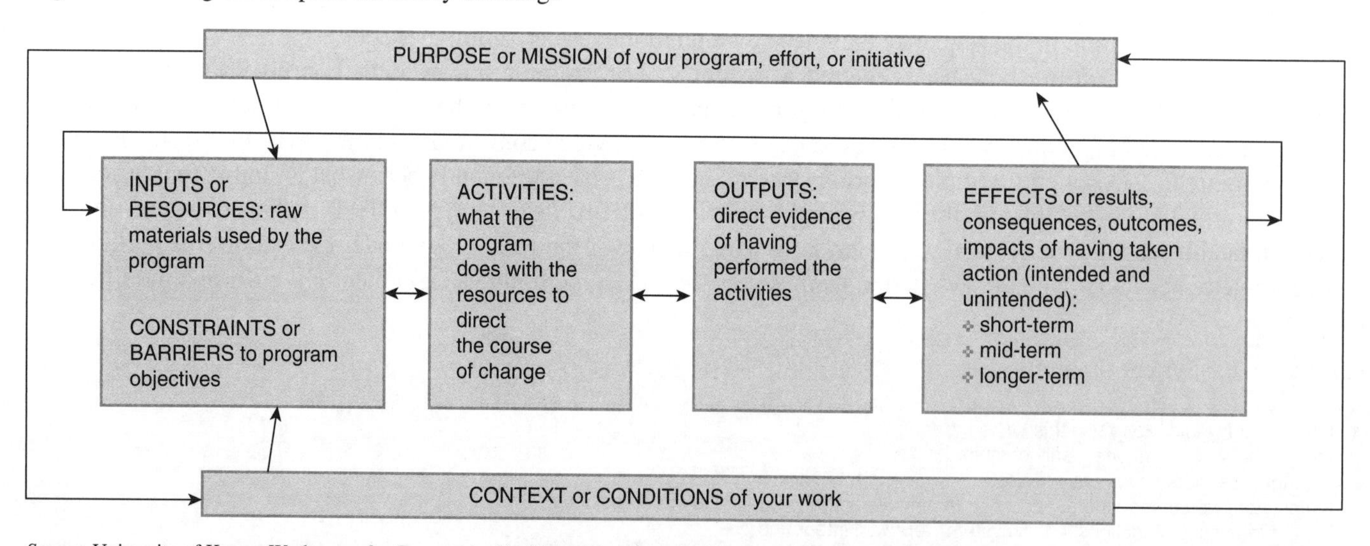

Source: University of Kansas Workgroup for Community Health and Development 2016. Reprinted with permission.

Returning to the example of beta blocker titration, the theory of change would be developed by working with stakeholders. A project team could create an initiative to increase the use of optimal doses of beta-blocker medication. A hypothetical theory of change in this scenario is "By developing a well-designed clinical reminder to guide decision support and clinical tasks, we will be able to increase in the number of patients on optimal doses of beta blocker medications." The team could also diagram the theory of change as a logic model, an example of which is shown in figure 6.4. The logic model depicts the input, activities, output, and outcomes in the project.

Figure 6.4 Logic model for beta-blocker project

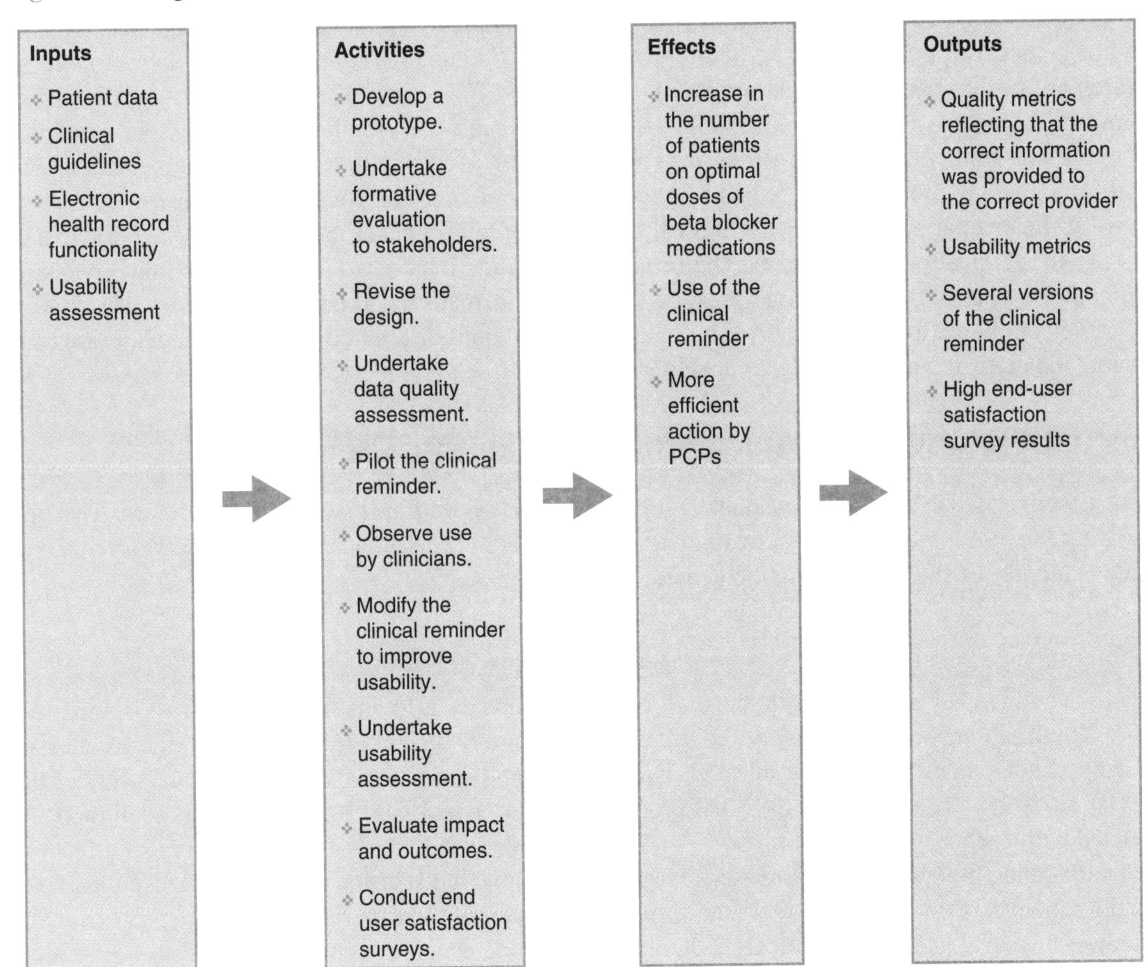

Evaluation Questions

Questions should be developed to guide the evaluation. The questions should be identified and answered based on the logic models and the critical activities. The data to be collected will need to answer these key questions and allow for the assessment of important aspects of the project. For example, evaluation questions about the development and implementation of a clinical reminder to prompt titration could be as follows:

- Were clinically relevant data and resources provided to PCPs to assist in setting optimal doses of beta-blocker medications for each eligible patient?
- Was the patient information provided at the right time in the clinical workflow?
- Did titration occur without adverse unintended consequences to the patient?
- Were the "five rights" present during the formative evaluation?
- Did the HIT incorporate good user centered design principals?

Evaluation Data Collection and Activities

Once the evaluation questions are determined, procedures are established to collect the data required to answer them. Quantitative and qualitative data can be collected through a variety of methods, including cross-sectional surveys, observation, semistructured interviews, focus groups, simulation, and analysis of existing data. The process of data collection should be feasible and the data accessible for collection. Cross-sectional surveys are used to capture information about a particular period in time, whereas observations ideally take place at multiple points in time. For example, the evaluator may want to determine how many times a provider has to search for information in another part of the medical record to obtain data about a patient. The purpose of observing and the data to be collected would be determined in advance.

A **semistructured interview** is undertaken by determining the research questions that we want to answer though the interview; it follows a guide but allows additional questions that seem appropriate or that are triggered by the participants' comments. Focus groups consist of purposefully assembled groups of individuals to whom questions related to a topic of evaluation or research are posed. For both semistructured interviews and focus groups, the interviews are recorded, with notes, audio-recording, or both. To undertake a simulation, evaluators can use a simulation laboratory or develop a prototype of the HIT to use in a simulated environment or in a simulated clinical care setting. Often, there is data that has already been collected for a given purpose. It may be possible to use the data to answer evaluation questions.

For example, to answer the evaluation questions listed for the titration of beta-blocker medication project, the evaluation team could observe the clinical processes, assess the possible EHR functionality to support the clinical decision support process, develop prototypes of the clinical reminder, and undertake formative evaluation through use of a clinical test script simulating patient care with the prototype. Additionally, the SUS could be applied during formative evaluation of iterative development, and after the final reminder is developed.

Examples of Evaluation Research Studies from the Scientific Literature

The following sections describe two examples of evaluation research studies found in the scientific literature. The first study evaluated the coding process to determine where sources of error occur. The second describes research related to clinical alerts. Both are examples of studies that provide generalizable knowledge.

Process Evaluation

O'Malley and colleagues examined key areas related to the use of clinical coded data. In this study, the process of inpatient coding was evaluated via multiple methods: a review of the scientific literature related to errors in coding, the creation of flow charts of the process of how codes for data are selected, interviews, and discussion with coders and the users of the coded data (O'Malley et al. 2005). By comparing the ideal process with the actual process, investigators identified the potential errors associated with each step in the coding process. The results showed that most of the factors that affect the coding process are not within the purview of the coding staff. Further, they showed that errors in coded data result from the variability inherent in the patient care processes as well as the variability of training and experience of coding professionals.

O'Malley and coauthors also evaluated the statistical method by which code accuracy is measured, and they provide a useful guide to how accuracy measures for coding can be calculated (O'Malley et al. 2005, 1). The most common statistics are sensitivity, specificity, positive predictive value, negative predictive value (discussed in chapter 12), and the Cohen's kappa (κ) coefficient (discussed in chapter 12). Although these statistics are simple to compute, determining what they mean is not a straightforward process. Interpretation of sensitivity and specificity statistics requires a gold standard, but O'Malley and associates note that there is no universal standard for the diagnostic labeling associated with coding. To create a standard, investigators could ask, "In medical chart reviews, how well do medical coders' ICD [International Classification of Diseases] code assignments match those of physicians?" With this question, the physicians' code assignments would function as the gold standard for medical presence of disease, and the researcher might use this standard to calculate specificity, sensitivity, and predictive values for the medical coders' ICD code assignments. However, the reliability of the physicians' medical diagnoses is not known. In their own research study, the authors estimate, in the context of medical chart review, the corroboration between physician and medical coders' ICD classifications.

This study illustrates a comparison of the ideal process of coding with the actual process of coding. It also illustrates that findings from an evaluation can provide details about constraints, such as communication between patients and clinicians, and what can be changed—for example the diligence in compiling information can be potentially improved.

Because computer-assisted coding is a method to identify all relevant information in a systematic way, many people expect that it will reduce error. This supposition could be tested by adapting the evaluation methods used by O'Malley's team to determine whether sources of error and error rates change when computer-assisted coding is used.

Goal-Based and Impact Evaluation

A computerized medication alert system was designed to decrease adverse events with medications. However, it was found that the alerts were often overridden because they lacked specificity and users experienced alert overload. Shah and coauthors redesigned the drug alerts to improve clinician acceptance (Shah et al. 2005, 1). Most importantly, they changed the system to use only a selective set of drug alerts that denoted the potential of a high-severity event, thereby minimizing interruptions to clinician workflow. The new design selected the alerts by using a commercial knowledge base modified to include a subset of only the most clinically relevant contraindications. The alerts were used with computerized prescribing in an EHR. The revised design was used in 31 Boston-area practices. During the use of this modified system, there were 18,115 drug alerts during the six-month study period. Of these, 5,182 (29 percent) were high-severity, and clinicians accepted (acted on) 67 percent of those alerts. The evaluation of the medication alert system revealed that the overarching goal of using clinical alerts to reduce adverse medication events was not being achieved due to the high rate of dismissal. Based on the findings of the first goal-based evaluation, the system was redesigned with user-centered design principals and evaluated a second time for impact. That impact evaluation reflected that high-severity medication alerts were accepted.

Outcome Evaluation

McCarren and colleagues (2013) have described how one healthcare organization evaluated an intervention to increase the desired outcome which was administration of beta blockers at optimal, maximally tolerated doses in patients with chronic heart failure. A multidisciplinary team, at the request of the chief of cardiology, began developing a clinical reminder to facilitate beta-blocker titration. Pharmacists were included in the team to determine how they could be involved in the clinical decision support for primary care providers. After a needs assessment was done, health IT developers, cardiologists, primary care providers, pharmacists, nurses, and a member of the nursing management team collectively determined that, to be effective, technology would need to be developed that included patient data, clinical guidelines, and actionable tools such as order sets for titration and to consult the pharmacists. They also determined that policies within the healthcare system would need to be modified to allow the clinical pharmacists to receive a consult through the clinical reminder to undertake titration (McCarren et al. 2013).

Additional Evaluation Resources in Health Informatics

One important resource for health informaticists is the EHR certification process provided by the Office of the National Coordinator for Health Information Technology (ONC). The certification is a voluntary process that specifies criteria for modules. Modules are then tested using scripts. The certification process is a kind of evaluation that provides assurance of functionality and consistency of the testing process (ONC 2016).

Another excellent resource for evaluating a wide range of HIT is the Agency for Health Research and Quality (AHRQ) Health IT Evaluation Toolkit, which provides a user-friendly, step-by-step guide to evaluating HIT. The toolkit helps in the development of evaluation goals, metrics, and methods to carry out the study. It also suggests that both quantitative and qualitative research methods be used to assess the technology (AHRQ 2009).

Review Questions

1. An HIT project team is implementing decision support software. After meeting with the software company, an initial configuration is developed. Clinical staff are asked to use the configuration and provide feedback for further modifications. What kind of evaluation is this? What might you undertake in the evaluation?
2. An HIM manager routinely measures the accuracy of computer-assisted-coding software used in the endoscopy suite to code records. What statistics should the manager consider using?
3. Following implementation of an HIT system, a project team determined that the system reduces the cost of medications. What kind of evaluation research is this?
4. Clinicians increased guideline-directed medical therapy for patients with chronic heart failure and readmissions were reduced. The research described is what type of evaluation research?
5. What do outcomes evaluation assess?
6. A multidisciplinary team of five researchers conducted observations and semi-structured interviews about a clinical reminder. The team wanted to assess the clinical content and workflow and communication. What model is likely being used by the researchers in their research?
7. What entity provides a step-by-step toolkit to evaluate health information technology?

8. The five rights for clinical decision support would include what five areas?
9. How is evaluation research different from an evaluation project?
10. What are the steps in an evaluation of health information technology?

Application Exercises

1. Obtain the SUS and undertake a usability assessment of a software program with 5 to 10 users. Calculate the average or mean of the SUS score for all the users.
2. Develop a set of semistructured interview questions to use in a mock formative evaluation project. Use the semistructured interview questions to gather information about how to improve a website of your choice by interviewing two or three classmates. Note the answers to the questions provided by participants during the interviews. Review the interview results and identify three improvements that could be undertaken to modify the website to make its design more user-centered.
3. Obtain the UNICEF (2014) theory of change methods brief. You are a program evaluator for your personal nutrition. Write a theory of change about eating more fruits and vegetables, and draw a logic model that includes the resources and activities that must be undertaken to increase consumption of vegetables and fruits.

References

Agency for Healthcare Research and Quality (AHRQ). 2009. Health IT Evaluation Toolkit. https://healthit.ahrq.gov/sites/default/files/docs/page/health-information-technology-evaluation-toolkit-2009-update.pdf.

Alkin, M.C. 2011. *Evaluation Essentials from A to Z.* New York: Guilford Press.

Baily, M.A., M. Bottrell, J. Lynn, and B. Jennings. 2006 (June–August). The ethics of using QI methods to improve health care quality and safety. *Hastings Center Report* special report:S1–S40. http://www.thehastingscenter.org/wp-content/uploads/The-Ethics-of-Using-QI-Methods.pdf.

Centers for Disease Control (CDC). 2013. Health Economics and Modeling Unit (HEMU). https://www.cdc.gov/ncezid/dpei/hemu/index.html.

Creatly. 2016. User Centered Design with Behavioral Marketing (blog post). http://creately.com/blog/marketing/user-centered-design-marketing.

Goldstein, M.K. 2008. Using health information technology to improve hypertension management. *Current Hypertension Reports* 10(3):201–207

Kaisler, S. and G. Madey. 2008. Complex Adaptive Systems: Emergence and Self-Organization. www3.nd.edu/~gmadey/Activities/CAS-Briefing.pdf.

Kannampallil, T.G., G.F. Schauer, T. Cohen, and V.L. Patel. 2011. Considering complexity in healthcare systems. *Journal of Biomedical Informatics* 44(6):943–947.

Kitson, A.L., J. Rycroft-Malone, G. Harvey, B. McCormack, K. Seers, and A. Titchen. 2008. Evaluating the successful implementation of evidence into practice using the PARIHS framework: Theoretical and practical challenges. *Implementation Science* 2008. 7(3). https://implementationscience.biomedcentral.com/articles/10.1186/1748-5908-3-1.

McCarren, M., E. Furmaga, C.A. Jackevicius, A. Sahay, T.L. Coppler, J. Katzianer, R.L. Griffiths, I. Tonnu-Mihara, and P. Heidenreich. 2013. Improvement of guideline β-blocker prescribing in heart failure: A cluster-randomized pragmatic trial of a pharmacy intervention. *Journal of Cardiac Failure*19(8):525–532.

McDaniel, R.R. Jr, H.J. Lanham, and R.A. Anderson. 2009. Implications of complex adaptive systems theory for the design of research on health care organizations. *Health Care Management Review* 34 (2):191–199

Miller, R.H., C. West, T.M. Brown, I. Sim, and C. Ganchoff. 2005. The value of electronic health records in solo or small group practices. *Health Affairs* 24(5):1127–1137.

New South Wales (NSW) Department of Environment and Conservation. 2004. Does Your Project Make a Difference? http://www.environment.nsw.gov.au/resources/community/projecteval04110.pdf.

Nilsen, P. 2015. Making sense of implementation theories, models and frameworks. *Implementation* 10:53.
Office of the National Coordinator for Health Information Technology (ONC). 2016. ONC Health IT Certification Program. https://www.healthit.gov/policy-researchers-implementers/about-onc-health-it-certification-program.
O'Malley, K.J., K.F. Cook, M.D. Price, K.R. Wildes, J.F. Hurdle, and C.M. Ashton. 2005. Measuring diagnoses: ICD code accuracy. *Health Services Research* 40(5):1625.
Pell Institute. 2016. Evaluation Toolkit: Evaluation Approaches and Types. http://toolkit.pellinstitute.org/evaluation-101/evaluation-approaches-types.
Prokopenko, M. 2009. Guided self-organization. *HFSP Journal* 3(5):287–289.
Rogers, P. 2014. Theory of Change. UNICEF Methodological Briefs: Impact Evaluation 2. https://www.unicef-irc.org/publications/747.
Shah, N.R., A.C. Seger, D.L. Seger, J.M. Fiskio, G.J. Kuperman, B. Blumenfeld, E.G. Recklet, D.W. Bates, and T.K. Gandh. 2005. Improving acceptance of computerized prescribing alerts in ambulatory care. *Journal of the American Medical Informatics Association* 13:5–11.
Sirajuddin, A.M., J.A. Osheroff, D.F. Sittig, J. Chuo, F. Velasco, and D.A. Collins. 2009. Implementation pearls from a new guidebook on improving medication use and outcomes with clinical decision support. Effective CDS is essential for addressing healthcare performance improvement imperatives. *J Healthcare Information Management* 23(4):38–45.
Sittig, D.F. and H. Singh. 2013. A red-flag-based approach to risk management of EHR-related safety concerns. *Journal of Healthcare Risk Management* 33(2):21–26.
Sittig, D.F. and H. Singh. 2010. A new sociotechnical model for studying health information technology in complex adaptive healthcare systems. *Quality and Safety in Health Care* 19(suppl):i68–i74.
University of Kansas Workgroup for Community Health and Development. 2016. Developing a logic model or theory of change. Section 1 in *The Community Tool Box*. http://ctb.ku.edu/en/table-of-contents/overview/models-for-community-health-and-development/logic-model-development/main.
University of Twente. 2016. Health Belief Model. https://www.utwente.nl/cw/theorieenoverzicht/Theory%20Clusters/Health%20Communication/Health_Belief_Model/.
US Department of Health and Human Services (HHS). 2017a. Usability.gov. Accessed February 2, 2017. https://www.usability.gov/what-and-why/user-centered-design.html.
US Department of Health and Human Services (HHS). 2017b. What and Why of Usability: System Usability Scale (SUS). Accessed 1/9/17. https://www.usability.gov/how-to-and-tools/methods/system-usability-scale.html.
Usabilitynet. 2006. Key Principles of User Centred Design. http://www.usabilitynet.org/management/b_design.htm.
Yancy, C.W., M. Jessup, B. Bozkurt, J. Butler, D.E. Casey, M.M. Colvin, M.H. Drazner, G. Filippatos, G.C. Fonarow, M.M. Givertz, S.M. Hollenberg, J. Lindenfeld, F.A. Masoudi, P.E. McBride, P.N. Peterson, L. Warner Stevenson, and C. Westlake. 2016. ACC/AHA/HFSA focused update on new pharmacological therapy for heart failure: An update of the 2013 ACCF/AHA guideline for the management of heart failure. *Circulation* 134(13):e282–293; erratum, e298.

Resources

Agency for Healthcare Quality and Research (AHRQ). 1999. Assessing the Quality of Internet Health Information. http://archive.ahrq. gov/research/data/infoqual.html.
American Evaluation Association. 2016. http://www.eval.org.
The Evaluators' Institute. 2016. http://tei.cgu.edu.
Flick, U. 2007. *The Sage Qualitative Research Kit*. 8 vols. Thousand Oaks, CA: Sage Publications.
UNICEF. 2014. Evaluation Methods Briefs. https://www.unicef-irc.org/KM/IE/impact_1.php.
UsabilityFirst. 2015. Introduction to User-Centered Design. http://www.usabilityfirst.com/about-usability/introduction-to-user-centered-design/.

7 Data Science and Data Mining

Ryan H. Sandefer, PhD

Learning Objectives

- Utilize technology for data collection, storage, analysis, and reporting of information.
- Apply knowledge of database querying and data exploration and mining techniques to facilitate information retrieval.
- Analyze statistical data for decision making.
- Recommend organizational action based on knowledge obtained from data exploration and mining.

Key Terms

Association rule mining
Clustering
Cross-industry process for data mining (CRISP-DM)
Data dictionary
Data mining
Data science
Data set
Data visualization
Database
Decision tree
Descriptive analytics
Distributed computing
Error rate
Exploratory data analysis (EDA)
Forecasting
Geospatial analysis
k-means clustering
Knowledge discovery in databases (KDD)
Logistic regression
Modeling
Multiple linear regression
Multiple logistic regression
Multinomial logistic regression
Predictive analytics
Predictive modeling
Prescriptive analytics
Simple linear regression
Trend analysis

The collection, management, analysis, and reporting of data and information have become important components for most professional disciplines, especially in healthcare. Professionals are asked to make decisions based on evidence, which is derived from the analysis of data. The Health and Medicine Division (formerly Institute of Medicine) of the National Academies of Science, for example, has developed core competencies for healthcare professionals. Those competencies include employing evidence-based practice, applying quality improvement, and utilizing informatics (Greiner and Knebel 2003, 46). To demonstrate these core competencies for health professionals, individuals must understand and use the growing base of evidence that exists in the published, scholarly literature. Additionally, professionals need to be able to use the data that are collected to make well-informed decisions related to issues of quality, access, and cost. The Health and Medicine Division's recommendations specify that health professionals should competently do the following:

- "Continually understand and measure quality of care in terms of *structure,* or the inputs into the system, such as patients, staff, and environments; *process,* or the interactions between clinicians and patients; and *outcomes*, or evidence about changes in patients' health status in relation to patient and community needs."

- "Assess current practices and compare them with relevant better practices elsewhere as a means of identifying opportunities for improvement."
- "Design and test interventions to change the process of care, with the objective of improving quality." (Greiner and Knebel 2003, 59)

The successful demonstration of these core competencies for health professionals requires effective use of data. The skills associated with working effectively with data comprise **data science**, which is the application of methods related to extracting value from existing data to solve problems, including analyzing existing data sets to identify patterns. The purpose of this chapter is to introduce data science methods, with an emphasis on **data mining**—the semiautomated and automated processes for exploring large databases and detecting relevant patterns and relationships (knowledge) in the data contained in those databases (Tufféry 2011, 4; Han and Kamber 2006, 5). Data mining is used in many industries, financial services, retailing, telecommunications, media, insurance, and healthcare (Linoff and Berry 2011, xxxvii). Examples of data mining in healthcare include identifying groups of patients, predicting patient volumes, and forecasting revenues, to name a few.

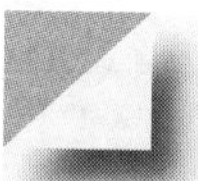

Real-World Case

Data science is used to address problems confronting healthcare delivery, such as the rise of healthcare-acquired infections (HAIs). According to estimates, HAIs are the fifth-leading cause of death in the United States, resulting in 75,000 deaths per year. The estimated annual cost of HAIs is approximately $45 billion (Reynolds and Canales 2016, S4).

Healthcare organizations and associated entities, such as third-party payers, have an interest in promoting data transparency to improve quality and control costs. More healthcare data than ever before are being published online and are accessible for analysis. The Centers for Medicare and Medicaid Services (CMS) has created Data.Medicare.gov, a portal for accessing data related to CMS-certified hospitals, nursing homes, physicians, home health agencies, dialysis facilities, and medical suppliers (CMS 2016a). This portal is an example of the Open Government Initiative, which requires every federal agency to publish high-quality data sets for the purpose of promoting research, transparency, and cost savings.

One of the files in CMS's Hospital Compare data set is titled "Healthcare Associated Infections," and the data in this data set provide information reported by hospitals through the National Healthcare Safety Network (NHSN) about infections that occur during inpatient stays in hospitals, including infections related to devices or those acquired through contact with other patients or surfaces (CMS 2016b). A **data set** is a file of related data, which are typically organized in rows and columns. It is different than a **database**, which is an organized collection of data and is typically represented by multiple tables that are connected by keys. In healthcare, data are typically stored in relational databases. The HAI data set included information on 4,628 US hospitals as of November 2016, and has data on 48 different measures of infection. Because each hospital reports on all measures of infection, the data set includes 222,144 observations. There are 16 columns in the dataset (see figure 7.1).

Figure 7.1 Healthcare associated infections dataset

	Provider ID	Hospital Name	Address	City	State	ZIP Code	County Name	Phone Number	Measure Name	Measure ID	Compared to National	Score	Footnote	Measure Start D	Measure End	Location
1	010001	SOUTHEAST ALABAMA MEI	1108 ROSS CLAR CIRC	DOTHAN	AL	36301	HOUSTON		(334) ; CLABSI: Lower Confidence Limit	HAI_1_CI_LOWER	Worse than the National Benchmark	1.667		01/01/2015	12/31/2015	
2	010001	SOUTHEAST ALABAMA MEI	1108 Address	N	AL	36301	HOUSTON		(334) ; CLABSI: Upper Confidence Limit	HAI_1_CI_UPPER	Worse than the National Benchmark	4.476		01/01/2015	12/31/2015	
3	010001	SOUTHEAST ALABAMA MEI	1108 Plain Text	N	AL	36301	HOUSTON		(334) ; CLABSI: Number of Device Days	HAI_1_DOPC_DAYS	Worse than the National Benchmark	7117		01/01/2015	12/31/2015	
4	010001	SOUTHEAST ALABAMA MEI	1108 API field name: address	N	AL	36301	HOUSTON		(334) ; CLABSI: Predicted Cases	HAI_1_ELIGCASES	Worse than the National Benchmark	5.681		01/01/2015	12/31/2015	
5	010001	SOUTHEAST ALABAMA MEI	1108 ROSS CLARK CIRC	DOTHAN	AL	36301	HOUSTON		(334) ; CLABSI: Observed Cases	HAI_1_NUMERATOR	Worse than the National Benchmark	18		01/01/2015	12/31/2015	
6	010001	SOUTHEAST ALABAMA MEI	1108 ROSS CLARK CIRC	DOTHAN	AL	36301	HOUSTON		(334) ; Central line-associated bloodstream infections (CLAB	HAI_1_SIR	Worse than the National Benchmark	2.816		01/01/2015	12/31/2015	
7	010001	SOUTHEAST ALABAMA MEI	1108 ROSS CLARK CIRC	DOTHAN	AL	36301	HOUSTON		(334) ; CAUTI: Lower Confidence Limit	HAI_2_CI_LOWER	Worse than the National Benchmark	1.595		01/01/2015	12/31/2015	
8	010001	SOUTHEAST ALABAMA MEI	1108 ROSS CLARK CIRC	DOTHAN	AL	36301	HOUSTON		(334) ; CAUTI: Upper Confidence Limit	HAI_2_CI_UPPER	Worse than the National Benchmark	3.313		01/01/2015	12/31/2015	
9	010001	SOUTHEAST ALABAMA MEI	1108 ROSS CLARK CIRC	DOTHAN	AL	36301	HOUSTON		(334) ; CAUTI: Number of Urinary Catheter Days	HAI_2_DOPC_DAYS	Worse than the National Benchmark	14326		01/01/2015	12/31/2015	
10	010001	SOUTHEAST ALABAMA MEI	1108 ROSS CLARK CIRC	DOTHAN	AL	36301	HOUSTON		(334) ; CAUTI: Predicted Cases	HAI_2_ELIGCASES	Worse than the National Benchmark	12.407		01/01/2015	12/31/2015	
11	010001	SOUTHEAST ALABAMA MEI	1108 ROSS CLARK CIRC	DOTHAN	AL	36301	HOUSTON		(334) ; CAUTI: Observed Cases	HAI_2_NUMERATOR	Worse than the National Benchmark	29		01/01/2015	12/31/2015	
12	010001	SOUTHEAST ALABAMA MEI	1108 ROSS CLARK CIRC	DOTHAN	AL	36301	HOUSTON		(334) ; Catheter-associated urinary tract infections (CAUTI) in	HAI_2_SIR	Worse than the National Benchmark	2.337		01/01/2015	12/31/2015	
13	010001	SOUTHEAST ALABAMA MEI	1108 ROSS CLARK CIRC	DOTHAN	AL	36301	HOUSTON		(334) ; SSI: Colon Lower Confidence Limit	HAI_3_CI_LOWER	Worse than the National Benchmark	1.116		01/01/2015	12/31/2015	
14	010001	SOUTHEAST ALABAMA MEI	1108 ROSS CLARK CIRC	DOTHAN	AL	36301	HOUSTON		(334) ; SSI: Colon Upper Confidence Limit	HAI_3_CI_UPPER	Worse than the National Benchmark	3.815		01/01/2015	12/31/2015	
15	010001	SOUTHEAST ALABAMA MEI	1108 ROSS CLARK CIRC	DOTHAN	AL	36301	HOUSTON		(334) ; SSI: Colon, Number of Procedures	HAI_3_DOPC_DAYS	Worse than the National Benchmark	Not Available	5 - Result	01/01/2015	12/31/2015	
16	010001	SOUTHEAST ALABAMA MEI	1108 ROSS CLARK CIRC	DOTHAN	AL	36301	HOUSTON		(334) ; SSI: Colon Predicted Cases	HAI_3_ELIGCASES	Worse than the National Benchmark	4.553		01/01/2015	12/31/2015	
17	010001	SOUTHEAST ALABAMA MEI	1108 ROSS CLARK CIRC	DOTHAN	AL	36301	HOUSTON		(334) ; SSI: Colon Observed Cases	HAI_3_NUMERATOR	Worse than the National Benchmark	10		01/01/2015	12/31/2015	
18	010001	SOUTHEAST ALABAMA MEI	1108 ROSS CLARK CIRC	DOTHAN	AL	36301	HOUSTON		(334) ; Surgical Site Infection from colon surgery (SSI: Colon)	HAI_3_SIR	Worse than the National Benchmark	2.196		01/01/2015	12/31/2015	
19	010001	SOUTHEAST ALABAMA MEI	1108 ROSS CLARK CIRC	DOTHAN	AL	36301	HOUSTON		(334) ; SSI: Abdominal Lower Confidence Limit	HAI_4_CI_LOWER	No Different than National Benchmark	Not Available	8 - The lo	01/01/2015	12/31/2015	
20	010001	SOUTHEAST ALABAMA MEI	1108 ROSS CLARK CIRC	DOTHAN	AL	36301	HOUSTON		(334) ; SSI: Abdominal Upper Confidence Limit	HAI_4_CI_UPPER	No Different than National Benchmark	2.154		01/01/2015	12/31/2015	
21	010001	SOUTHEAST ALABAMA MEI	1108 ROSS CLARK CIRC	DOTHAN	AL	36301	HOUSTON		(334) ; SSI: Abdominal, Number of Procedures	HAI_4_DOPC_DAYS	No Different than National Benchmark	Not Available	5 - Result	01/01/2015	12/31/2015	
22	010001	SOUTHEAST ALABAMA MEI	1108 ROSS CLARK CIRC	DOTHAN	AL	36301	HOUSTON		(334) ; SSI: Abdominal Predicted Cases	HAI_4_ELIGCASES	No Different than National Benchmark	1.301		01/01/2015	12/31/2015	
23	010001	SOUTHEAST ALABAMA MEI	1108 ROSS CLARK CIRC	DOTHAN	AL	36301	HOUSTON		(334) ; SSI: Abdominal Observed Cases	HAI_4_NUMERATOR	No Different than National Benchmark	0		01/01/2015	12/31/2015	
24	010001	SOUTHEAST ALABAMA MEI	1108 ROSS CLARK CIRC	DOTHAN	AL	36301	HOUSTON		(334) ; Surgical Site Infection from abdominal hysterectomy (	HAI_4_SIR	No Different than National Benchmark	0.000		01/01/2015	12/31/2015	
25	010001	SOUTHEAST ALABAMA MEI	1108 ROSS CLARK CIRC	DOTHAN	AL	36301	HOUSTON		(334) ; MRSA Lower Confidence Limit	HAI_5_CI_LOWER	No Different than National Benchmark	0.162		01/01/2015	12/31/2015	
26	010001	SOUTHEAST ALABAMA MEI	1108 ROSS CLARK CIRC	DOTHAN	AL	36301	HOUSTON		(334) ; MRSA Upper Confidence Limit	HAI_5_CI_UPPER	No Different than National Benchmark	1.730		01/01/2015	12/31/2015	
27	010001	SOUTHEAST ALABAMA MEI	1108 ROSS CLARK CIRC	DOTHAN	AL	36301	HOUSTON		(334) ; MRSA Patient Days	HAI_5_DOPC_DAYS	No Different than National Benchmark	83773		01/01/2015	12/31/2015	
28	010001	SOUTHEAST ALABAMA MEI	1108 ROSS CLARK CIRC	DOTHAN	AL	36301	HOUSTON		(334) ; MRSA Predicted Cases	HAI_5_ELIGCASES	No Different than National Benchmark	4.719		01/01/2015	12/31/2015	
29	010001	SOUTHEAST ALABAMA MEI	1108 ROSS CLARK CIRC	DOTHAN	AL	36301	HOUSTON		(334) ; MRSA Observed Cases	HAI_5_NUMERATOR	No Different than National Benchmark	3		01/01/2015	12/31/2015	
30	010001	SOUTHEAST ALABAMA MEI	1108 ROSS CLARK CIRC	DOTHAN	AL	36301	HOUSTON		(334) ; Methicillin-resistant Staphylococcus Aureus (MRSA) B	HAI_5_SIR	No Different than National Benchmark	0.636		01/01/2015	12/31/2015	
31	010001	SOUTHEAST ALABAMA MEI	1108 ROSS CLARK CIRC	DOTHAN	AL	36301	HOUSTON		(334) ; C.diff Lower Confidence Limit	HAI_6_CI_LOWER	Better than the National Benchmark	0.459		01/01/2015	12/31/2015	
32	010001	SOUTHEAST ALABAMA MEI	1108 ROSS CLARK CIRC	DOTHAN	AL	36301	HOUSTON		(334) ; C.diff Upper Confidence Limit	HAI_6_CI_UPPER	Better than the National Benchmark	0.896		01/01/2015	12/31/2015	
33	010001	SOUTHEAST ALABAMA MEI	1108 ROSS CLARK CIRC	DOTHAN	AL	36301	HOUSTON		(334) ; C.diff Patient Days	HAI_6_DOPC_DAYS	Better than the National Benchmark	81130		01/01/2015	12/31/2015	
34	010001	SOUTHEAST ALABAMA MEI	1108 ROSS CLARK CIRC	DOTHAN	AL	36301	HOUSTON		(334) ; C.diff Predicted Cases	HAI_6_ELIGCASES	Better than the National Benchmark	56.348		01/01/2015	12/31/2015	
35	010001	SOUTHEAST ALABAMA MEI	1108 ROSS CLARK CIRC	DOTHAN	AL	36301	HOUSTON		(334) ; C.diff Observed Cases	HAI_6_NUMERATOR	Better than the National Benchmark	37		01/01/2015	12/31/2015	

Source: CMS 2016b.

The HAIs dataset can be analyzed using methods of data science. Numerous analyses could be conducted with this data. For example, data analysis can determine state-level geographic differences in HAI rates. Figure 7.2 presents information regarding each state's likelihood of being above the national average. The odds ratios and 95 percent confidence intervals that are in boldface are statistically significant. The information demonstrates clearly that there are geographic differences among hospitals that are better or worse than the national benchmark. For example, as of November 2016, hospitals in New Hampshire and Hawaii were over six times more likely than hospitals in other states to have lower HAI rates than the national average. This finding could lead to specific hypotheses and research questions being developed about quality outcomes in individual states. The purpose of data mining is to continuously explore these sorts of questions.

Figure 7.2 Results of logistic regression analysis for hospital-acquired infections in US hospitals as of November 2016

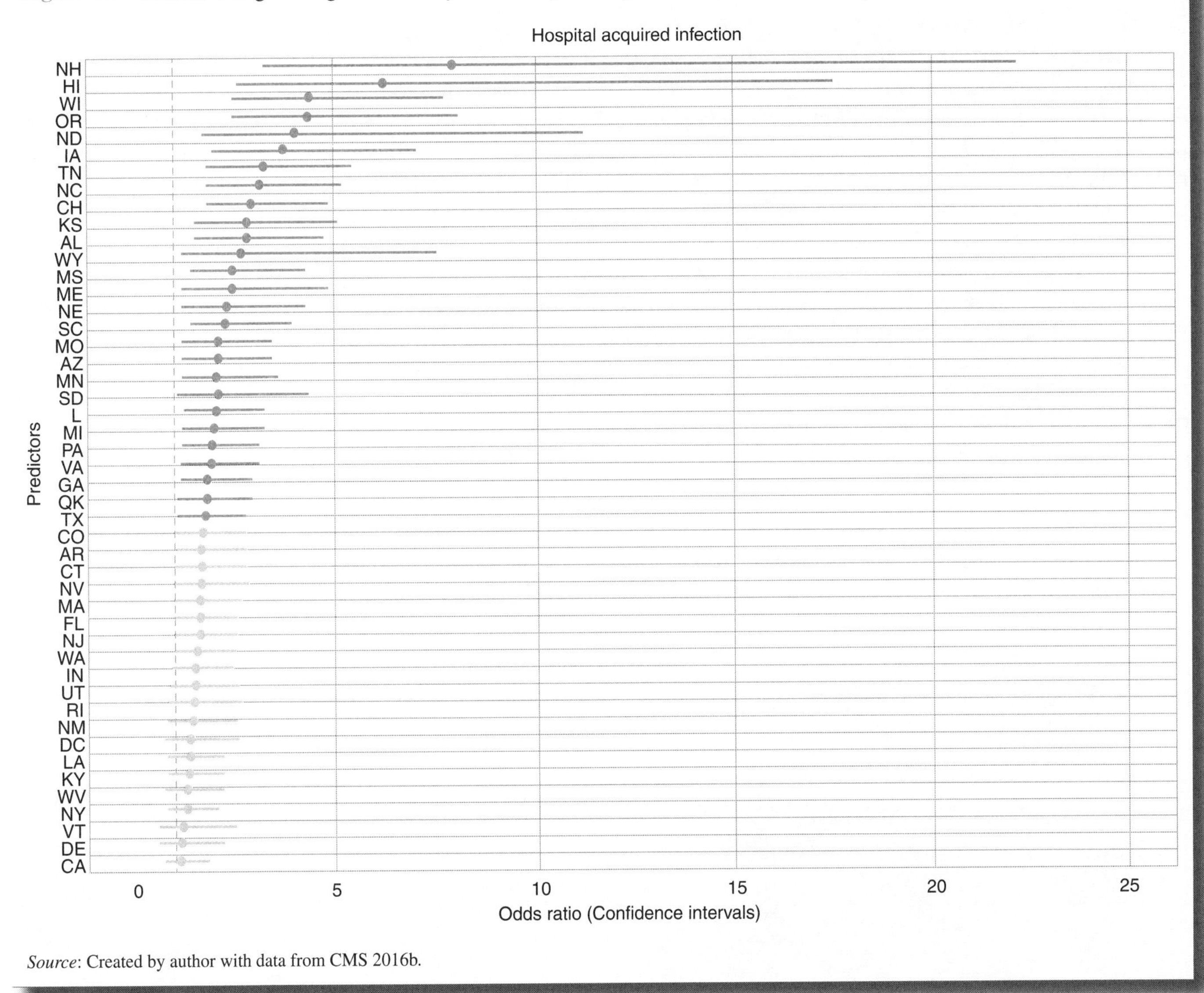

Source: Created by author with data from CMS 2016b.

Data Science

Data science focuses on addressing problems. It involves multiple phases: understanding the background to the issue at hand (including the data), preparing the data for analysis, analyzing data, evaluating results, and deploying the findings. For this reason, data science has been described as "managing the process that can transform hypotheses in to actionable predictions" (Zumel et al. 2014, xix). To apply data science, researchers combine knowledge of statistics, data mining, and computer science with subject matter expertise in a domain such as healthcare. Data science involves a variety of analytic techniques, including descriptive, predictive, and prescriptive analytics.

- **Descriptive analytics** summarize data into meaningful charts and reports. For example, descriptive analytics can be used for financial data such as budgets, sales, revenues, or costs.
- **Predictive analytics** provide forecasts for the future based on analysis of past performance as demonstrated in historical data. Researchers use predictive analytic methods to detect patterns or relationships in these data and then extrapolate these relationships forward in time.
- **Prescriptive analytics** are used to identify the best alternatives to minimize or maximize some objective. (Evans and Lindner 2012, 6)

According to some experts, "more than anything, what data scientists do is make discoveries while swimming in data" (Davenport and Patil 2012). The amount of data being generated today is almost beyond comprehension. IBM has estimated that 2.5 quintillion bytes of data are produced globally every day; 10 million Blu-ray discs would be needed to hold that many data (IBM 2016). The level of monthly data traffic is expected to grow from approximately 90,000 terabytes per month in 2009 to over 11 million terabytes per month in 2017 (Letouzé and Jütting 2015). Data are being created at a remarkable pace across many sectors of the economy, and healthcare has been identified as a sector that could potentially add value to services through data science. However, not enough professionals have the requisite skills to collect, process, cleanse, model, visualize, and present the data—by 2018, there may be a shortage of nearly 200,000 data scientists with the knowledge, skills, and abilities to meet the demand (Manyika et al. 2011).

This chapter will focus on one model for approaching data science problems, the **cross-industry process for data mining (CRISP-DM)**, which breaks the process of data mining into six distinct phases that apply to any project: business understanding, data understanding, data preparation, modeling, evaluation, and deployment (see figure 7.3) (IBM 2016). The CRISP-DM process is the focus because it is a widely accepted model for data mining across industries. Other data science models not covered in this chapter include the Sample, Explore, Modify, Model, and Assess (SEMMA) model and Predictive Data Mining Markup Language (PMML) (Zumel et al. 2014). The CRISP-DM provides a step-by-step framework for approaching data mining projects. This chapter will provide an overview of each step in the process.

Figure 7.3 The cross-industry process for data mining (CRISP-DM) model

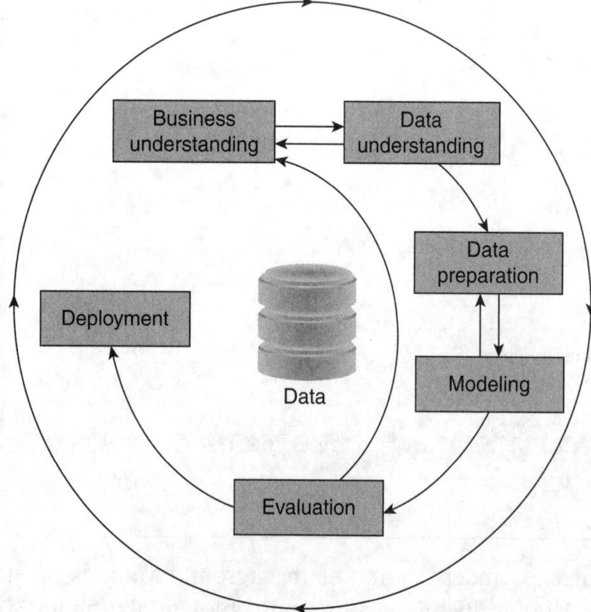

The phases of the CRISP-DM will be discussed in the following sections.

Business Understanding

The first step in a data science project is developing a business understanding regarding the problem that the project is attempting to solve. As was previously noted, data science, by its nature, uses data and data analytic techniques to answer questions and, potentially, to improve outcomes. To accomplish this objective, data scientists research the topic, define project goals and objectives, and specify quantifiable measures related to the project goals. This stage in the process likely involves conversations with project sponsors and organizational stakeholders, as well as a review of the literature. Ultimately, this phase of the project informs data scientists regarding the practical relevance of potential findings from an analysis.

The following are questions that a researcher might ask to gather a business understanding of a data science project:

- What is the organization doing to address the issue? How are current efforts working?
- How is the organization measuring the issue? Is the process working? Why or why not?
- What data are being used to assess the issue? What is the quality of the data that are being used?
- What does the organization hope to gain from the analysis?
- What barriers or challenges are related to the issue? What would address the challenges or barriers?

The ultimate purpose of this phase of the project is to understand the context surrounding the issue being researched. By asking relevant questions such as those listed here, data scientists may improve their approach to solving the problem.

Data Understanding

Once researchers obtain a proper understanding of the business case, the next step in a data science project is to gain an understanding of the data that will be used to address the problem. *Data understanding* generally refers to obtaining data and getting familiar with how they are collected and formatted. This step is a major part of any data science project. As has been mentioned, organizations are collecting more data than ever before, and the volume and complexity of the data collected and stored can make data access challenging. For the purpose of data integrity and for the purpose of the quality of any data utilization, researchers must understand the data that are currently being collected, the frequency of collection, how data are stored, the quality of the data, and any potential issues about working with the data.

In the data understanding phase, researchers require direct access to the data. The methods for accessing the data vary greatly depending on the source—different sources may use different technologies or programming languages, and the data may be stored in different formats. In healthcare, databases efficiently store massive amounts of clinical or administrative data. These data can be accessed and analyzed through computer applications, but working with these databases is challenging because of their potential scope. Healthcare organizations often have many large databases, and data scientists rely on tools to help them understand the structure, the format of the data, and the location of the data. One tool is the **data dictionary**, which is "a descriptive list of names (also called 'representations' or 'displays'), definitions, and attributes of data elements to be collected in an information system or database. … A data dictionary promotes clearer understanding, helps users find information, promotes more efficient use and reuse of information, and promotes better data management" (Bronnert et al. 2011). Data dictionaries are a critical asset for data scientists to use when working with existing data because they provide clear definitions of each data element, the location of each data element, and information about the format of the data element. Figure 7.4 shows the data dictionary for the CMS inpatient limited data set (LDS) database. This data dictionary includes a number for each variable, a short name for the data field, a long name for the data field, a label (description) of the data field, the data type, and the length of the data element. There are 256 data elements included in this LDS related to CMS claims (CMS 2016c).

Figure 7.4 CMS limited data set data (LDS) inpatient dictionary

No.	Field Short Name	Field Long Name	Label	Type	Length
			Base Claim File		
1	DSYSRTKY	DESY_SORT_KEY	LDS Beneficiary ID	NUM	9
2	CLAIMNO	CLAIM_NO	Claim number	NUM	12

(Continued)

Figure 7.4 *(Continued)*

No.	Field Short Name	Field Long Name	Label	Type	Length
			Base Claim File		
3	PROVIDER	PRVDR_NUM	Provider Number	CHAR	10
4	THRU_DT	CLM_THRU_DT	Claim Through Date (Determines Year of Claim)	DATE	8
5	RIC_CD	NCH_NEAR_LINE_REC_IDENT_CD	NCH Near Line Record Identification Code	CHAR	1
6	CLM_TYPE	NCH_CLM_TYPE_CD	NCH Claim Type Code	CHAR	2
7	QUERY_CD	CLAIM_QUERY_CODE	Claim Query Code	CHAR	1
8	FAC_TYPE	CLM_FAC_TYPE_CD	Claim Facility Type Code	CHAR	1
9	TYPESRVC	CLM_SRVC_CLSFCTN_TYPE_CD	Claim Service classification Type Code	CHAR	1
10	FREQ_CD	CLM_FREQ_CD	Claim Frequency Code	CHAR	1
11	FI_NUM	FI_NUM	FI Number	CHAR	5
12	NOPAY_CD	CLM_MDCR_NON_PMT_RSN_CD	Claim Medicare Non Payment Reason Code	CHAR	2
13	PMT_AMT	CLM_PMT_AMT	Claim Payment Amount	NUM	12
14	PRPAYAMT	NCH_PRMRY_PYR_CLM_PD_AMT	NCH Primary Payer Claim Paid Amount	NUM	12
15	PRPAY_CD	NCH_PRMRY_PYR_CD	NCH Primary Payer Code	CHAR	1
16	ACTIONCD	FI_CLM_ACTN_CD	FI Claim Action Code	CHAR	1
17	PRSTATE	PRVDR_STATE_CD	NCH Provider State Code	CHAR	2
18	ORGNPINM	ORG_NPI_NUM	Organization NPI Number	CHAR	10
19	AT_UPIN	AT_PHYSN_UPIN	Claim Attending Physician UPIN Number	CHAR	12
20	AT_NPI	AT_PHYSN_NPI	Claim Attending Physician NPI Number	CHAR	12
21	OP_UPIN	OP_PHYSN_UPIN	Claim Operating Physician UPIN Number	CHAR	12
22	OP_NPI	OP_PHYSN_NPI	Claim Operating Physician NPI Number	CHAR	12
23	OT_UPIN	OT_PHYSN_UPIN	Claim Other Physician UPIN Number	CHAR	12
24	OT_NPI	OT_PHYSN_NPI	Claim Other Physician NPI Number	CHAR	12
25	MCOPDSW	CLM_MCO_PD_SW	Claim MCO Paid Switch	CHAR	1
26	STUS_CD	PTNT_DSCHRG_STUS_CD	Patient Discharge Status Code	CHAR	2
27	PPS_IND	CLM_PPS_IND_CD	Claim PPS Indicator Code	CHAR	1
28	TOT_CHRG	CLM_TOT_CHRG_AMT	Claim Total Charge Amount	NUM	12
29	ADMSN_DT	CLM_ADMSN_DT	Claim Admission Date	DATE	8
30	TYPE_ADM	CLM_IP_ADMSN_TYPE_CD	Claim Inpatient Admission Type Code	CHAR	1
31	SRC_ADMS	CLM_SRC_IP_ADMSN_CD	Claim Source Inpatient Admission Code	CHAR	1
32	PTNTSTUS	NCH_PTNT_STATUS_IND_CD	NCH Patient Status Indicator Code	CHAR	1
33	PER_DIEM	CLM_PASS_THRU_PER_DIEM_AMT	Claim Pass Thru Per Diem Amount	NUM	12
34	DED_AMT	NCH_BENE_IP_DDCTBL_AMT	NCH Beneficiary Inpatient Deductible Amount	NUM	12
35	COIN_AMT	NCH_BENE_PTA_COINSRNC_LBLTY_AM	NCH Beneficiary Part A Coinsurance Liability Amount	NUM	12

Source: CMS 2016c.

Another tool used by data scientists is the entity relationship diagram (ERD), which depicts the relationships among multiple tables connected within a database. An ERD shows the primary and foreign keys (these are the data attributes that link one database table to another) for each table, as well as each additional attribute contained in each table. Figure 7.5 presents an ERD with a few tables.

Figure 7.5 Example of an entity relationship diagram (ERD)

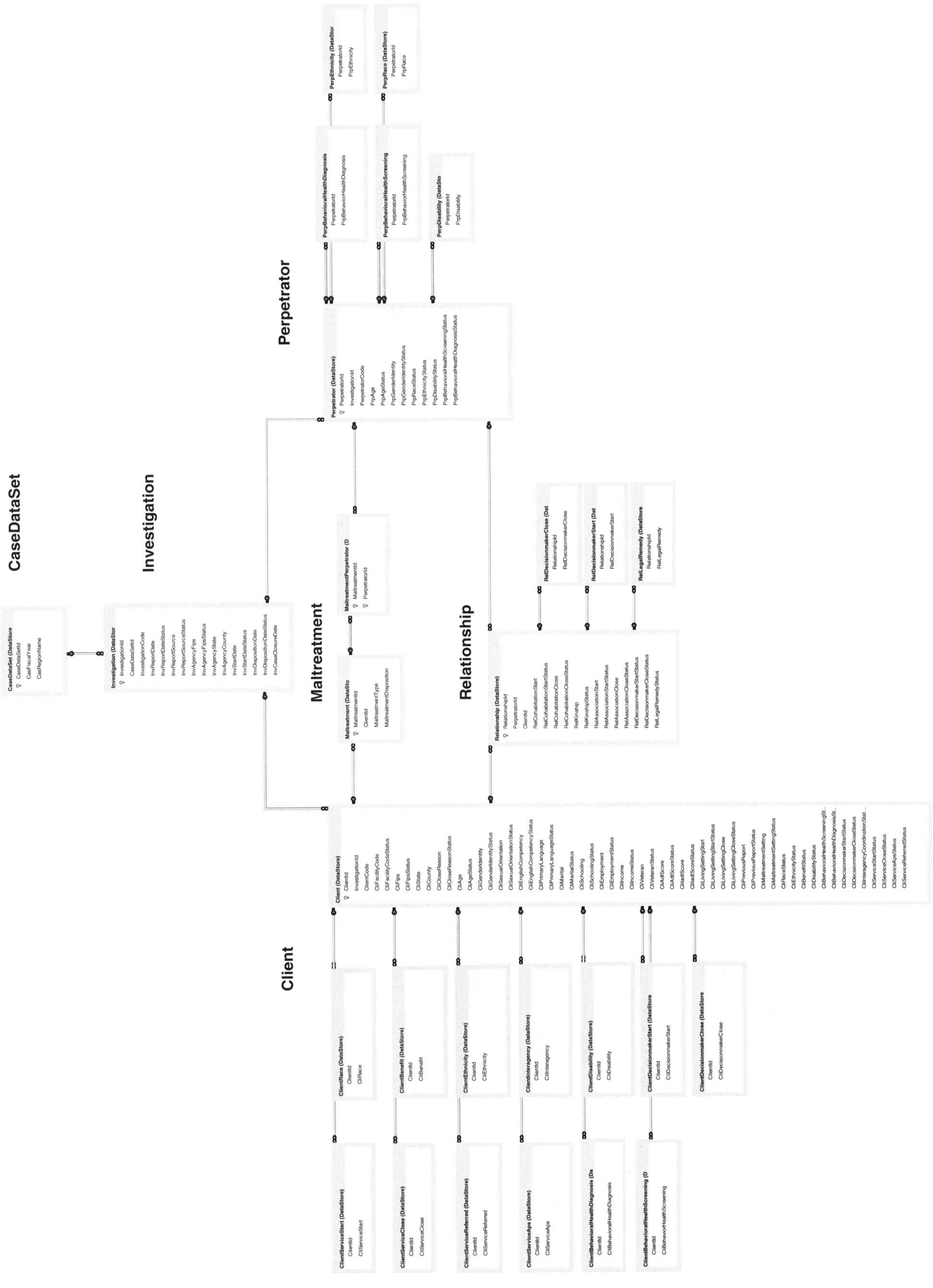

Source: HHS 2015, 63.

When vast amounts of data are to be analyzed, data scientists employ various data processing techniques. Traditional methods of data storage and extraction, such as SQL (structured query language), are used, and other techniques, such as NoSQL (none SQL), offer an alternative for relational databases. SQL is a standard programming language for working with databases. NoSQL is a method used with databases that distribute data in other ways than relational tables (relational tables are simply datasets linked together through common identifiers), such as using key values to spread data across many databases to reduce storage inefficiency and improve processing capacity. NoSQL is simply one example of methods used to process large amounts of data quickly. Other examples involve distributed processing—spreading computing processes across multiple computers to increase efficiency. For example, Apache Hadoop is a set of tools to facilitate distributed processing of data across multiple systems, which could include up to thousands of disparate computers. **Distributed computing** spreads data and analytics tasks equally across many computers to speed processing time. In this way, distributed computing helps overcome the shortcomings of legacy systems for data collection, which are usually much more efficient of collecting and storing data than extracting and analyzing it. For example, "Imagine if we had 100 drives, each holding one hundredth of the data. Working in parallel, we could read the data in under two minutes," as opposed to two and a half hours if it was stored on one system (White 2012, 3).

Data understanding can include **exploratory data analysis (EDA)**, which "involves getting a basic understanding of a dataset through numerous variable summaries and visual plots" (Williams 2011, 99). EDA can suggest potential issues related to data quality, such as issues with the distribution of data. It can also assist in identifying patterns in data, and therefore directly focus on particular areas that would have otherwise gone unnoticed by the data scientist.

Researchers can use a variety of techniques to conduct EDA. For example, **geospatial analysis** uses geographical maps to illustrate differences in data across variables. For example, figure 7.6 illustrates a breakdown of each US state based upon the proportion of physicians who have adopted certified electronic health record (EHR) systems (ONC 2015), and figure 7.7 presents information related to the proportion of physicians who have adopted the capability to exchange secure electronic messages with patients. Together, these figures illustrate a wide disparity between the adoption of EHRs and the use of secure messaging systems, which are a feature of EHR systems, to engage patients. While the adoption of EHR systems among physicians is over 60 percent in every US state, adoption of secure messaging capabilities is much lower. In fact, only five states report more than 75 percent of physicians with this capacity. This information could be useful for proposing hypotheses related to technology adoption among physicians.

Figure 7.6 Proportion of physicians that have adopted certified electronic health records

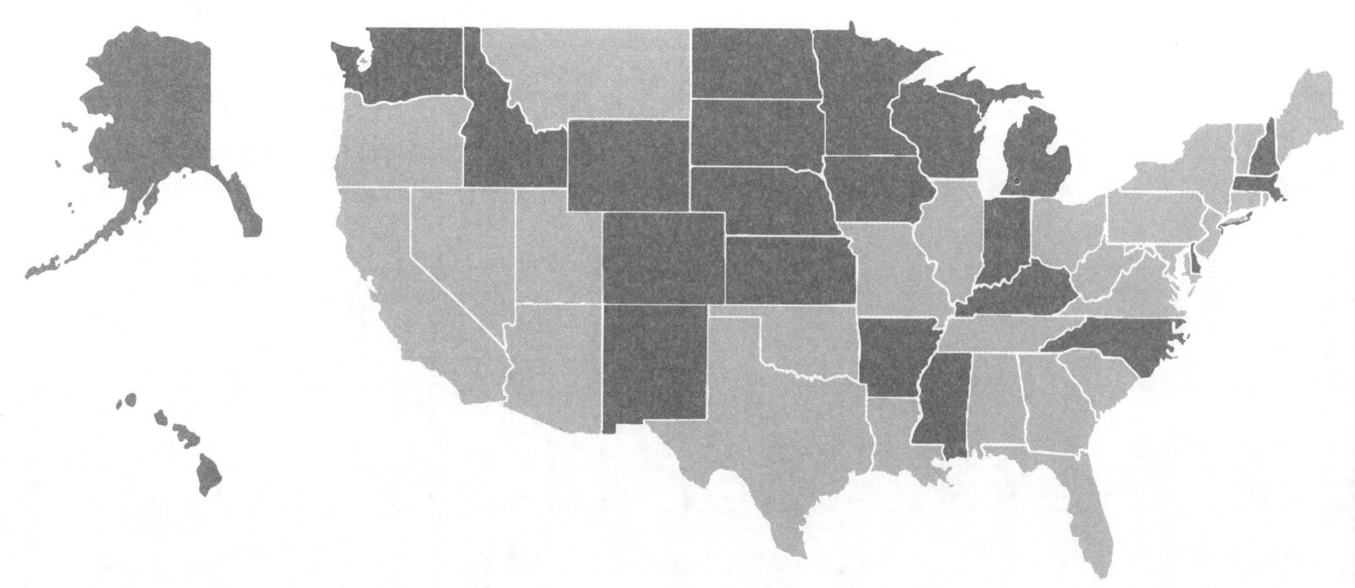

Source: ONC 2015.

Figure 7.7 Proportion of physicians with capability to send secure messages with patients

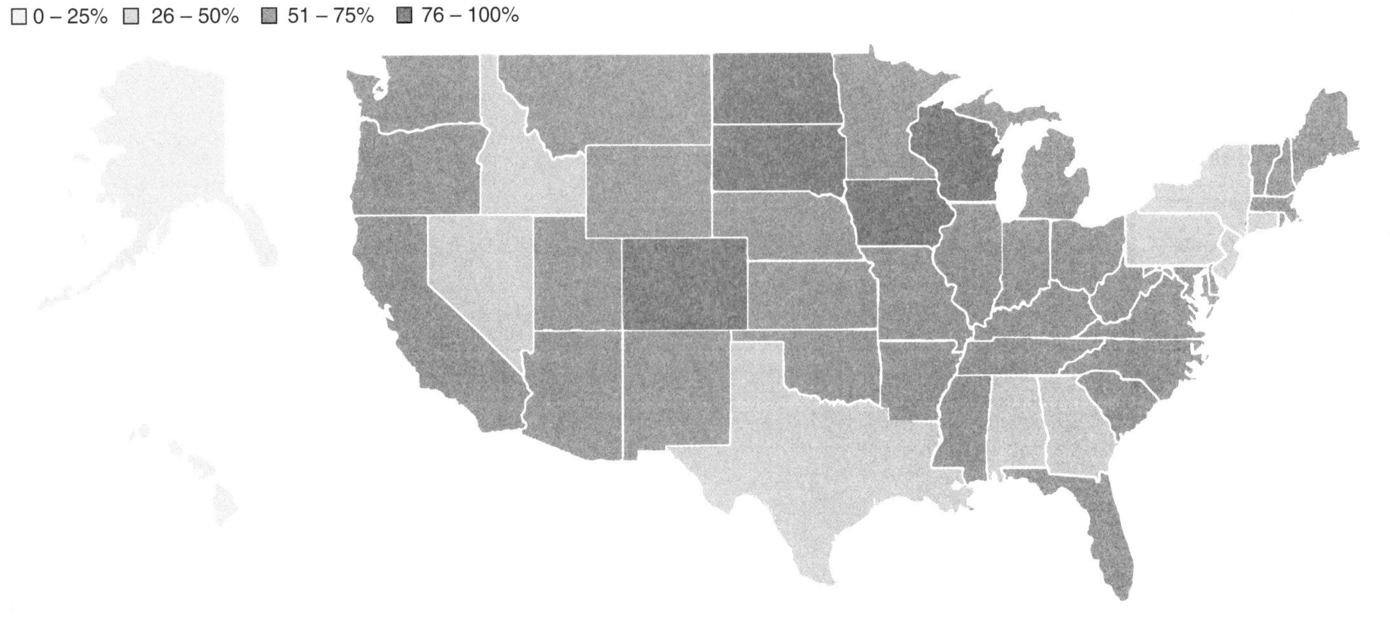

Source: ONC 2015.

EDA can use graphs to analyze data. For example, figure 7.8 displays the percentage of nonfederal acute-care hospitals reporting adoption of EHRs between 2009 and 2014 (ONC 2016), and figure 7.9 shows the EHR adoption rate for office-based physicians for the same time period (ONC 2016). A researcher comparing these figures might ask why EHR adoption has been advancing more rapidly among nonfederal acute-care hospitals than office-based physicians.

Figure 7.8 Percentage of non-federal acute care hospitals with a basic electronic health record (EHR), 2009–2014

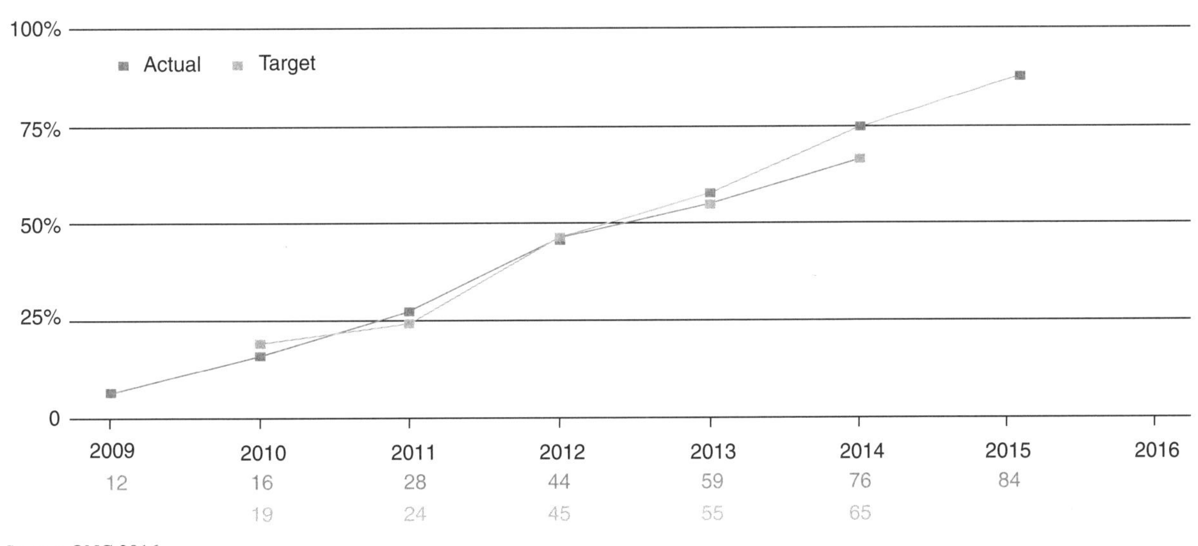

Source: ONC 2016.

Figure 7.9 Percentage of office-based physicians with a basic electronic health record (EHR), 2009–2014

Office of the national coordinator for health IT budget performance measure
Percent of office-based physicians who have adopted a basic EHR

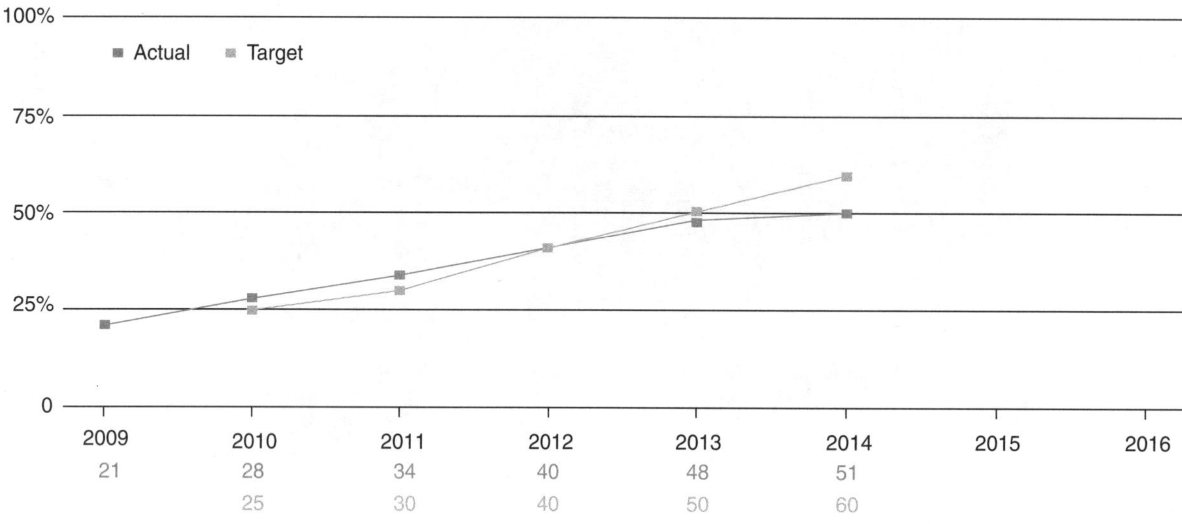

Source: ONC 2016.

Another EDA technique is the use of tables to display information. Figure 7.10 is a CMS dashboard presenting data on Medicare drug spending by drug in 2015. The last column in the table presents the annual change in average cost per unit of the drug. One drug, Vimovo, is reported to have had a 543 percent increase in cost per unit since 2013. Another drug, Targretin, reported a 123 percent increase in average cost per unit, and reported one of the top-20 highest average annual costs that the beneficiary had to pay out of pocket (CMS 2016d). This type of analysis suggests multiple research questions related to increases in drug prices and their impact on consumers. For example, were the increases in reported drug costs related to increases in specific diagnoses over the same time period—in other words, is there an association between the cost of drugs and the demand for them?

Figure 7.10 Medicare drug spending in 2015

MEDICARE DRUG SPENDING DASHBOARD 2015

S - Drug selected due to high total program spending.
B - Drug selected due to high annual spending per user.
U - Drug selected due to large increase in average cost per unit.

MEDICATIONS LIST | INFORMATION

			Brand Name	Generic Name	Coverage Type	Total Spending	Beneficiary Count	Total Annual Spending Per User	Average Annual Beneficiary Cost Share*	Annual Change in Average Cost Per Unit**
S			Abilify	Aripiprazole	Part D	$1,572,428,343	322,582	$4,875	$520	14%
	B		Abraxane	Paclitaxel Protein-Bound	Part B	$276,806,046	17,828	$15,526	$3,141	1%
		U	Accuneb: Albuterol Sulfate	Albuterol Sulfate	Part B	$20,603,233	516,660	$40	$10	26%
S			Advair Diskus	Fluticasone/Salmeterol	Part D	$2,270,015,726	1,321,483	$1,718	$288	7%
	B		Afinitor	Everolimus	Part D	$393,806,656	7,661	$51,404	$3,253	12%
S			Alimta	Pemetrexed Disodium	Part B	$547,767,946	21,948	$24,958	$4,733	1%
S			Aranesp	Darbepoetin Alfa In Polysorbat	Part B	$294,317,556	58,290	$5,049	$1,034	8%
	B		Atripla	Efavirenz/Emtricitab/Tenofovir	Part D	$589,704,409	28,135	$20,960	$1,603	7%
S			Avastin	Bevacizumab	Part B	$1,117,896,685	208,450	$5,363	$1,011	4%
		U	Brovana	Arformoterol Tartrate	Part B	$178,698,319	68,624	$2,604	$553	17%
		U	Carbamazepine	Carbamazepine	Part D	$89,715,056	172,550	$520	$96	131%
		U	Chlorpromazine HCl	Chlorpromazine HCl	Part D	$112,990,177	51,416	$2,198	$104	128%
	B		Cimzia	Certolizumab Pegol	Part B	$174,852,795	9,983	$17,515	$3,581	4%
		U	Clobetasol Propionate	Clobetasol Propionate	Part D	$389,702,537	998,291	$390	$44	151%
S			Copaxone	Glatiramer Acetate	Part D	$1,382,386,515	27,621	$50,048	$3,730	-32%
S			Crestor	Rosuvastatin Calcium	Part D	$2,883,122,484	1,733,071	$1,664	$328	14%
		U	Cyanocobalamin Injection	Cyanocobalamin (Vitamin B-12)	Part B	$6,925,115	574,137	$12	$3	39%
		U	Depo-Medrol: Methylprednisolone Acetate	Methylprednisolone Acetate (40 mg)	Part B	$9,771,022	1,235,507	$8	$2	19%
		U	Depo-Medrol: Methylprednisolone Acetate	Methylprednisolone Acetate (80 mg)	Part B	$11,505,875	962,804	$12	$3	16%
		U	Econazole Nitrate	Econazole Nitrate	Part D	$118,587,925	289,022	$410	$28	276%
		U	Enalapril Maleate	Enalapril Maleate	Part D	$124,592,962	798,422	$156	$41	104%
S			Enbrel	Etanercept	Part D	$1,385,143,655	51,081	$27,117	$1,590	19%
	B		Erbitux	Cetuximab	Part B	$244,141,566	8,800	$27,743	$5,630	1%
S			Eylea	Aflibercept	Part B	$1,813,496,828	180,020	$10,074	$2,053	0%
	B		Faslodex	Fulvestrant	Part B	$186,300,193	15,240	$12,224	$2,496	2%
	B		Forteo	Teriparatide	Part D	$430,210,944	35,902	$11,983	$1,156	29%
	B		Gammagard Liquid	Immun Glob G (IGG)/Gly/Iga 50+	Part B	$264,248,241	11,713	$22,560	$4,549	-1%

*The Average Annual Beneficiary Cost Share is the average amount that beneficiaries using the drug paid out of pocket during the year; for Part D drugs, the amount displayed here is based only on Part D beneficiaries without a Low Income Subsidy (LIS).

**For Part D drugs, this measure accounts for unit cost changes for different strengths and dosage forms of a drug and presents a weighted average of these percent changes.

CMS *Produced by the CMS/Office of Enterprise Data & Analytics (OEDA), September 2016*

Source: CMS 2016d.

Data Preparation

The next step in the CRISP-DM process is to prepare the data for formal analysis. Once the data are identified and explored, researchers use a variety of techniques to process them to ensure they are useful for analysis. For data to be useful, they typically require recoding, transforming, and cleansing. This phase of the project is likely to be the most time-consuming (Assunção et al. 2015, 4; Ordonez and Chen 2012, 1). For example, the data may be in a text format (such as hospital names), but researchers may want to analyze them in numerical format (or vice versa). The data element may be numerical (such as age), but it is often more useful to recode the data into categories for analysis (such as age ranges). Data can also be disorganized and "dirty"—there may be erroneous values, such as "NA" (not available), or filler values, like 9999, that need to be removed prior to analysis. There may also be outliers (extreme values) in the data set, and it may be necessary to exclude these values from the data to avoid skewing of the results. Table 7.1 summarizes some of the most common methods used to prepare data for analysis.

Table 7.1 Methods of data preparation

Method	Description	Example
Transform	Changing the value of an observation through a calculation	Natural log of numerical variable
Recode	Creating new variables from existing data	Creating three age categories (young adult, adult, elderly) from the numerical variable of age in years (15–80 years)
Normalize	Rescaling data that have a wide numerical spread	To address extreme values in age, the value can be normalized to have mean value of 0 and standard deviation of 1
Remove	Deleting data of poor quality	Deleting data that is redundant, erroneous, or errant, such "NA" (not available).

Modeling

In the modeling phase of the CRISP-DM process, researchers use various techniques or procedures to gather insights from data. **Modeling** is the process of using existing data to construct an explanation of how they were created. Some of the most common modeling techniques are also known as *data mining procedures*. Data mining is also called **knowledge discovery in databases (KDD)** and has been defined as the "algorithmic means by which patterns are extracted and enumerated from data" (Chimieski and Ribeiro Fagundes 2013, 45). KDD has been described as the "non-trivial process of identifying valid, novel, potentially useful, and ultimately understandable patterns in data" (Fayyad et al. 1996, 6). KDD is interdisciplinary, involving researchers from statistics, computer science, and business and uses an array of techniques, such as database management, machine learning, pattern recognition, and artificial intelligence. KDD also relies heavily on **data visualization**, which is the "use of graphics to examine data" (Zumel et al. 2014, 41). KDD is a multiphase process that involves selecting data, preparing data, analyzing data, and interpreting results. Experts emphasize that these phases, which can be both automated and nonautomated, result in the retrieval, investigation, and creation of *usable* knowledge (Norton 1999, 10–11).

Predictive modeling is the use of models to forecast from existing data whether an event will occur. Predictive modeling separates variables into two categories or classes, the target (also referred to as the *response, outcome,* or *dependent variable*) and the input (also referred to as *independent variables, predictors, covariates, observed variables,* or *descriptive variables*). The purpose of predictive modeling is to create models that predict the target variables based upon the terms of the input variables. The target variable typically is binary (for example, "yes" or "no") or has classes. Input variables can have multiple levels (for example, "strongly disagree," "disagree," "neutral," "agree," and "strongly agree"). Multiple algorithmic techniques fall under the umbrella of predictive modeling, including classification, regression, clustering, and association rule mining, to name a few. Some of these techniques are discussed in depth in the next sections of this chapter.

Classification and Decision Trees

Classification uses an existing rule or characteristic to generalize about data and fit new data into a predefined category (class). For example, a rule classifies new e-mail messages as legitimate e-mail or as "spam." Decision trees are one of the most common classification techniques used in data mining. A **decision tree** is a machine-learning technique used to predict categorical or numerical variables by creating rules from training data that result in the best performance of the model. Decision-tree analysis uses branching logic to make predictions, categorizing data using a tree-like model that groups decisions based on responses. Decision trees are a "way to model a complex decision process as a tree with branches representing all possible intermediate states or final outcomes of an event. The probabilities of each intermediate state or final outcome and the perceived utilities of each are combined to attach expected utilities to each outcome. The science of drawing decision trees and assessing utilities is called decision analysis" (Wyatt and Sullivan 2005, 40). The purpose of the decision tree is to develop a model that best predicts an outcome variable based on historical data. The variables that construct the tree are called *nodes*. The initial node in the tree is called the *root*, and all other nodes are called *leaves*. The paths between nodes are referred to as *rules*. Decision tree models represent the decision rules that lead to the most predictive outcome. Figure 7.11 provides a simple illustration of a decision tree for predicting uses for personal health records (PHRs) for accessing health information online. The target is PHR use ("yes" or "no"). The root node is related to education level (college education or no college education). In this example, the decision tree shows the importance of specific variables for predicting the outcome of PHR use. College education, socioeconomic status (poverty and foreign travel), and health condition (allergies) are important nodes in determining the outcome of PHR use. Among individuals with a college education who reported traveling to foreign countries in the past year, 75 percent report using a PHR. In contrast, 12 percent of people who report that they do not have a college education and live in poverty and 40 percent of individuals who report not having a college education and not being in poverty report PHR use.

Figure 7.11 Example of a decision tree to predict who uses a personal health record (PHR)

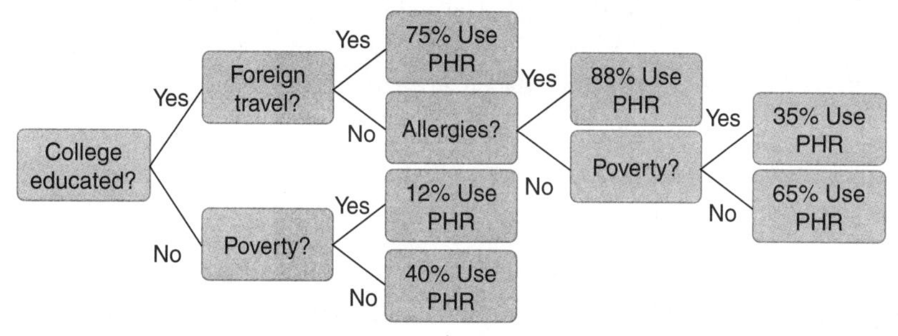

Source: Minnesota Population Center 2016.

Among the numerous applications of decision-tree modeling in healthcare is the creation of evidence-based guidelines to improve treatment decisions. Decision-tree modeling is used to identify clinically significant predictors of treatment outcomes, and results are used to create decision support rule systems (Williams 2011, 99). Decision-tree models have also been used to show the association between variables and onset of chronic disease (Koh and Tan 2011, 66).

Regression

Regression is another common predictive modeling technique. Its purpose is to identify whether there is a statistical relationship or correlation between numerical variables. **Simple linear regression** aims to predict an outcome (dependent variable) based upon a single predictor (independent variable). Researchers use **multiple linear regression** when multiple predictors are used to predict the outcome. **Logistic regression** aims to predict a categorical target, which is a dependent variable that is qualitative and falls into groups. The predictor variables used can be categorical or numerical. If the target variable has more than two levels, **multinomial logistic regression** is used. If the target variable is binary the regression method is called **multiple logistic regression**. (See also discussions of regression in chapters 5 and 9.) Figure 7.12 shows the results of a simple linear regression. The *x*-axis and *y*-axis reflect two quantitative variables (typically, the dependent variable is plotted on the *y*-axis), and the points are plotted on a scatterplot. Hypothetically, the *y*-axis could represent the total cost of patient care and the *x*-axis could represent patient length of stay. The dots reflect the data and the line reflects the regression line. The distance between the line and the data points reflect the residuals.

The slope of the line indicates the correlation between the two variables. A line that rises from left to right indicates a positive relationship between the two variables. A line that falls from left to right indicates a negative relationship. The slope of the line determines whether it is a strong or weak correlation. (See also discussion of linear associations in chapter 9.)

Figure 7.12 Example of a simple linear regression showing correlation between patient length of stay (LOS) and total cost of patient care

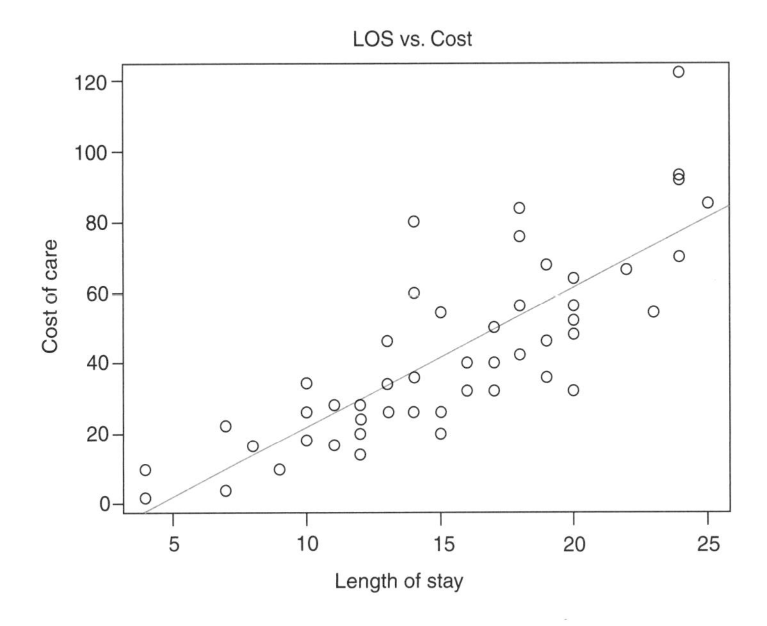

Regression techniques have many applications and are often used in healthcare research. Because data science typically aims to create models that have predictive ability, data scientists often analyze specific variables on a time continuum. Trend analysis involves collecting data over time to determine changes, trends, or patterns in the data that can be used for forecasting (predicting outcomes at a date in the future). A variety of statistical methods are used for trend analysis, including simple linear regression. In one study, researchers used simple linear regression to evaluate hospitalization and mortality rates associated with severe sepsis. Their results showed the rates of severe sepsis more than doubled in an 11-year period, and the rates increased faster than previously predicted (Dombrovskiy et al. 2013, 1246). Numerous healthcare studies have employed logistic regression analysis to develop predictive models. For example, researchers have evaluated the financial impact of health information exchange (HIE) systems on emergency department care, and their results indicate a statistically significant reduction in hospital admissions, head computed tomography (CT) use, body CT use, and laboratory test ordering. Annually, HIE use saved nearly $2 million dollars (Frisse et al. 2012, 331).

Clustering

Clustering, or *segmentation,* groups data objects within the database that are similar to each other and are dissimilar to data objects in other groups. The groups created are determined by what is meaningful to the analyst. For example, a healthcare organization could use clustering to identify a group of patients who could benefit from nutrition education and alert those patients to the opportunity.

k-means clustering is an algorithm for partitioning a data set into multiple groups (clusters) and systematically analyzing the data to identify observations that are similar based on multiple characteristics (Zumel et al. 2014, 88). The ultimate goal is to use the existing data to create clusters of data that are more similar to each other than to data in any other cluster. For example, *k*-means clustering has been used to analyze breast cancer datasets to cluster subtypes based upon gene expression (Lehmann et al. 2011). Figure 7.13 displays the results of a *k*-means clustering analysis and illustrates how the analysis has separated the observations into three distinct clusters based on the data. Hypothetically, the results could represent response to a specific medication based upon three distinct age groupings.

Figure 7.13 Example of *k*-means clustering

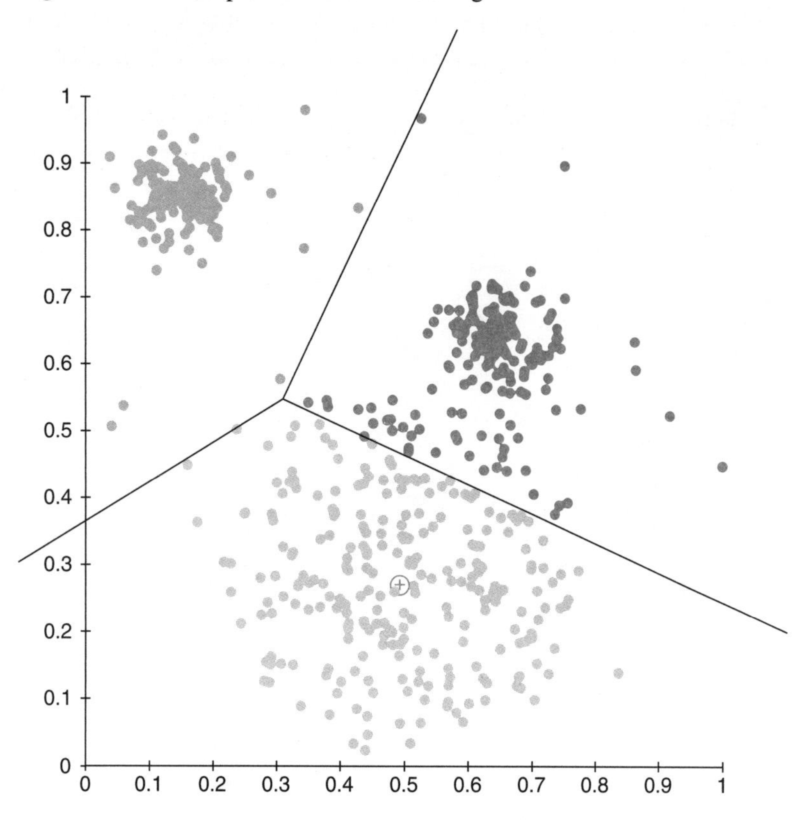

Association Rule Mining

Association rule mining, or *dependency modeling,* is a data-mining technique that analyzes identifying attributes that frequently occur together in a data set. Association rule mining has been described as "efficiently discovering frequent sets in data" (Manyika et al. 2011). The model is structured as a two-part statement (if-then statements), with an antecedent (if) and a consequent (then), that describes significant and often hidden relationships (dependencies) among data (variables) in a database. For example, if the results for a specific test are between a certain range, then the patient is at an increased risk for a specific diagnosis. This general class of modeling is also known as "market basket analysis" because retailers use information about items often purchased together to make suggestions to customers about additional potential purchases. For an example from health informatics, data analysts could describe relationships among diseases that are common for patients age 65 years and older, but uncommon for patients ages 50 to 64 years, and for the set of former cases describe the frequent comorbidities (Lu et al. 2009, 17). This information could be used to design educational outreach programs and internal continuing education programs. Association rule mining has also been used for detecting factors associated with attention deficit hyperactive disorder (ADHD) (Tai et al. 2009, e77), HAIs (Reynolds et al. 2016, S4), and heart disease (Nahar et al. 2013, 1086).

Evaluation

The purpose of data science is to answer questions about a variety of problems, and the CRISP-DM process emphasizes the critical nature of evaluating the results of analytic projects. Evaluation can include data visualization, descriptive statistics, inferential statistics, and more. As we have discussed, data mining uses algorithms to create models for predicting outcomes. The measures used to evaluate predictive accuracy include the error rate, which is the number of observations the model incorrectly predicts divided by the actual number of observations. Prediction can also be evaluated by a variety of other measures, including sensitivity (true positive), specificity (true negative), positive predictive value (precision), negative predictive value, and accuracy (true positives divided by total population). These concepts are defined and discussed in chapters 5 and 12.

Prediction can also be evaluated through the receiver operator characteristic (ROC), which is used to generate an area under the curve (AUC). The AUC is a visualization of model quality measured by plotting the model's positive predictive value (see chapter 12 for more information). For example, researchers could plot the AUC value for a predictive model related to identifying heart disease among a specific population. Plotting the AUC (true positive rate over the false positive rate) for this example with a hypothetical value of 0.88 visualizes the usefulness of the model compared to chance.

Deployment

The last phase in the data science process is deployment—applying the models and findings in some ongoing basis. Because data science projects aim to address real-world problems, it is hoped that the information and knowledge gained through these projects will be implemented in some capacity. Deployment may involve implementing a new algorithm as a function of decision support. For example, using several key factors, researchers developed a predictive model that identifies patients at high risk of being readmitted to the hospital, and this model can be used to help providers advise patients and reduce the number of hospitals readmissions (Billings et al. 2006, 327). The means of deployment may be a formal or informal report to a department, funding agency, or other entity, or researchers may add to the literature by publishing findings in a peer-reviewed academic journal.

Review Questions

1. What organization considers understanding evidence related to healthcare practice to be a core competency of healthcare professionals?
2. What term is defined as the total number of incorrectly classified observations divided by total correctly classified observations?
3. What classification models aim to group observations with others that are similar?
4. Multiple logistic regression is limited to how many predictor variables?
5. What do decision trees use to create predictive models?
6. Plotting data on a map is an example of what technique?
7. Which type of analytics involves summarizing data into meaningful charts or reports?
8. Parallel processing is considered a form of what?
9. What is a descriptive list of names (also called "representations" or "displays"), definitions, and attributes of data elements to be collected called?
10. What is the term for managing the process of what can transform hypotheses into actionable predictions?

Application Exercises

1. Access the Medicare data analysis website (CMS 2016a) and create an analysis using the built-in data visualization tools. Click one of the Compare tabs (such as Hospital or Physician) and click one of the datasets (such as Complications or Healthcare Associated Infections). On the top bar, there is are buttons called "Filter" and "Visualization." Click "Filter." Identify multiple variables to filter. Then click "Sort and roll up." Group the data as needed. Click "Visualization." Select the appropriate visualization to display the data. This dashboard provides end-users the capability of choosing data sets, as well as conducting multiple types of analysis including geospatial analysis (map) and other types of charts (bar, pie, and so on).
2. Locate and read an article focused on telling stories with data. Based on the article, write an explanation of how data story-telling is critical to data science–related projects in health informatics and information management.
3. The Office of the National Coordinator for Health Information Technology (ONC) Health IT Dashboard provides a variety of interactive data tools. Access the ONC Health IT Dashboard (2016a). Choose one of the dashboards by clicking "View Dashboard." Using the dashboard, create a new graphic visualization by selecting appropriate filters related to the dashboard. For example, click the dashboard title "EHR Vendors Reported by Office-Based Providers Demonstrating Meaningful Use." Select "Epic Systems Incorporated" in the drop-down menu. Ensure that the radio buttons for "Market Share," "2014 Reporting Year," and "Display All Office-based Providers with This Vendor" are selected. Drag the upper percentage range to 33. Select the box that states: "Click to Display Data Labels." Once you have created a visualization, explain what it shows.

References

Assunção, M.D., R.N. Calheiros, S. Bianchi, M.A.S. Netto, and R. Buyya. 2015. Big Data computing and clouds: Trends and future directions. *Journal of Parallel and Distributed Computing* 79:3–15.

Billings, J., J. Dixon, T. Mijanovich, and D. Wennberg. (2006). Case finding for patients at risk of readmission to hospital: Development of algorithm to identify high risk patients. *BMJ* 333(7563): 327.

Bronnert et al. 2011. *Health Data Analysis Toolkit*. Chicago: AHIMA. http://library.ahima.org/PdfView?oid=103453.

Centers for Medicare and Medicaid Services (CMS). 2016a. Data.Medicare.gov. https://data.medicare.gov/.

Centers for Medicare and Medicaid Services (CMS). 2016b. Healthcare Associated Infections. https://data.medicare.gov/data/hospital-compare.

Centers for Medicare and Medicaid Services (CMS). 2016c. LDS Inpatient Data Dictionary, version J. https://www.cms.gov/Research-Statistics-Data-and-Systems/Files-for-Order/LimitedDataSets/Downloads/InpatientVersionJ2011.pdf.

Centers for Medicare and Medicaid Services (CMS). 2016d (December). Medicare Drug Spending Dashboard 2014. https://www.cms.gov/Research-Statistics-Data-and-Systems/Statistics-Trends-and-Reports/Dashboard/Medicare-Drug-Spending/Drug_Spending_Dashboard.html.

Chimieski, B.F. and R.D. Ribeiro Fagundes. 2013. Association and classification data mining algorithms comparison over medical datasets. *Journal of Health Informatics* 5(2).

Davenport, T.H. and D. Patil, D. 2012 (October). Data scientist: The sexiest job of the 21st century. *Harvard Business Review* 90. https://hbr.org/2012/10/data-scientist-the-sexiest-job-of-the-21st-century.

Dombrovskiy, V.Y., A.A. Martin, J. Sunderram, J., and H.L. Paz. 2007. Rapid increase in hospitalization and mortality rates for severe sepsis in the United States: A trend analysis from 1993 to 2003. *Critical Care Medicine* 35(5):1244–1250.

Evans, J.R. and C.H. Lindner. 2012. Business analytics: The next frontier for decision sciences. *Decision Line* 43(2):4–6.

Fayyad, U., G. Piatetsky-Shapiro, and P. Smyth. 1996. From data mining to knowledge discovery in databases. *AI magazine* 17(3):37.

Frisse, M. E., K.B. Johnson, H. Nian, C.L. Davison, C.S. Gadd, K.M. Unertl, P.A. Turri, and Q. Chen. 2012. The financial impact of health information exchange on emergency department care. *Journal of the American Medical Informatics Association* 19(3):328–333.

Greiner, A.C. and E. Knebel. 2003. *Health Professions Education: A Bridge to Quality*. Washington, DC: National Academies Press.

Han, J. and M. Kamber. 2006. *Data Mining: Concepts and Techniques*. 2nd ed. San Francisco, CA: Morgan Kaufmann Publishers.

IBM. 2016. Bringing Big Data to the Enterprise: What Is Big Data? Accessed 22 August 2016. https://www-01.ibm.com/software/data/bigdata/what-is-big-data.html.

Koh, H.C. and G. Tan. 2011. Data mining applications in healthcare. *Journal of Healthcare Information Management* 19(2):64–72.

Lehmann, B. D., J.A. Bauer, X. Chen, M.E. Sanders, A.B. Chakravarthy, Y. Shyr, and J.A. Pietenpol. 2011. Identification of human triple-negative breast cancer subtypes and preclinical models for selection of targeted therapies. *Journal of Clinical Investigation* 121(7):2750–2767.

Letouzé, E. and J. Jütting. 2015. Official statistics, Big Data and human development. Data-Pop Alliance White Series Paper. https://www.paris21.org/sites/default/files/WPS_OfficialStatistics_June2015.pdf.

Linoff, G.S. and M.J.A. Berry. 2011. *Data Mining Techniques*. 3rd ed. Indianapolis, IN: Wiley Publishing, Inc.

Lu, D.F., W.N. Street, F. Currim, R. Hylock, and C. Delaney. 2009. A data modeling process for decomposing healthcare patient data sets. *Online Journal of Nursing Informatics* 13(1).

Manyika, J., M. Chui, B. Brown, J. Bughin, R. Dobbs, C. Roxburgh, and A.H. Byers. 2011 (May). Big Data: The Next Frontier for Innovation, Competition, And productivity. McKinsey Global Institute. http://www.mckinsey.com/business-functions/digital-mckinsey/our-insights/big-data-the-next-frontier-for-innovation.

Minnesota Population Center and State Health Access Data Assistance Center. 2016. Integrated Health Interview Series. Version 6.21. Minneapolis: University of Minnesota. https://ihis.ipums.org/ihis/index.shtml.

Nahar, J., T. Imam, K.S. Tickle, and Y.P.P. Chen. 2013. Association rule mining to detect factors which contribute to heart disease in males and females. *Expert Systems with Applications* 40(4):1086–1093.

Norton, M.J. 1999. Knowledge discovery in databases. *Library Trends* 48(1):9–21.
Office of the National Coordinator for Health Information Technology (ONC). 2016. ONC Budget Performance Measures. Health IT Dashboard. http://dashboard.healthit.gov/dashboards/onc-budget-performance-measures.php.
Office of the National Coordinator for Health Information Technology (ONC). 2015. Office-Based Physician Health IT Adoption. Health IT Dashboard. http://dashboard.healthit.gov/dashboards/physician-health-it-adoption.php.
Ordonez, C. and Z. Chen. 2012. Horizontal aggregations in SQL to prepare data sets for data mining analysis. *IEEE Transactions on Knowledge and Data Engineering* 24(4):678–691.
Reynolds, K.A. and R.A. Canales. 2016. Quantitative risk modeling of healthcare acquired infections and interventions using baseline data and simple models. *American Journal of Infection Control* 44(6):S4–S5.
Tai, Y. M. and H.W. Chiu. 2009. Comorbidity study of ADHD: Applying association rule mining (ARM) to National Health Insurance Database of Taiwan. *International Journal of Medical Informatics* 78(12):e75–e83.
Tufféry, S. 2011. *Data Mining and Statistics for Decision Making*. Chichester, UK: John Wiley and Sons Ltd.
US Department of Health and Human Services (HHS). 2015. *Development of a National Adult Protective Services Data System: NAMRS Pilot Final Report.* Vol. 2, *System Documentation.* https://aspe.hhs.gov/sites/default/files/pdf/187561/NAMRSpilot-V2.pdf.
White, T. 2012. *Hadoop: The Definitive Guide,* 3rd ed. Sebastopol, CA: O'Reilly Media.
Williams, G. 2011. *Data Mining with Rattle and R: The Art of Excavating Data for Knowledge Discovery*: New York: Springer Science and Business Media.
Wyatt, J.C. and F. Sullivan. 2005. ABC of health informatics: What is health information? *BMJ* 331(7516):566.
Zumel, N., J. Mount, and J. Porzak. 2014. *Practical Data Science with R.* Shelter Island, NY: Manning.

Resources

Pieczkiewicz, D. 2015. Exploratory data analysis and data visualization of MS-DRGs. In *Data Analytics in Healthcare Research: Tools and Strategies*. Edited by D. Marc and R. Sandefer. Chicago: AHIMA Press.
Wyatt, J. and J. Liu. 2002. Basic concepts in medical informatics. *Journal of Epidemiology and Community Health* 56(11):808–812.

8 Systematic Reviews and Meta-Analyses

Leming Zhou, PhD, DSc; Dilhari DeAlmeida, PhD, RHIA; and Valerie Watzlaf, PhD, MPH, RHIA, FAHIMA

Learning Objectives

- Explain the steps and techniques for performing systematic reviews and meta-analysis.
- Determine research questions, databases, inclusion and exclusion criteria, quality appraisal methods, and data analysis methods used in published systematic reviews and meta-analyses.
- Create a report about research results.
- Discuss the application of research findings in published systematic reviews and meta-analyses.

Key Terms

Cochrane Collaboration tool
Exclusion criteria
Fixed-effects model
Forest plot
Funnel plot
GRADE (Grading of Recommendations, Assessment, Development, and Evaluation) system
Grey literature
Hand search
Inclusion criteria
Literature review
Meta-analysis
Meta-regression
Newcastle-Ottawa scale (NOS)
PICOS
Preferred Reporting Items for Systematic Review and Meta-Analysis Protocols (PRISMA-P)
PROSPERO
Publication bias
Quality appraisal
Random-effects model
Research protocol
Research question
Risk of bias
Screening process
Sensitivity analysis
Subgroup analysis
Systematic review

When seeking to review state-of-the art research, students and researchers in the field of health informatics may become overwhelmed by the enormous quantity of published articles that they could potentially read. There were approximately 28,100 active peer-reviewed English-language journals in 2014, and the annual growth rate of science-related journal articles between 1960 and 2006 was at least 4.7 percent (Ware and Mabe 2015, 6). In recent years, about 2.5 million journal articles have been published annually; this number includes contributions via the open-access movement (the worldwide effort to provide free online access to scientific and scholarly research literature) and articles in online-only journals (Ware and Mabe 2015, 6). The volume of available research is significantly larger when conference proceedings (particularly in the field of computer science and information science), open-access paper archives such as arXiv and bioRxiv, and in-house publications, such as personal websites, are also considered. The PubMed database alone "comprises more than 26 million citations for biomedical literature from MEDLINE, life science journals, and online books" (NCBI 2016). This chapter explains various review strategies to help cope with the massive amount of possible information sources and to find the information most relevant to a specific research question or project.

A **literature review** is an approach to examining published information on a topic or field. A typical literature review is used to create a foundation and justification for one's research or to demonstrate knowledge on the current state of a field. In one literature review, multiple studies that used computational modeling (computer programs that can simulate the development of disease) on atherosclerosis in the past 10 years, and the conclusions were drawn based on the analysis of these models (Parton et al. 2016, 562).

In a typical literature review, the reviewers select a number of articles according to a certain standard (determined by the reviewers), such as the quality of journals and the reputation of authors, and then summarize the results in those articles. In many cases, this type of literature review is performed by an expert in the field of study. The reviewer alone determines which articles are appropriate selections according to his or her own experience and preferences. This practice can be convenient, but it can easily lead to biases in the review. For example, the literature reviewer may prefer to review articles published in certain journals, or papers published by certain authors.

A **systematic review** uses a predetermined plan to search, evaluate, and synthesize the results on a topic area. Conducting a systematic review is often a quicker and more cost-effective way than a randomized controlled trial (RCT) to answer a primary research question. It can provide the researcher with high-quality evidence on their hypothesis or research question. (Systematic review is also discussed in chapter 10.) **Meta-analysis** is the statistical arm within the systematic review; it combines both quantitative and qualitative research studies to arrive at a statistically sound conclusion.

A research team typically performs the systematic review, which is based on a research question that is also established by the researchers. All the articles related to this research question are collected and evaluated, regardless of the journal, author, or institutional affiliations of the authors. The review has specific inclusion and exclusion criteria, and the entire systematic review process is explicitly presented and strictly followed. Therefore, the result is more objective than the typical literature review performed by one person or a few experts in one field.

The systematic review has been applied in most research fields and is highly important in the health sciences. When researchers in the health sciences publish the results of a study, they primarily describe their study subjects and only report the results obtained from these study subjects. These results are limited by the study design and scope. For example, the subjects might be from one hospital or one healthcare network, have a specific disease, or live in a rural or urban environment. In contrast, when a research team conducts a systematic review, they come up with a specific research question, collect similar types of research articles according to the research question, extract relevant data from these articles (the relevance is determined by the research question), combine the data together, and summarize the results (systematic review alone) or perform a statistical data analysis (meta-analysis) on the data collected from those research articles. Hence, the results from the systematic review and meta-analysis may be useful for developing clinical practice guidelines because they can determine which studies are reliable, which ones are generalizable, and which results should be used under what circumstances. The guidelines that are developed may then lead to higher quality healthcare services and better health outcomes. As a result, systematic review and meta-analysis are able to exceed randomized controlled studies, cohort studies, case reports, expert opinions, animal studies, and in vitro studies to provide the highest quality evidence for evidence-based medicine (Hoyt and Hersh 2014, 327). This is demonstrated in an evidence pyramid shown in figure 8.1. In the evidence pyramid, evidence is sequenced from least to most clinically relevant bottom to top.

Figure 8.1 Clinical relevance of evidence

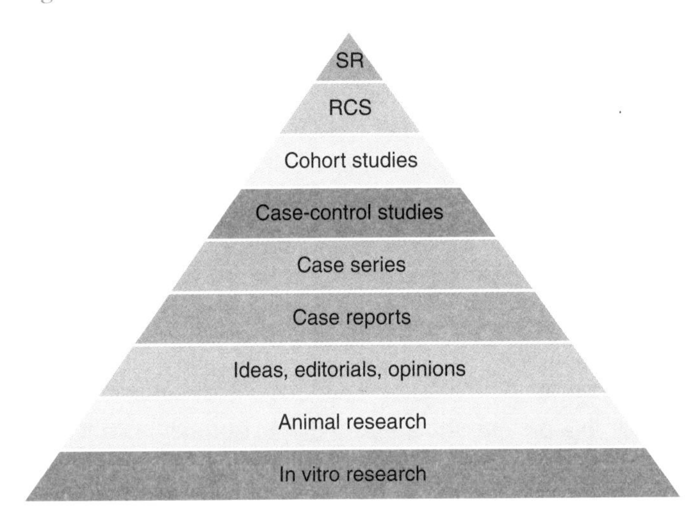

In health informatics, many questions need to be answered. Is a clinical decision support system helpful for reducing medical errors? Does the work efficiency of small-scale clinics improve after they adopt electronic health record (EHR) systems? Are the security features in mobile health applications sufficient for protecting patients' privacy? Can health information technology (HIT) improve the quality of cancer care and chronic disease management? There are many studies on these topics and other important health informatics questions, and different research teams have offered answers based on their studies. However, like the health sciences studies mentioned earlier, the results from these health informatics studies are not consistent and each study has its own limitations. To obtain a convincing answer to each of these questions and guide the decision for the next step, a systematic review and meta-analysis can often be used to systematically select, evaluate, and analyze the data in these studies.

In the following sections, the description of a step-by-step procedure for conducting a systematic review is provided, starting from an overview, then moving on to defining research questions, searching research articles in journal article indexing databases, selecting articles based on the research question and inclusion and exclusion criteria, extracting data from selected articles, and finally analyzing data and reporting results.

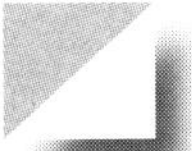

Real-World Case

Among the large number of available mobile health apps are many created to encourage individuals to be more physically active and lose weight. Flores Mateo and colleagues were interested in determining the effectiveness of these mobile health apps. More specifically, they asked, "Do mobile apps that promote weight loss and increase physical activity actually help users achieve these goals?" To answer this question, the research team performed a systematic review and meta-analysis to evaluate the efficacy of mobile phone apps to promote weight loss and increase physical activity (Flores Mateo et al. 2015). Their research will be used as an example throughout this chapter.

Steps in Conducting a Systematic Review

There are typically nine steps in conducting a systematic review:

1. Defining the research question(s)
2. Creating the systematic review protocol
3. Identifying the terms of the project
4. Defining the inclusion and exclusion criteria
5. Performing searches in databases
6. Selecting articles according to inclusion and exclusion criteria
7. Reviewing articles and extracting data from the articles
8. Conducting quality appraisal and data analysis (meta-analysis)
9. Writing a final report

Each step will be described in more detail in the following sections. Throughout the discussion of these steps, we will refer to two sample research studies that used a systematic review and meta-analysis and provide a step-by-step guide on how to conduct a systematic review and meta-analysis. In the real-world case above, Flores Mateo and colleagues performed a systematic review and meta-analysis to evaluate the efficacy of mobile phone apps to promote weight loss and increase physical activities and compared them with other interventions (Flores Mateo et al. 2015, e253). In another study, Tarver and Menachemi used a systematic review and meta-analysis to examine the impact of HIT in cancer care at different levels of the care continuum (Tarver and Menachemi 2016, 420–427).

Step 1: Defining the Research Question(s)

A **research question** is an explicit statement of the question a research team wants to answer in a research project. Defining this question is critically important in a systematic review because all the other steps in the review are closely related to the definition. For instance, the research question helps determine which articles and papers are relevant to the review and which are not. If the research question is to evaluate the efficacy of mobile phone apps to promote weight loss and increase physical activity, as in the study by Flores Mateo and associates, research related to physical activity mobile apps will be included, and studies about physical activity without mobile apps involved will be excluded. The selection of citation databases to be searched and the data analysis strategy will also be specific to this research question. Therefore, it is recommended that the research team spend sufficient time discussing and refining their research question(s) before they move forward.

Because the research question for a systematic review (or other type of research) may not be completely clear at the beginning of the study, revisions at later points in the research process may take place before the final research question is defined. For instance, a research team may initially want to know whether mobile health apps are beneficial in improving healthcare outcomes, but this is a large topic and the different kinds of health outcomes (such as weight, blood pressure, or blood glucose control) may not be comparable. For one specific type of healthcare outcome, there are multiple possible approaches to measuring the outcome and implementing the mobile health app. Therefore, the research team might narrow the research question to focus on the impact of smartphone-based mobile health apps on weight loss and physical activity, as Flores Mateo and colleagues did. The procedure is shown in figure 8.2. A general rule of thumb for determining the final research question is that the question should be specific to a particular topic and the research team should be able to identify a sufficient but manageable number of articles for the systematic review in the later steps. Further guidance on determining a systematic review research question can be found in the resources list.

Figure 8.2 Steps in defining a research question

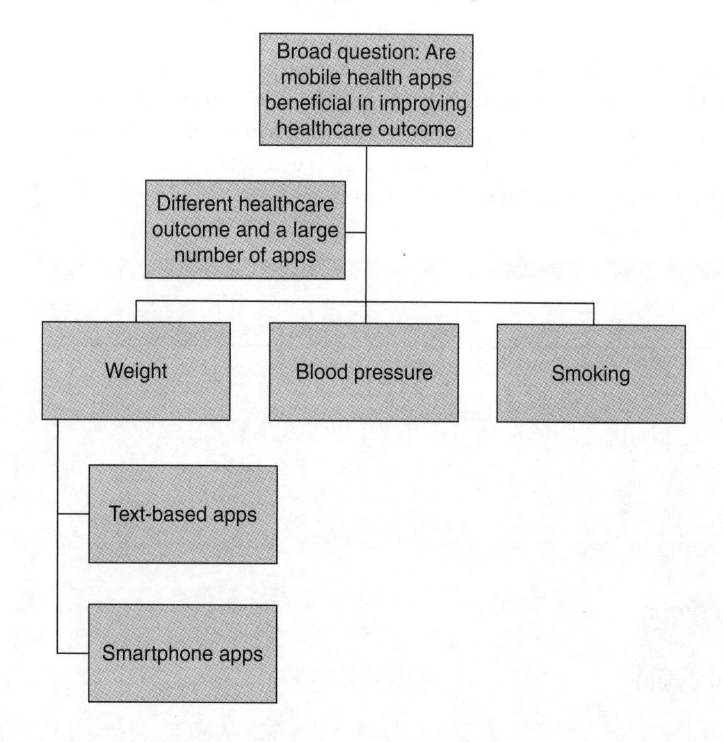

Additionally, many mobile apps have been designed to promote weight loss and increase physical activity, and multiple research studies have investigated change in physical activity levels and body mass index (BMI) before and after the use of certain mobile apps. The various studies used different research approaches, targeted different populations, and had different sample sizes (typically small ones). Therefore, it is not surprising that these studies offer conflicting conclusions. In one RCT with 41 young adults using mobile health interventions for weight management, the change in BMI associated with mobile phone app interventions was insignificant (Hebden et al. 2014, 322–332). In contrast, in a randomized controlled pilot study, researchers worked with 68 overweight and obese men and women for 6 months and observed a significant change in body weight associated with mobile phone interventions (Allen et al. 2013). Which conclusion should be trusted? It is hard to make the decision only based on these two studies. A systematic review and meta-analysis can help obtain a better idea about the efficacy of mobile phone interventions to promote weight loss and increase physical activity because the conclusion will be based on the analysis of data and results from multiple and similar type of studies. Therefore, the research question for this systematic review is narrowed to "how efficacious are mobile phone interventions in promoting weight loss and increasing physical activity?"

The question of whether HIT is important in the management of cancer also needs to be refined to serve as a meaningful research question to guide a systematic review. Multiple studies have been done on the impact of HIT on cancer care, especially at specific stages of cancer (such as cancer prevention and diagnosis) and different activities in cancer treatment (such as behavior-change interventions and decision making). However, there is no clear answer about the impact of HIT in cancer care across all levels of the care continuum (risk assessment, prevention, detection, diagnosis, treatment, survivorship, and end-of-life care). Therefore, Tarver and Menachemi defined the research question for their systematic review and meta-analysis as follows: "What is the impact of HIT on cancer care across the continuum of care?"(Tarver and Menachemi 2016, 420).

Step 2: Creating the Systematic Review Protocol

A systematic review **research protocol** defines the detailed steps the research team should follow to conduct the research. A systematic review typically takes several months, and can take more than a year. Therefore, it is a good idea to have the protocol created before the search for papers so that the protocol can consistently guide the research team through the entire review process. Refer to Watzlaf et al. (2015) for an example of a systematic review protocol.

It is recommended that the construction of a systematic review protocol be based on the **Preferred Reporting Items for Systematic Review and Meta-Analysis Protocols (PRISMA-P)** (Moher et al. 2015). The PRISMA-P includes the following 17 items that are considered essential, minimum components to include in systematic reviews and meta-analyses:

- Title of the systematic review protocol
- Registration number if the protocol is registered at one specific registry, such as PROSPERO
- The names, institutional affiliations, and e-mail addresses of all authors who conduct the systematic review study, and the mailing address of the corresponding author. Sometimes, the contributions of protocol authors are also mentioned.
- Amendments to a previously released systematic review protocol if changes have been made on the protocol, or a statement about using amendments to document changes on the protocol
- Financial support sources and sponsor for the review
- Rationale for conducting the systematic review
- Objectives: An explicit statement of the research question and the corresponding study participants, interventions, comparators, and outcomes
- Eligibility criteria for making selections on research studies that will be included or excluded in the systematic review
- Information sources for the systematic review study, such as citation databases, websites, and authors of published articles
- Search strategy for the systematic review study, such as the names of citation databases and keywords used for the database search
- A plan to manage, select, and process the research studies collected by using the search strategy
- Data items that will be extracted from those studies. The data simplification steps can also be presented if applicable
- Outcomes from which data will be extracted, and prioritization of main and additional outcomes

- The methods for assessing risk of bias in individual studies
- The methods for qualitatively and quantitatively synthesizing data, and planned summary measures, including additional statistical analyses if applicable
- The planned methods for assessing meta-bias, such as publication bias across studies and selective reporting within studies
- The planned methods for assessing the cumulative evidence

In the following sections, we will provide detailed descriptions of many of these items. Self-explanatory items, such as title, registration, author information, financial support, and amendments, are not addressed.

After the systematic review protocol is created, the research team may choose to publish the protocol in a journal or in a protocol database such as **PROSPERO**, an international prospective register of systematic reviews. Once the protocol is created, the review team should strictly follow the protocol to conduct the systematic review and meta-analysis. If the investigators need to make any changes in the systematic review after the protocol is released to the public, they should create amendments for the protocol, instead of making changes directly on the protocol.

Step 3: Identifying the Terms of the Project

PRISMA-P recommends that each systematic review include detailed eligibility criteria using **PICOS**, which stands for *participants, interventions, comparisons, outcome(s),* and *study design* of the systematic review reporting system. Because these items are closely related to the research question of the systematic review study, it is also recommended that the systematic review research question includes these components (Shamseer et al. 2015, g7647).

The following is the PICOS for the 2015 study by Flores Mateo and coauthors on mobile physical activity and weight management apps:

- P: The study participants are study subjects in the selected mobile health app studies on weight loss and physical activity promotion.
- I: The interventions are recent mobile health apps.
- C: The comparisons are other approaches to promote weight loss and increase physical activity, such as in-person coaching and telemedicine.
- O: The outcome is the changes of weight and physical activity level, compared to other approaches. In certain cases, there are primary outcomes and secondary outcomes. Primary outcomes are the most important outcomes for this systematic review. Secondary outcomes are any additional outcomes that are to be addressed with the systematic review. In many cases, there are only primary outcomes.
- S: The study designs included are RCTs, case-control studies, and matched case-control trials.

In addition to PICOS, time frame and setting are often stated when the terms of the systematic review are identified. (See chapter 10 for how PICO[TS] is used in developing key questions for the systematic review.) In the 2015 mobile phone apps study done by Flores Mateo and associates, the authors only set the upper limit of the time frame, August 2015, and did not include a restriction on the setting. With regards to the time frame, the final selection results show that the selected articles were from 2010 through 2015. The reason for the time frame is that mobile phone apps were developed mainly after 2008, and it took roughly two years to perform the designed studies, analyze the data, and then publish the findings. Therefore, although the authors did not specifically set the lower limit as 2010, the database search result reflected the historical circumstances. Generally speaking, if a research topic has a much longer history—for instance, the impact of technology on the management of health records—the authors will need to carefully choose the time frame according to the history of the research field and the specific research question.

Step 4: Defining Inclusion and Exclusion Criteria

Inclusion criteria are the criteria used to keep articles in the study, and the **exclusion criteria** are the criteria used to remove articles from the study. These criteria are used to screen articles obtained in the database search, which will be described in step 5. The inclusion and exclusion criteria are mainly determined by the terms of the project and the research question. Some level of redundancy may be seen in some components. In some cases, there is no restriction at all in certain components.

The following are the inclusion and exclusion criteria used in the 2015 mobile phone app study done by Flores Mateo and associates (2015):

- **Participants**
  - Inclusion criteria: Study subjects who participated in physical activity and weight management mobile app studies, and who had no other disease except for obesity
  - Exclusion criteria: Study subjects who did not participate in mobile app studies
- **Interventions**
  - Inclusion criteria: Sophisticated mobile physical activity and weight management app
  - Exclusion criteria: Studies of subjects who did not use mobile physical activity app; mobile app interventions that were based on text messaging; use of personal digital assistants (PDAs) to deliver the intervention
- **Comparators**
  - Inclusion criteria: Studies that compared the intervention group to a control group whose subjects did not use a mobile app
  - Exclusion criteria: Studies that used a mobile app or did not have a control group.
- **Outcomes**
  - Inclusion criteria: Change of weight–related health measures (such as body weight, BMI, or waist circumference) or measures of physical activity level
  - Exclusion criteria: No measures of weight-related parameters
- **Study design**
  - Inclusion criteria: All types of studies that used a control group comparison to evaluate mobile app intervention for weight management and physical activity promotion, such as randomized and nonrandomized controlled trials, case-control studies, and matched case-control trials
  - Exclusion criteria: Case reports and case series, studies without a control group, reviews, editorials, and non-research letters
- **Time frames**
  - Inclusion criteria: Studies published up to August 2015
  - Exclusion criteria: Studies performed prior to 2010 (not explicitly stated in the article but implied in other selection criteria, such as the exclusion of text messaging intervention and no involvement of PDAs)
- **Setting**
  - Inclusion criteria: Any setting
  - Exclusion criteria: None
- **Language**
  - Inclusion criteria: Any language
  - Exclusion criteria: None

Step 5: Performing Searches in Databases

To perform searches in databases, investigators must decide on two components: the keywords that will be used in the database search and the databases used to perform the search. In some studies, the keywords can be easily determined by reading the research question. For instance, in the mobile app study, the research question is to evaluate the efficacy of mobile apps to promote physical activity level and weight loss, and therefore the keywords are "mobile application", "apps", "smartphone", "physical activity", "exercise", "weight", "obesity", "body mass index", and "body weight". These keywords can be organized with "AND" and "OR" to form a search statement. In this study, the keyword search statement, using MeSH terms, in PubMed was as follows: ("mobile application" OR apps OR smartphone) AND ("physical activity" OR exercise OR activity OR inactivity OR weight OR obesity OR "body mass index" OR "waist circumference" OR "body weight") AND humans (Flores Mateo et al. 2015, e253).

In some studies, researchers cannot obtain all search keywords from the research question alone and therefore need to take additional steps to build the keyword list and database search statement. For example, in the impact of HIT on cancer care study, the research question was to determine the impact of HIT on cancer care across the continuum of care (Tarver and Menachemi 2016, 420). A few keywords can be identified from this research question, such as "health information technology," "cancer care," and "continuum." However, these keywords are broad terms and many irrelevant articles would be obtained if just these keywords are used to conduct the database search. Therefore, the keywords need to be more specific.

For example, "electronic health records", "patient Internet portals", "personal health records", "electronic medical records", "clinical decision support", and "clinical reminders" are more specific types of HIT systems; similarly, terms such as "neoplasm", "tumor", "preventive services", "tobacco use", "cancer diagnosis", "cervical smear", "screening", "colonoscopy", "mammography", "pap smear", and "survivorship" are specific terms closely related to cancer care. As in the previous example, these keywords are linked by "AND" and "OR" to form a keyword search statement. When using the same keywords to perform searches in different databases, the search statements need to be designed specifically for each database.

In biomedical research, PubMed is one choice for a citation database because it includes a vast number of citations in biomedical research. Depending on the specific research project, other databases may be selected in addition to or instead of PubMed. In their 2015 mobile app study, Flores Mateo and colleagues also used Scopus (started in 1960) and the Cumulative Index to Nursing and Allied Health Literature (CINAHL, started in 1960). In the impact of HIT on cancer care study, the selected databases were PubMed, CINAHL, and PsycINFO (Tarver and Menachemi 2016, 421). There are many other indexing databases available for keyword searches, such as Sociology Abstract, Cochrane Central Database of Controlled Trials (CENTRAL), Applied Social Sciences Index and Abstracts (ASSIA), British Education Index (BEI), ERIC, IEEE Xplore, EMBASE, Compendex, Web of Science, ACM Digital Library, and INSPEC. The systematic review research team should carefully choose databases that are suited to their research question and provide relevant content. If a database does not have the citations of relevant articles, it should be excluded from the list of the databases to search.

After the keywords and databases are determined, investigators can issue the keyword search statements to the corresponding databases. In certain cases, researchers need to search the **grey literature**, which is the body of publications that is available in print, electronically, or both, but is not published in easily accessible publications, such as journals (Eden et al. 2011, 98–99). Examples of grey literature can include conference proceedings, research registries, and reports in databases and other suitable resources. Sometimes, researchers also need to perform a **hand search** in journals (visit the website of journals and perform keyword search there) to account for studies missed due to the imperfections of indexing, search strategies, and database compilation. Occasionally, investigators may need to contact the authors of a study to obtain certain articles or supplementary materials.

The search strategy can be executed by the systematic review research team or a reference librarian. After the screening of articles is completed, an investigator may also go through the reference list of each selected article and identify relevant articles from those references.

All the search results can be exported into a reference management program, such as Reference Manager, EndNote, or Mendeley, which can be used to remove duplicate citations from the list. The database search is shown in the top portion of figure 8.3. In some cases, study authors must be contacted to clarify whether the same data set was used in multiple studies so that the same data and results are not used multiple times in the systematic review and meta-analysis, which would introduce bias into the final conclusion. If the authors cannot be reached and the study reports do not specify whether the data sets are identical, the systematic review team needs to take efforts to compare the published works from the same authors or groups and come up their own conclusion.

Figure 8.3 Flow chart summarization of database search and data extraction

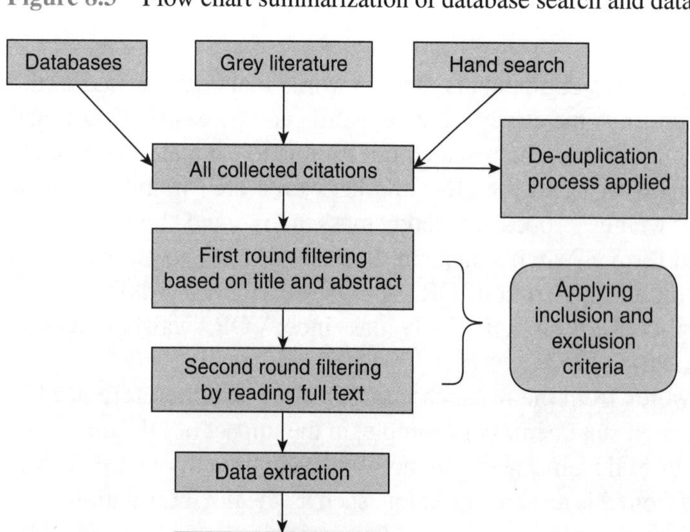

Step 6: Selecting Articles According to Inclusion and Exclusion Criteria

After the database search result is available, a screening process—the process of selecting (filtering) articles according to predetermined inclusion and exclusion criteria—can be conducted. The screening process is typically done in two or more rounds. In the first round, at least two independent reviewers in the research team should evaluate the database search results (or article records). These search results used in this round only include the article titles, years, and abstracts. The reviewers cannot see information such as author names, institutions, and journals. The two reviewers need to be familiar with the inclusion and exclusion criteria and strictly follow them to select articles. Each reviewer independently labels each article with "Yes" or "No" and a brief reason for the label. If both reviewers label an article with "Yes," this article will move to the next round of selection. If both reviewers label one article with "No," this article will be removed from the systematic review study. If one reviewer labels the article with "Yes" and the other reviewer labels it with "No," the two reviewers need to discuss the difference and resolve discrepancies by consensus. During the discussion, the recorded reasons for the label should be retained for future use. The two reviewers may also seek the opinion of a third independent reviewer if one is available. In this case, the discrepancies still need to be resolved by discussion and consensus among all reviewers.

It is recommended that the two independent reviewers first go through a relatively small number of articles (for instance, 30 to 50 articles), compare their labeling results, and conduct the discussion and resolve discrepancies. This initial process may help them to determine whether they have a different understanding on the inclusion and exclusion criteria. Once the two reviewers share a common view of the eligibility criteria, they may then evaluate all the search results.

Typically, before the first round of screening (or filtering), the database search results include a few hundred to several thousand articles. After the first round of filtering, the number of articles may be dramatically reduced, usually to the range of 30 to a few hundred. After all, numerous keyword search results may not be relevant to the specific systematic review research question.

In the next step, the full texts of selected articles obtained in the first round of filtering should be downloaded from the journal websites or requested from libraries. In the second round of filtering, the two reviewers read the full texts of these articles and follow the inclusion and exclusion criteria to label these articles again with "Yes" or "No" and a brief reason for the label. The selection process is the same as in the first round of filtering, and the research team eventually has a list of articles to include in the systematic review study. As mentioned earlier, in some cases, the research team may choose to go through the reference lists of these selected articles and identify additional relevant articles. The final list of articles included in this systematic review study is obtained after these two rounds of filtering. The full texts of these selected articles may be stored in a shared account, such as a secure cloud-based storage tool in which the research team can share large documents as well as collaborate. The middle part of figure 8.3 shows the two rounds of article filtering (the screening process).

In these two rounds of article filtering, inter-reviewer reliability can be evaluated using Cohen's kappa (κ) coefficient, which measures the agreement between two reviewers who each classify multiple items into two mutually exclusive categories ("Yes" or "No"). The equation for kappa is:

$$\kappa = \frac{\Pr(o) - \Pr(e)}{1 - \Pr(e)}$$

Where $\Pr(o)$ is the observed agreement between two reviewers, and $\Pr(e)$ is the probability of random agreement. If the two reviewers are in complete agreement, then kappa is 1.

To understand how to calculate a kappa coefficient, consider the following example: Two reviewers (1 and 2) independently label 100 articles with "Yes" or "No," and the agreements and disagreements are counted as shown in table 8.1). Note that the sum of the agreements and disagreements must be the same as the number of labeled articles (100 in this example).

Table 8.1 Reviewer agreement and disagreement count data

		Reviewer 2	
		Yes	No
Reviewer 1	Yes	50	10
	No	5	35

- First, the observed agreement is calculated. This is the total number of articles labeled "Yes" or "No" by both reviewers out of all articles. In this example, 50 articles were labeled "Yes" by both reviewers, and 35 articles were labeled "No" by both reviewers. Therefore, the observed agreement is $\Pr(o) = (50 + 35)/100 = 0.85$.
- Reviewer 1 assigned "Yes" to 60 articles (50 + 10; the total of the numbers in the "Yes" row). In other words, reviewer 1 assigned "Yes" 60 percent of the time (60/100 = 0.60).
- Reviewer 2 assigned "Yes" to 55 articles (50 + 5; the total of numbers in the "Yes" column). Thus, reviewer 2 assigned "Yes" 55 percent of the time (55/100 = 0.55).
- Hence, the probability that both reviewers would assign "Yes" *randomly* is $0.60 \times 0.55 = 0.33$.
- Reviewer 1 assigned "No" to 40 articles (5 + 35; the total of numbers in the "No" row). In other words, reviewer 1 assigned "No" 40 percent of the time (40/100 = 0.40).
- Reviewer 2 assigned "No" to (10 + 35) = 45 articles (the total of numbers in the "No" column). Thus, reviewer 2 assigned "No" 45 percent of the time (45/100 = 0.45).
- Hence, the probability that both reviewers would assign "No" *randomly* is $0.40 \times 0.45 = 0.18$.
- Therefore, the probability of random agreement is $\Pr(e) = 0.33 + 0.18 = 0.51$. We obtain the following kappa coefficient:

$$\kappa = \frac{\Pr(o) - \Pr(e)}{1 - \Pr(e)} = \frac{0.85 - 0.51}{1 - 0.51} = 0.69$$

This kappa (κ) coefficient is calculated during the article selection phase of review to ensure the inter-reviewer reliability is at or above a chosen threshold (for instance, 0.8). If the kappa (κ) coefficient falls below the chosen threshold (0.8), inter-reviewer reliability is insufficient and the two reviewers need to discuss the selection procedure until agreement is reached. A kappa value of 0.61 or higher is substantial; a value of 0.81 or higher is considered as almost perfect (Landis and Koch 1977, 159–174).

In the 2015 mobile app study, Flores Mateo and coauthors identified 1,122 articles through database searching. They also identified two additional articles from review and reference lists. After they removed duplicated records, they had 946 records in total. In the first round of filtering, they excluded 903 articles by reviewing the titles and abstracts. They reviewed the full texts of 43 articles in the second round of filtering and excluded 31 articles by applying their inclusion and exclusion criteria, such as the participants, intervention, comparators, outcomes, and study design. Therefore, 12 articles were used in the systematic review and meta-analysis (Flores Mateo et al. 2015, e253).

In their 2016 impact of HIT on cancer care study, Tarver and Menachemi searched four databases and obtained 3,355 citations. After they removed 1,428 duplicates, there were 1,927 unique titles. In the first round of filtering, the authors excluded 1,834 articles based on titles and abstracts. In the second round of filtering, they excluded 8 articles based on the full texts of 93 articles. The researchers then identified 37 additional articles through review of reference lists of the selected articles. In the end, 122 articles were used for the systematic review and meta-analysis. In some articles, multiple study outcomes were reported and each outcome represented an individual analysis (Tarver and Menachemi 2016, 421). Therefore, this meta-analysis incorporated a total of 156 individual analyses. A systematic review report typically includes a flow diagram, such as figure 8.4, which shows the article selection process.

Figure 8.4 Sample flow diagram for article selection

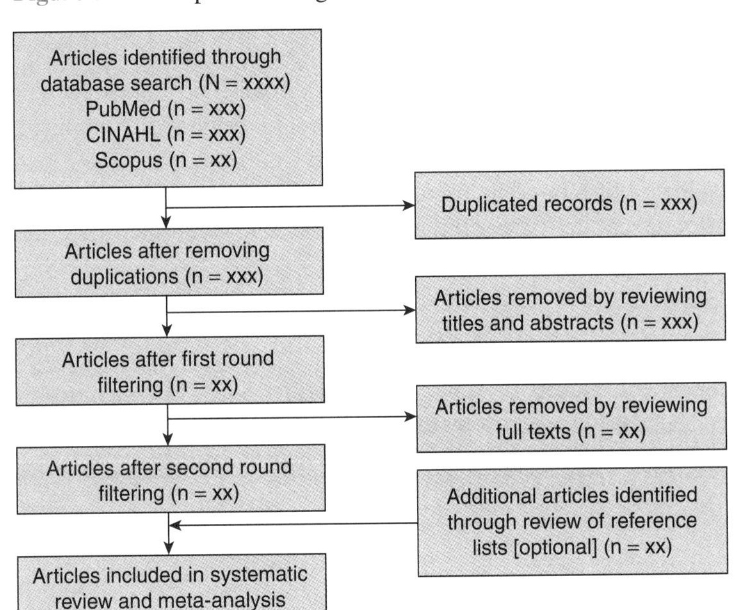

Some software programs are specifically designed for systematic review data management. For example, Distiller Systematic Review (DistillerSR) software is an Internet-based software program that facilitates collaboration among reviewers during the study selection process. Eppi-Reviewer is another web-based software for systematic review data management program. The database search results and full text PDF files can be imported into these programs. They may reduce data entry errors during the data extraction process because they can directly extract data from those papers into precreated data extraction forms. The extracted data can also be exported directly into statistical analysis software. This type of program can also facilitate the creation of the flow diagram (as shown in figure 8.3) once the screening process is completed. While all the steps described in this chapter can be done without the use of these software programs, they can make certain steps easier.

Step 7: Reviewing and Extracting Data from Articles

After the articles to be used for review and meta-analysis are determined, the next step is to review those articles and extract data from them. There are various approaches to reviewing these articles. Some research teams choose to split the articles into a few groups, and each reviewer processes one group of articles. This strategy is typical when the number of selected articles is large (for example, more than 100 articles). When the number of articles is relatively small (such as in the range of 30 to 50), the research team may review those articles together, or each member can review the articles while the team works as a group to extract the desired data.

To achieve a high-quality systematic review and meta-analysis, two or more reviewers in the team should independently review all the selected articles, follow the same approach to extract data from those articles, and use standard forms to report the extracted data. At the end of this process, these data forms are merged together. If there are discrepancies in data items, they should be resolved via discussion. It is also recommended that the reviewers perform calibration exercises before they start the review and data extraction. If it is not feasible to have more than one person review all the articles and extract data independently, another reviewer should at least randomly choose a few articles after the data extraction and verify the accuracy of the extracted data by following the same procedure used by the original reviewer. The research team always should explicitly report their data extraction approach in their final report.

Data extraction can be complicated, especially if the targeted topic is complex. For instance, in the 2016 HIT impact to cancer care study includes many different types of HIT systems, such as EHR systems, personal health record systems, clinical decision support systems, computer-assisted diagnosis systems, and reminder systems, to name just a few. Additionally, the study covers many different types of cancer (such as breast cancer, cervical cancer, lung cancer, prostate cancer), multiple cancer care continuum levels (risk assessment, prevention, detection, diagnosis, treatment, survivorship, and end of life care), various intervention focuses (such as patient, provider, and both), and multiple study outcomes (such as behavior change, decision making, education, pain management, psychosocial, and screening rates) (Tarver and Menachemi 2016, 422). It is a complicated task to accurately extract all these data items from 122 research articles. Therefore, it is recommended that the data extraction forms be developed carefully a priori and documented in the review protocol.

Table 8.2 shows a simple example of a data form, which can be easily created by various software programs such as Microsoft Excel and Microsoft Word. One may also choose to use the aforementioned systematic review data management program, such as DistillerSR, to create the data form. In the HIT impact to cancer care study, a coding sheet was developed to systematically extract information from all selected articles. The extracted information includes the study design; cancer continuum level; setting; HIT intervention focus; cancer type; HIT intervention; and outcome of studies (Tarver and Menachemi 2016, 421–422).

Table 8.2 Sample data form

Study	Setting	Study Design	Sample Size	Cancer Type	Continuum Level	HIT Intervention	HIT Intervention Focus	Outcomes

In the mobile app study, two reviewers independently reviewed the 12 selected articles and extracted data from them. They resolved discrepancies by consensus. The authors developed a data form in Microsoft Word to track the extracted data items, including author, country where study took place, age of participants, length of follow-up, sample size, and study outcomes, such as the mean and standard deviation of body weight, BMI, waist circumference, and physical activity. When the same cohort authored multiple publications, Flores Mateo and coauthors did not use all the data; instead, they chose to use only the data from the study from the cohort with the longest follow-up period. When the follow-up periods were equivalent, they selected the study with the largest number of cases, the study that used internal comparisons, or the most recent study (Flores Mateo et al. 2015, e253). These decisions are very reasonable for this specific study. Typically, a larger sample size will provide a more reliable the statistical result than a smaller sample. Also, changes in body weight are more meaningful when measured at the end of a study with a long follow-up period (short-term studies do not show differentiate between people who initially lose weight and keep it off and those who lose weight and then regain it). Studies with a control group available can remove a lot of uncertainty about whether the intervention and outcomes are related. Finally, recent studies usually have a better study design than older ones, or the implementation of recent mobile apps can be assumed to be better than those that were first released, which in turn may lead to more trustworthy research results.

In certain cases, selected articles omit information that is needed for the systematic review. When this happens, reviewers need to contact the authors of the articles to obtain those data items. For instance, let us suppose a research team is conducting a systematic review about the security features in telemedicine systems, and one article provides detailed descriptions about their major security features but only briefly mentioned their encryption approaches. Without more information about encryption, the data from this article may not fit the systematic review criteria. The reviewers can contact the authors and ask for further clarification about their encryption algorithms. However, if one article missed many desired items, it may be removed from the systematic review study and meta-analysis.

Another issue that arises during the review and data extraction is the language of the articles. In many cases, the research team only chooses to process articles written in certain languages (typically the native languages of the research team members). After all, if no one in the research team has the knowledge of a particular language, it is very unlikely that the team can extract correct information from articles written in that language. Some research teams may choose to use human or computer language translation services. All choices (only one language, a few languages, or all languages) are acceptable. The major focus is the accuracy of the extracted data, which may be affected by the need to translate articles.

Step 8: Conducting Quality Appraisal and Data Analysis (Meta-Analysis)

After the desired data are extracted from the selected papers, the next step is a **quality appraisal**, the assessment of the quality of selected studies. This assessment can be done at the outcome or study level, or both. Several different systems are used in healthcare research to evaluate literature. The **GRADE (Grading of Recommendations, Assessment, Development and Evaluation) system** is often used to judge the quality of evidence in healthcare literature and evidence-based research (Guyatt et al. 2008). In the GRADE system, quality-of-evidence criteria for systematic reviews include study limitations (risk of bias), indirectness of evidence, inconsistency of results, imprecision of results, and publication bias (Guyatt et al. 2011a, 407; Guyatt et al. 2011b, 1277; Guyatt et al. 2011c, 1283; Guyatt et al. 2011d, 1294; Guyatt et al. 2011e, 1303). **Risk of bias** is the chance that a systematic error or deviation from the truth exists in results or inferences (AHRQ 2012). **Publication bias** results when researchers or scientific journal editors treat studies that demonstrate positive results differently from studies that demonstrate negative results. Researchers may not submit negative or inconclusive results for publication, and editors may prefer to publish positive results in their journals. In other words, although those individual studies are valid and the results from those studies are reasonable, because of a biased publishing approach, the conclusion obtained from the systematic review and meta-analysis by using these individual studies may be misleading.

Researchers can assess the overall quality of evidence for every important outcome using the GRADE 4-point ranked scale: (4) high; (3) moderate; (2) low; and (1) very low. Typically, researchers may obtain reliable results based on high- or moderate-quality evidence. The results obtained from low- or very low–quality evidence have some uncertainty. The systematic review research team should explicitly indicate the evidence the team used to assess individual studies and the reasons for identifying the rank. In the five GRADE quality-of-evidence criteria, indirectness of evidence, inconsistency of results, and imprecision of results are self-explanatory. In the following paragraphs, further details will be provided for the evaluation of risk of bias and publication bias.

To evaluate the risk of bias for the selected studies, reviewers may collect information using the **Cochrane Collaboration tool**, which covers sequence generation, allocation concealment, blinding, incomplete outcome data, and selective outcome reporting (Higgins et al. 2011). In an RCT, a random sequence is generated for patient allocation. Allocation concealment means that the person enrolling patients is unaware of the group to which they will be allocated. Insufficient blinding means patients, caregivers, outcome recorders, or data analysts know the arm (for example, treatment versus control group) to which patients are allocated. The two reviewers will make an independent judgment whether the possible risk of bias, as indicated in the extracted data from each study, is "high risk" or "low risk." If information in the study is insufficient for making this judgment, the reviewers may rate the domain as "unclear." In this case, the research team may contact the authors of the study to obtain further information or clarification so that the team can have an accurate rate of risk of bias. The two reviewers discuss their disagreements and resolve them by consensus or by consulting a third reviewer. The final risk of bias needs to be evaluated within and across studies.

The Cochrane Effective Practice and Organization of Care group developed multiple resources for systematic review. For instance, the group provides one tool for assessing the risk of bias in quasi-experimental designs. The **Newcastle-Ottawa scale (NOS)**, an assessment tool designed for evaluating the quality of nonrandomized studies, can be used to assess the quality of case-control and cohort studies. It can also be adapted to assess observational studies or cross-sectional studies. Using the NOS, the quality of studies can be rated from 1 to 9. The studies rated 1 through 3 are at high risk of bias; 4 through 5 indicates medium risk; and 6 through 9 indicates low risk (Wells et al. 2014).

Reviewers can draw a funnel plot, a graph designed to check for the existence of publication bias, on the collected data from the selected studies. A **funnel plot** is a scatter plot of the intervention effect estimated from individual studies against some measure of each study's size or precision. Typically, the effect estimates are plotted on the horizontal axis and the study sizes are plotted on the vertical axis. In general, effect estimates from small scale studies scatter widely at the bottom of the graph, and the spread narrows as the sample size becomes bigger. In the absence of publication bias, the larger-scale studies are plotted near the mean and the smaller scale studies are spread evenly on both sides of the mean (symmetric distribution), forming a roughly funnel-shaped distribution. Deviation from this shape can indicate publication bias in the selected studies; a bias toward positive findings is most common, because articles with positive results are more likely to be published than articles with negative results (Guyatt et al. 2011b, 1277). Funnel plots can be created with many tools, such as Microsoft Excel, R, SPSS, SAS, and Stata.

Figure 8.5 is an example of a funnel plot of publication bias for 100 articles. The *x*-axis is a coefficient used for indicating the reported results in different studies and the *y*-axis is the sample sizes. This funnel plot shows that the values of the measure are widely spread to an expected value (vertical line) when the sample sizes are small, but they get closer to the expected value when the sample sizes are larger. The plot is slightly shifted to the left-hand side, which indicates a slight publication bias in the selected articles.

Figure 8.5 A publication-bias funnel plot created from a simulated data set of 100 articles

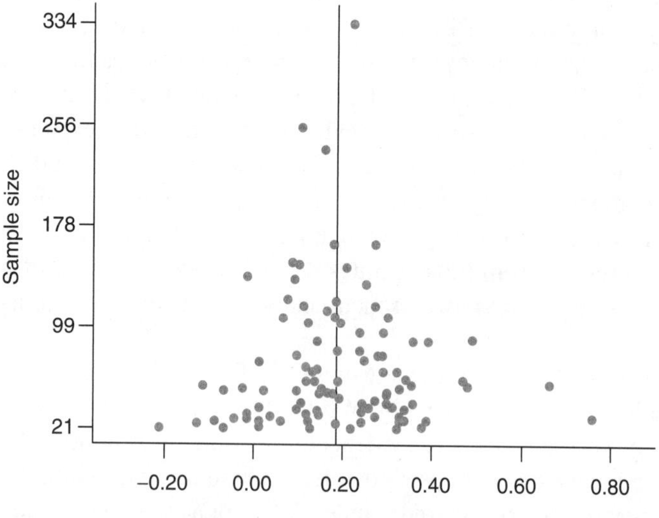

When serious positive publication bias is identified, the systematic review team may want to consider including more publications from grey literature (articles posted on websites, preprint archives, blogs, theses, dissertations, technical reports) since they may provide negative results on the same topic. The team may also consider excluding results from studies with small sample sizes.

In their 2015 health effects of mobile app study, Flores Mateo and coauthors assessed the risk of bias following Cochrane's recommendation. They considered random sequence generation, allocation concealment, blinding of participants and personnel, blinding of outcome assessment, incomplete outcome data, and selective reporting. They categorized each criterion as "clear yes," "not sure," or "clear no." In their assessment, the randomization was considered adequate in most of the chosen studies in this meta-analysis, but the blinding was not done sufficiently in those studies. The risk of reporting bias was low since there were no discrepancies between the outcomes that authors intended to measure and those reported in the study. Overall, the risk of bias was high in most of the selected studies, mainly because the blinding was done insufficiently and because the study participant dropout rate during the clinical trial was large. The authors also assessed publication bias by using funnel plots. Their funnel plot for clinical trials of mobile apps for weight loss shows reasonable symmetry, which means there is no evidence of publication bias in the selected studies.

After the quality appraisal on the selected studies and extracted data items is complete, the research team can begin performing qualitative and quantitative analyses on the extracted data.

Qualitative Analysis

In a systematic review study, the investigators may choose to only perform qualitative analyses rather than qualitative and quantitative analyses. The outcomes of selected studies can be summarized and compared qualitatively, or comparisons can also be done for specific parts of different studies. Comparative content analysis (CCA) can be employed to determine themes across the qualitative data. NVivo software is excellent software to use to organize and analyze qualitative data for CCA.

However, qualitative analyses are limited by subjectivity—that is, different reviewers may draw different conclusions from qualitative analyses. Qualitative analysis is inherently interpretive, and the data are not intended to lead to generalized conclusions (Bearman and Dawson 2013). For example, research teams typically perform focus group studies before they design a mobile app for targeted patients. These teams can choose to directly report the feedback collected from the participants of those focus group studies. When a qualitative analysis is performed on these focus group study results, different researchers may have different ways to categorize these results and come up with their own interpretations.

Quantitative Analysis

In most cases, a systematic review includes quantitative analyses of the collected data. The analyses can be as simple as some descriptive statistics, such as the frequency of one specific conclusion occurring in selected studies, the percentage of agreements among studies on certain items, or the average and variations of certain numerical values inside one study or multiple studies. One can also perform more systematic and sophisticated statistical analysis on all selected studies; this more advanced approach is the meta-analysis.

Meta-analysis offers a quantitative way of synthesizing the results of multiple studies with the same study design or similar study designs. The rationale behind meta-analysis is that a larger sample collected from multiple similar studies will cancel out biases inherent in any single study. Therefore, the obtained results will be more robust or generalizable. Before the research team performs the meta-analysis, team members need to use the results obtained in the study appraisal to choose reliable data items or outcomes to perform the meta-analysis. Otherwise, the obtained results from the meta-analysis will likely be misleading.

After the desired data is extracted from the selected articles and evaluated, the research team can use various statistical analysis methods to process the data. For example, for binary data (such as improved or not improved; disease or no disease), commonly computed statistics are odds ratios, relative risks, and the risk difference (see chapter 5 and chapter 12 for more details about these statistics). For continuous data, such as weight or blood pressure measurements, commonly computed statistics include the Pearson product-moment correlation and measures of effect, such as Cohen's *d* or Glass's delta (see chapters 9 and 12 for additional information about these measures).

The specific meta-analysis steps include the following (Forrestal 2014, 230):

1. Quantitatively standardize the results of all the selected studies by calculating a common summary statistic so that these studies are comparable. For example, one research study may report height of subjects and their weight change before and after an intervention, whereas another research study may report the change of BMI before and after a similar intervention. To compare the results of these two studies, the researcher needs to convert the height and weight in the first study into BMI (BMI equals weight in kilograms divided by the square of height in meters).
2. Determine whether to use a fixed-effects model or a random-effects model. A **fixed-effects model** calculates a pooled effect estimate by assuming all the variations among studies are caused by chance (Cochrane Collaboration 2016). A **random-effects model** calculates the effect estimate by assuming there are other sources of variation among included studies (Cochrane Collaboration 2016). The selection of the model is determined by the studies included in the meta-analysis. If the studies in the meta-analysis are generally similar and the variations among studies are from random chance, a fixed-effects model should be used. If the selected studies are heterogeneous and there is additional source of variations among studies beyond random chance, a random-effects model should be used.
3. Statistically integrate studies by calculating the overall estimate of effect of the studies' intervention.
4. Perform sensitivity analysis, subgroup analysis, or meta-regression. **Sensitivity analysis** is used to determine whether a study's (such as meta-analysis) results change if assumptions, statistical techniques, inputs, or other elements of a research plan are varied. One approach is to perform the meta-analysis multiple times while varying some assumptions or data/studies and observing how the meta-analysis result changes. If one specific study dramatically changes the result of meta-analysis, this meta-analysis is problematic. **Subgroup analysis** evaluates data representing subsets of participants or studies. In the former case, all participants in the selected studies are split into subgroups according to certain features such as sex, age, or race, and the results for these subgroups are compared. In the latter case, the selected studies are categorized into subgroups, either randomly or according to the type of the studies (RCTs or case-control studies), and the results for these subgroups can be compared to determine whether they are consistent or not. The sample size in individual studies is typically too small to conduct subgroup analysis, but this method can be applied in meta-analysis; for example, subgroups of the same sex, age, race, geographic location might be used. **Meta-regression** is a regression analysis of the data from multiple studies. Meta-regression is typically used when the number of selected studies is large (> 10).

In this chapter, we use two examples to explain these meta-analysis steps. Before we describe the meta-analysis performed in the two examples, it is necessary to discuss the forest plot, which is widely used in reporting meta-analysis results.

A **forest plot** is a graphical display of estimated results from multiple studies on the same topic, the amount of variation, and the overall estimate of the effect (Lalkhen and McCluskey 2008, 143). It is often used to visually present the result of meta-analysis. In a forest plot, there is a row for each study and rows for the overall result. There are multiple columns of information in one forest plot. The following list demonstrates what might be found in a typical forest plot:

- Column 1 is the list of studies included in the meta-analysis. Some authors arrange the studies in alphabetic order by the first authors' last names; other authors arrange the studies in chronological order with the oldest at the top; and still other authors arrange the studies using factors such as sex, age, intervention, and research design to order of studies. One can determine the proper order of studies by the research purpose and the situation of the selected studies. The order for the remaining columns is flexible and may not always align with the numbers used in this discussion. However, the information they contain will resemble what we describe below.

- Columns 2 and 3 list the results from the experimental and control groups in each study. In some cases, the forest plot provides just one simple number per study in each group; and in other cases, the forest plot includes multiple numbers per study in each group, such as mean, standard deviation, and total.
- Column 4 notes the weight of each study in the meta-analysis. The weight is typically determined by the sample size of each study.
- Column 5 shows the final result of each study and the overall outcome of the meta-analysis, including the 95 percent confidence interval. For continuous data, this column could be a weighted mean difference or a standardized effect size. For binary data, this column could be the odds ratio, relative risk, or risk difference.
- Column 6 is a visualization of the information in column 5. As shown in figure 8.5, the solid vertical line represents the line of no effect; in other words, along this line, the experimental and control groups have similar results. For binary data, this vertical line locates at value 1. For continuous data, the vertical line locates at value 0. For each study, there is one box with a line representing the results of the study. The length of the line is the confidence interval of the study. The size of the box is proportional to the precision of the study's estimate and its weight in the meta-analysis (Lalkhen and McCluskey 2008, 143). For example, the size of the box can be proportional to the inverse of variance of the weighted mean difference in continuous data set. A diamond, instead of a box, is used to show the overall results of the meta-analysis. The width of the diamond is used to show the 95 percent confidence interval. If the meta-analysis has multiple groups, there will be one diamond for each group.
- In certain cases, there is one more column used to show the quality of each study.

At the bottom left corner of the forest plot, the results of the test for heterogeneity (difference of studies, I^2 statistics) are shown. If the meta-analysis has multiple groups of studies, a set of heterogeneity test results is presented for each group, and typically placed below the list of studies in that group. If the I^2 statistic is greater than 50 percent, the meta-analysis is considered high in heterogeneity.

Figure 8.6 shows one example of a forest plot for a binary data set in a meta-analysis about the effectiveness of antipsychotics in adults (Abou-Setta et al. 2012, J-1). Column 1 is a list of five studies included in the meta-analysis. Columns 2 and 3 are the adverse event results for two different medications. Column 4 is the weight of each study in the meta-analysis. Column 5 is the risk ratio of individual studies and the overall meta-analysis, including 95 percent confidence intervals. Column 6 is the visual representation of the data in column 5. The heterogeneity test result is shown at the bottom left corner, and the I^2 value (34 percent) means the heterogeneity of the included studies was not high.

Figure 8.6 Example of a forest plot

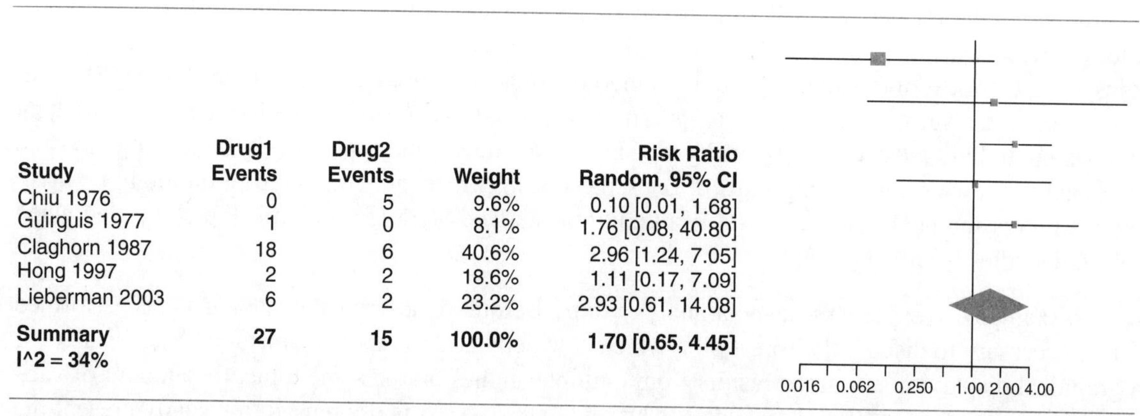

Source: Adapted from Abou-Setta et al. 2012.

As mentioned earlier in this section, Flores Mateo and colleagues evaluated the quality of their 12 selected articles on the health effects of mobile phone app interventions and determined that there was no evidence of publication bias. There were 10 RCTs and 2 nonrandomized controlled trials. In the 10 RCTs, one study did not report body weight; therefore, 9 studies were included in a meta-analysis of the net change in body weight associated with mobile phone app intervention (Flores Mateo et al. 2015, e253).

- In the first step of the meta-analysis, the common result of all selected studies was the net change of the body weight in kilograms, which was expressed as the weight change during mobile phone intervention minus the weight change during the control diet. The mean and standard deviation of the net change of body weight were calculated.
- In the second step of the meta-analysis, a random-effects model was chosen because in the selected studies, the size of samples, the country of the studies, the age of subjects, the study durations, and the outcome measures were highly different. Therefore, it is very likely that the variations of these studies were from sources beyond random chance.
- In the third step of the meta-analysis, the random-effects model was used to calculate the mean difference, the weight of each study in the meta-analysis, and the overall meta-analysis result.
- In the fourth step of the meta-analysis, a sensitivity analysis was performed and one study was excluded from the meta-analysis because it was not a randomized study and there was no intervention in the control group. The meta-analysis result was not changed after this study was excluded. In other words, the selection of the studies was proper and this meta-analysis result was robust.

Flores Mateo and associates did not perform a subgroup study because of the small number of studies included in the meta-analysis, the small number of subjects, and the heterogeneity of those studies (as noted, a random-effects model was used to perform the meta-analysis). The meta-analysis indicated that mobile phone app interventions resulted in significant decreases in body weight, compared to the control group. The same analysis on BMI produced a similar conclusion. However, when the meta-analysis was performed on physical activity, the result indicated an insignificant difference in physical activity between the mobile app intervention and control groups. The authors used multiple forest plots to present their meta-analysis results.

In the HIT impact on cancer care study, Tarver and Menachemi performed multiple subgroup analyses and meta-regressions because of the large number of studies (122 articles and 156 individual analyses in those studies). They used a chi-square statistic to investigate differences in study characteristics and built logistic regression models to identify study characteristics associated with reporting beneficial results. The authors performed bivariate analysis to determine the impact of HIT on patients and healthcare providers, and the impact of HIT on decision making, behavioral change, and psychosocial outcomes. The authors also performed a multivariate analysis by controlling for different study characteristics such as sample size, study design, the type of HIT application, HIT target population, continuum level, and study outcomes. From these analyses, the authors concluded that the beneficial impact of HIT differed across the cancer continuum. A beneficial outcome was less likely in HIT interventions targeted at patients than HIT interventions targeted to physicians. Also, studies that assessed the impact of HIT on behavioral change were less likely to find a beneficial effect (Tarver and Menachemi 2016, 422–426).

Step 9: Writing a Final Report

In the final report of the systematic review and meta-analysis, the research team should report all the details that were obtained during the process, including the study's research question, the location of the study protocol, the keywords for the database search, the search strategies, the software used to manage the collected citations, the details of inclusion and exclusion criteria, the article screening procedure (including a flow diagram of the selection), the data extraction process (including the corresponding data forms and software used), the quality appraisal steps and results, details of study selection for data analysis and meta-analysis procedure, and the findings from the systematic review and meta-analysis study.

The research team also needs to provide a discussion about the issues found during the study, such as the limitations in the study (for example, a low number of studies, high risk of bias, control groups missing in multiple studies, or any biases from reviewers), any surprising results, and the reasons for these issues. The research team may also provide recommendations about the practical application of the research. After all, this is one of the major purposes for conducting a systematic review and meta-analysis.

Overall, the final report of the systematic review and meta-analysis should make it possible for other researchers to reproduce the study by following all the steps described in the report.

Review Questions

1. What are the steps in a systematic review?
2. What is the difference between a systematic review and a meta-analysis?
3. Aside from the examples mentioned in this chapter, what are some HIM or informatics areas where investigators could use the systematic review to answer a research question(s)?
4. What are exclusion and inclusion criteria, and why are they important in performing a systematic review?
5. What is a database search strategy and how is it created?
6. What are the methods used to screen articles obtained in the database search?
7. How does one perform quality appraisals on selected articles?
8. What methods can be used to extract data from selected articles?
9. What is the difference between qualitative analysis and quantitative analysis?
10. After researchers extract data from selected articles, what steps should generally be taken to analyze the data?

Application Exercises

1. Go to the journal website for *Briefs in Bioinformatics* and find an article related to your field of study. For example, you can use "Computational models for predicting drug response in cancer research" (Azuaje 2016). Read through the article and try to determine these items: the research question of the review, keywords used to search databases, inclusion and exclusion criteria, quality appraisal steps, and summary of review results. Report your findings.
2. Go to the website of *Journal of the American Medical Informatics Association* and search for systematic review articles by typing "systematic review" in the Search Articles field. Choose a recently published systematic review article, such as "Electronic tools to support medication reconciliation—a systematic review" (Marien et al. 2016). Read through the article and determine the following items: the research question of the review study, keywords used to search databases, databases used for the search, inclusion and exclusion criteria, quality appraisal steps, and summary of review results. Report your findings.
3. Go to the website of *Journal of the American Medical Association* and search for systematic review and meta-analysis articles by typing "systematic review AND meta-analysis" in the article search field. Choose a recently published systematic review and meta-analysis article, such as "Prevalence of depression and depressive symptoms among resident physicians: A systematic review and meta-analysis" authored by D. Mata and colleagues and published in 2015. Read through the article and determine the following items: the research question of the review study, keywords used to search databases, databases used for the search, inclusion and exclusion criteria, quality appraisal steps, data extraction steps, data analysis methods, and summary of review results. Report your findings.

References

Abou-Setta, A.M., S.S. Mousavi, C. Spooner, J.R. Schouten, D. Pasichnyk, S. Armijo-Olivo, A. Beaith, J.C. Seida, S. Dursun, A.S. Newton, and L. Hartling. 2012. First-generation versus second-generation antipsychotics in adults: Comparative effectiveness.*Comparative Effectiveness Reviews* 63(12) https://www.ncbi.nlm.nih.gov/books/NBK107254/pdf/Bookshelf_NBK107254.pdf.

Agency for Healthcare Research and Quality (AHRQ). 2012(March). Assessing the risk of bias of individual studies in systematic reviews of health care interventions. http://effectivehealthcare.ahrq.gov/index.cfm/search-for-guides-reviews-and-reports/?pageaction=displayproduct&productid=998.

Allen, J. K., J. Stephens, C.R. Dennison Himmelfarb, K.J. Stewart, and S. Hauck. 2013. Randomized controlled pilot study testing use of smartphone technology for obesity treatment. *Journal of Obesity* 2013:151597. https://www.hindawi.com/journals/jobe/2013/151597.

Bearman, M. and P. Dawson. 2013. Qualitative synthesis and systematic review in health professions education. *Medical Education* 47(3):252–260.

Cochrane Collaboration. 2016. Glossary. http://community-archive.cochrane.org/glossary.

Eden, J., L. Levit, A. Berg, and S. Morton, eds. 2011. Finding What Works in Health Care: Standards for Systematic Reviews. Washington, DC: The National Academies Press.

Flores Mateo, G., E. Granado-Font, C. Ferre-Grau, and X. Montana-Carreras. 2015 (November). Mobile phone apps to promote weight loss and increase physical activity: A systematic review and meta-analysis. *Journal of Medical Internet Research* 17(11):e253. http://www.jmir.org/2015/11/e253/.

Forrestal, E. 2014. Foundation of evidence-based decision making for health care managers—Part II: Meta-analysis and applying the evidence. *Health Care Management* 33(3):230–244.

Guyatt, G.H., A.D. Oxman, G.E. Vist, R. Kunz, Y. Falck-Ytter, P. Alonso-Coello, H.J. Schunemann, and GRADE Working Group. 2008. GRADE: An emerging consensus on rating quality of evidence and strength of recommendations. *British Medical Journal* 336(7650): 924–926.

Guyatt, G.H., A.D. Oxman, G. Vist, R. Kunz, J. Brozek, P. Alonso-Coello, V. Montori, E.A. Akl, B. Djulbegovic, Y. Falck-Ytter, S.L. Norris, J.W. Williams, Jr., D. Atkins, J. Meerpohl, and H.J. Schunemann. 2011a. GRADE guidelines: 4. Rating the quality of evidence—study limitations (risk of bias). *Journal of Clinical Epidemiology* 64(4):407–415.

Guyatt, G.H., A.D. Oxman, V. Montori, G. Vist, R. Kunz, J. Brozek, P. Alonso-Coello, B. Djulbegovic, D. Atkins, Y. Falck-Ytter, J.W. Williams, Jr., J. Meerpohl, S.L. Norris, E.A. Akl, and H.J. Schunemann. 2011b. GRADE guidelines: 5. Rating the quality of evidence—publication bias. *Journal of Clinical Epidemiology* 64(12):1277–1282.

Guyatt, G.H., A.D. Oxman,, R. Kunz, J. Brozek, P. Alonso-Coello, D. Rind, P.J. Devereaux, V.M. Montori, B. Freyschuss, G. Vist, R. Jaeschke, J.W. Williams, Jr., M.H. Murad, D. Sinclair, Y. Falck-Ytter, J. Meerpohl, C. Whittington, K. Thorlund, J. Andrews, and H.J. Schunemann. 2011c. GRADE guidelines: 6. Rating the quality of evidence—imprecision. *Journal of Clinical Epidemiology* 64(12):1283–1293.

Guyatt, G.H., A.D. Oxman, R. Kunz, J. Woodcock, J. Brozek, M. Helfand, P. Alonso-Coello, P. Glasziou, R. Jaeschke, E.A. Akl, S. Norris, G. Vist, P. Dahm, V.K. Shukla, J. Higgins, Y. Falck-Ytter, H.J. Schunemann, and GRADE Working Group. 2011d. GRADE guidelines: 7. Rating the quality of evidence—inconsistency. *Journal of Clinical Epidemiology* 64(12):1294–1302.

Guyatt, G.H., A.D. Oxman, R. Kunz, J. Woodcock, J. Brozek, M. Helfand, P. Alonso-Coello, Y. Falck-Ytter, R. Jaeschke, G. Vist, E.A. Akl, P.N. Post, S. Norris, J. Meerpohl, V.K. Shukla, M. Nasser, H.J. Schunemann, and GRADE Working Group. 2011e. GRADE guidelines: 8. Rating the quality of evidence—indirectness. *Journal of Clinical Epidemiology* 64(12):1303–1310.

Hebden, L., A. Cook, H.P. van der Ploeg, L. King, A. Bauman, and M. Allman-Farinelli. 2014. A mobile health intervention for weight management among young adults: A pilot randomised controlled trial. *Journal of Human Nutrition and Diet* 27(4):322–332.

Higgins, J.P., D.G. Altman, P.C. Gotzsche, P. Juni, D. Moher, A.D. Oxman, J. Savovic, K.F. Schulz, L. Weeks, and J.A. Sterne. 2011. The Cochrane Collaboration's tool for assessing risk of bias in randomised trials. *British Medical Journal* 343:d5928. http://www.bmj.com/content/343/bmj.d5928.

Hoyt, R. and W.R. Hersh. 2014. Evidence Based Medicine and Clinical Practice Guidelines. Chapter 14 in *Health Informatics: Practical Guide for Healthcare and Information Technology Professionals*. Edited by R. Hoyt and A. Yoshihashi. 6th ed. Lulu Press.

Lalkhen, A.G. and A. McCluskey. 2008. Statistics V: Introduction to clinical trials and systematic reviews. *Continuing Education in Anaesthesia and Critical Care Pain* 8(4):143–146.

Landis, J.R., and G.G. Koch. 1977. The measurement of observer agreement for categorical data. *Biometrics* 33:159–174.

Moher, D., L. Shamseer, M. Clarke, D. Ghersi, A. Liberati, M. Petticrew, P. Shekelle, L.A. Stewart, and PRISMA-P Group. 2015. Preferred reporting items for systematic review and meta-analysis protocols (PRISMA-P) 2015 statement. *Systematic Reviews* 4:1. http://systematicreviewsjournal.biomedcentral.com/articles/10.1186/2046-4053-4-1.

National Center for Biotechnology Information (NCBI). 2016. PubMed.gov. https://www.ncbi.nlm.nih.gov/pubmed.

Parton, A., V. McGilligan, M. O'Kane, F.R. Baldrick, and S. Watterson. 2016. Computational modelling of atherosclerosis. *Briefings in Bioinformatics* 17(4):562–575.

Shamseer, L., D. Moher, M. Clarke, D. Ghersi, A. Liberati, M. Petticrew, P. Shekelle, L.A. Stewart, and PRISMA-P Group. 2015. Preferred reporting items for systematic review and meta-analysis protocols (PRISMA-P) 2015: Elaboration and explanation. *British Medical Journal* 349:g7647.

Tarver, W.L. and M. Menachemi. 2016. The impact of health information technology on cancer care across the continuum: A systematic review and meta-analysis. *Journal of the American Medical Informatics Association* 23(2):420–427.

Ware, M. and M. Mabe. 2015. *The STM Report: An Overview of Scientific and Scholarly Journal Publishing.* International Association of Scientific, Technical and Medical Publishers. http://www.stm-assoc.org/2015_02_20_STM_Report_2015.pdf.

Watzlaf, V., D. DeAlmeida, L. Zhou, and L. Hartman. 2015. Protocol for systematic review in privacy and security in telehealth: Best practices for healthcare professionals. *International Journal of Telerehabilitation* 7(2): 15–22.

Wells, G.A., B. Shea, D. O'Connell, J. Peterson, V. Welch, M. Losos, and P. Tugwell. 2014. The Newcastel-Ottawa Scale (NOS) for Assessing the Quality of Nonrandomised Studies in Meta-analysis. http://www.ohri.ca/programs/clinical_epidemiology/oxford.asp.

Resources

Azuaje, F. 2016(July). Computational models for predicting drug response in cancer research. *Briefings in Bioinformatics.* http://bib.oxfordjournals.org/content/early/2016/07/20/bib.bbw065.full.

Cochrane. 2016. Cochrane. http://epoc.cochrane.org/resources.

Cold Spring Harbor Laboratory. 2016. bioRxiv. http://biorxiv.org.

Cornell University Library. 2016. arXiv. http://lanl.arXiv.org.

Counsell, C. 1997. Formulating questions and locating primary studies for inclusion in systematic reviews. *Annuals of Internal Medicine* 127(5):380–387.

Elsevier. 2016. Scopus. https://www.scopus.com/.

Marien, S., Krug, B., Spinewine, A. 2016. Electronic Tools to Support Medication Reconciliation—A Systematic Review. *Journal of the American Medical Informatics Association*, 24(1): 227–240. http://jamia.oxfordjournals.org/content/24/1/227.long.

SUNY Downstate Medical Center. The evidence pyramid. http://library.downstate.edu/EBM2/2100.htm.

PART

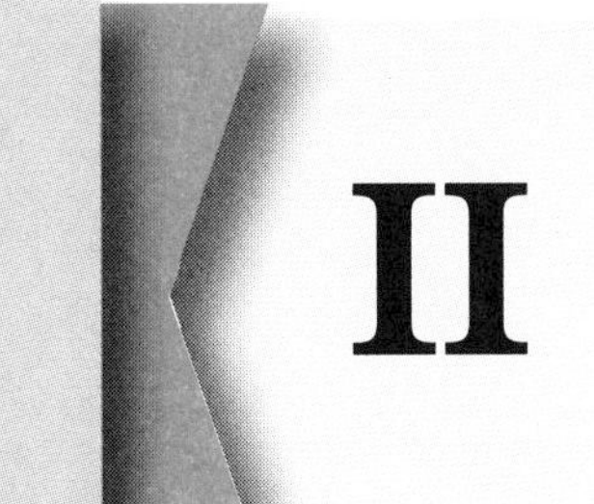

Research Process

9 Applied Statistics

10 Defining the Research Question and Performing a Literature Review

11 Selecting the Research Design and Method and Collecting Data

12 Analyzing Data and Presenting Results

9 Applied Statistics

Elizabeth J. Forrestal, PhD, RHIA, CCS, FAHIMA

Learning Objectives

- Select descriptive and inferential statistics appropriate to the research question, the type of data, and other aspects of the population or the research design.
- Choose parametric or nonparametric statistical tests appropriately.
- Justify the selection of a statistical analytic test.
- Use key terms associated with quantitative statistical tests appropriately.

Key Terms

2×2 table
Bar chart
Bivariate
Box-and-whisker plots
Categorical data
Contingency table
Continuous data
Curvilinear associations
Dependent sample
Descriptive statistics
Discrete data
Frequency distribution
Histogram
Independent sample
Inferential statistics
Interquartile range (IQR)
Interval data
Kurtosis
Line graph
Mean
Measures of central tendency
Measures of dispersion
Median
Metric data
Mode
Multivariate
Nominal data
Nonparametric data
Nonparametric test
Normal (bell) curve
Normal distribution
Ordinal data
Parametric data
Parametric test
Pie chart
Proportion
Range
Ratios
Ratio data
Robust
Scatter graph
Skewness
Standard deviation
Statistics
Stem-and-leaf diagram
Target population
Unit of analysis error
Univariate

Health informatics and HIM researchers, healthcare personnel, and the general public use **statistics**, the science of collecting, classifying, displaying, analyzing, and interpreting numerical data, to benefit from and make sense of the numerical data that surround them. *Biostatistics* is a specialized branch of statistics that applies statistical tests to biological data, such as the data obtained from experiments on humans and animals. In healthcare, examples of numerical data include laboratory test results in electronic health records (EHRs), productivity data in administrative records, and diagnostic and procedural codes in claims data. This chapter presents information on the use of statistics in health informatics and HIM research and provides examples from published studies.

The purpose of this chapter is to familiarize the reader with commonly encountered statistical tests and the language of statistics. The emphasis of the chapter is on application—matching the appropriate statistical test to the goal of the researcher—rather than on mathematical proofs and computations. The formulas can be found in statistical textbooks, such as the textbooks and online statistical resources listed in the resources at the end of this chapter. The reader may also want to consult with a statistician if he or she is planning to conduct a quantitative study. This chapter covers goals of quantitative researchers, level of data, factors in selecting a statistical test, descriptive statistics, inferential statistics, and the misuse of statistics.

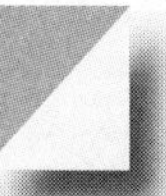

Real-World Case

Researchers at the American Health Information Management Association (AHIMA) conducted a study to "examine employers' and educators' perceptions of graduate preparedness among health information [management] students joining the workforce" (Jackson et al. 2016). Data collection was performed through a telephone survey of a stratified random sample of employers and educators. The survey contained a total of six questions. The first two questions were rated on a scale of 1 through 5 with 1 being "not important" and 5 being "critically important." The following three subitems were rated in the first question: professional and technical skills, leadership skills, and employability skills (Jackson 2016). The second question concerned the importance of experiential learning with three rated subitems: professional practice experience or internship, apprenticeship, and other (such as previous employment or volunteering). The third and fourth questions collected yes-or-no data with "no" being assigned "1" and "yes" being assigned "2." The third question asked whether a disconnect existed between graduate preparation and employers' needs. The fourth question asked whether the respondent believed that the federal government could assist in better preparing students to meet employers' needs. The fifth question was open-ended, allowing the respondents to make free-form comments about how employers and educators could work together to better prepare graduates for employers' needs. The sixth question had three subitems regarding respondents' demographic information. The research data were presented in four tables. The researchers found a statistically significant difference between the perceptions of employers and educators in their assessment of graduates' preparation in the areas of professional and technical skills, leadership skills, and employability skills. Educators noted higher levels of student preparedness with regard to professional and technical skills and leadership skills than employers did. Both employers and educators "noted a need for improved employability skills (e.g., communication skills and workplace etiquette). No difference was found between the two groups with regard to the need to increase apprenticeships and professional practice experience to cover this gap in formal training. Finally, when asked how the federal government might assist with preparing students, more than half of the respondents noted the importance of apprenticeships and funding for these opportunities" (Jackson et al. 2016, 1). Based on the analysis of their data, the researchers concluded that "academic programs should promote real-world experience through professional practice," apprenticeship programs, or both (Jackson et al. 2016, 4).

Goals of Quantitative Researchers

Two goals for quantitative researchers are to be able to state that their intervention contributed to or was the cause of the change in the dependent variable and to be able to state that their findings can be generalized to a population. Processes connected to probability and random sampling support those goals.

Probability

Probability is the heart of statistics. Statistical tests attempt to separate chance from contributing factors and causes (Wissing and Timm 2012, 126). Chance exists because researchers cannot be absolutely assured that their small group of subjects (random sample) is very similar to the larger population. By random chance—a fluke—the sample could be, for example, older on average than the population or particularly computer-savvy. This random difference could affect the research study's results. Consequently, statistics involves probability; that is, how probable (likely) is the outcome? Have we separated chance from the contributing factor or cause?

Random Sampling

Random sampling is the unbiased selection of subjects from the population of interest (sampling is discussed in greater detail in chapters 2 and 11). Unbiased selection means that each member of the population has an equal chance of being selected. The population of interest is known as the **target population**. Examples of populations include all healthcare managers, all academic health centers, all adolescent patients with asthma, and so forth. However, collecting data from entire populations is impractical in terms of cost, time, and resources. Therefore, researchers collect data from a representative subset of the target population, known as a *random sample*. Statistics are numerical characteristics of samples, such as the mean and standard deviation. Statistics from random samples are used to estimate parameters—the population's numerical characteristics. When the sample is representative of the population, then it is assumed that the researcher's findings can be generalized to the entire population. These aspects of statistics—estimation and assumptions—make uncertainty an element of statistics. Some people may feel uncomfortable about this element of statistics, especially when numbers seem so black and white. This discomfort may be lessened when estimates and assumptions are based on knowledge gained during the literature review (chapter 10).

Level of Data

The level of data affects the statistical test that can be applied. Researchers and research methodologists use other expressions to refer to level of the data or *data levels*. These expressions for data level include the *scale* of the data, as in chapter 2; the *type* of the data; the *level of measurement;* and the *scale of measurement*. Additionally, the word *data* is sometimes replaced with *variable,* as in the phrase *type of variable*. This section includes descriptions of the data levels with examples, a discussion of some of the other terms associated with data levels that readers may encounter in publications of research, information about parametric and nonparametric data, and a review of associations among variables.

Nominal, Ordinal, Interval, and Ratio Data

Research methodologists describe four levels of data. From the lowest level to the highest level, these levels are nominal, ordinal, interval, and ratio. The levels are hierarchical because at each level, nominal to ratio, the amount of information contained in the data increases. Additionally, more sophisticated statistical analyses can be applied as the data level moves from low to high. The four levels are described as follows:

- **Nominal data** are values or observations that can be named or labeled. Examples of nominal data include sex (male or female), state of residence (New York, Virginia, and so forth), and job title (administrator, supervisor, and so forth). Nominal data can be numbers, such as a Zip code or Social Security number. Zip codes label certain areas. Social Security numbers represent people. Neither Zip codes nor Social Security numbers can have mathematical operations (addition, subtraction, multiplication, and division) applied to them. Sometimes, for convenience, nominal data are coded with numbers, such as Male = 0 and Female = 1, or No = 1 and Yes = 2. Nominal data may be described as dichotomous, binary, or binomial when there are only two categories, such as improved or not improved, alive or dead, or true or false. Representing the lowest level of data, nominal data cannot be ranked nor measured.
- **Ordinal data** represent values or observations that can be ranked (ordered). Ranking scales or rating scales are common examples of ordinal data. Ordinal data convey more information than nominal data because ordinal data show relationships in terms of a sequence of rankings. An example of ordinal data is students' level of standing, as freshman, sophomore, junior, and senior. A frequently encountered ranking scale is the Likert scale (see chapter 11). Examples of the use of ranking scales are as follows:

  - Patients are asked to indicate the severity of their pain on a scale from 1 to 10.
  - Physicians are asked to rank their satisfaction with the new alert system on a scale from 1 to 5.
  - Consumers are asked to rate the usability of a patient portal on a scale from 1 to 7.

  However, because these rankings are subjective, the difference in satisfaction between 2 and 3 may be much less than the difference between 4 and 5. Similar to nominal data, ordinal data cannot have mathematical operations applied to them.
- **Interval data** represent values or observations that occur on an evenly distributed scale that does not begin with a true zero. For example, time in years is an evenly distributed scale that does not begin with a true zero. The interval

between 1985 and 1990 is the same as the interval between 2011 and 2016, but zero is unknown. Temperature in Fahrenheit is another example of interval data because the intervals between the degrees are evenly distributed, but the scale does not begin at a true (absolute) zero (the Kelvin temperature scale does). The mathematical operations of addition, subtraction, and multiplication may be applied to interval data. However, without a true zero, division cannot be done be applied (40 degrees Fahrenheit is not half as warm as 80 degrees) (Alreck and Settle 2004, 261).

- **Ratio data** represent values or observations that occur on an evenly distributed scale that begins at a true zero. Height, weight, and length are examples of ratio data. All mathematical operations may be applied to ratio data.

The type of data depends on the way the variable is measured, not some inherent attribute of the variable. For example, as ratio data, height can be measured in inches; however, as nominal data, height can be categorized as short or tall. Therefore, researchers should be careful to collect data in the form that matches their intended statistical test.

Other Terms Associated with Level of Data

Readers of research publications may also encounter terms associated with levels of data other than nominal ordinal, interval, and ratio. These other terms are described as follows:

- **Discrete data versus continuous data**—**Discrete data** are separate and distinct values or observations that can be measured across a set of fixed values, such as the number of visits or number of children. Patients in the hospital represent discrete data because each patient can be counted. **Continuous data** represent values or observations that have an infinite number of points along a continuum. For example, measurements made with a ruler can be a foot, an inch, a half-inch, a quarter-inch, an eighth-inch, to infinity.
- **Numerical data versus categorical data**—*Numerical data* can have mathematical operations applied. Numerical data are interval data and ratio data. Numerical data include discrete data and continuous data. **Categorical data** are data that can be grouped, such as by race or age group (youth or adult). Categorical data are nominal data and ordinal data.
- **Quantitative data versus qualitative data**—*Quantitative data* include interval data and ratio data. Quantitative data may be discrete or continuous. *Qualitative data* include categorical (norminal and ordinal) data.
- **Metric data versus nonmetric data**—**Metric data** are interval and ratio data. *Nonmetric data* are nominal or ordinal data.

Understanding these terms helps researchers select the appropriate statistical test and ways of presenting the data.

Parametric Data Versus Nonparametric Data

Parametric data are continuous data, interval data, and ratio data. Their distributions are assumed to be normal (normal curves). (See next section for a discussion of distributions.) **Nonparametric data** are discrete data, nominal data, and ordinal data. No assumptions are made about their distributions. Different statistical tests are used for parametric data and nonparametric data.

Associations among Variables

Associations among variables can be linear or nonlinear. Linear and nonlinear associations require different statistical tests. Figure 1.3 in chapter 1 shows two linear associations and a nonlinear association.

Linearly associated variables cluster around a straight line when they are graphed. This straight-line association is known as a *linear association* or a *linear relationship*. This characteristic of the data is called *linearity*. As described in chapter 1, linear associations can be either positive or negative. In a positive (direct) linear association, the values of the variables move in the *same* direction. When the value of one variable increases, the value of the other variable also proportionately increases (figure 1.3a). Conversely, when the value of one variable decreases, the value of the other variable also proportionately decreases. In both cases, the variables are proportionately moving in the same direction—as one increases so does the other *or* as one decreases so does the other. In a negative (inverse) linear association, the values of the variables move in *opposite* directions. When the value of one variable increases, the value of the other variable proportionately decreases (figure 1.3b). Conversely, as the value of one variable decreases, the value of the other variable proportionately increases. In both cases, the variables are proportionately moving in the opposite directions—as one increases, the other decreases *or* as one decreases, the other increases. Linear associations are frequently found in research.

Nonlinear associations also exist. Curvilinear is a common nonlinear association. **Curvilinear associations** are named for their shapes, such as *s*-curves, *j*-curves, and *u*-curves. Figure 1.3c is an *s*-curve. Graphing the rate of adoption of a new technology over time typically results in an *s*-curve (also called *sigmoid function*) because adoption usually begins slowly, then shows rapid growth, and finally tapers off. Not illustrated in figure 1.3 are *j*-curves and *u*-curves. An example of a *j*-curve is the association between blood pressure and mortality (Tsika et al. 2014, 126). High blood pressure levels are associated with higher mortality from cardiovascular disease. Also, while less common, very low blood pressure is also associated with higher morality. A *u*-curve was found between age and financial costs for end-stage renal disease, with the youngest and oldest groups of adults 18 years and older incurring the most costs and the groups in the middle the fewest costs.

Factors in Selecting a Statistical Test

Multiple statistical tests can be applied to research data, and researchers often analyze their data using more than one test. In selecting tests, researchers consider several factors because the appropriate tests vary by these factors. These factors, which will be discussed in the subsequent sections, arc as follows:

- Purpose of the research (research design)
- Type of variable(s)
- Number of variables
- Nature of the target population
- Number, size, and independence of the groups

Table 9.1 summarizes this information as a decision table to assist readers in selecting the appropriate descriptive and inferential test(s).

Table 9.1 Decision table for selecting a statistical test*

Purpose	Type of Variables		Assumptions**	
	Independent Variable	**Dependent Variable**	**Parametric** • **Normal distribution** • **Homogeneity of variance** • **Independent samples**	**Nonparametric** • **Any distribution** • **Any variance** • **Any samples**
Description				
Describe group(s)	0	Nominal		Mode, bar chart
Describe group(s)	0	Ordinal		Median, mode, interquartile range, bar chart
Describe group(s)	0	Continuous	Mean, median, mode, range, interquartile range, standard deviation, histogram	Median, inter-quartile range for nonnormal
Inferential Difference				
Compare one group to hypothetical value	0	Ordinal or nonnormal continuous		One-sample median test
Compare one group to hypothetical value	0	Normal continuous	Independent one-sample *t*-test	
Compare proportions of one group to hypothetical value	0	1 nominal		Chi-square goodness of fit

(*Continued*)

Table 9.1 (*Continued*)

Purpose	Type of Variables		Assumptions**	
	Independent Variable	**Dependent Variable**	**Parametric** ✧ **Normal distribution** ✧ **Homogeneity of variance** ✧ **Independent samples**	**Nonparametric** ✧ **Any distribution** ✧ **Any variance** ✧ **Any samples**
Compare two independent groups	Dichotomous and nominal	Normal continuous	Independent-measures *t*-test	
Compare two independent groups	Dichotomous and nominal	Ordinal or nonnormal continuous		Mann-Whitney *U* test
Compare two independent groups	2-level nominal (>5 per level)	Nominal		Chi-square test of independence (Fisher exact test for cells ≤5)
Compare two matched groups or pairs	Nominal	Normal continuous	Paired *t*-test	
Compare two matched groups or pairs	Nominal	Ordinal or continuous		Wilcoxon signed-rank test
Compare three or more independent groups	Nominal and 3 or more levels	Normal continuous	One-way ANOVA	
Compare three or more independent groups	Nominal and 3 or more levels	Ordinal or nonnormal continuous		Kruskal-Wallis test
Compare three or more independent groups	2 nominal with 2 or more levels	Normal continuous	Two-way ANOVA	
Compare three or more dependent (matched, paired) groups	2 nominal with 2 or more levels	Normal continuous	One-way repeated measures ANOVA	
Compare three or more dependent (matched, paired) groups	2 nominal with 2 or more levels	Nominal or ordinal or nonnormal continuous data		Friedman test
Compare three or more independent groups of adequate size	2 nominal with 2 or more levels	More than one normal continuous	MANOVA	
Compare two or more independent groups	2 or more at least at the nominal with 2 or more levels and a normal continuous covariate	Normal continuous	ANCOVA	
Inferential Association				
Quantify the linear relationship between two variables	Normal continuous	Normal continuous	Pearson product-moment correlation coefficient	

(*Continued*)

Table 9.1 (*Continued*)

Purpose	**Type of Variables**		**Assumptions****	
	Independent Variable	**Dependent Variable**	**Parametric** ✣ **Normal distribution** ✣ **Homogeneity of variance** ✣ **Independent samples**	**Nonparametric** ✣ **Any distribution** ✣ **Any variance** ✣ **Any samples**
Quantify the monotonic*** relationship between two variables	Ordinal or nonnormal continuous	Ordinal or nonnormal continuous		Spearman rank order correlation
Predict value of dependent variable based on value of linearly related independent variable	1 normal continuous	1 normal continuous	Simple regression	
Predict value of dependent variable based on value of linearly related independent variables	2 or more nominal or normal continuous	1 normal continuous	Multiple regression	

*Not all statistical tests in the table are discussed in the text, and not all statistical tests discussed in the text are in the table.
**Statistical tests may have other specific assumptions; be sure to check a general statistics textbook or consult a statistician.
****Monotonic* means that (1) as one variable increases, the other variable increases; or (2) as one variable decreases, the other variable decreases; the relationship may or may not be linear.

As each factor is discussed in this chapter, an example from table 9.1 is referenced to show how the elements of the table guide the selection of statistical tests. Statistical tests may also have other specific assumptions that factor into their selection; be sure to check a general statistics textbook or consult with a statistician.

Purpose of the Research

Researchers match the purpose of their research and their statistical test. Researchers whose purpose is to test hypotheses that propose differences between groups use statistical tests, such as the chi-square test of independence, paired *t*-test, the Wilcoxon signed-rank test, and analysis of variance (ANOVA). On the other hand, researchers whose purpose is to investigate relationships between groups or variables use statistical tests, such as Pearson product-moment correlation coefficient, Spearman rank order correlation, and simple and multiple regression. For example, in table 9.1, under Inferential Association, see the purpose, "Quantify the linear relationship between two variables"; reading across the row, one learns that when the independent and dependent variables are normal continuous, the appropriate statistical test is the Pearson product-moment correlation coefficient.

Type of Variable

The type of variable in terms of its data level affects the selection of descriptive and inferential statistical tests. For example, in table 9.1, under the purpose of Description, see the first row. In that row, there is no independent variable ("0"); however, the dependent variable is nominal. The appropriate descriptive statistics are noted as mode and bar chart.

Number of Variables

The number of variables also affects the choice of statistical test. For example, in table 9.1, in the bottom two rows, the simple regression has one independent variable and one dependent variable. However, the multiple regression has two or more independent variables and one dependent variable.

Nature of the Target Population

The nature of the target population also affects the choice of statistical test. **Parametric tests** are used when a target population's parameters (characteristics, such as mean and standard deviation) are assumed to be normally distributed (see discussion of bell curve later in the chapter) and meet or nearly meet the following assumptions:

- Random selection of samples from population
- Independent selection of samples from population
- Normal distribution of variable in population
- Interval or ratio level of measurement
- Homogeneity of variances
- Unrestricted range
- Linearity

Several of the concepts associated with these assumptions, such as random selection, level measurement (data), and linearity have been discussed earlier in the chapter. The independence of selection is discussed in the following subsections. Two assumptions that are not detailed in this chapter are homogeneity of variance and unrestricted range. *Homogeneity of variance* is the assumption that two or more groups have equal variances (variations from the mean). *Unrestricted range* means the population has not been limited to some selected criterion or to a narrow range of possible values. Parametric tests are said to be **robust** when they are relatively unaffected by deviations from the assumptions and are still able to produce accurate, unbiased results.

In addition to the seven previously listed assumptions, adequate sample sizes are required to use parametric tests (such as ≥30 or ≥100, depending on the purpose). Examples of parametric tests are the independent measures *t*-test, ANOVA, and Pearson product-moment correlation coefficient.

Nonparametric tests generally make no assumptions about the distribution of the population's parameters. Nonparametric tests are used for the following:

- Samples that do not meet the underlying assumptions for parametric tests
- Sample sizes that are small
- Nominal or ordinal data

Nonparametric tests are also known as *parameter-free tests* or *distribution-free tests*. Examples of nonparametric tests are the chi-square test and the Spearman rank order correlation. For example, on table 9.1, under the purpose of Inferential Difference, see the first row. In the row, there is no independent variable ("0"); however, the dependent variable is ordinal or nonnormal continuous. In the last column, "Assumptions," the assumption is nonparametric and the choice of statistical test is one-sample median test.

Number, Size, and Independence of Groups

The selection of statistical test also depends on the number of groups (samples), the comparative sizes of the groups, and the independence of the groups. In many instances, researchers want to compare two groups, such as the experimental group and the control group. However, in other types of studies, researchers may want to compare results from 10 different communities or from all 50 states.

Researchers must take into account unequal sizes of groups. This inequality could result in violation of homogeneity of variance (Huck 2012, 438). However, some statistical tests are quite robust and can handle differences in sizes. For example, in many instances, ANOVA can handle unequal group sizes.

The independence of the samples is a factor. **Independent samples** have no effect on one another and are not correlated. They can be from the same population or from different populations. Often, the control group and experimental group are independent samples. **Dependent samples** are matched or paired samples or are repeated measures. In matched samples, the researcher purposefully creates pairs, such as matching a graduate with his or her externship supervisor. Through this matching, the academic program could compare the graduates' perspectives on the quality of the education and the supervisors' perspectives on the graduates' capabilities. Pairs can also occur naturally, such as IQs of twins. In repeated measures, the same variable is measured twice, under different circumstances, on each subject, such as a pretest, multiple interim tests, and a posttest. For example, on table 9.1 under the purpose of Inferential Difference, see the fourth and seventh rows. For the fourth row, the purpose is "compare two independent groups," and the choice of statistical test is independent measures *t*-test. For the seventh row, the purpose is "compare two matched groups or pairs," and the choice of statistical test is paired *t*-test.

Descriptive Statistics

Descriptive statistics describe "what is" by classifying, organizing, and summarizing numerical data about a particular group of observations (Ravid 2011, 29). Descriptive statistics are also called *summary statistics.* This section discusses the purpose of descriptive statistics, frequency distributions, ratios and proportions, measures of central tendency, measures of dispersion, and some correlations.

Purposes of Descriptive Statistics

The purposes of descriptive statistics are to examine the raw data, summarize the data, and conduct exploratory data analysis. Descriptive statistics are **univariate**, meaning they analyze one variable. Researchers begin with descriptive statistics to verify the accuracy of the data entry. They then can assess whether the data are normally distributed or whether the data are nonnormal.

Frequency Distributions

A **frequency distribution** is the frequency with which values of a variable occur in a sample or population. These occurrences can be presented as counts or percentages in tables. Frequency distributions can also be displayed as tables and graphics, such as bar graphs and histograms. In a graph of a distribution, all the possible values are listed along the *x*-axis (horizontal axis or abscissa) and the frequency with which a value occurs is listed along the *y*-axis (vertical axis or ordinate).

In the next subsections, concepts associated with frequency distributions will be addressed. These concepts include the normal distribution; the properties of the normal distribution; the properties of nonnormal distributions; tables; and bar charts, histograms, and other graphical displays.

Normal Distribution

Many variables in research have a normal distribution. A normal curve shows the distribution of measurements of a variable. In a **normal distribution**, when the frequencies of a variable's values are graphed, they form a bell-shaped curve (figure 9.1). Other terms for a normal distribution are *Gaussian distribution* and *normal bell curve.*

Properties of the Normal Distribution

Properties of the **normal (bell) curve** underlie many statistical tests. See figure 9.1, the normal bell curve. A normal distribution is determined by its mean and standard deviations. The bell is symmetrical and extends to infinity in both directions. Note that the curve never actually touches the x-axis at either end. The mean, median, and the mode are all the same. The mean is the middle, vertical line that divides the curve into equal halves. The mean, being the most frequent value, is the highest point of the curve. The area under the normal curve equals 1.0 and accounts for 100 percent of cases,

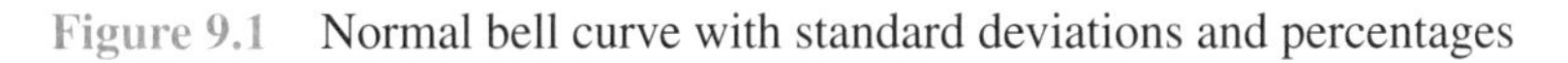

Figure 9.1 Normal bell curve with standard deviations and percentages

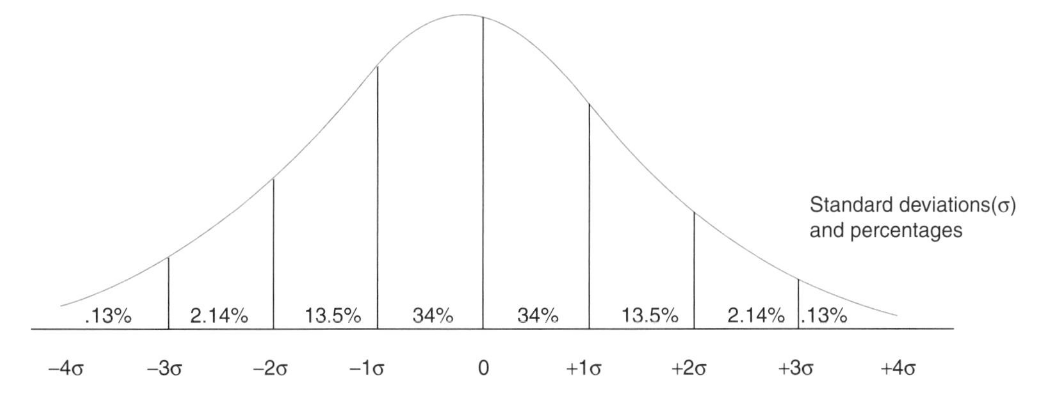

such as responses. One standard deviation on either side of the mean includes more than 68 percent of values. Two standard deviations on either side of the mean include more than 95 percent of values. Three standard deviations of either side of the mean include more than 99 percent of values. The further a value is from the middle, the more increasingly uncommon it is. Uncommon values or extremes are outliers and are in the tails (positive and negative) of the normal curve.

Properties of Nonnormal Distributions

Kurtotic, skewed, bimodal, and multimodal are types of nonnormal distributions. **Kurtosis** is a measure of the heaviness of both tails of a frequency distribution. The value of a normal kurtosis statistic is zero. Kurtotic distributions with negative kurtosis statistics are "heavy" in their tails; they appear overly broad (flattened). Known as *platykurtic distributions,* the values are overly represented in the tails of the curve. See figure 9.2a. Kurtotic distributions with positive kurtosis statistics are "light" in their tails; they appear overly tall (peaked). Known as *leptokurtic distributions,* the values are clustered in the middle of the distribution. See figure 9.2b.

Figure 9.2 Nonnormal distributions

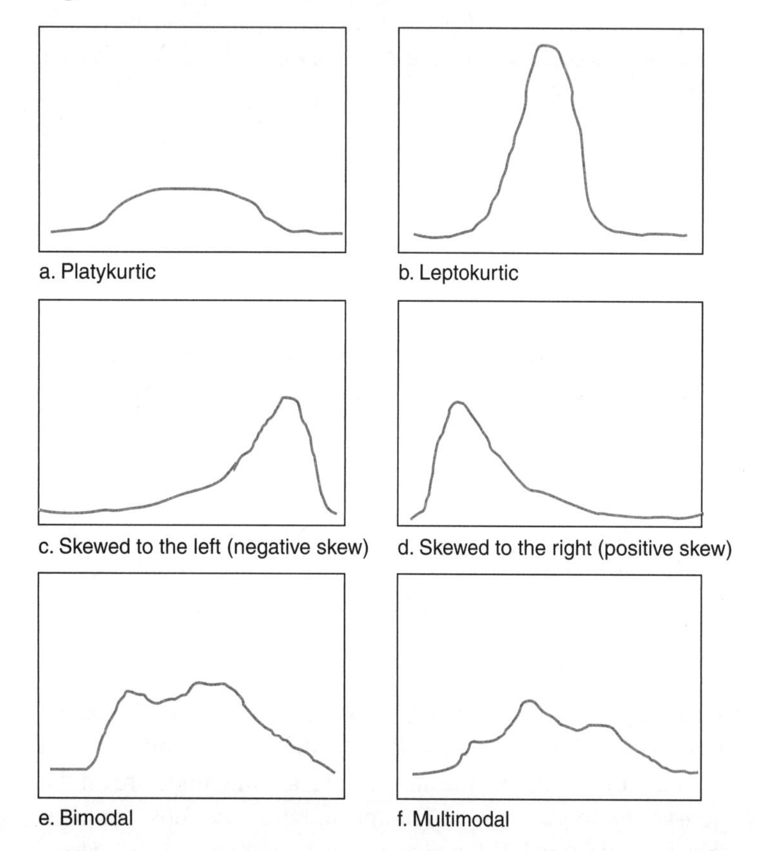

Skewness is the nonsymmetrical slant or tilt of the distribution. It occurs when values are overly represented in one of the tails of the distribution. Therefore, the mean, median, and mode are different values. When values cluster in the left tail, the distribution is negatively skewed or "skewed to the left." See figure 9.2c. When values cluster in the right tail, the distribution is positively skewed or "skewed to the right." See figure 9.2d.

Bimodal means that a frequency distribution of values has two modes. The classic example is the heights of all adults; there is one mode for women and a second mode for men. See figure 9.2e. *Multimodal* means that a frequency distribution of values has three or more modes. See figure 9.2f. Hospital readmissions show a multimodal distribution because reasons for readmissions, such as poor nutrition, wound breakdown, or noncompliance with medications, take varying lengths of time to occur (Morrow 2016, 27–28).

Tables

Tables, also known as *tabular presentations,* show numerical or descriptive data in a grid of rows and columns. Researchers generate tables for several reasons. Tables allow researchers to record, describe, examine, compare and contrast, and see the relationships among their data. Researchers also generate tables as an initial step in data analysis because tables allow researchers to organize and view their data and to identify potential trends or data entry errors. Tables can also be purely informative, such as a table showing the sociodemographic profile of a sample. The level of data affects how they are presented in tables.

Nominal, ordinal, interval, and ratio data are presented in frequency distributions. Frequency distributions summarize the frequency with which the values of a variable occur in a data set. The variable numbers should be listed in columns, not rows. The values can be presented as raw counts, percentages, or both. Nominal data are presented as frequencies and percentages. Ordinal data are presented as medians, percentages, and ranges. Interval and ratio data can be presented in the ways that nominal and ordinal data are presented and can also presented as means, standard deviations, and variance.

Tables that present data about one variable are univariate. Table 9.2 is univariate. In a hypothetical study, a researcher collected data on the variable of "sex" from a sample of health informatics professionals attending a conference. The table presents the frequencies of male and female attendees in terms of raw count and percentage.

Table 9.2 Univariate frequency distribution of health informatics professionals at a conference

Sex	Number (%)
Female	35 (52.2)
Male	32 (47.8)

Bivariate frequency distributions, which describe two variables, can also be presented as a table. The table has a set of values for one variable across the top (one row) and a set of values for a second variable down the side (column). For example, table 9.3 is an expansion of table 9.2. Table 9.3 shows, in addition to the sex of the hypothetical sample, the frequency distribution of the academic backgrounds of the health informatics professionals. In this sample, the academic backgrounds were computer science, health informatics, medicine, and nursing. For this hypothetical study, the frequency distribution shows the prevalence of clinicians in health informatics (39 males and females in medicine and nursing to 28 males and females in computer science and health informatics).

Table 9.3 Bivariate frequency distribution of health informatics professionals at a conference

Sex	Academic Background			
	Computer Science	Health Informatics	Medicine	Nursing
Female	4	8	9	14
Male	8	8	12	4

A **contingency table** visually presents information on two or more variables. Contingency tables are also known as *frequency tables, cross-tabulation tables,* and *cross-classification tables.* The number of cells in a contingency table depends on the number of variables and the number of values that the variables can have. In health informatics and HIM, researchers often have dichotomous variables. Dichotomous variables have two values: yes or no, hit or no-hit, improved or not-improved, and so forth.

Table 9.4 is a contingency table for the results of a hypothetical preliminary study on the ability of a decision support system to predict sepsis. Table 9.4 is also known as a **2×2 table** because there are two variables (system prediction of sepsis and actual health outcome of sepsis) and each variable has two values (sepsis and no sepsis). There are four cells ($2 \times 2 = 4$). At this stage of its development, the decision support system had 17 "hits" (true positives [A]), 9 "false alarms" (false positives [B]), 3 "misses" (false negatives [C]), and 6 "correct rejections" (true negatives [D]) for a total of 35 predictions. The decision support system made correct predictions 66 percent of the time (17 true positives plus 6 true negatives equals 23 correct predictions; 23 divided by 35 is 0.66). (For other examples of a contingency tables, see the 2×2 tables in chapter 5.)

Table 9.4 Example of contingency table (2×2 table)

Decision Support System's Prediction	Actual Health Outcome		Totals
	Sepsis	No Sepsis	
Sepsis	17 (A)	9 (B)	26 (A + B)
No sepsis	3 (C)	6 (D)	9 (C + D)
Totals	20 (A + C)	15 (B + D)	35 (A + B + C + D)

A = Number of cases of with sepsis and correct system prediction
B = Number of cases system predicted to have sepsis who did not have sepsis
C = Number of cases predicted to have no sepsis who did have sepsis
D = Number of cases of no sepsis and correct system prediction
A + C = Total number of cases with sepsis
B + D = Total number of cases without sepsis
A + B = Total number of cases system predicted to have sepsis
C + D = Total number of cases system predicted not to have sepsis

Contingency tables may also have more than two variables, such as a three-way table. Three-way tables are also known as 2×2×2 tables and have eight cells ($2 \times 2 \times 2 = 8$). The researchers of the hypothetical decision support system to predict sepsis reworked their decision algorithms. At this stage, the system's predictive ability improved; however, the improvement varied by the patient's sex. Table 9.5 shows a three-way table with three variables (system prediction of sepsis, actual health outcome of sepsis, and sex) and each variable has two values (sepsis and no sepsis). The decision support system's overall ability to predict sepsis was 91 percent (78 true positives plus 13 true negatives equals 91 correct predictions; 91 divided by 100 is 0.91). The hypothetical decision support system's ability to predict sepsis was better for female patients than male patients. For males, the system's ability was 87.5 percent (40 true positives plus 2 true negatives equals 42 correct predictions; 42 divided by 48 is 0.875). For females, the system's ability was 94.2 percent (38 true positives plus 11 true negatives equals 49 correct predictions; 49 divided by 52 is 0.942).

Table 9.5 Example of three-way contingency table (2×2×2 table)

Decision Support System's Prediction	Actual Health Outcome				Totals
	Sepsis		No Sepsis		
	Male	Female	Male	Female	
Sepsis	40	38	5	2	85
No sepsis	1	1	2	11	15
Totals	41	39	7	13	100

Total number of true positives (40 + 38) = 78
Total number of false positives (5 + 2) = 7
Total number of false negatives (1 + 1) = 2
Total number of true negatives (2 + 11) = 13
Total males (41 + 7) = 48
Total females (39 + 13) = 52

Bar Chart, Histogram, and Other Graphical Displays

Researchers graph their data to describe variables, compare and contrast them, and see relationships among them. Many types of graphical displays exist, such as the normal and nonnormal curves shown in the previous subsection. This subsection first presents bar charts, histograms, line graphs, scatter graphs, and pie charts. Then, the subsection presents information on stem-and-leaf diagrams and box-and-whisker plots.

Principles of good graphic design increase the clarity of the information in charts, histograms, and graphs. In these graphical displays for descriptive studies, all the possible values are listed along the *x*-axis (horizontal axis or abscissa) and the frequency with which a value occurs is listed along the y-axis (vertical axis or ordinate). In studies with independent and dependent variables, the independent variable is graphed along the x-axis and the dependent variable along the y-axis. Explanations of other principles, specific to particular to this set of graphical displays are as follows:

- **Bar charts** visually present data by showing comparisons between and among variables and illustrating major characteristics in the distribution of data. The height of the bar corresponds to the frequency of the value's occurrence. Bar charts show comparisons between and among nominal or ordinal data, such as sexes, grades, or rankings. As figure 9.3c shows, bar charts can have gaps between the bars. Figure 9.3a shows median patient satisfaction scores (ordinal data) by quarter. Bar charts can become complex, such as multiple bar charts and stacked bar charts.

Figure 9.3 Example of bar chart, histogram, line graph, scatter graph, and pie chart

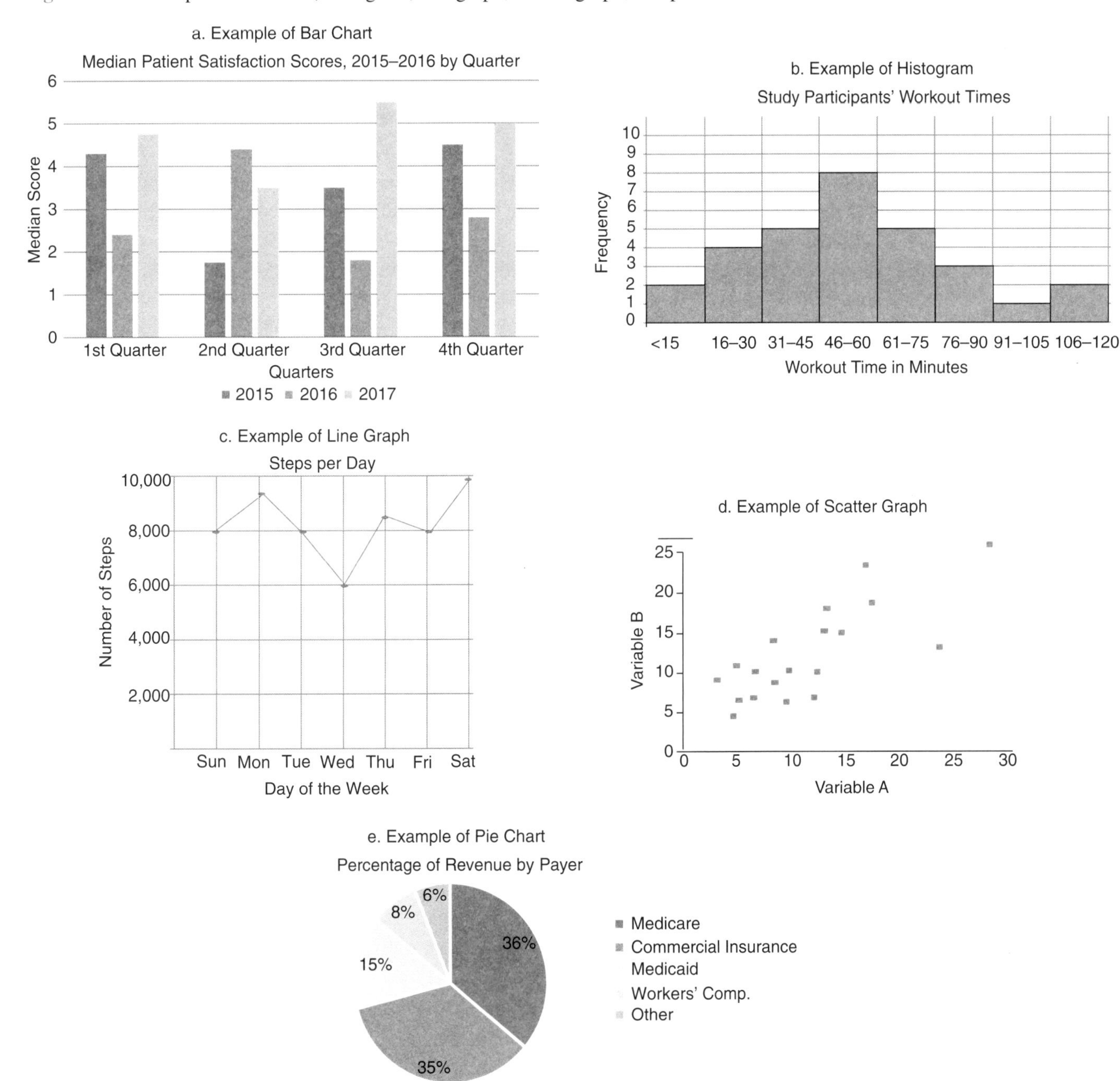

- **Histograms** show major characteristics in the distribution of data and summarize data about variables whose values are numerical and measured on an interval or ratio scale (continuous data). The data are divided into ranges called *bins* or *class intervals*. No simple rule exists to calculate the width of bins. Determining the bin width requires some trial and error. The bins should include the smallest and largest values and be equally sized. Generally, the number of bins varies from 5 to 20, depending upon the situation (Dos Passos 2010, 310). Smaller data sets tend to have fewer bins than larger data sets.

  In a histogram, as in a bar chart, the height of the bar corresponds to the frequency of the value's occurrence; however, in a histogram, the bars are adjoining with no gaps between the bars. Figure 9.3b is a histogram summarizing the frequency of participants' workout times. As figure 9.3b shows, the bars of histograms are adjoining with no gaps. The bars cannot be rearranged without losing meaning.
- **Line graphs** show trends for one variable over time. As figure 9.3c shows, the *x*-axis represents time and the *y*-axis represents the frequency of an event. Line graphs can also compare trends for multiple variables. In line graphs for multiple variables, each variable has its own line.
- **Scatter graphs** (plots or diagrams) show the association between two variables. The clustering or dispersion (scattering) of the data points shows the association between the two variables. The association can be linear or nonlinear. Figure 9.3d shows a positive linear association between variable a and variable b.
- **Pie charts** visually show the proportions (percentages) of a variable in each value, relationships among the values, and the whole. As figure 9.3e shows, the proportions are pie slices and the whole is the whole circle of the pie. For example, if the variable is source of revenue and the values are Medicare, commercial insurance, Medicaid, workers'compensation, and other, then each value, such as Medicare or Medicaid, is a slice of the pie. Adding the percentages of all the values should equal 100 and the "slices" create a complete "pie."

In descriptive statistics, other ways to display data include stem-and-leaf diagrams (plots) and box-and-whisker plots (box plots). These graphical displays show the raw data and the range and distribution of scores (results or observations) and make outliers visible. These types of displays are also techniques of exploratory data analysis.

Stem-and-leaf diagrams summarize data while maintaining all the individual data points. Diagram A in figure 9.4. shows the following data set, sorted into numerical order: 62, 66, 67, 71, 74, 75, 75, 81, 82, 82, 83, 93, 94, 101, 101, 103, 105. The "stem" column is the unique elements of the data set after removing last digit(s). The "leaves" column is the final digits placed in a row next to the appropriate stem column. Therefore, the row "7|1455" represents the values: 71, 74, 75, 75.

Figure 9.4 Stem-and-leaf diagram

Stem	Leaves
6	267
7	1455
8	12223
9	34
10	1139

A

Leaves	Stem	Leaves
267	6	
45	7	15
123	8	22
4	9	3
	10	1139

B

Diagram B in figure 9.4 represents the same data set split into halves. This format, known as the *back-to-back stem and leaf plot,* would be used if the researcher wanted to make comparisons. For example, the researchers could compare pretest and posttest observations or could compare scores from two different subpopulations. All the data points are still displayed with the pretest observations on the left side and the posttest observations on the right side. The row "45|7|15" still represents the values: 71, 74, 75, 75.

Box-and-whisker plots (box plots) display variation in a data set and summarize its key features (see figure 9.5). These features of the data set are the median, the upper and lower quartiles, the largest and smallest values (range), and the outliers. Box-and-whisker plots are used to (1) compare multiple data sets or (2) analyze or convey a data set's key features, rather than the detail (AHRQ 2017).

Figure 9.5 Box-and-whisker plot for risk-standardized mortality rates by proportion of African-American patients in the hospital—Medicare fee-for service beneficiaries age 65 years and older

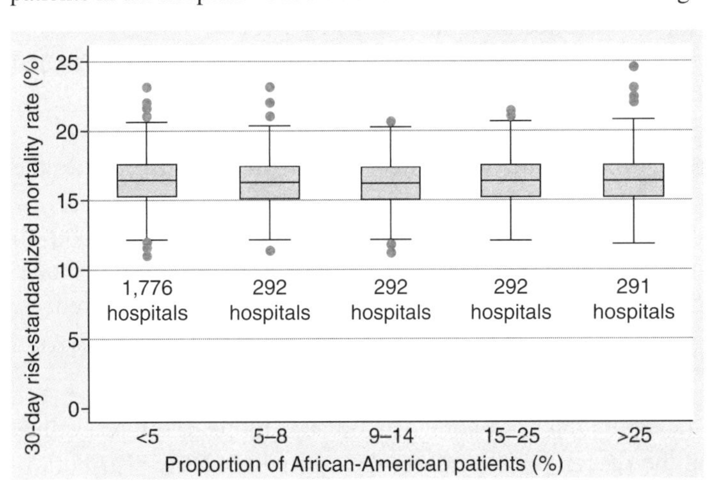

Source: CMS 2010, 14.

Box-and-whisker plots are constructed by finding, within a data set, the median, the upper and lower quartiles (quarters), the largest and smallest values, the interquartile range (IQR, defined later in this chapter, under measures of dispersion), and the outliers. The median line is in the center of a box formed by the upper and lower quartiles. The "whiskers" extend to the largest and smallest values, excluding outliers. Outliers are 1.5 times (standardized multiplier) the IQR on each end. The outliers are indicated with asterisks (dots in figure 9.5). Box-and-whisker plots are analyzed by looking at the location of the median, the range of the data (length of the "whiskers"), the data set's symmetry, and the existence of outliers. For example, skewness in the data set is indicated when the median is not centered in the middle of the box. The data sets shown in figure 9.5 are not skewed because the medians are centered in the boxes.

Ratios and Proportions

Ratios and proportions are known as *frequency measures*. They compare one part of a frequency distribution to another part or to the entire distribution. Frequency measures are all calculated by dividing a numerator (top number) by a denominator (bottom number) and multiplying the result by a power of ten (1; 10; 100; 1,000, and so on). Nominal and ordinal data are usually summarized with ratios and proportions. Metric data can also be expressed as ratios and proportions, but they may first need to be grouped (CDC 2012, 2-8–2-15).

Ratios are comparisons of two values. The values can be unrelated. To calculate a ratio, one value is divided by the other value; the result can be 1, greater than 1, or less than 1. Ratios are written as the numerator followed by a colon and then the denominator. Using data from table 9.3 as an example, the ratio of male health informatics professionals with a computer science background to female health informatics professionals with a computer science background is 8:4. The convention is to standardize the statement to 2:1 (which is derived by dividing both numbers by the lower number, in this case, 4).

Proportions are comparisons of a part to the whole. A proportion is a type of ratio in which the numerator's quantity is included in the denominator. Proportions can be expressed as a decimal, a fraction, or a percentage (CDC 2012, 3-4–3-6). In the case of percentages, the quotient is multiplied by 100. Using data from table 9.3 as an example, the proportion of female health informatics professionals with a medical background (9) to all the conference attendees (67) is 13.4 percent.

Measures of Central Tendency

The **measures of central tendency** represent the clustering of the majority of a data set's values around its middle value. They are also known as *measures of location*. The measures of central tendency are the mean, the median, and the mode and are described as follows:

- **Mean:** Average calculated by adding up all the values and dividing by the number of values. Calculating the mean is only appropriate for metric data. (The mean described here is the arithmetic mean; other types of means include the geometric mean and the trimmed mean.)

For example: For the set [42, 47, 42, 43, 42, 45, 43, 50, 42], the sum of the numbers is 396; there are 9 values in the set, and the mean is 44 [396/9 = 44].
Note: The mean is sensitive to outliers; in other words, that the mean can be skewed by outliers.

- **Median:** Middle value when all the values are placed in numeric order. Half of the values are above the median and half of the values are below the median. Medians may be calculated for ordinal data and metric data.
For example: For the set [42, 42, 42, 42, 43, 43, 45, 47, 50], the number at the center of the values is 43.
Note: When there are an even number of values, the mean of the middle two numbers is calculated and becomes the median.
- **Mode:** Value that occurs most frequently. A mode is commonly used for nominative data, but it can be used for all levels of data. The mode is determined by listing all the values in numerical order and finding the most common one.
For example: For the set [42, 42, 42, 42, 43, 43, 45, 47, 50], the most commonly occurring value, at four occurrences, is 42.
Note: As previously described in nonnormal distributions, a data set may have more than one mode.

In a normal distribution, the mean, median, and mode are the same value. In nonnormal distributions, the three values vary. The selection of mean, median, or mode depends upon the researcher's purpose, the normality of the distribution, and the presence of outliers. For example, selecting the mean as the measure of central tendency when the data set contains outliers may misrepresent the data because the value of the mean can be distorted by outliers. Therefore, means are used with normal distributions and medians for kurtotic or skewed distributions (CDC 2012, 2-16).

Measures of Dispersion

Measures of dispersion show the distribution of observations away from the central value. They show the variability of the data. The measures of dispersion are also known as the *measures of spread* because they show the spread of the variable's values. The measures of dispersion include the range, the interquartile range, the standard deviation, and the normality of the distribution.

- **Range:** Difference between greatest and smallest value.
For example: For the set [42, 42, 42, 42, 43, 43, 45, 47, 50], the greatest value is 50 and the smallest value is 42. The difference is calculated by subtracting 42 from 50, which results in a range of 8 [50 – 42 = 8].
Note: Ranges can be calculated for ordinal and metric data.
- **Interquartile range:** Range within which the middle 50 percent of values fall. Interquartile ranges can be calculated for ordinal and metric data.
- **Standard deviation:** Average distance from the mean that each value lies. The standard deviation shows how concentrated or dispersed values are from the distribution's center. Standard deviations can only be calculated for metric data.
- **Normality of distribution:** Normal distribution has the greatest frequency of values in the middle of the curve. Nonnormal distributions have curves with kurtosis or skewness.

The selection of a measure of dispersion depends upon the normality of the distribution. Generally, standard deviations are used with means and ranges whereas interquartile ranges are used with medians (CDC 2012, 2-53).

Correlation

Correlations can be descriptive statistics when the researcher's purpose is to describe the association. Correlations describe the strength and nature of an association. Statistical tests that involve two variables are called **bivariate**. **Multivariate** correlational tests involve multiple dependent (outcome) variables. Pearson product-moment correlation coefficient is often calculated when correlations are used descriptively. Correlations are discussed in more detail in the section on Inferential Statistics.

Inferential Statistics

Inferential statistics allow investigators to detect differences or associations between groups and to generalize those findings from the sample to the entire population of interest. Inferential statistics are based on probability theory (Singleton and Straits 2010, 509) and have two purposes. The first purpose of inferential statistics is to make predictions (inferences) about the population's characteristics (parameters) from the sample's characteristics. The second purpose is to test hypotheses—the researcher's measurable suppositions. This section builds on the information provided in the previous section, explaining some of the commonly encountered inferential statistical tests that were briefly described in table 9.1 and helping readers choose the appropriate inferential statistical test by matching the selection factors to the features of an individual study.

Independent One-Sample *t*-Test

The independent one-sample *t*-test is used to detect differences when (1) the dependent variable is continuous (interval or ratio) and normally distributed, and (2) the data are independent observations. There is no independent variable. The independent one-sample *t*-test detects differences between a group's mean and a "hypothesized value." The independent one-sample *t*-test is also known as the *one-sample* t-*test*. Examples of "hypothesized values" include a mean derived from previous research or the literature, a mean based on theory, a benchmark, a historical value, or a known population mean. For example, a health information coding supervisor could compare the coding productivity—minutes per record—of the integrated delivery system's 32 coding professionals against a benchmark productivity standard—minutes per record—published in the literature.

Independent-Measures *t*-Test

The independent-measures *t*-test is used to detect differences in means when (1) the independent variable is dichotomous (for example, gender: male or female; educational level: high school or university) and nominal, (2) the dependent variable is normally distributed and continuous (interval or ratio), and (3) the two samples are independent. The independent-measures *t*-test is also known as the *independent* t-*test,* the *independent-samples* t-*test,* the *two-sample* t-*test,* the *unpaired* t-*test,* and the *Student's* t-*test*. For example, researchers used an independent-measures t-test to compare the e-health literacy among users and nonusers of social media for health information (Tennant et al. 2015, 4). The independent-measures *t*-test is often used to detect whether outcomes differ between the experimental group and the control group.

Mann-Whitney *U* Test

The Mann-Whitney *U* test has the same purpose as the independent measures *t*-test, except the Mann-Whitney *U* test detects differences in two groups' medians and the test is nonparametric. The Mann-Whitney *U* test is used when (1) the independent variable is dichotomous (male-female) and nominal, (2) the dependent variable is ordinal or nonnormally distributed continuous (interval or ratio), and (3) the two samples are independent. Other names for the Mann-Whitney *U* test are the *Mann–Whitney–Wilcoxon (MWW),* the *Wilcoxon rank-sum test,* or the *Wilcoxon–Mann–Whitney test.*

A Mann-Whitney *U* test could be used, for example, to compare opinions of seminar participants at two different professional meetings who attended an expert's "Big Data" session (which used the same content and slides at both meetings). The two groups of participants ranked their agreement on the value of the session to their work on a Likert scale (strongly agree = 5, agree = 4, neutral = 3, disagree = 2, strongly disagree = 1). The expert could use the Mann-Whitney *U* test to compare the two sessions' median rankings by the two groups of seminar participants.

Chi-Square Test

The chi-square test is used to compare results when (1) the dependent variable is nominal or ordinal and there is no independent variable *or* both the independent and dependent variables are nominal or ordinal, (2) the samples are independent, and (3) the cells contain more than five responses (see the boxes in table 9.6 for examples of cells). *Chi* stands for the 22nd letter of the Greek alphabet—similar to *X* in English—and is sometimes shown as χ; thus, chi-square is sometimes designated as χ^2 in journal articles. There are two applications of the chi-square: chi-square goodness of fit and the chi-square test of independence. Both are nonparametric tests.

- The chi-square goodness of fit is used to determine whether the distribution of subjects' responses is significantly different from the "hypothesized" distribution. The single variable is dichotomous (for example, gender: male chief information officers versus female chief information officers). The researchers could be interested in whether the actual proportion of male and female chief information officers is significantly different from the hypothesized proportions. In the chi-square goodness of fit test, the proportions can be equal or unequal. The chi-square goodness of fit is also called the *one-sample goodness-of-fit test* and the *Pearson's chi-square goodness-of-fit test*.

- The chi-square test of independence is used to determine whether significant differences exist when (1) there are two nominal or ordinal dependent variables, (2) the independent variable is nominal or ordinal and the dependent variable is ordinal or nominal, and (3) the samples are independent. Other names for the chi-square test of independence are just *chi-square,* the *Pearson chi-square test,* and the *chi-square test of association*. The chi-square test of independence can also be used to as a probe to determine whether an association exists between nominal and ordinal variables. However, the chi-square test does not show the strength of the relationship (association).

Table 9.6 Example of cells in contingency table

	Rural Hospitals	**Urban Hospitals**
Adequate access to behavioral health services	3	10
Inadequate access to behavioral health services	17	10

For example, researchers conducted a study in which they retrospectively reviewed a convenience sample of EHRs from one home health agency. Using the chi-square test of independence, comparisons were made by age categories, gender, and ethnicity for the frequency of prescribed medication categories and polypharmacy (concurrent prescriptions of more than 4 prescriptions). Statistically significant differences in prescription frequency of cardiovascular agents were found when comparing (1) patients 65 years or older and patients younger than 65 years, and (2) female patients and male patients. Additionally, statistically more white patients than African-American patients met the criterion of polypharmacy (Arena et al. 2015, 98–100).

Fisher Exact Test

The Fisher exact test is used rather than the chi-square test if one of the data cells in the contingency table is 5 or less. For example, in the hypothetical contingency table (table 9.6), the value in the cell for "Rural Hospitals–Adequate access to behavioral health services" is 3, which means the Fisher exact test could be used.

Paired *t*-Test

The paired *t*-test is used to detect differences in means when (1) the independent variable is nominal, (2) the dependent variable is continuous, and (3) the samples are dependent, such as the same group with two observations, dyads (supervisor-employer, husband-wife), or matched groups (Cohen 2013, 341–343, 354–355). Several terms are used for this statistical test, depending upon the exact composition of the groups: *dependent* t-*test, paired-samples* t-*test, related-samples* t-*test, matched-samples* t-*test, within-persons* t-*test,* and *repeated measures* t-*test*. For example, researchers used the paired *t*-test to evaluate providers' knowledge of driving safety for older adults in terms of the providers' self-assessed preparedness as well as their documentation of assessment and management. Embedded in the EHR was a driving clinical support tool. Providers' self-assessed preparedness and their documentation were evaluated before and after training on the tool. The posttraining evaluation showed significantly increased self-assessed preparedness and improved documentation (Casey et al. 2015, S136).

Wilcoxon Signed-Rank Test

The Wilcoxon signed-rank test is used to detect differences in medians when (1) the independent variable is nominal, (2) the dependent variable is ordinal or continuous, and (3) the samples are dependent, such as two observations on the same subject. As a hypothetical example, leaders of an integrated delivery system asked the Big Data expert to present a two-day seminar on Big Data applications to its supervisory personnel. At the beginning of the first day of the seminar, the expert had the participants rank their agreement on the value of Big Data to their work on a Likert scale (strongly agree = 5, agree = 4, neutral = 3, disagree = 2, strongly disagree = 1). At the end of the seminar's second day, the expert again had the participants rank the value of Big Data to their work on the same Likert scale. The expert then conducted a Wilcoxon signed-rank test to understand whether the participants' rating of the value of Big Data to their work changed after they attended the two-day seminar. Note, that while the names are similar, the Wilcoxon *signed-rank* test and the Wilcoxon *rank-sum* test are not the same. The former is used when the samples are *dependent* (paired, matched, same subject, and such); the latter (see Mann-Whitney U test) is used when the samples are *independent*.

Analysis of Variance

Analysis of variance (ANOVA) is a family of statistical tests to detect differences in means between groups. ANOVAs allow simultaneous comparisons between groups. Types of ANOVAs include one-way ANOVA, two-way ANOVA, repeated-measures ANOVA, multivariate ANOVA (MANOVA), and analysis of covariance (ANCOVA).

One-Way ANOVA

One-way ANOVA is similar to the independent-measures *t*-test except that ANOVA is used when the independent variable has three or more groups. (Technically, ANOVA could be used for two groups, but typically the independent-measures *t*-test is used in that situation because it is easier to conduct.) ANOVA is used to detect differences between the means of groups when (1) the one independent variable is nominal with three or more levels, (2) the dependent variable is normally distributed and continuous (interval or ratio), and (3) the samples (groups) are independent. In a one-way ANOVA, one variable is varied. For example, if researchers have three or more levels of a nominal variable (such as level of type of intervention: for example, online module, face-to-face seminar, and none) and are considering running a series of independent-measures *t*-tests between all the pairs of levels, they can simplify their process by running the one-way ANOVA because the one-way ANOVA analyzes all the data in one calculation. Moreover, one-way ANOVA is desirable because running multiple independent-measures *t*-tests increases the type I error (false positive) rate (see chapter 12).

For example, researchers noted that healthcare insurers have encouraged patients to receive surgical operations at Centers of Excellence. Retrospectively reviewing EHRs, these researchers examined whether, within a regionalized healthcare system, travel distances to receive major cancer surgery varied by sociodemographic factors. Using one-way ANOVA, the researchers made comparisons between age, race, cancer type, and hospital of destination. Significant differences in travel patterns were found by age, race, and cancer surgery type.Younger patients, white patients, or patients receiving esophageal or pancreatic resections were more likely to travel further within the regional system to receive major cancer surgery. In comparison, African-American patients were less likely to travel further than other racial or ethnic groups to receive major cancer surgery (Smith et al. 2015, 99–102).

The nonparametric alternative of the one-way ANOVA is the Kruskal-Wallis test, which is used when the dependent variable is ordinal or the dependent variable's distribution is nonnormal. Other names for the Kruskal-Wallis test are the *Kruskal-Wallis* H *test* (*H* is the test statistic), the *Kruskal-Wallis test by ranks,* and the *one-way ANOVA on ranks*.

Two-Way ANOVA

The two-way ANOVA is used to detect differences between the means of groups when (1) the two independent variables are nominal and have two or more levels, (2) the dependent variable is continuous (interval or ratio), and (3) the samples (groups) are independent. For example, a researcher could investigate the effect of level of physical activity (low, moderate, high) and of sex (male, female) on weight loss. Two-way ANOVA helps to show whether there is an interaction between the two independent variables (physical activity and sex in this case) in how they affect the dependent variable (weight loss in this case).

One-Way Repeated Measures ANOVA

One-way repeated measures ANOVA is used to detect differences between the three or more groups means when (1) the two independent variables are nominal and have two or more levels, (2) the dependent variable is continuous (interval or ratio) and normally distributed, and (3) the samples (groups) are dependent. For example, one-way repeated measures ANOVA would be used to understand whether there is a sustained difference in coding speed among coding professionals after a two-day seminar on circulatory anatomy and physiology. Observations of coding speed are made three times: immediately before the seminar, one month after the seminar, and six months after the seminar. Coding speed is the dependent variable. The independent variable is time period: immediately before, post–one month, and post–six months. The measures are dependent (repeated) because the same individuals' coding speeds are being measured three times.

The Friedman test is the nonparametric alternative to the repeated-measures ANOVA. The two-way repeated-measures ANOVA is used when there are two independent measures (such as time period and on-site versus teleworker).

Multivariate ANOVA (MANOVA)

Multivariate ANOVA (MANOVA) is used when there is more than one dependent variable. For example, in a study of post–hospital discharge Medicare beneficiaries, researchers used MANOVA when examining the differences between beneficiaries who were subsequently rehospitalized and beneficiaries who were admitted to a skilled nursing facility during the study's follow-up period. The independent variables in the MANOVA were being readmitted to a hospital and being admitted to a skilled nursing facility, and the dependent variables were age, gender, function, number of diagnoses, number of nursing visits, number of medications, and evidence of depression (Carew and Resnick 2015, 52).

Analysis of Covariance (ANCOVA)

Analysis of covariance (ANCOVA) tests whether means are statistically different and is used when the independent variable is strongly and linearly correlated (covarying) with the dependent variable or when other linearly covarying factors are involved. For example, depression and cardiovascular disease are strongly associated (Renoir et al. 2013, 1), so the two variables are said to covary. ANCOVA accounts for the "noise" (confusion) of the covariance. The two or more independent variables are nominal or normally distributed continuous, and the dependent variable is continuous with a normal distribution. A third variable, the covariate variable, is the control variable (Huck 2012, 347). ANCOVA is a sophisticated test that combines analysis of variance and linear regression analysis (Ritz et al. 2015, 166).

Pearson Product-Moment Correlation Coefficient

The Pearson product-moment correlation coefficient is used detect relationships when (1) both the independent and dependent variables are continuous (interval or ratio), (2) the relationship is linear, and (3) the observations are independent. The Pearson product-moment correlation coefficient is "used to evaluate both the statistical significance of the relationship and the magnitude and direction of the relationship" (Allua and Thompson 2009, 170). The Pearson product-moment correlation coefficient "ranges from –1.0 to +1.0: a +1.0 indicates a perfect direct (positive) relationship, and a –1.0 indicates a perfect inverse (negative) relationship" (Allua and Thompson 2009, 170). Other terms for the Pearson product-moment correlation coefficient are Pearson's *r*, correlation coefficient, linear correlation coefficient, and Pearson correlation.

Researchers used the Pearson product-moment correlation coefficient in a study to explore the accessibility of Internet mobile health and rehabilitation (iMHere) apps for individuals with spina bifida. The purposes of the iMHere apps are to support self-care and adherence to self-care regimens for individuals who are vulnerable to secondary complications, such as people with spina bifida and other complex conditions. Participants completed 108 multistep tasks using the apps. The Pearson product-moment correlation coefficient revealed a slightly negative statistically significant correlation between the order of tests and the completion time. A significant positive correlation was found between (1) the time to complete a task and the steps to complete tasks, (2) the steps to complete tasks and the mistakes encountered by participants, and (3) the time to complete a task and the mistakes encountered by participants (Yu et al. 2015, 3–4).

Spearman Rank Order Correlation

The Spearman rank order correlation is the nonparametric alternative to the Pearson product-moment correlation coefficient. The independent and dependent variables are ordinal. A Spearman rank order correlation may also be used for continuous data that are not normally distributed, are nonlinear, or have significant outliers (violations of the assumptions for the Pearson product-moment correlation coefficient). The Spearman rank order correlation is also called the *Spearman correlation,* the *Spearman's correlation,* the *Spearman rank order* r, the *Spearman rank* r, the *Spearman* rho, or the *Spearman ρ. Rho* or ρ is the 17th letter of the Greek alphabet (the same as *r* in the English alphabet). For example, the Spearman rank order correlation would be performed if either the independent or dependent variables were collected using a Likert scale or other ranking scale. If the sample size is very small, the alternative to the Spearman rank order correlation is the Kendall's tau-b (τ_b) correlation coefficient (also known as *Kendall's* tau-b).

Simple Regression

The simple regression is used to detect relationships when (1) the one independent (predictor, explanatory) variable is continuous (ratio or interval) with a normal distribution, (2) the one dependent (outcome) variable is continuous with a normal distribution, (3) the samples are independent, and (4) the variables have a linear relationship. Other terms for the simple regression are simple linear regression or linear regression. For example, researchers conducted a study to test the associations between categories of body mass index and other factors among a sample of Mexicans ages 50 years and older. Simple regression revealed that among older adults, body mass index seemed to have a significant relationship with physical activity, age, sex, income, and marital status (Rivas-Marino et al. 2015, 329–330).

Multiple Regression

Multiple regressions are used to detect relationships when (1) two or more independent variables are nominal or continuous (ratio or interval), (2) the dependent variable is continuous (ordinal data require ordinal regression), and (3) the samples are independent. Regression models are used to do the following:

- Explain causes of outcomes
- Predict relationships among factors (independent or predictor variables) and outcomes (dependent variables)
- Adjust for imbalances among predictor variables between groups
- Make comparisons between and among groups
- Detect interactions among predictor variables

Similar to ANOVA, multiple regression is a family of statistical tests including multiple linear regression, hierarchical regression, logistical regression, and Poisson regression.

Multiple regression is commonly used in health-related research. When reading articles, be aware of the specific language that researchers use when describing regressions. *Multivariate* tests involve multiple dependent (outcome) variables (Hidalgo and Goodman 2013, 39). *Multivariable* tests involve multiple independent and multiple dependent variables.

The use of theory-driven regression models, such as hierarchical regression, should be prioritized over the use of step-wise regression models because step-wise regression models may compound type I (false positive) errors (Norman and Streiner 2014,158–160). In theory-driven regression models, the investigator determines and sets the order of the variables based on theory and information in the literature. In step-wise regression, the computer builds the model by successively adding or removing variables based on their power to explain additional variance.

In the study in which the researchers were investigating e-health literacy among users and nonusers of social media, which was previously mentioned in the section on the independent-measures *t*-test, the investigators also used multiple regression analyses. Multiple regression analyses were used to determine associations between sociodemographics (such as age and gender), social determinants (such as education and income), and electronic device use (such as desktop computer or mobile phone) on self-reported e-health literacy and social media use for seeking and sharing health information (Tennant et al. 2015).

Complex variations of multiple regression exist, such as mixed-effects models. Mixed-effects models are sophisticated extensions of regressions used as tools to analyze grouped data. Grouped data result from longitudinal studies, repeated measurements, blocked designs, and multilevel (hierarchical) or clustered structures. Examples of studies that would use mixed-effects models are as follows:

- Longitudinal studies that analyze change over time, such as survival studies, time-to-event outcomes, and responses to treatments. In these studies, the data are collected multiple times at specific periods. The collected data are called *repeated measurement data, longitudinal measurement outcomes,* or *serial observations* (Asar et al. 2015, 334; Johnson 2015, 69).
- Studies that collect clustered data, such as clinic patients clustered by physician or hospital patients in a multihospital integrated delivery system clustered by hospital. These two clustering examples could also be considered multilevel (hierarchical) structures.

There are two major categories of mixed-effects models: linear models and nonlinear models.

Standardized language for the mixed-effects models has not been established. Variations of the mixed-effects models are also called *hierarchical (multilevel) models, mixed models, random effects models, random coefficient models, covariance components models,* and *variance components models.* Variations also occur within the categories, such as hierarchical linear models that are also known as *multi-level linear models, nested models, mixed linear models,* and *covariance components models*. The profusion of terms for these models can be confusing; however, readers can determine that the analysis is using a mixed-effects model by focusing on the purpose of the study and the grouping of the data.

Other Tests and Terms

In addition to the commonly used tests in inferential statistics, a general awareness of some other inferential statistical tests and terminology may assist readers in understanding the health literature and determining whether an article's findings would be applicable to their healthcare organization. Readers may encounter sensitivity analyses, the Cox (proportional hazard regression) model, the hazard rate, the Poisson regression, and the Bonferroni correction in the methods, results, and discussion sections of articles.

Sensitivity analyses are analytic techniques to determine whether a study's results change if assumptions, statistical techniques, inputs, or other elements of a research plan are varied. Sensitivity analyses have many uses, such as the following:

- To check the impacts of outliers, of cut-off points, or of different ways of handling missing data.
- To gauge whether a study's results are the same for all subgroups, such as groups by patient type, gender, age category, race or ethnicity, insurance or socioeconomic status, or other subpopulation characteristic. Sensitivity analyses can answer questions such as, "Does the intervention have the same effects for women and men (or computer-savvy users and computer-illiterate users)?"
- To check, in meta-analyses, whether one study's outcomes are unduly influencing the overall measure of effect (Thabane et al. 2013, 2, 3–8)

When the results of analyses are consistent or unchanged by testing variations in the plan's elements, the results are said to be robust (Delaney and Seeger 2013, 145). Decision makers' confidence in using the conclusions and inferences from robust results is increased. Sensitivity analyses should be a part of the plan for statistical analysis. Clinicians, administrators, policymakers, and other leaders are interested in knowing an intervention's varying effects on subgroups. Providing this information makes the research meaningful to users. (Note that sensitivity analyses are *not* the same as sensitivity and specificity that were discussed in chapter 5.)

Examples of other inferential statistics tests include:

- **Cox (proportional hazards regression) model:** Relates covariates or risk factors to outcome. Often used with hazard rates (death, life expectancy)
- **Hazard (function) rate:** Proportion of subjects who die in an increment of time, starting a one point in time, who had survived to that point (in other words, the probability of dying in a specified interval). Outcomes other than death can be studied
- **Poisson regression:** Statistical test for data that are discrete counts of independent events occurring in a certain time period and being small in number compared to the entire population (based on Poisson distribution). An example of such data in healthcare would be the number of hospital admissions per day

Finally, when reviewing the literature, one might encounter the term Bonferroni correction, which is an adjustment made when multiple hypothesis tests are made on the same set of data; sets likelihood of falsely rejecting a hypothesis at a value (α = value and k = number of tests; Bonferroni correction = α/k).

Misuse of Statistics

Misuse of statistics can be accidental or intentional. For example, statistics are accidentally misused when the wrong statistical test is unintentionally used or some other mistake is made. As a consequence, the study's reported results and conclusions are untrustworthy. Statistics are intentionally misused when researchers deliberately disguise their actual results by writing in confusing language or glossing over their undesirable or insignificant findings. An undesirable side effect of the misuse of statistics is that some people and policymakers distrust research. Types of accidental and intentional misuse of statistics include invalid statistics, lying with statistics, unit of analysis error, and confusing correlation with causation.

Invalid Statistics for Ordinal Data

Ignorance sometimes leads researchers to treat ordinal data like metric data. Unlike metric data, ordinal data do *not* have true numerical value. The rankings (scales, ratings) are conceptual, subjective differences; they are not actual differences. As such, means and standard deviations should not be calculated for ordinal data. Although the rankings are presented as numbers, researchers should avoid the temptation of performing these calculations (see also discussion in chapter 2).

Lying with Statistics

In 1954, Huff published his landmark book on how to lie with statistics. Lying with statistics can be achieved by using biased samples, distorting graphics, selecting the wrong statistical test, failing to check whether the test's assumptions are met, and other methods (De Veaux and Hand 2005, 231). Sometimes, the researchers are not deliberately lying, but they misrepresent data to obscure errors or undesirable results so that their research is published. Sometimes, they overdramatically present research results to get attention, or journalists and advocates of a particular viewpoint take the statistics from a research study out of context.

Costs, lengths of stay, mortality rates, and treatment effects are often presented in the most dramatic way possible. Bamboozling the reader is especially easy with percentages, proportions, and ratios because the reader does not have a frame of reference to adequately interpret the numbers. For example, in a study, the risk of error was 2 percent for the experimental group and 1 percent for the control group. The researcher calculated a relative risk: 1 percent divided by 2 percent equals 50 percent. The researcher could have calculated an absolute risk: 2 percent minus 1 percent equals 1 percent. However, 50 percent seems to be a much more notable outcome than 1 percent (example based on ACP 2000). Researchers can provide the greatest clarity by reporting including actual, raw data as well as their statistical manipulations.

Unit of Analysis Error

Researchers can also unintentionally make a procedural error, known as a unit of analysis error. A unit of analysis is the study's focus that is being examined and for which data have been collected. The unit of randomization reflects the researchers' focus—individuals, groups, objects, and other phenomenon. A **unit of analysis error** is a mismatch between the unit of randomization and the data (measurements or observations) that are used for statistical tests (Huck 2012, 249). A unit of analysis error occurs when the unit of randomization and the unit of analysis differ. For example, suppose that the researchers' question is the effects of an educational module on the functioning of a group practice as a whole; the study is not supposed to investigate the module's effects on the individual clinicians. Based on their question, the researchers randomize 15 group practices. However, the researchers gather data on the effects of the module on the individual clinicians. Then, to conduct the statistical tests for the unit of analysis, the entire group practice, the researchers must aggregate their data. To do this, they might use the practices' means, rather than the individuals' means. A useful tip to avoid this error is that the number of observations (measurements) being analyzed should match the number of units that were randomized (Deeks et al. 2011).

Unit of analysis errors have occurred in health informatics research. Holt and colleagues did a systematic review and meta-analysis of 42 research articles on the influence of EHR reminder systems on clinicians' processes, such as conducting screenings, and on clinical outcomes, such as blood pressure control, and found that 28 studies were affected by unit of analysis errors. The researchers of the original studies had randomized at the level of the clinician or clinical team, but they had analyzed patient outcome data (Holt et al. 2012, 980).

Confusing Correlation with Causation

Researchers may unintentionally or through ignorance confuse correlation with causation. Correlations cannot prove causation. Correlations only demonstrate associations or relationships among variables. Correlations cannot establish the cause and the effect. (See also discussion of these concepts in chapter 1.) Terms such as *prove, cause,* and their variants (*proves, causes,* and so forth) must be avoided when presenting results of correlation studies and any other nonexperimental study.

Review Questions

1. In a negative linear association, as the value of one variable moves in a negative direction (decreases), the value of the other variable also proportionately moves in a negative direction (decreases). Is this statement true or false? Why?
2. What are at least three purposes of descriptive statistics?
3. What are at least three characteristics of a normal curve?
4. A student's roommate gave her the following tip on how to determine whether a distribution is skewed to the right or skewed to the left: Look at the curve's highest point or peak. If the peak is nearer to the right side of the curve, the distribution is skewed to the *right*; if the peak is nearer to the left side of the curve, the distribution is skewed to the *left*. Should the student use this tip? Why or why not?
5. A chart has gaps between the bars. What type of chart is it, and what type of data would it display?
6. Which graphical display would a researcher use to show the variation, potential skewness, and the potential existence of outliers in a data set? What is your justification for your answer?
7. What are three measures of central tendency? What are three measures of dispersion?
8. Consider the following situation: The data set does *not* meet the underlying assumptions of parametric tests. Your purpose is to compare the proportions of one group to a hypothesized distribution. The only dependent variable is nominal, and there is no independent variable. Which statistical test should you would choose for this situation? What is your justification for your answer?
9. Consider the following situation: The data set meets the assumptions of parametric tests. Your purpose is to compare the performance of clinician pairs (physician and his or her physician assistant) before and after the enhancement of the embedded decision support tool (two observations). The independent variable is nominal, and the dependent variable is continuous. Which statistical test should you choose for this situation? What is your justification for your answer?
10. Consider the following situation. You want to quantify the association between stress and lack of confidence. Your data set meets the assumptions of parametric tests, and your independent and dependent variables are continuous. Which statistical test should you choose for this situation? What is your justification for your answer?

Application Exercises

1. Answer the following questions based on the real-world case at the beginning of the chapter.
   a. What type of data resulted from the respondents' ratings of the health information graduates in the first and second questions?
   b. What type of data resulted from the respondents' answers to the third and fourth questions?
   c. As a student, what take-aways does the article give you that you could use to improve your employability postgraduation?
2. Healthcare organizations often place educational materials on websites. Researchers evaluated the readability, content, and quality of educational materials related to preeclampsia (a complication of pregnancy associated with high blood pressure and damage to kidneys) (Lange et al. 2015, 383). Researchers searched the websites of US obstetrics and gynecology residency programs for patient education materials. The readability, content, and quality of these materials were assessed. The readability data were continuous and normally distributed. To evaluate the online materials' readability level, the researchers compared online materials' mean readability level against the recommended sixth-grade reading level (Lange et al. 2015, 385–386). The researchers found that the online materials' mean readability level was above the recommended sixth–grade reading level. Which statistical test did the researchers use and why?
3. Researchers conducted a study to evaluate users' experiences in using secure e-mail messaging (Haun et al. 2015, e282, 1–12). To collect data, the researchers surveyed patients who had registered for the Veteran Health Administration's web-based patient portal, My HealtheVet, and had opted to use secure messaging. The paper-based

survey collected sociodemographic data; assessed health and computer literacy (BRIEF Health Literacy Screening Tool); assessed common computer skills (Computer-Email-Web [CEW] Fluency Scale); assessed knowledge and skills to find, evaluate, and apply electronic health information (eHealth Literacy Scale [eHEALS]); and collected information on use and perceptions of secure messaging.

a. The researchers stated that survey's instruments to collect data on health and computer literacy were Likert scales. What type of data level did the researchers collect with these instruments? Based on the chapter, what descriptive statistics could be applied to these data?
b. Based on the information in the chapter, which descriptive statistical methods could the researchers perform on the gender, ethnicity, and marital status data collected from the respondents? What types of tables and graphics could the researchers use to present these data?
c. In the study, respondents were asked to rank the frequency of their use of secure messaging use as: *never use*, *few times per month or less*, *at least once a week*, and *every day*. Based on the information in the chapter, what statistical test did the researchers perform to assess differences in the frequency of using secure messaging between sex, ethnicity, and marital status? What reasons support your answer?

References

Agency for Healthcare Research and Quality (AHRQ). 2017. Box and Whisker Plot. Accessed January 7, 2017. http://healthit.ahrq.gov/health-it-tools-and-resources/workflow-assessment-health-it-toolkit/all-workflow-tools/box-and-whisker-plot.

Allua, S. and C.B. Thompson. 2009. Inferential statistics. *Air Medical Journal* 28(4):168–171.

Alreck, P.L. and R.B. Settle. 2004. *The Survey Research Handbook,* 3rd ed. New York: McGraw-Hill/Irwin.

American College of Physicians (ACP). 2000 (January–February). Primer on absolute vs. relative differences. *Effective Clinical Practice.* http://ecp.acponline.org/janfeb00/primer.htm.

Arena, S.K., A. Bacyinski, L. Simon, and E.L. Peterson. 2015. Medications and fall risk indicators among patients case-managed by physical therapists. *Home Healthcare Now* 33(2):96–102.

Asar, Ö., J. Ritchie, P.A. Kalra, and P.J. Diggle. 2015. Joint modelling of repeated measurement and time-to-event data: An introductory tutorial. *International Journal of Epidemiology* 44(1):334–344.

Carew, A.P. and B. Resnick. 2015. Outcomes of the Maryland Person-Centered Hospital Discharge Program: A pilot targeting decreasing long-term care use and hospital readmissions. *Care Management Journals* 16(1):48–58.

Casey, C.M., K. Salinas, and E. Eckstrom. 2015. Electronic health record tools to care for at-risk older drivers: a quality improvement project. *Gerontologist* 55(Suppl 1):S128–S139.

Centers for Disease Control and Prevention (CDC). 2012. *Principles of Epidemiology in Public Health Practice: An Introduction to Applied Epidemiology and Biostatistics,* 3rd ed. Atlanta, GA: Centers for Disease Control and Prevention, Self-Study Course SS1978. https://www.cdc.gov/ophss/csels/dsepd/ss1978/ss1978.pdf.

Centers for Medicare and Medicaid Services (CMS). 2010 (September 29). Medicare Hospital Quality Chartbook 2010: Performance Report on Outcomes Measures for Acute Myocardial Infarction, Heart Failure, and Pneumonia. https://www.cms.gov/Medicare/Quality-Initiatives-Patient-Assessment-Instruments/HospitalQualityInits/Downloads/HospitalChartBook.pdf.

Deeks, J.J., J.P.T. Higgins, and D.G. Altman. 2011. Unit-of-Analysis Issues. Unit 9.3.1 in *Cochrane Handbook for Systematic Reviews of Interventions Version 5.1.0.* Edited by Higgins, J.P.T. and S. Green. http://handbook.cochrane.org/.

Delaney, J.A.C. and J. Seeger 2013. Sensitivity Analysis. Chapter 11 in *Developing a Protocol for Observational Comparative Effectiveness Research: A User's Guide.* Edited by Velentgas, P., N.A. Dreyer, P. Nourjah, S.R. Smith, and M.M. Torchia. Rockville, MD: Agency for Healthcare Research and Quality: 145–160. http://www.effectivehealthcare.ahrq.gov/search-for-guides-reviews-and-reports/?pageaction=displayproduct&productid=1166.

De Veaux, R.D. and D.J. Hand. 2005. How to lie with bad data. *Statistical Science* 20(3):231–238.

Haun, J.N., N.R. Patel, J.D. Lind, and N. Antinori N. 2015. Large-scale survey findings inform patients' experiences in using secure messaging to engage in patient-provider communication and self-care management: A quantitative assessment. *Journal of Medical Internet Research* 17(12):e282(1–12).

Hidalgo, B. and M. Goodman. 2013. Multivariate or multivariable regression? *American Journal of Public Health* 103(1):39–40.

Holt, T.A., M. Thorogood, and F. Griffiths. 2012. Changing clinical practice through patient specific reminders available at the time of the clinical encounter: Systematic review and meta-analysis. *Journal of General Internal Medicine* 27(8): 974–984.

Huck, S.W. 2012. *Reading Statistics and Research*, 6th ed. Boston: Pearson.

Huff, D. 1954. *How to Lie with Statistics*. New York: Norton.

Jackson, K. 2016. Personal communication with the author, April 18, 2016.

Jackson, K., C.L. Lower, and W.J. Rudman. 2016 (Spring). Crossroads between workforce and education. *Perspectives in Health Information Management*: 1–11.

Johnson, W. 2015. Analytical strategies in human growth research. *American Journal of Human Biology* 27(1)1:69–83.

Lange, E.M., A.M. Shah, B.A. Braithwaite, W.B. You, C.A. Wong, W.A. Grobman, and P. Toledo. 2015. Readability, content, and quality of online patient education materials on preeclampsia. *Hypertension in Pregnancy* 34(3):383–390.

Morrow, R. 2016. *Leading High-Reliability Organizations in Healthcare*. Boca Raton, FL: CRC Press.

Norman, G.R., and D.L. Streiner. 2014. *Biostatistics: The Bare Essentials*, 4th ed. Shelton, CT: People's Medical Publishing House.

Ravid, R. 2011. *Practical Statistics for Educators*, 4th ed. Lanham, MD: Rowman & Littlefield.

Ritz, C., A.R. Kniss, and J.C. Streibig. 2015. Research methods in weed science: Statistics. *Weed Science* 63(special issue):166–187.

Rivas-Marino, G., J. Negin, A. Salinas-Rodríguez, B. Manrique-Espinoza, K.N. Sterner, J. Snodgrass, and P. Kowal. 2015. Prevalence of overweight and obesity in older Mexican adults and its association with physical activity and related factors: An analysis of the study on global ageing and adult health. *American Journal of Human Biology* 27(3):326–333.

Singleton, R.A., Jr. and B.C. Straits. 2010. *Approaches to Social Research,* 5th ed. New York: Oxford University Press.

Smith, A.K., N.M. Shara, A. Zeymo, K. Harris, R. Estes, L.B. Johnson, and W.B. Al-Refaie. 2015. Travel patterns of cancer surgery patients in a regionalized system. *Journal of Surgical Research* 199(1):97–105.

Tennant, B., M. Stellefson, V. Dodd, B. Chaney, D. Chaney, S. Paige, and J. Alber. 2015. eHealth literacy and Web 2.0 health information seeking behaviors among baby boomers and older adults. *Journal of Medical Internet Research* 17(3):e70(1–16).

Thabane, L., L. Mbuagbaw, S. Zhang, Z. Samaan, M. Marcucci, C. Ye, M. Thabane, L. Giangregorio, B. Dennis, D. Kosa, V. Borg Debono, R. Dillenburg, V. Fruci, M. Bawor, J. Lee, G. Wells, and C.H. Goldsmith. 2013. A tutorial on sensitivity analyses in clinical trials: The what, why, when and how. *BMC Medical Research Methodology* 13:92(1–12).

Tsika, E.P., L.E. Poulimenos, K.D. Boudoulas, and A.J. Manolis. 2014. The *j*-curve in arterial hypertension: Fact or fallacy? *Cardiology* 129(2):126–135.

Wissing, D.R. and D. Timm. 2012. Statistics for the nonstatistician: Part I. *Southern Medical Journal* 105(3):126–130.

Yu, D.X., B. Parmanto, B.E Dicianno, and G. Pramana. 2015. Accessibility of mHealth self-care apps for individuals with spina bifida. *Perspectives in Health Information Management* 1–19. http://perspectives.ahima.org/accessibility-of-mhealth-self-care-apps-for-individuals-with-spina-bifida/#.VpJv88tIiUk.

Resources

Brase, C.H., and C.P. Brase. 2017. *Understandable Statistics: Concepts and Methods, Enhanced,* 11th ed. Stamford, CT: Cengage Learning.

Campbell, M.J. 2006. *Statistics at Square Two: Understanding Modern Statistical Applications in Medicine*, 2nd ed. Malden, MA: Blackwell Publishing.

Campbell, M.J., and T.D.V Swinscow. 2009. *Statistics at Square One,* 11th ed. Hoboken, NJ: John Wiley & Sons.

Campbell, M.J., and T.D.V. Swinscow. 1997. *Statistics at Square One,* 9th ed. London, England: BMJ Publishing Group. http://www.bmj.com/about-bmj/resources-readers/publications/statistics-square-one.

Chernick, M.R. 2011. *The Essentials of Biostatistics for Physicians, Nurses, and Clinicians*. Hoboken, NJ: John Wiley and Sons.

Gerstman, B.B. 2015. *Basic Biostatistics: Statistics for Public Health Practice,* 2nd ed. Burlington, MA: Jones and Bartlett Learning.

Horton, L. 2016. *Calculating and Reporting Healthcare Statistics,* 5th ed. Chicago: AHIMA.

Leigh, J.P. 1988. Assessing the importance of an independent variable in multiple regression: Is stepwise unwise? *Journal of Clinical Epidemiology* 41(7):669–677.

McKillup, S. 2012. *Statistics Explained: An Introductory Guide for Life Scientists,* 2nd ed. New York: Cambridge University Press.

Motulsky, H. 2014. *Intuitive Biostatistics: A Nonmathematical Guide to Statistical Thinking,* 3rd ed. New York: Oxford University Press.

Scott, I., and D. Mazhindu. 2014. *Statistics for Healthcare Professionals: An Introduction,* 2nd ed. Thousand Oaks, CA: Sage Publications.

Westfall, P.H. 2014. Kurtosis as peakedness, 1905–2014. R.I.P. *American Statistician* 68(3):191–195.

White, S. 2016. *A Practical Approach to Analyzing Healthcare Data,* 3rd ed. Chicago, IL: AHIMA.

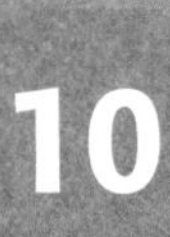

Defining the Research Question and Performing a Literature Review

Elizabeth J. Forrestal, PhD, RHIA, CCS, FAHIMA

Learning Objectives

- Formulate research questions for topics in health informatics and HIM.
- Articulate clear hypotheses related to research questions.
- Search knowledge bases such as bibliographic databases.
- Extract essential information from information sources.
- Use key terms associated with research questions, hypotheses, and literature reviews appropriately.

Key Terms

Abstract
Alternative hypothesis
Annotated bibliography
Annual review
Bibliographic database
Hypothesis
Null hypothesis
One-tailed hypothesis
Operational definition
Operationalize
PICO(TS)
Problem statement
Purpose statement
Two-tailed hypothesis

This chapter begins part II's exploration and study of the research process. Chapter 9, Applied Statistics begins this part on the research process because decisions in this chapter on defining the research question and decisions in the next two chapters are often related to the selected statistical tests. For example, the statistical test affects decisions about the level of data collected, such as categorical or continuous. To support their purpose, quantitative researchers seek to align their statistical methods with how they define their research question, the selection of a research design and methods, and the collection and analysis of, and the reporting of their findings.

In chapter 1, research was defined as a systematic process of inquiry aimed at discovering or creating new knowledge about a topic; confirming or evaluating existing knowledge; or revising outdated knowledge. This systematic process consists of the following six components:

- Defining the research question
- Performing a literature review
- Selecting a research design and method
- Collecting data
- Analyzing the data
- Presenting results

Purpose drives decisions in each of these components of the research process. For example, purpose affects how the researcher decides to define the research question. If the researcher's purpose is to identify relationships, the research question includes terms such as "related" or "associated." Other terms would be used in the research question if the researcher's purpose was to compare results.

This chapter presents information on the first two components of the research process: defining the research question and performing the literature review. The remaining two chapters in this part each present two components. Chapter 11 presents information on selecting the research design and method and collecting data, and chapter 12 presents information on analyzing data and presenting results. This chapter explains how to develop and refine a research topic and to conduct and write a literature review.

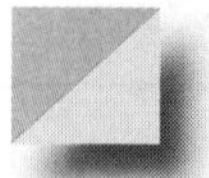

Real-World Case

"Big Data" have the potential to improve the health of individuals and of entire populations by providing "new insights from the growing volumes and sources of data with the goal of answering business, operational, and clinical questions in near-real time" (Fernandes et al. 2012, 39). However, Stephan Kudyba, the founder of a data analytics company and author of a book on Big Data and analytics explains that organizational plans for Big Data can fail if managers and leaders do not ask the right questions (Kudyba 2015). Kudyba terms the issue a "gap problem," which means the problem to be analyzed has been misidentified.

Tortorella and colleagues have outlined four steps in a general problem-solving framework that can help managers and leaders ask the right questions and correctly identify the problem needing analysis (Tortorella et al. 2015, 234). Derived from product development processes, the framework involves senior managers who provide objectives and purpose as well as focus groups of people who are involved in the problem. The researchers detail the framework's processes. For example, the second problem-identification step, current scenario analysis, incorporates four stages: observation of the workplace, collection of quantitative data, collection of qualitative data from focus groups, and triangulation to compare and contrast the quantitative and qualitative findings. The researchers also list appropriate tools for each step, such as graphics tools and fish-bone diagrams. Applying their framework in a study, the researchers found that the framework's qualitative stage allowed different views and perspectives to be considered in understanding the problem and enhanced and validated hypotheses made based on quantitative data.

Development and Refinement of a Research Topic

Research begins within a topic. Students in their academic programs may find research topics that pique their interest when writing papers for their courses. Health informatics and HIM researchers and practitioners may find their research topics in their work activities, such as the following:

- Designing information systems to support decision making for clinicians, administrators, policy makers, researchers, patients and clients, and consumers
- Maximizing the functioning of information technologies and systems through their design, implementation, or use
- Creating and modeling systems to standardize, capture, store, organize, search, process, analyze, share, and communicate health data, information, and knowledge
- Understanding how individuals, organizations, and societies interact with systems and technologies and how they use health data, information, and knowledge

Once they have chosen a topic, researchers define the research question or problem. A research question is a clear statement in the form of a question about the specific issue within a topic that a researcher wishes to study. This chapter uses the term *research question* to include research problems (areas of concern in either practice or literature). Table 10.1 lists potential research questions related to the health informatics and HIM topics previously listed. These potential research questions will be referred to by number in the following subsections that explain how to develop and refine a research topic. These subsections are the development of the research question, the problem statement, the hypothesis, and the purpose statement.

Table 10.1 Examples of research topics in health informatics and HIM and their potential research questions

No.	Research Topic	Potential Research Question
1.	Interoperability and exchange of information among healthcare organizations, accrediting bodies, regulatory agencies, and other authorized entities	What is the effect of health information exchange on Medicaid costs in states with higher levels of managed care penetration versus states with lower levels of managed care penetration?

(*Continued*)

Table 10.1 (*Continued*)

No.	Research Topic	Potential Research Question
2.	Findings of evaluation studies of health information systems and technology	How comprehensive is an evaluation framework when it is used in evaluations of health information technologies (HITs) in settings different from those in which the framework was originally developed? (Sockolow et al. 2015, 406)
3.	Information technology and improvement of clinicians' performance, clinical care, and health outcomes	Does the greater use of HIT at *nonhospital facilities* improve pregnancy outcomes at *hospitals* in the same network? (Deily et al. 2013, 70–71)
4.	Factors in the adoption and use of HITs and systems	What factors are associated with federally qualified health centers' adoption of electronic health record (EHR) systems after the Health Information Technology for Economic and Clinical Health (HITECH) authorized federal investments in health information technologies? (Jones and Furukawa 2014, 1255)
5.	Standards for reporting on studies in health informatics and health information management	What comprehensive set of elements and standardized structure for refereed journal articles can be used to report the results of qualitative studies that will improve the quality of the published articles and subsequently facilitate the inclusion of their results in systematic reviews and guidelines to inform health information practice? (Pearson et al. 2015, 671)
6.	Access use, quality, and types of consumer e-health initiatives	What factors influence patients' acceptance and use of consumer e-health applications in primary healthcare settings? (Zhang et al. 2015, 2)
7.	Classifications, terminologies, coded data, and structured reports	What are the strengths and weaknesses of health data management and reporting systems that capture and transfer routine monitoring and evaluation data from the point of generation at the health facility or community level to the point of incorporation into national health statistics as related to the five functional components of a data management system? (Ledikwe et al. 2014, 2)

Source: Adapted from Forrestal 2016a, Application Exercise No. 1.

Development of a Research Question

The development of a research question begins with purpose, or the aim of the research. Investing time and effort in developing the research question is crucial. In developing a research question, researchers may use the mnemonic FINER as well as quantitative or qualitative processes that specify and refine their question.

FINER

FINER is a mnemonic that captures the characteristics of well-developed research questions (Cummings et al. 2013, 17–19). FINER stands for the following criteria:

- Feasible: Sufficient numbers of subjects exist; the researcher has the expertise, time, and resources; and the question's scope is manageable.
- Interesting: The question is interesting to the researcher, and is interesting (as evidenced in the literature) to practitioners, policy makers, funding agencies, the public, the field in general, or a combination of these stakeholders.
- Novel: Answering the question confirms, challenges, or advances the field's current knowledge.
- Ethical: The study is capable of being conducted without harming subjects or participants.
- Relevant: The study's results advance scientific knowledge, evidence-based practice, or both.

These characteristics are general aspects of a well-developed research question. Researchers can check their research question against these criteria to see whether they have a question that will lead to a successful research study. It is important write well-developed research questions because they guide the literature review and the selection of the research design.

Quantitative Process Versus Qualitative Process

Researchers conduct *quantitative* investigations to generate objective information. When developing a quantitative research question, they follow a linear process. As described in the next subsection, this process focuses the question to be researchable and specific. By the onset of a quantitative study, the research question is clearly defined.

Researchers conduct *qualitative* investigations to interpret or understand phenomena. When developing a qualitative research question, they follow an iterative or cyclical process. As described in the next subsection, this process refines an initial, preliminary question during the study. A qualitative study, therefore, may begin with ambiguity in the research question.

Process of Developing the Research Question

Development of the research question continues, for both quantitative and qualitative researchers, by identifying specific questions and, for quantitative researchers, by formatting this specific question.

Sources of Questions Sources of research questions include research models, recommendations of previous researchers, gaps in the body of knowledge, problematic areas, and organizations' problems. The contributions of these sources are described as follows:

- **Research models:** Research models show the factors and relationships in a theory. Researchers can select one or two factors that other researchers have raised questions about or have found problematic. For example, figure 1.1 in chapter 1 shows the eight dimensions of the sociotechnical model (Sittig and Singh 2010, i69). A researcher interested in patients' use of portals would refer to the model's dimension of "human-user interface" and, specifically, the relationship between patients and portals.
- **Recommendations of previous researchers:** In journal articles, conference proceedings, theses, and dissertations, researchers make recommendations for additional research based on the results of their own research. Researchers suggest additional variables that could be the focus of the next study on this research topic. They also suggest other populations or subpopulations or settings in which subsequent research could be conducted. Researchers might also identify unintentional flaws in their own study that researchers could address in a replication study.
- **Gaps in the body of knowledge:** Published as journal articles, systematic reviews, and meta-analyses of the literature on a topic identify gaps. (See chapter 8 on systematic reviews and meta-analyses.) These review articles can be examined for research questions. Researchers should determine whether these gaps can be filled by descriptions, relationships, or differences. This knowledge helps researchers select the appropriate research design, such as descriptive research, correlational research, or quasi-experimental research.
- **Problematic areas:** In systematic reviews and annotated bibliographies, authors identify problematic areas. An **annotated bibliography** is a list of citations, each with a paragraph that summarizes the issues that the citation addressed, its main contentions or claims, and its methodological soundness. Problematic areas can include controversial issues upon which researchers do not agree, contradictory or ambiguous findings, methodological flaws or limitations, and unquestioned assumptions.
- **Organizations' problems:** Organizations, such as healthcare organizations or health-related agencies, may need assistance in solving managerial problems, answering operational questions, implementing new systems, or improving existing communications and technologies. For example, as mentioned in the real-world case at the start of this chapter, healthcare organizations are using Big Data to answer their business, operational, and clinical questions. Remember, though, the "gap problem" discussed in that case. It is important to identify the right problem; otherwise, the data analytics will fail to solve it (Fernandes et al. 2012, 39).

Usually, a research question will address a recurring or widespread problem. However, the singular importance of a sentinel event (an unexpected serious occurrence, such as death resulting from medication error) or the attitude of one or two influential leaders, such as heads of health agencies or healthcare organizations, may justify a research study.

Refinement of the Research Question Researchers refine their research question by narrowing its focus to a manageable scope and a researchable question. This refinement relates back to feasibility in the FINER mnemonic. Refinement of the research question can also reveal the amount of time and work the research study is likely to require. For example, in refining their question, researchers may learn that a problem involves many more factors than they had originally thought. Comprehensively studying the backgrounds of all these factors would require more time than the researchers have. Thus, they would refine their question to focus on one or two factors. Refinement continues during the literature review as researchers learn more details about their topic.

Scope relates to the breadth of the question. A broad question has a wide scope, such as the whole population of a nation, the entire healthcare sector, or all aspects of an EHR. A wide scope is unmanageable because it requires researchers to cover too many aspects of a topic and is beyond their time and financial resources. Instead, researchers narrow their scope. For example, rather than studying the entire healthcare sector, researchers could narrow their scope to a subpopulation of primary care physicians in rural clinics or to a specific setting in the healthcare sector, such as clinics, hospitals, nursing homes, or health maintenance organizations. In a different scenario, researchers could narrow the scope of a study on the EHR to the use of one feature of a decision support system or to the feature's use in one setting, such as a solo physician practice.

A researchable question is one that can be empirically studied. It involves observable phenomena. For example, researchers can observe whether nurses are using a medication-delivery decision support system in an intensive care unit. Researchers can ask patients about their perceptions of a patient portal. Nonresearchable questions are ones for which the researchers cannot make observations. Examples of nonresearchable questions are philosophical questions or impossible questions. For example, the question "Is technology causing the decline of society?" rests on abstractions—has a decline even been established? And the question "What would health technology be like if there had been no Renaissance?" starts with a hypothetical situation that cannot be tested—undeniably, there *was* a Renaissance.

As a part of refining the questions, researchers quantify the scale of the question. *Scale* is the extent or pervasiveness of the issue, such as the number of sites, patients, practitioners, or technologies that are involved. Another aspect of scale is the amount of time or money that is involved.

PICO(TS) PICO(TS) is an acronym that stands for the elements of a well-developed, manageable research question. Taking into account the elements, PICO(TS), helps researchers formulate research questions. The elements of PICO(TS) are described as follows:

- **P**atient, population, or problem of interest includes the condition, subpopulation, and other characteristics or demographics.
- **I**ntervention is broadly defined as the treatment, program, exposure, or other independent variable manipulated in the study.
- **C**omparison (or control) is the alternative to the intervention, such as status quo (no intervention) or existing technology or treatment against which the effect of the study's intervention is being compared or checked.
- **O**utcome is the specific result of interest, such as weight loss, increased use of a decision support system, or another dependent variable. The outcome should be specific, measurable, and related to the question.
- **T**iming is time frame of the study or the duration of the outcome of interest, such as glycemic control or a disease. Timing is optional because it is not applicable in all studies.
- **S**etting is the context of interest, such home or primary care clinic. Setting is also optional because it is not applicable in all studies (AHRQ 2014)

Often, based on the research topic, researchers use only some of the elements of PICO(TS). In those cases, the researchers refer to the acronym by the elements that they are using, such as PICO, PICOT, or PICOS. For example, see how PICOS was used in chapter 8 to determine eligibility criteria and to focus the research question for a systematic review.

Expert researchers provide templates to formulate PICO(TS)-framed research questions. The templates are for research questions related to an intervention, a prognosis or prediction, a diagnosis or diagnostic test, an etiology, and a meaning (Fineout-Overholt and Stillwell 2015, 30). These templates can be matched to a research design. For example, the template for an intervention matches the study design for randomized controlled trials (RCTs), and the template for meaning matches the study design for qualitative studies. The templates are available from the American Academy of Ambulatory

Care Nursing (2006) and may be used for educational and research purposes without permission. The following sentence revises the potential research question number 1 in table 10.1 as a PICO(TS)-framed research question:

> *In states with higher levels of managed care penetration, how does health information exchange, compared to states with lower levels of managed care penetration, affect Medicaid costs?*

- **P**opulation is "states with higher levels of managed care penetration."
- **I**ntervention is "health information exchange."
- **C**omparison is "states with lower levels of managed care penetration."
- **O**utcome is "Medicaid costs."

In this case, **T**iming and **S**etting are omitted. However, the researchers could, if they desired, add the considerations of a time period, such as 2010 through 2015, and a setting, such as inpatient hospital.

As another example, the following sentence revises potential research question number 2 in table 10.1 as a PICO(TS)-framed research question about the Health Information Technology Reference-Based Evaluation Framework (HITREF):

> *In healthcare settings different from those where HITREF was originally developed, what is the effect of using HITREF compared to its use in the original settings on comprehensiveness?*

- **P**opulation is "healthcare settings different from those where HITREF was originally developed."
- **I**ntervention is "using HITREF."
- **C**omparison is "original settings."
- **O**utcome is "comprehensiveness."

Again, in this case, **T**iming and **S**etting are omitted. However, the researchers could add time periods, such as 2005 through 2009 versus 2010 through 2014, and context (setting), such as tier-one research journals.

PICO(TS)-framed questions are often associated with RCTs; however, they are also applicable to other types of research, such as descriptive research, quasi-experimental studies, and systematic reviews and meta-analyses.

Not all research questions lend themselves to the full use of PICO(TS). For example, question number 3 in table 10.1, "Does the greater use of HIT at *nonhospital facilities* improve pregnancy outcomes at *hospitals* in the same network?" does not include a comparison. However, the researchers have defined their populations (P) as "nonhospital facilities" and "hospitals in the same network," their intervention (I) is "greater use of HIT," and the outcome (O) is "pregnancy outcomes." Question number 4 in table 10.1, in which the researchers are identifying factors, has no intervention (I), comparison (C), or outcome (O); however, the population (P) is stated as "federally qualified health centers."

Writing research questions, even when using the PICO(TS) format to formulate them, takes practice. Generally, though, formulating the research question using the PICO(TS) format, or at least considering its elements, helps researchers perform their literature review, determine their research design and method (Riva et al. 2012, 169), and improve the quality of the reporting of their study (Rios et al. 2010, 3).

Problem Statement

Researchers continue to refine their research question by writing a **problem statement**, a single sentence with an action verb, such as *explore* or *compare,* that specifically and succinctly states what the researcher will be doing to investigate the problem or question (Colling 2003, 226). An example of a problem statement is "This study explores the documentation of race/ethnicity before and after the physician group practice's implementation of the updated version of the EHR." The problem statement also limits the study's scope by setting its boundaries—aspects of the problem or question that the researcher will *not* be investigating. In this example, documentation of the administration of influenza, pneumonia, and other vaccines is outside the study's boundaries. Finally, the action verb in the problem statement indicates the study's research design. For example, using the verb *explore* indicates that the researchers will be conducting a descriptive or qualitative study.

Quantitative researchers **operationalize** their problem statement, which means that they formulate the problem statement using operational definitions obtained during their literature review (literature reviews are covered in the second part of this chapter). **Operational definitions** are terms from the literature (the body of published studies and authoritative books) that are measurable and capable of generating data. The following is an example of a problem statement related to topic number 1 in table 10.1 and the corresponding PICO(TS) we constructed earlier:

> *This study compares the effects of health information exchange on Medicaid costs in states with managed care penetration greater than the national percentage of penetration with states with managed care penetration less than the national percentage of penetration.*

Notice that in the problem statement the researchers have operationalized "higher levels of managed care penetration" and "lower levels of managed care penetration" as "managed care penetration greater than the national percentage of penetration" and "managed care penetration less than the national percentage of penetration." Moreover, the researchers have used the action verb *compare,* thereby telling the reader that they will be comparing effects.

In qualitative research, the problem statement is a tentative supposition. As a working possibility, the problem statement guides initial data collection and is revised during the study based on the data obtained.

Hypothesis

Writing the hypothesis is the researchers' next step in the process of the research study. A **hypothesis** is a statement of the researchers' predictions on the outcome of the study. Researchers base their hypothesis on a theory, a model, an observation, or an expectation from their analysis and interpretation of studies in the literature.

Both quantitative and qualitative researchers use hypotheses. Quantitative researchers clarify their hypotheses as they are performing the literature review. Qualitative researchers clarify their hypotheses as they collect and analyze their data.

Quantitative Hypotheses Versus Qualitative Hypotheses

In a quantitative study, a hypothesis is an explicit, testable statement that describes a research question in operational definitions and measurable terms. It predicts the effect or impact that the independent variable will have on the dependent variable and reflects the intent of the study. Therefore, the four components of a quantitative hypothesis are as follows:

- Variables as operationalized in the literature
- A prediction of a difference or an association
- A computable measurement
- The study's intention

Including these four components helps researchers write clear, testable, and measurable hypotheses and avoid writing ambiguous or untestable hypotheses. Examples of quantitative hypotheses are shown in table 10.2.

Table 10.2 Examples of pairings of alternative hypothesis and null hypothesis

Hypothesis	Symbol	Sample Text
Alternative (one-tailed)	H1	The use of the prescribing decision support system in the group of clinicians receiving the tailored alerts will be 10 percent higher than the use of the system in the group receiving the generic alerts.
Null	H0	There is no difference in the use of the prescribing decision support system between the group of clinicians receiving the tailored alerts and the group receiving the generic alerts.
Alternative (two-tailed)	H1	There will be a 10 percent difference in the levels of use of voice recognition software between the group of physicians receiving the training and the group not receiving it.
Null	H0	There is no difference in the levels of use of voice recognition software between the group of physicians receiving the training and the group not receiving it.

Hypotheses are written prior to (a priori) data collection and analysis because the statement of the hypothesis leads to setting the significance level and power and selecting the statistical test. (These concepts are discussed in greater detail in chapter 12.) A priori hypotheses not only are a part of a study's logical flow but also are believed to minimize the "cherry-picking" of positive or interesting outcomes (Berger et al. 2014, 149). It should be noted, however, that some exploratory research, such as data mining, is conducted without a priori hypotheses.

Qualitative researchers write tentative or working hypotheses rather than testable hypotheses. As the researchers gather and analyze data, they revise their working hypotheses and create new ones. Therefore, the researchers work in a cycle beginning with a working hypothesis, collecting data, revising hypotheses, and creating new working hypotheses, and then collecting more data about those new hypotheses. Figure 3.6 in chapter 3, illustrates this iterative process. An example of a qualitative hypothesis is "Employers place more emphasis on industry-related credentials and certifications than on formal academic attainment" (Rudman et al. 2016, 2).

Alternative Hypothesis and Null Hypothesis

When writing their hypothesis statement, quantitative researchers include alternative hypotheses and null hypotheses. These hypotheses are written as matched pairs.

Quantitative researchers state what they predict in alternative hypotheses. The **alternative hypothesis** states that there is a difference or an association between the independent and dependent variables. The properties of statistical tests do not allow the direct testing of alternative hypotheses. An example of an alternative hypothesis follows:

> *There will be a 10 percent difference in level of use of the patient portal between the experimental group in the interactive online community and the control group in the online diary feature.*

Alternative hypotheses are symbolized as H1 (or HA) for the first alternative hypothesis, H2 (or HB) for the second alternative hypothesis, and so on.

Researchers write the null hypothesis to conduct statistical testing. The word *null* means none. The **null hypothesis** states that there is no difference or there is no association between the independent variable and the dependent variable. Statistical tests are designed to test the null hypothesis. An example of a null hypothesis follows:

> *There is no difference in the level of use of a patient portal between the experimental group in the interactive online community and the control group in the online diary feature.*

The null hypothesis is symbolized as H0.

The alternative hypothesis is formulated first. After the alternative hypothesis is formulated, its matching null hypothesis is formulated. The alternative and null hypotheses are mutually exclusive and incorporate all possible outcomes of the research. Additional examples of paired alternative and null hypotheses are shown in table 10.2.

Direction of the Alternative Hypothesis

Alternative hypotheses are one-tailed or two-tailed (see table 10.2 for examples). In a **one-tailed hypothesis**, the researcher predicts the direction of the results as being more or less (greater or smaller, higher or lower). The direction is one way. On the other hand, in a **two-tailed hypothesis**, the researcher makes no prediction about the direction of the results. The researcher does not state whether the difference or association is "more or less," or "higher or lower." In two-tailed hypotheses, the researchers simply state that a difference or an association exists. For each alternative hypothesis, researchers choose whether they will use a one-tailed hypothesis or a two-tailed hypothesis. They do not use both.

The choice of a one-tailed hypothesis or a two-tailed hypothesis depends upon the theory or model that the researcher is using, the previous results that the researcher found in the literature, or the type of study, such as non-inferiority trial in which the question is whether the new treatment is not appreciably worse than an existing treatment (Streiner 2015, 629). A one-tailed hypothesis is also called a *one-tailed test* and a two-tailed hypothesis is also called a *two-tailed test*. The word *tailed* in one-tailed and two-tailed hypotheses refers to the bell-shaped (normal) curve as demonstrated in figure 10.1.

Two-tailed hypotheses have tails on both ends of the bell-shaped normal curve. One-tailed hypotheses contain a tail only on one end.

Figure 10.1 Tails of hypotheses

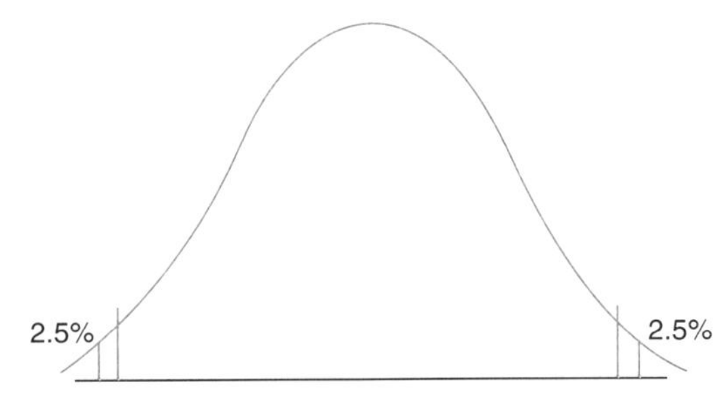

5% probability in two-tailed test

The alternative hypothesis about the patient portal presented in the last section is a two-tailed hypothesis. The hypothesis states that "there will be a 10 percent difference." The hypothesis did not give the hypothesis a direction, meaning that the alternative hypothesis did not state whether the use of the portal would be higher or lower. An example of one-tailed hypothesis in the previous example is as follows:

> *The level of use of the patient portal will be 10 percent higher in the experimental group in the interactive online community than in the control group in the online diary feature.*

Two-tailed hypotheses are more conservative than one-tailed hypotheses because one-tailed hypotheses only test in one direction, not both directions. The one-tailed hypothesis provides a greater ability to detect a difference or an association because it only tests the effect on one side of the bell curve. Selecting a two-tailed test or a one-tailed test affects how the significance level is set. As discussed in chapter 12, significance levels are often set at 0.05. This level is for the two-tailed hypothesis (two-tailed hypothesis is the default for many statistical software packages). The equivalent of 0.05 for a one-tailed test is 0.10 (0.05 multiplied by 2). Another common significance level for two-tailed hypotheses is 0.01; its equivalent for one-tailed hypotheses is 0.02 (0.01 multiplied by 2).

Purpose Statement

The **purpose statement** is a declarative sentence that summarizes the specific topic and goals of the research study. It clearly states what the researchers are attempting to achieve. The purpose statement is placed near the beginning of an article or grant proposal to explain the reason for the study, engage the reader, or both. The purpose should make clear how the research will advance the goals or knowledge of the reader, audience, or funding agency. An example of a purpose statement is as follows:

> *The purpose of this article is to explain "the facility closure process for HIM [health information management] professionals, to describe the impact on revenue cycle operations ... and to advance the HIM body of knowledge for practice. (Lail et al. 2016, 2)*

Journals and funding agencies may use other terms for the purpose statement, such as *aims, objectives,* and *goals.* Researchers use the term that is required by the journal to which they intend to send their manuscript (unpublished article) or funding agency to which they intend to send their research proposal. For example, the US Department of Health and Human Services' Public Health Service (PHS) 398 Grant uses the term *specific aims* (HHS 2016). Other funding agencies require both goals and objectives, with the objectives being measurable and time-limited. Finally, the purpose statement may reflect the researcher's overarching goal if there are no external requirements. As a result, the purpose statement may be broader than the research question.

Literature Review

A *literature review* is the systematic acquisition, analytic examination, critical evaluation, and synthesis of the important information about a topic (*critical* in this context means judicious, such as in "critical thinking"). The research question guides the literature review.

Good literature reviews are comprehensive and relevant. They trace the development of the accepted knowledge base on a topic and identify gaps in that body of knowledge. Moreover, literature reviews identify both competently conducted research and inadequately conducted research. Additionally, good literature reviews exclude irrelevant or tangential studies and are focused only on information pertinent to the research question. As a result, after completing a thorough literature review, researchers have a synthesis of current, important information about a topic.

This information helps researchers improve their research question and refine their hypotheses. During the literature review, they can return to the questions and hypotheses to revise them based on the information that they are collecting, such as operational definitions and other researchers' results.

The term *literature review* is used with three meanings, which are defined as follows:

- Meaning 1: *Process* of identifying, reading, summarizing, analyzing, and synthesizing the writings of recognized scholars and experts.
- Meaning 2: *Dependent product,* which is the introduction to a manuscript or an article in which researchers explain how they arrived at their research question.
- Meaning 3: *Independent product,* in which the introduction of meaning 2 is expanded and refined into an entirely separate, independent, and peer-reviewed article, book chapter, or book. Known as a *systematic review* or *meta-analysis,* this literature review is a specialized type of research and is discussed in greater detail in chapter 8. In addition to the systematic review and meta-analysis explained in chapter 8, there are two other types of systematic reviews whose definitions are based on their purpose:
  - *Scoping systematic reviews* are exploratory reviews that map the range, extent, and breadth of relevant evidence and literature and other available information resources on a topic.
  - *Rapid reviews* are simplified, less-comprehensive reviews that generally conceptualize questions and are conducted when decision makers or policymakers need information within one to six months. **Annual reviews** are entire journals or books on recently published research articles on a topic.

See table 10.3 for general descriptions and examples of these three uses of the term *literature review*.

Table 10.3 Three meanings of *literature review*

Meaning	General Description	Definition or Examples
1	*Process*	Identifying, reading, summarizing, analyzing, and synthesizing the writings of recognized scholars and experts.
2	*Dependent product* Grant proposal (1 to 2 paragraphs) Journal article (1 to 5 paragraphs) Master's thesis or doctoral dissertation (1 chapter) Poster presentation (1 to 3 paragraphs) Proceedings or conference paper (1 to 5 paragraphs)	Excerpt from research article by Rudman et al. (2016): Evolving economic and technological advances have affected the work environment and the workforce, including the health information management profession. Finding a competent person for each job is more critical than ever. "Almost one half of new hires fall short of expectations, predominantly because of fit issues, rather than technical competence."[1] A survey by a Washington-based research firm showed that approximately 46 percent of 20,000 new hires failed within the first 18 months.[2] Research has shown that finding the right person to fit the right job is a difficult process. Costs surrounding a bad hire have been calculated at 50 to 200 percent of the first-year salary, while the costs of an employee who leaves within the first year may reach 162 percent of the first-year salary.[3] For example, costs associated with an employee earning $35,000 per year ($16 per hour) could reach $56,700 per year if the placement is unsuccessful—with this cost being exclusive of the cost of bringing on a replacement for the position. Additional findings suggest that failure to succeed is often linked to soft skills, such as the lack of coachability (26 percent), low levels of emotional intelligence (23 percent), motivation problems (15 percent), and temperament issues (17 percent), while a mere 11 percent of failures are attributed to a lack of technical or professional competence.[4]

(*Continued*)

Table 10.3 (*Continued*)

Meaning	General Description	Definition or Examples
	Term research paper for a course (3 to 25 pages)	The present study employed the Appreciative Inquiry approach to identify respondents' definitions of competency and the methods used in the hiring process to assess the competency of potential employees.
3	*Independent product* (separate entire work)	Note: Citations of reviews as independent products in bibliographic databases include the publication type [Review].
	Systematic review article (7 to 30 pages)	Otte-Trojel, T., A. de Bont, T.G. Rundall, and J. van de Klundert. 2016. What do we know about developing patient portals? A systematic literature review. *Journal of the American Medical Informatics Association* 23(e1):e162–e168.
	Meta-analysis article (7 to 30 pages)	Baysari, M.T., E.C. Lehnbom, L. Li, A. Hargreaves, R.O. Day, and J.I. Westbrook. 2016. The effectiveness of information technology to improve antimicrobial prescribing in hospitals: A systematic review and meta-analysis. *International Journal of Medical Informatics* 92:15–34.
	Annual review (Entire book 150 to 200 pages)	Wiederhold, B.K. and G. Riva. 2014. *Annual Review of Cybertherapy and Telemedicine 2014: Positive Change: Connecting the Virtual and the Real*. Studies in Health Technology and Informatics, vol. 199. Fairfax, VA: IOS Press.

[1-4]Superscripts appear as in original article. See original article (Rudman et al. 2016) for references.

The next sections guide the reader to understanding the purpose of the literature review, its development, acquiring the information for it, and writing it.

Purposes of the Literature Review

Literature reviews have the following three purposes:

- To orient readers to the issue and to persuade them of the necessity of the research study;
- To assure the reader that the researcher has conducted a thorough review of all aspects of the topic
- To build the researcher's knowledge in the topic

The literature review should guide the reader to conclude that the logical and necessary next step is the research proposed by the researchers. The thoroughness of the literature review lends credibility to the study. Researchers, as a result of their literature review, come to a complete understanding of the topic and can demonstrate the competencies listed in figure 10.2. Researchers who can apply these competencies are able to clearly explain their research topic and are more likely to conduct a research study that yields accurate and meaningful evidence that can be used in practice.

Figure 10.2 Competencies resulting from a strong knowledge base

- Outline a historical overview of a topic, including turning points, trends, and controversies.
- Describe research frames and approaches in the topic.
- Explain the evolution of major theories and differentiate between accepted theories and those outside the mainstream.
- Relate leading theorists and researchers to their ideas and findings.
- Determine applicable models, appropriate research designs and methods, worthwhile interventions, and pertinent and confounding factors.
- Clarify concepts, identify relevant variables and main outcome measures with their operational definitions, and describe expected results.
- State advantages and disadvantages of various research methods.
- Identify sources of data, populations, and sampling techniques.
- Cite the strengths and weaknesses of commonly used instruments.
- Select appropriate analytic techniques.
- Assess the thoroughness of literature reviews in published studies.
- Identify competently conducted research and inadequately conducted research.
- Detect unexplored issues, gaps, or discrepancies in the body of knowledge that his or her research can investigate, fill, or resolve.

Source: Forrestal 2016b, p. 569.

Process of the Literature Review

A literature review is a systematic process requiring critical thinking skills. Researchers use these skills during all four steps of the process, which are as follows:

1. Identify sources of information for the literature review.
2. Seek and retrieve the literature.
3. Collect and record information underlying the competencies (listed in figure 10.2).
4. Analyze, evaluate, and synthesize the information obtained in the previous step.

Each of these four steps are covered in the following sections of the chapter.

Sources of Information

In the first step, the researcher identifies sources of information. Sources exist in various formats, including printed works, such as articles in peer-reviewed journals and in magazines, books, book chapters, conference papers, and government documents. Typically, the authors of the articles, books, and other documents are recognized researchers, scholars, and experts on the topic. However, sources of information are not limited to printed works. As figure 10.3 shows, many other types of sources exist, such as audiovisual media and electronic media. The credibility of the creators of these other information sources should be determined as described in a following subsection. Usually, a literature review is mostly based on published literature. However, for some research methods, other information sources may be important; for example, audiovisual media may useful for the qualitative approach. Therefore, consideration should be given to identifying all the potential information sources for the literature review.

Figure 10.3 Sources of information

Periodicals
Abstract
Annual review
Cartoon
Journal
Magazine
Monograph
Newsletter
Newspaper

Books, brochures, and book chapters
Book
Book chapter
Brochure
Dictionary
Encyclopedia
Legal citation
Manual
Map or chart
Pamphlet
Product insert
Published or archived letter

Legal, technical, and research reports
Government bulletin
Government report
Industry report
Issue brief
Monograph
Nongovernment agency report
Position paper
Reference report
University report
White paper
Working paper

Proceedings of meetings
Conference
Meeting
Poster session
Symposium
Unpublished proceeding paper

Doctoral dissertations and master's theses
Abstract of dissertation
Abstract of thesis
Dissertation
Thesis

Unpublished works
Submitted manuscript
Unpublished letter
Unpublished manuscript
Unpublished raw data

Reviews
Book
Film
Video

Audiovisual media
Address
Audiotape
Chart
Film
Lecture
Music recording
Performance
Published interview
Recorded interview
Slide
Speech
Television broadcast and transcript
Television series and transcript
Unpublished interview
Work of art

Electronic media
Computer program
Computer software
Electronic database
Online abstract
Online book
Online journal
Press release
Social media
Software manual
Website

Many of the sources of information identified in figure 10.3 are available to health informatics and HIM researchers through libraries or through reciprocal agreements between the researchers' employers and educational institutions. Practitioners may be able to access sources of information and databases through their workplaces. Healthcare organizations often have their own libraries or may have arrangements with institutions that provide access to libraries. Additionally, members of professional associations and societies, such as the American Health Information Management Association (AHIMA), have access to information resources offered by those organizations. Once researchers have identified a source, they consider its credibility and whether it is grey literature or a primary or secondary source.

Credibility of Sources The credibility of information sources should be appraised. Information from peer-reviewed (refereed) journals, also called *research journals* or *academic journals,* is more credible than information from popular (trade) magazines. Peer-reviewed journals are a type of professional or scientific journal for which content experts evaluate articles for quality and relevance prior to publication. This evaluation, called *peer review*, seeks to ensure that the information reported in the journal is of the highest quality (Dine et al. 2015, 8). Some bibliographic databases, such as CINAHL (Cumulative Index of Nursing and Allied Health Literature), identify journals as being peer-reviewed. Other bibliographic databases, such as the US National Library of Medicine's MEDLINE, do not. If it is unclear whether a journal is peer-reviewed, researchers can ask a librarian or consult Ulrichsweb, an online directory of publications ("serials") available through a library's licensed resources. Examples of peer-reviewed journals are *Perspectives in Health Information Management, Journal of the American Medical Informatics Association, Journal of the American Medical Association, New England Journal of Medicine,* and *Science*. Popular magazines, such as *Scientific American* and *Computerworld,* are not peer-reviewed.

The credibility of information sources other than journals can be appraised by using the following AACODS mnemonic (Tyndall 2010):

- **A**uthority: Authors should be associated with a reputable organization, such as a university or a government agency.
- **A**ccuracy: The document should state the research method and show that the protocol has been followed. There should be a reference list.
- **C**overage: The document should state its inclusion and exclusion criteria (as discussed in chapter 8).
- **O**bjectivity: The document should present all sides of an issue.
- **D**ate: The document should have a date indicating when it was created or published.
- **S**ignificance: The document should provide relevant and timely information.

Other methods of appraising the credibility of an information source include contacting experts in the topic and obtaining their opinions and searching articles to see whether the source has been cited by other researchers. Additionally, exploring the websites of authors, publishers, and organizations may show whether their documents are nonpartisan or have political or social agendas.

Grey Literature For health informatics researchers, an important information source is *grey literature*. Grey literature is produced by government agencies, such as the Health and Medicine Division of the National Academies of Sciences, Engineering, and Medicine; academic institutions; or companies like Deloitte LLP and RAND Corporation, and it can provide relevant, timely information that is otherwise unavailable. Examples of grey literature include technical reports, technology assessments, pamphlets, and product inserts. Many of these documents are available on the Internet. The citation for PICO(TS) in this chapter is an example of grey literature published online (AHRQ 2014). Once obtained, the grey literature's credibility should be appraised using the previously discussed AACODS mnemonic or other methods.

Primary Sources Versus Secondary Sources Information sources can be either primary or secondary sources. *Primary sources* are first-hand sources of which there are many types. For example, in historical research design, a type of primary source is an original document. In a literature review, a primary source could be the original published study, such as research-based articles in *Educational Perspectives in Health Informatics and Information Management*, *Journal of Medical Internet Research*, or *International Journal of Medical Informatics*. *Secondary sources* are second-hand sources, such as summaries of the original research studies. For literature reviews, primary sources are generally preferable to secondary sources. See the historical research design section and table 1.3 in chapter 1 for more information about types of primary and secondary sources and their uses in research.

Search and Retrieval of Information Sources

In the second step of a literature review, researchers seek and retrieve information sources from knowledge bases, such as bibliographic databases and digital collections (see table 10.4). **Bibliographic databases** collect publication data about published literature such as journals, magazines, newspaper articles, books, book chapters, and other information sources; these databases are structured so that the information can be easily accessed and managed. The databases' scopes vary depending on the type of information source indexed and by academic disciplines covered. For example, some databases only index peer-reviewed journals whereas others also index conference proceedings and book chapters. Also, in terms of scope, some databases focus on indexing publications from certain academic disciplines, such as health sciences, whereas others are multidisciplinary. Multisubject, interdisciplinary search engines allow researchers to concurrently search across multiple databases making use of all of a library's database subscriptions. *Digital collections* extend the search and retrieve functions beyond text materials to other forms of electronic media, such as audio and video recordings. Digital collections are managed like bibliographic databases and their holdings are available online. The Centers for Medicare and Medicaid Services (CMS) and the AHRQ offer online digital collections.

Table 10.4 Selected bibliographic databases and other digital collections

Bibliographic Database or Digital Collection	Types of Sources Collected or Indexed
ABI/INFORM Complete	Journals, dissertations, working papers, business newspapers, trade publications, business and economics magazines, and country- and industry-focused reports in business, health services and information management, accounting, and finance
ACM Digital Library (Association for Computing Machinery)	Journals, magazines, and conference proceedings in computer science and engineering
AHRQ's "Effective Health Care Program Library of Resources" and "Research Tools and Data"	PowerPoint presentations, full research reports, summaries of evidence-based research, educational materials, and other resources on healthcare interventions and treatment options for a variety of health conditions
	Statistical data on healthcare delivery and summaries and full reports of research findings and technology assessments
AHIMA HIM Body of Knowledge	Articles from the *Journal of the American Health Information Management Association* and *AHIMA Advantage*; proceedings from AHIMA's Annual Convention and Exhibit; AHIMA practice briefs, toolkits, leadership models, position statements, reports, guidelines, and white papers; and government publications, such as the *Federal Register* and documents from the US Department of Health and Human Services
Business Source Complete	Journals and books covering business, management, economics, banking, finance, accounting, and other topics
CINAHL	Journals and publications in nursing, biomedicine, health sciences librarianship, consumer health, and allied health disciplines
CMS Research, Statistics, Data, and Systems	Broad range of quantitative resources, summary information, and research reports on Medicare and Medicaid programs, demonstration projects, health expenditures, and key statistics
Federation of American Scientists Office of Technology Assessment Archive	US Office of Technology Assessment's reports, background papers, and contractor papers analyzing scientific and technical policy issues of the 1970s–1990s
Google Scholar	Journals, dissertations, books, abstracts, and court opinions covering multiple fields from academic publishers, professional societies, online repositories, universities, and other websites

(*Continued*)

Table 10.4 *(Continued)*

Bibliographic Database or Digital Collection	Types of Sources Collected or Indexed
IEEE Xplore (Institute of Electrical and Electronics Engineers)	Transactions, journals, magazines, and conference proceedings in computer science and engineering
JSTOR (Journal Storage)	Journals in the humanities, social sciences, and sciences
LexisNexis Academic	Foreign and domestic newspapers, magazines and trade journals, federal and state cases and statutes, law reviews, company financial information, medical news, and state and nation profiles in accounting, marketing, business, and law
MEDLINE/PubMed	Citations, abstracts, and sometimes full articles from journals and other publications in medicine, nursing, allied health, dentistry, veterinary medicine, healthcare system, and preclinical sciences such as chemical sciences, and bioengineering
National Information Center on Health Services Research and Health Care Technology (NICHSR)	Publications and web materials, such as data, funding announcements, reports, and links to websites, produced by the National Library of Medicine and other organizations that are of interest to the health services research community
New York Academy of Medicine Library's *Grey Literature Report*	Medical and public health topics not indexed in academic databases

Source: Adapted from Forrestal 2016b, p. 572.

Researchers must create and follow a systematic plan to identify the databases and collections to search as well as all the terms used to query the databases. Although the digitization of library holdings puts these resources at the researchers' fingertips, they need to have the information skills to fully delve into the holdings and capture all relevant information. Researchers can build their skills in querying bibliographic databases and digital collections and in using reference management software (see examples in next section). Libraries often offer workshops or tutorials on these topics.

Students and instructors have access to sources of information and bibliographic databases through the holdings of their educational institutions' libraries. Libraries purchase licenses that allow their users access to the various databases. Just as different libraries have purchased different books, different libraries have purchased different licenses.

Health informatics and HIM researchers need to search a variety of databases because health informatics and HIM are multidisciplinary, meaning that the information resources do not reside in one bibliographic database or search engine. (A *search engine* is a computer program, such as Google or Bing, that is designed to use keywords or other characters to search, identify, and retrieve documents, images, or other items in bibliographic databases or on the Internet.) Moreover, relying only on the output of multisubject, interdisciplinary search engines is unwise because not all databases are included in these large search engines. Searching multiple databases is necessary because the databases' contents vary. For example, an article about data mining to identify signals of adverse drug reactions from different data sources, such as spontaneous reporting databases, electronic health records, and the medical literature was published in *ACM Computing Surveys* (Karimi et al. 2015). *ACM Computing Surveys* is indexed in the computer science databases, but not in MEDLINE. Researchers accustomed to searching MEDLINE for articles on mining health data would have missed this article if they did not search other databases. Similarly, MEDLINE indexes *IEEE/ACM Transactions on Computational Biology and Bioinformatics*, but CINAHL does not, so a search of CINAHL only would miss articles from that source. Therefore, to ensure that all relevant articles are captured, researchers should search interdisciplinary search engines and multiple discipline-specific bibliographic databases.

Many documents of the grey literature are not referenced in bibliographic databases. Yet, this information source is important because so many technical reports from government and private industry are in the grey literature. A few tools to search the grey literature exist. These tools include the National Technical Reports Library of the US Department of Commerce (2016), the New York Academy of Medicine's *Grey Literature Report* (2016), and others (see the resource list at the end of the chapter).

Collection and Recording of Information Sources

The third step in a literature review is to collect and record information from the sources. To organize and manage information sources, researchers use reference management software, such as Reference Manager, EndNote, RefWorks, BiblioExpress, Zotero, and others. These software packages allow researchers to do the following:

- Create their own bibliographic databases.
- Use the packages' search engines to directly download citations and full-text articles into their personal bibliographic databases.
- Import the contents of databases into word-processing software.
- Transform bibliographic entries into the required style of the journal, using style editor tools.

The following procedure describes a way to search for and retrieve peer-reviewed journal articles:

1. Generate a list of key terms and synonyms. In the health and medical databases, these terms are known as *medical subject headings (MeSH).*
2. Generate a list of target databases.
3. Enter queries using the key terms and synonyms, and focus the queries using limits, such as publication type (refereed journal), language (English), and time periods.
4. Scan the abstracts of the retrieved articles to determine their relevance and identify pivotal articles. **Abstracts** are brief summaries of the major parts of a research study.
5. Save the articles that are available electronically. (Note: The researcher should digitally scan or photocopy articles that are unavailable electronically. Although it might be convenient to only use online articles, the resulting literature review would be incomplete and biased.)
6. Run new queries on the databases or retrieve additional articles based on information obtained while scanning abstracts and articles initially retrieved, such as previously unretrieved articles written by leading theorists or researchers, references cited at the end of the pivotal articles, and new terms based on the MeSH headings of the pivotal articles.

Be sure to capture complete citation data as listed in figure 10.4. Also, collect and record all the information that forms a strong knowledge base (refer to figure 10.2).

Figure 10.4 Citation data required for various style guides

- Full names of the authors, including first names and middle initials or middle names and in the order listed by the publication. Also, note the names of editors for books and compilations, and be aware that some entries in websites have authors.
- Full title and subtitle of the article and journal; chapter and book; video; or website.
- Complete information about dates of publication, including the year, month, day, and season. (Be aware that some entries in websites are dated.)
- Complete name and location (city, state, country) of the publisher (for books and videos).
- Inclusive page numbers (for an article or chapter).
- Volume number and issue number for journals, multivolume books, and periodicals (sometimes, these data are only on the front of the publication).
- Accurate URL and access date (for Internet sources).
- Accurate DOI (Digital Object Identifier) for all documents that have them. The DOI is a unique, stable identifier for articles and other documents in an online environment. The DOI is alphanumeric, beginning with the number 10, then a prefix (four or more digits representing the publisher), a forward slash, and a suffix (numbers assigned to the article by the publisher).

Researchers should recap the research of previous scholars and researchers and record key information from this recap in a summary table that lists each study in a row, with columns displaying its features, such as author; publication year; research question and hypothesis; research design and method; time frame, sample, and response rate; analytical techniques; and key findings, limitations, and recommendations, as shown in table 10.5. Capturing data and recording information initially during the first reading of the information source will help to reduce rework when the research report or article is written.

Table 10.5 Summary table of the information from peer-reviewed journal articles or other information sources

Author and Year	Research Question and Hypothesis	Research Design and Method	Time Frame, Sample, and Response Rate	Analytic Techniques	Key Findings, Limitations, and Recommendations
X 2016	How are after-visit summaries (AVSs) being used in primary care offices and what are patients' perceptions of the AVS? Hypothesis not stated.	❖ Mixed methods ❖ Descriptive ❖ Interview survey	❖ Time frame not stated ❖ Convenience sample of 209 patients ❖ Participation rate not stated	❖ Percentages ❖ Thematic analysis of participants' comments	❖ Goal of AVS as a communication tool to engage and support patients is often unmet. ❖ Limitation of convenience sample at two primary care clinics. ❖ Recommends survey sent to larger group of participants and studies on physicians' perceptions about using random sample of AVSs.
L, M, and N 2015	What is the relationship among physicians using an online tool, clinical outcomes for diabetes patients, and team cohesion? It is predicted that the use of the online tool will be associated with improved clinical outcomes and that team cohesion will be a moderator.	❖ Quantitative ❖ Quasi-experimental ❖ Cohort study	❖ 3 years ❖ 565 physicians in year 1; 678 physicians in year 2; and 626 physicians in year 3 ❖ 48%, 62%, and 61%, respectively	Multivariate linear regression	❖ Use of the tool improved clinical outcomes for patients with diabetes, and team cohesion was a significant positive moderator of the effect. ❖ Limitation of study's setting: primary care in one integrated delivery system. ❖ Recommends additional study of the effects of team cohesion.

Source: Adapted from Forrestal 2016b, p. 573.

Analysis, Evaluation, and Synthesis of Information Sources

The fourth and last step of the literature review process requires the most time. Researchers now analyze, evaluate, and synthesize the information they have captured and recorded in the third step. The summary table, created in the third step, can act as an analytic and evaluative tool by identifying and emphasizing features, common characteristics, trends, and gaps in the published literature or other information sources (table 10.5). Merely chronicling a long series of descriptions of previous studies is inadequate. Instead, in synthesis, researchers compare similarities and contrast differences among the previous studies, critically evaluate the previous studies' methods and analytic tools, interpret the findings, and draw conclusions about the information from the previous studies. Synthesis makes sense of all the information that has been captured (see meaning 2 in table 10.3 for an example).

Experts suggest the following four guidelines to assist researcher-writers in analyzing, evaluating, and synthesizing the information from their sources (Gastel and Day 2016, 62):

- *Describe the nature and scope of the problem.* For example, in the meaning 2 example in table 10.3, the authors summarize key information from two sources: "Almost one half of new hires fall short of expectations, predominantly because of fit issues, rather than technical competence,[1]" and "A survey by a Washington-based research firm showed that approximately 46 percent of 20,000 new hires failed within the first 18 months[2]" (superscripts in original document lead to the references cited). The authors are both capturing the readers' interest and describing the nature of the problem (new hires falling short) and its scope (46 percent of 20,000 new hires failed within the first 18 months).

Further describing the problem's scope, in their next paragraph, the authors provided information on the costs of this problem (Rudman et al. 2016, 1).

- *Review the current knowledge about the problem.* For example, the authors quoted in table 10.3 gave readers the following information: "Additional findings suggest that failure to succeed is often linked to soft skills, such as the lack of coachability (26 percent), low levels of emotional intelligence (23 percent), motivation problems (15 percent), and temperament issues (17 percent), while a mere 11 percent of failures are attributed to a lack of technical or professional competence[4]" (superscript in original document). The experts also identify the specific gap in knowledge that the researcher-writers are trying to fill.
- *Identify the researchers' objective, such as research question, problem statement, or hypotheses.* For example, the authors quoted in table 10.3 wrote that their objective was "to identify respondents' definitions of competency and the methods used in the hiring process to assess the competency of potential employees."
- *State the method of the study.* In the article quoted in table 10.3, the authors stated that they "employed the Appreciative Inquiry approach." They later defined the Appreciative Inquiry approach in the methods section of their article.

Additional resources to assist researcher-writers in composing their literature review are listed in Resources at the end of the chapter.

Development of the Literature Review

After completing the literature review process, researchers develop the introduction to their paper or write their review article. These two documents—the introduction or the review article—are literature review products. The characteristics of a well-developed literature review include the following:

- Comprehensive coverage that is also relevant and focused
- Concise statement of what is known and unknown about a topic
- Logical and succinct summary of the research question or problem, using mostly primary sources
- Critical analysis and evaluation of important sources that includes strengths, weaknesses, limitations, and gaps
- Synthesis

In sum, good literature reviews deliver concentrated knowledge to the reader.

In writing literature reviews, researchers are guided by conventions, such as transparency, organizational structure, progression, equitable coverage, pertinence, and style. These conventions are discussed in the following paragraphs.

Transparency

Literature reviews are transparent. In research, transparency means providing enough information so that someone else could replicate the researchers' process. Therefore, researchers briefly describe the strategy used to identify the literature. In addition, they explain the scope of the literature review by explicitly stating both their inclusion and exclusion criteria. (See chapter 8 for information on inclusion and exclusion criteria.)

Organizational Structure

An organizational structure helps readers follow the researchers' reasoning. Explicitly stating the order helps to guide the reader. A literature review can be organized by the research model with each component being discussed in turn. The components of the model directly related to the researchers' study are discussed in greater detail. A literature review can also be organized thematically by issues in the topic. Chronology is yet another organizing function. A coherent and logical order adds to the clarity of the literature review.

Progression

Literature reviews follow a progression. Researchers begin with a broad, general question and then gradually narrow the topic into a problem statement or hypothesis. For example, the researchers might begin the description of the problem as a general societal concern. Supporting citations could come from popular magazines and opinion articles. Then, they focus the discussion by explaining how this problem or question affects health informatics and HIM professionals.

Researchers then describe research studies related to the research question. Supporting citations here come from scholarly journal articles, technical government reports, or other credible, scientific papers. The review of studies is chronological, moving from older studies to more current studies. The review ends at the problematic or ambiguous findings, the unresolved problem, or the issue that the researchers' study specifically addresses. This progression results in readers understanding the need for the study.

Equitable Coverage

Equitable coverage means that the literature review includes opinions contrary to those of the researchers. Convincing literature reviews are unbiased. Therefore, researchers include important studies that support of their beliefs as well as those that are contrary to their beliefs. Readers could interpret the absence of the contradictory studies as bias. Evidence of bias detracts from the credibility of the literature review. However, the researchers might suggest explanations of the contradictory findings based on their evaluation and analysis.

Pertinence

Studies included in the research study should be pertinent. Pertinent studies include research studies that advance the topic, add new variables, or direct the topic to new areas of investigation. Researchers should provide enough information about these studies, such as the features listed in the summary given in table 10.5, that their quality can be assessed. The review should describe key studies in greater detail than replication or duplicative studies. Research studies that have the same findings and variables can be described together.

If tangentially related studies are included in the review, their pertinence is explicitly stated. Researchers discuss previous studies that were conducted inadequately or resulted in gaps or conflicts, especially if the researchers are rectifying the error. To justify their study, researchers specifically point out the inadequacies, gaps, or conflicting results that their study is addressing.

The analogy of a funnel is useful. Being a wide tube at the top and narrowing at the bottom, the funnel guides liquid into a small opening. Similarly, the literature review begins broadly by discussing the studies that are generally related to the researchers' question. The review then funnels down by discussing the studies that are progressively more closely related. Finally, at the very end, the literature review has guided the reader to believe that the researchers' proposed study is necessary.

Style

Verb tense matters. Tradition and logic demand that researchers pay close attention to verb tense when they write literature reviews. Verb tenses situate the event or idea in time. Present tense is used to express truths, accepted theories, and facts. Present tense is also used to explain recent, valid studies. The past tense, with the relevant date, is used to describe past studies with continued historical significance. Examples are:

- *Accepted theory:* Specific goals motivate employees more than vague goals.
- *Recent study:* Johnson's results illustrate the importance of specific goals.
- *Study of historical importance:* In 1972, the study of Smith and colleagues showed the importance of expectancy in motivation.

Generally, the safest rule is to use present tense for published studies and theories. Finally, the literature review concludes with a Problem Statement. In quantitative studies, the conclusion also includes a hypothesis.

Review Questions

1. What is FINER and how can it help you write a well-developed research question?
2. What are five sources of research questions? How can each source contribute to the development of significant research questions or problems?
3. Consider the following statement: "Researchers should write broad research questions so that they appeal to greatest possible number of stakeholders, such as physicians and legislators." What are your reasons for agreeing or disagreeing with this statement?
4. Identify PICO(TS) in the following sentence: "Among primary care physicians, how does a face-to-face training module, compared to an on-demand module, affect meaningful use of alerts within six months?"

5. Write the following question in PICO(TS) format, remembering that (TS) is optional: "In university students with asthma, what is the effect of an online, interactive social community on adherence to asthma medication versus an online diary in which students record daily their use of inhaled corticosteroid preventer?"
6. A researcher wants to investigate how chief financial officers' decision-making is affected by an executive dashboard that draws real-time data from the patient management information system (components such as admission-discharge-transfer and patient census), the patient accounting system, and the general ledger. What bibliographic databases, digital collections, or other information sources that the researcher could search? Name at least five resources.
7. How does the problem statement indicate the study's research design?
8. What is a hypothesis in a quantitative study?
9. What is the difference between one-tailed hypotheses and two-tailed hypotheses? Which type of hypothesis is more conservative?
10. How does the analogy of a funnel apply to the writing of the literature review?

Application Exercises

1. Conduct a series of searches to find publications in PubMed (NLM 2016). Begin by reading PubMed's *Quick Start Guide* under Using PubMed. Be sure to note that the *Quick Start Guide* provides information on general searches, searching by author and journal name, and other common strategies. Near the bottom of "Section Contents," click on "I need further assistance and training." In this section, under "Search Field Descriptions and Tags," you see all fields upon which you can conduct a search. Pay particular attention to how to search field descriptions and tags as you complete the following exercises.
   - Find publications written by people at your academic institution. In "Search Field Descriptions and Tags," "Affiliation" is PubMed's term for academic institutions, employers, and other organizations with which authors may be associated ("affiliated"). As a trial, find a publication at the University of Pittsburgh by Watzlaf. First, return to the PubMed home page. Click "Advanced" under the Search box at the top of the page. Second, in the PMC Advanced Search Builder, click the left box in the top row and select "Affiliation." Enter "University of Pittsburgh" in the right box. Third, in the "Builder," click on the left box in lower row, and select "Author." Enter "Watzlaf" (this field can be "autocomplete"). Click "Search." Click one of the article titles returned in the search, and expand "Author Information" to verify the affiliation of the article's authors. Then, find publications written by authors from your academic institution. You may either enter specific authors, names or you may omit any entries in the second row to find all authors.
   - Find systematic reviews published in *Perspectives in Health Information Management* (*PHIM*) and the *Journal of the American Medical Informatics Association* (*JAMIA*). Which journal has published more systematic reviews?
   - Find publications about clinical trials of EHRs in the time period, January 1, 2015, through December 31, 2016, using "Topic-Specific Queries" under "PubMed Tools."
2. In PubMed, find three clinical trials that use EHRs to manage the care of patients with diabetes mellitus. Complete a summary table of the information from peer-reviewed journal articles or other information sources (see table 10.5 in this book). You may want to review in the PubMed tutorial how to combine searches in your search history.
3. Return to chapter 9's real-world case. Write a research question about the case and a two-tailed alternate hypothesis and a null hypothesis for the question.

References

Agency for Healthcare Research and Quality (AHRQ). 2014 (February). Research Questions and PICO(TS). Appendix C in *The Effective Health Care Program Stakeholder Guide.* Rockville, MD: Agency for Healthcare Research and Quality. http://www.ahrq.gov/research/findings/evidence-based-reports/stakeholderguide/appendixc.html.

American Academy of Ambulatory Care Nursing. 2006. Template for Asking PICOT Questions. https://www.aaacn.org/sites/default/files/documents/misc-docs/1e_PICOT_Questions_template.pdf.

Berger, M.L., B.C. Martin, D. Husereau, K. Worley, J.D. Allen, W. Yang, N.C. Quon, C.D. Mullins, K.H. Kahler, and W. Crown. 2014. A questionnaire to assess the relevance and credibility of observational studies to inform health care decision making: An ISPOR-AMCP-NPC good practice task force report. *Value in Health* 17(2):143–156.

Colling, J. 2003. Demystifying nursing research: Defining the problem to be studied. *Urologic Nursing* 23(3):225–226.

Cummings, S.R., W.S. Browner, and S.B. Hulley. 2013. Conceiving the Research Question and Developing the Study Plan. Chapter 2 in *Designing Clinical Research,* 4th ed. Edited by Hulley, S.B., S.R. Cummings, W.S Browner, D.G. Grady, and T.B. Newman. Philadelphia, PA: Lippincott Williams & Wilkins:14–22.

Deily, M.E., T. Hu, S. Terrizzi, S-Y. Chou, and C.D. Meyerhoefer. 2013. The impact of health information technology adoption by outpatient facilities on pregnancy outcomes. *Health Services Research* 48(1):70–94.

Dine, C.J., A.S. Caelleigh, and J.A. Shea. 2015. Selection and Qualities of Reviewers. Chapter 2 in *Review Criteria for Research Manuscripts,* 2nd ed. Edited by Durning, S.J., and J.D. Carline. Washington, DC: Association of American Medical Colleges.

Fernandes, L., M. O'Connor, and V. Weaver. 2012. Big data, bigger outcomes. *Journal of AHIMA* 83(10):38–44.

Fineout-Overholt, E. and S.B. Stillwell. 2015. Asking Compelling, Clinical Questions. Chapter 2 in *Evidence-Based Practice in Nursing and Healthcare: A Guide to Best Practice,* 3rd ed. Edited by Melnyk, B.M. and E. Fineout-Overholt. Philadelphia, PA: Wolters Kluwer: 24–39.

Forrestal, E. 2016a. Instructor Manual. Research Methods. Chapter 19 in *Health Information Management: Concepts, Principles, and Practice,* 5th ed. Edited by P.K. Oachs and A.L. Watters. Chicago: AHIMA Press.

Forrestal, E. 2016b. Research Methods. Chapter 19 in *Health Information Management: Concepts, Principles, and Practice,* 5th ed. Edited by P.K. Oachs and A.L. Watters. Chicago: AHIMA Press.

Gastel, B. and R.A. Day. 2016. *How to Write and Publish a Scientific Paper,* 8th ed. Santa Barbara, CA: Greenwood.

Jones, E.B. and M.F. Furukawa. 2014. Adoption and use of electronic health records among federally qualified health centers grew substantially during 2010–12. *Health Affairs* 33(7):1254–1261.

Karimi, S., C. Wang, A. Metke-Jimenez, R. Gaire, and C. Paris. 2015(July). Text and data mining techniques in adverse drug reaction detection. *ACM Computing Surveys* 47(4):1–39.

Kudyba, S. 2015(April 7). Tackling Common Analytics Problems. International Institute for Analytics. http://iianalytics.com/research/tackling-common-analytics-problems.

Lail, P.L., S.S. Laird, K. McCall, J. Naretto, and A. York. 2016 (Fall). Facility closure: How to get in, get out, and get what is important. *Perspectives in Health Information Management:* 1–11.

Ledikwe, J.H., J. Grignon, R. Lebelonyane, S. Ludick, E. Matshediso, B.W. Sento, A. Sharma, and B. Semo. 2014. Improving the quality of health information: A qualitative assessment of data management and reporting systems in Botswana. *Health Research Policy and Systems* 12:7(1–10).

New York Academy of Medicine. 2016. *Grey Literature Report*. http://www.greylit.org.

Pearson, A., Z. Jordan, C. Lockwood, and E. Aromataris. 2015. Notions of quality and standards for qualitative research reporting. *International Journal of Nursing Practice* 21(5):670–676.

Rios, L.P., C. Ye, and I. Thabane. 2010. Association between framing of the research question using the PICOT format and reporting quality of randomized controlled trials. *BMC Medical Research Methodology* 10(11):1–8.

Riva, J.J., K.M.P. Malik, S.J. Burnie, A.R. Endicott, and J.W Busse. 2012. What is your research question? An introduction to the PICOT format for clinicians. *Journal of the Canadian Chiropractic Association* 56(3):167–171.

Rudman, W., S.S. Hart-Hester, J. Richey, and K. Jackson. 2016 (Summer). Hiring for competency: Hiring to not fail vs. hiring to succeed. *Perspectives in Health Information Management:* 1–6.

Sittig, D.F. and H. Singh. 2010. A new sociotechnical model for studying health information technology in complex adaptive healthcare systems. *Quality and Safety in Health Care* 19(Suppl3):i68–i74.

Sockolow, P.S., K.H. Bowles, and M. Rogers. 2015. Health Information Technology Evaluation Framework (HITREF) comprehensiveness as assessed in electronic point-of-care documentation systems evaluations. *Studies in Health Technology and Informatics* 216:406–409.

Streiner, D.L. 2015. Statistics commentary series: Commentary #12—one-tailed and two-tailed tests. *Journal of Clinical Psychopharmacology* 35(6):628–629.

Tortorella, G.L., S. Viana, and D. Fettermann. 2015. Learning cycles and focus groups: A complementary approach to the A3 thinking methodology. *Learning Organization* 22(4):229–240.

Tyndall, J. 2010. *The AACODS Checklist*. Archived by Flinders Academic Commons. http://dspace.flinders.edu.au/xmlui/bitstream/handle/2328/3326/AACODS_Checklist.pdf?sequence=4.

US Department of Commerce. 2016. National Technical Information Service. National Technical Reports Library. https://ntrl.ntis.gov/NTRL.

US Department of Health and Human Services (HHS) Public Health Service. 2016. Grants Application. PHS 398, OMB No. 0925-0001. https://grants.nih.gov/grants/funding/phs398/398_forms.pdf.

Wiederhold, B.K. and G. Riva. *Annual Review of Cybertherapy and Telemedicine 2014: Positive Change: Connecting the Virtual and the Real*. Studies in Health Technology and Informatics, vol. 199. Fairfax, VA: IOS Press.

Zhang, X., P. Yu, J. Yan, and I.A.M. Spil. 2015. Using diffusion of innovation theory to understand the factors impacting patient acceptance and use of consumer e-health innovations: A case study in a primary care clinic. *BMC Health Services Research* 15:71(1–15).

Resources

American Psychological Association. 2016. PsychEXTRA. http://www.apa.org/pubs/databases/psycextra/index.aspx.

Canadian Agency for Drugs and Technologies in Health (CADTH). 2015. Grey Matters: A Practical Tool for Searching Health-Related Grey Literature. http://www.cadth.ca/en/resources/finding-evidence-is/grey-matters.

Durning, S.J. and J.D. Carline, eds. 2015. *Review Criteria for Research Manuscripts,* 2nd ed. Washington, DC: Association of American Medical Colleges. https://members.aamc.org/eweb/upload/Review%20Criteria%20For%20Research%20Manuscripts.pdf.

Dynarski, M. and E. Kisker. 2014. *Going Public: Writing about Research in Everyday Language*. Washington, DC: U.S. Department of Education, Institute of Education Sciences, National Center for Education Evaluation and Regional Assistance, Analytic Technical Assistance and Development. http://ies.ed.gov/pubsearch/pubsinfo.asp?pubid=REL2014051.

Garrard, J. 2017. *Health Sciences Literature Review Made Easy: The Matrix Method,* 5th ed. Burlington, MA: Jones & Bartlett Learning.

Hamilton Lopez M., R. Singer Cohen, and E. Holve. 2012 (December 13). Building the informatics infrastructure for comparative effectiveness research (CER): A review of the grey literature. EDM Forum, AcademyHealth. http://repository.edm-forum.org/cgi/viewcontent.cgi?article=1008&context=edm_briefs.

Toledo, A.H., R. Flikkema, and L.H. Toledo-Pereyra. 2011. Developing the research hypothesis. *Journal of Investigative Surgery* 24(5):191–194.

US National Library of Medicine (NLM). 2014. Health Services Research Projects in Progress (HSRProj). http://wwwcf.nlm.nih.gov/hsr_project/home_proj.cfm.

US National Library of Medicine (NLM). 2016. PubMed Central. https://www.ncbi.nlm.nih.gov/pubmed/.

Washington, L. 2008. Analyzing workflow for a health IT Implementation: An often short-shrifted step is essential in successful IT deployments. *Journal of AHIMA* 79(1):64–65.

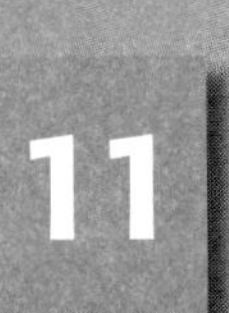

11 Selecting the Research Design and Method and Collecting Data

Elizabeth J. Forrestal, PhD, RHIA, CCS, FAHIMA

Learning Objectives

- Select a research design and method appropriate to the research question.
- Articulate the processes of data collection.
- Identify a data collection instrument appropriate to the research question.
- Determine standard and suitable tools and techniques to collect data.
- Select a sampling technique appropriate to the research question.
- Explain how data collection procedures affect studies' timelines and the quality of their collected data.
- Use key terms associated with instruments, sampling, samples, and data collection appropriately.

Key Terms

Categorical items
Concurrent validity
Constructs
Content validity
Content validity index (CVI)
Content validity ratio (CVR)
Convergent validity
Coverage error
Discriminant (divergent) validity
Elicitation
Heterogeneity
Instrument
Internal consistency reliability
Interrater reliability
Intrarater reliability
Likert scale
Nonrandom (nonprobability) sampling
Numerical items
Purposive sampling
Quota sampling
Rater reliability
Response bias
Sample size calculation
Sample survey
Sampling
Sampling error
Sampling frame
Saturation
Scale
Semantic differential scale
Semistructured question
Snowball sampling
Structured question
Subject matter expert (SME)
Survey
Theoretical sampling
Unstructured question

The topics of this chapter are selecting a research design and method and collecting data. Some of the concepts presented in this chapter were introduced in earlier chapters as methods of conducting research were discussed. This chapter builds upon those previous discussions.

The chapter begins by examining the impact of the research's purpose as well as other key factors on the selection of the research study's design and method. It then discusses factors affecting the selection of instruments, techniques, and tools to gather data. Issues related to sampling and sample size are then reviewed. The chapter concludes with a list of procedures that researchers should consider prior to collecting data. The following real-world case discusses an area of research, population health, that is gaining importance.

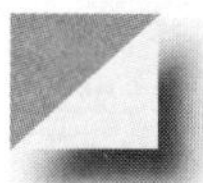

Real-World Case

Population health is a popular topic in the healthcare sector. However, a consensus about what *population health* means is lacking. Experts provide different definitions. One is that population health is collecting and analyzing patient data from a broad range of information sources, segmenting patient populations by their disease risks and other risk factors, and creating actionable information and clinical workflows that improve patient outcomes and financial results (Dowding 2016). A much simpler definition is that population health is improving the health outcomes for a defined population in a specific geographic area (HIMSS Analytics 2015).

In 2015, the Health Research and Educational Trust (HRET) partnered with the American Hospital Association (AHA) and the Public Health Institute (PHI) to survey 6,365 hospitals about the hospitals' approaches to population health, and 22 percent of the hospitals responded. Of these responding hospitals, 85 percent reported a "strong" or "total" commitment to population health or had population health in their vision statement (HRET 2015, slide 4). Another survey of nearly 200 healthcare executives reported similar results (HIMSS Analytics 2015). Population health is more than just an initiative in the private sector. Government agencies, such as the Centers for Medicare and Medicaid Services (CMS) and the Agency for Healthcare Research and Quality (AHRQ), are also interested in promoting population health (Kaplan et al. 2015). For example, improving population health is in the mission of CMS (2016a, 3).

Research has an important role in population health, as can be seen by the first definition's emphasis on "collecting and analyzing patient data from a broad range of information sources." However, Douglas B. Fridsma, president and chief executive officer of the American Medical Informatics Association (AMIA), has pointed out that the challenge is to "find the patterns" in the data (Dowding 2016). He explains that some of the most important data in population health management are not structured; although they do not "fit neatly inside columns, rows, and tables," unstructured data "can be every bit as important" as structured data (Dowding 2016). For example, key data about population health are in the physicians' free text progress notes or in the patients' descriptions of their illness. In these human narratives is "where the hidden gems and associations will be found as we look ahead to population health" (Dowding 2016). Finding and capturing these hidden gems and associations will require that researchers select the appropriate research design and method—a topic of this chapter.

Selecting a Research Design and Method

The selection of the appropriate research design and method increases the likelihood that the data collected are relevant, high quality, and directly related to the research question. Researchers weigh multiple factors when selecting the design and method of a research study. The purpose of the research is considered first. Researchers then weigh issues associated with internal and external validity and the impact of these issues on their design and method. Finally, the researchers consider other factors, such as their own skills and resources. Each of these factors is described in this section.

Purpose of the Research

The most important factor in selecting a research design and method is the purpose of the research. This purpose is reflected in the research question and problem statement. For example, if the researchers' purpose is to establish a causal relationship, they will select an experimental research design and a matching method, such as a randomized controlled trial (RCT). If the researchers' purpose is to explore a poorly understood area of practice, they will select a descriptive, observational, or correlational design and a method matching one of those designs, such as a survey or a case study. In table 1.2 in chapter 1, readers can see seven research designs with methods that are potential matches.

Internal Validity and External Validity

Two types of validity, internal validity and external validity, are associated with selecting the research design and method. *Internal validity* is the extent to which the researchers' design and processes are likely to have prevented bias and increased accuracy in their results. As explained in chapter 4, a research study is considered internally valid if it shows that only the independent variable caused the effect on the dependent variable and excludes any possible effect by a confounding variable. Certain factors, however, may threaten internal validity. These factors are potential sources of bias and error that may contaminate the study's results. These factors, also known as *threats,* are described in detail in chapter 4. *External validity* is the extent to which a study's results can be generalized (applied) to other settings, populations, or other phenomena. External validity becomes important when researchers want their results applied in the workplace or to other similar phenomena and when practitioners consider whether they can apply the researchers' results in their own settings.

Both internal validity and external validity are key considerations for researchers. However, achieving both internal and external validity becomes a balancing act for researchers as they design their studies. Studies high in internal validity may not reflect the external environment; thus, their external validity is compromised. On the other hand, to achieve external validity, researchers give up the control necessary for internal validity. In the final assessment, however, internal validity weighs more heavily than external validity because internal validity is related to the accuracy of the data.

Other Factors in Selecting a Research Design and Method

Researchers establish a match among the research design and method, internal and external validity, and other factors. These other factors, associated with the researchers' expertise and resources, are as follows:

- **Skills:** Can the researcher conduct the laboratory experiments, moderate the discussions, or perform the analytic techniques necessary for the research?
- **Time:** Does the researcher have the time to devote to conducting the research, such as in the case of a longitudinal study over a period of 10 years?
- **Money and resources:** Can the researcher afford the equipment and other costs of the research, such as setting up a simulation laboratory or paying the fees for proprietary software or a survey instrument?
- **Potential subjects:** Are sufficient numbers of subjects available, and are they willing to participate, given their busy schedules?

By realistically assessing these factors and making sound decisions based on that assessment, researchers improve the odds that they can successfully complete the research study. The following section introduces the next process of a research study, collecting data.

Planning to Collect Data

The processes of data collection support the quality of the data, and the general quality of the research study. Data collection includes planning, selecting an instrument (data collection tool), determining techniques and tools for data collection, deciding on a sampling strategy and sample, performing precollection procedures, and then, finally, actually collecting data.

Researchers write data collection plans for both quantitative and qualitative studies. The data collection plan includes what data will be collected, by whom the data will be collected, how the data will be collected, and when the data will be collected. In addition to timelines for the actual data collection, the plan includes timelines for the procedures involved in data collection, such as obtaining appropriate approvals, training data collectors, and performing a pilot study (discussed later in the chapter). High-quality research depends on a carefully conceived plan and its flawless execution. Researchers document the procedures of and adherence to the plan for the methods section of the study, which reports the plan's execution in detail so that other researchers can replicate the study. A lack of attention to detail in the planning and execution of the data collection may cast doubt on the soundness of the study's results. While plans are written for both quantitative and qualitative studies, the plans differ as described in the following paragraphs.

Quantitative Plan for Data Collection

Prior to beginning any data collection, quantitative researchers write a step-by-step plan that considers every logistical detail. This plan is written in conjunction with the statistical analysis plan (discussed in chapter 12). As the researchers work on these two components of the overall plan for the study, they compile a complete list of all the data elements required for each statistical test that they plan to perform. Then, prior to collecting data, researchers ensure that their data collection strategies will obtain all of the required data elements. Additionally, researchers determine the number of cases needed to run the statistical tests. This detail is particularly important when there are subgroups of unequal size in the sample. For example, researchers may want to investigate various clinicians' views of an alert system in an integrated delivery system (IDS). For these researchers, the umbrella term "clinicians" could include family nurse practitioners (FNPs), primary care physicians, and physician assistants. If the IDS had few FNPs, a lack of sufficient of data related to the FNPs could limit the statistical tests that could be performed. Executing the plan exactly as written is important because deviating from the plan could jeopardize the study's internal validity.

Qualitative Plan for Data Collection

The plans for qualitative studies are less structured than the plans for quantitative studies. The level of structure "depends on the time available, how much already is known about the phenomena under study, the instruments already available, and the analysis that will be made" (Miles et al. 2014, 19). When researchers experienced in qualitative techniques study topics about which little is known, new field sites and potential participants may emerge as the researchers learn more about their research question during their research study. However, when the research addresses topics or concepts that are well-defined, or when the researchers are beginners, many details about field sites and potential participants should be predetermined. Qualitative researchers meticulously document the procedures of their study as they execute it. This documentation becomes the means by which other researchers can replicate the study and its results as well as the basis of the study's conclusion validity (the conclusions' reasonableness, discussed in chapter 12).

Selection of an Instrument

In the context of research, an **instrument** is a standardized, uniform way to collect data. Examples of instruments include checklists, coding schemes and manuals, clinical screenings and assessments, educational tests, index measures, interview guides (schedules), personality tests, projective techniques, psychological tests, questionnaires, rating scales, scenarios, and vignettes, among others. Using a well-designed instrument minimizes bias and maximizes the certainty of the independent variable's (treatment's) effect on the dependent variable (outcome). This section discusses sources of instruments, validity and reliability of instruments, and other factors in selecting an instrument.

Sources of Instruments

Researchers can find standardized instruments in electronic databases. These databases provide descriptions of instruments, often with their validity and reliability (see next section). Examples of electronic databases that health informatics and health information management (HIM) researchers could use to begin their search for an appropriate instrument include the following:

- Health IT Survey Compendium (AHRQ 2017)
- Human Factors: Workbench Tools (FAA 2017)
- HaPI (Health and Psychosocial Instruments) (BMDS 2015)
- Mental Measurements Yearbook with Tests in Print (Buros Center for Testing 2016)

Researchers can also find standardized instruments during their literature review as they read articles. (See chapter 10 for more information on the literature review.)

Validity of Instruments

Validity, as it relates to instruments, means the extent to which the instrument measures what it is intended to measure. (*Validity* for instruments is different than *internal validity* that was discussed in chapter 4.) In other words, as stated in chapter 2, validity indicates that "the right thing was measured." The four types of validity related to instruments that are discussed in the following sections are face validity, content validity, construct validity, and criterion validity. Chapter 2 introduced these types of validity; here, they are discussed in greater depth.

Face Validity

Face validity is the extent to which the instrument appears to measure what it says it measures. For example, an instrument on HIM departmental policies and procedures for release of information would lack face validity if the instrument had no items on verifying the identity of people who pick up the information in person. Face validity is related to the instrument's items apparently covering all aspects of a topic based on a subject matter expert review. **Subject matter experts (SMEs)** are authorities in the instrument's domain, topic, or field. For example, SMEs for the release-of-information policy and procedure instrument would include HIM department managers and release-of-information supervisors. SMEs read the items of an instrument to evaluate whether the content appears to measure the phenomenon sought. In evaluating face validity, SMEs make intuitive and subjective judgments about an instrument's merit. The connotation of *face* in face validity is that, upon probing the instrument in depth, this appearance may not be true. Technically, face validity is superficial and is a weak measure of validity.

Content Validity

The content of a topic or domain is represented by the instrument's items. *Content validity,* as defined in chapter 2, is when an instrument includes all of a topic's content that it is supposed to contain. More specifically, content validity is the rigorous determination that the instrument's content represents all the relevant aspects of a topic and does not include aspects that are extraneous and unrelated (irrelevant) to its topic. The items in the instrument have operationalized the topic or domain. Both relevance and irrelevance are considered. For example, an instrument about usage of the components of an electronic health record (EHR) should contain items about each component of an EHR and should not contain items about electronic insurance claims.

One way to assess an instrument's content validity is to have SMEs review it and provide their opinions. In his classic article, Lawshe provides a method to quantify the SMEs' opinions (1975, 567–569). In Lawshe's method, researchers ask each SME to independently score the essentiality of each item on the instrument, as one of the following:

- Essential
- Useful but not essential
- Not necessary

The next step is to calculate the **content validity ratio (CVR)**—the ratio of the number of items that the SMEs scored as essential and the total number of SMEs, adjusted for 50 percent agreement (Lawshe's assumption) (Lawshe 1975, 567). Thus, the CVR focuses on how essential the SMEs viewed an item. For each item, the CVR represents the SMEs' level of agreement in numerical terms, as calculated in figure 11.1. Lawshe's minimally acceptable values for CVRs are listed in table 11.1.

Figure 11.1 Content validity ratio (CVR) formula and examples

$$CVR = \frac{n_e - (N/2)}{(N/2)}$$

n_e = number of subject matter experts indicating "essential"
N = total number of subject matter experts

Example 1

$n_e = 9$
$N = 14$

$$CVR = \frac{9 - (14/2)}{(14/2)}$$

$$CVR = \frac{9 - 7}{7}$$

$$CVR = \frac{2}{7}$$

$$CVR = 0.28$$

Example 2

$n_e = 15$
$N = 20$

$$CVR = \frac{15 - (20/2)}{(20/2)}$$

$$CVR = \frac{15 - 10}{10}$$

$$CVR = \frac{5}{10}$$

$$CVR = 0.5$$

Source of formula: Lawshe 1975, 567.

Table 11.1 Minimum values of content validity ratio (CVR)*

No. of SMEs**	Minimum CVR value***
5	0.99
6	0.99
7	0.99
8	0.75
9	0.78
10	0.62
11	0.59
12	0.56
13	0.54
14	0.51
15	0.49
20	0.42
25	0.37
30	0.33
35	0.31
40	0.29

*Two-tailed test, α = 0.05; one-tailed test, α = 0.025 [Wilson et al.'s correction of "one-tailed test, α = 0.05" (per Lawshe)].
**Subject matter experts.
3***The discontinuity between 5–7 SMEs and 8 SMEs and the anomaly between 8 SMEs and 9 SMEs remain unexplained. Regarding the discontinuity, Wilson and colleagues suggest that Schipper (Lawshe's statistician) required a stricter congruence for fewer SMEs. The anomaly between 8 SMEs and 9 SMEs may be a typographical or typesetting error in the original article.
Source: Lawshe 1975, 568; Wilson et al. 2012, 200–202.

The underlying concept of this method is that the greater the strength of the SMEs' consensus on items' essentiality, the greater the content validity.

The following paragraph demonstrates how the CVR and minimum value work. Example 1 in figure 11.1 has a CVR of 0.28 and 14 total experts. Checking the minimum value in table 11.1 for 14 experts shows that the minimum CVR value should be 0.51. Therefore, example 1 does not meet the minimum value and needs to be deleted from the instrument (or revised and its CVR rechecked). On the other hand, example 2 in figure 11.1 has a CVR of 0.50 and 20 total experts. Checking the minimum value in table 11.1 for 20 experts shows that the minimum CVR is 0.42. This item meets the minimum and should be retained in the instrument.

The next step is to calculate the overall content validity of the instrument. The **content validity index (CVI)** is a numerical representation of the SMEs' aggregate level of agreement for the entire instrument (Lawshe 1975, 572–573). One way to determine the CVI is to calculate the mean (average) of the individual item's CVRs. Table 11.2 shows an overall CVI for a 10-item instrument. The CVI was calculated by adding the individual CVRs of items 1 through 10 (bottom row of table) and dividing by 10, the number of items.

Table 11.2 Calculation of content validity index (CVI): Sample ratings on a 10-item instrument by 14 subject matter experts (SMEs)

SME	Item 1	Item 2	Item 3	Item 4	Item 5	Item 6	Item 7	Item 8	Item 9	Item 10	Overall CVI
A		x							x	x	
B	x	x	x	x	x	x	x	x	x	x	

(*Continued*)

Table 11.2 (*Continued*)

SME	Item 1	Item 2	Item 3	Item 4	Item 5	Item 6	Item 7	Item 8	Item 9	Item 10	Overall CVI
C	x	x	x	x	x	x	x	x	x	x	
D	x	x	x	x	x	x	x	x	x	x	
E		x	x	x	x	x	x		x	x	
F	x	x	x	x	x	x	x	x	x	x	
G	x	x	x	x	x	x	x	x	x	x	
H	x	x	x	x	x	x	x	x	x	x	
I		x	x	x	x	x	x		x	x	
J	x	x	x	x	x	x	x	x	x	x	
K	x	x	x	x	x	x	x	x	x	x	
L		x	x	x	x	x	x		x	x	
M		x	x	x	x	x	x		x	x	
N	x		x	x	x	x	x	x	x		
No. in Agreement	9	13	13	13	13	13	13	9	14	13	
CVR	0.29	0.86	0.86	0.86	0.86	0.86	0.86	0.29	1	0.86	**0.76 (mean of CVRs)**

x = rated as "essential"
Source of process: Lawshe 1975, 572–573.

Finally, the instrument's acceptability is determined by comparing it to criteria. The criteria take into account all the items' individual CVRs and the instrument's overall CVI. The criteria for an instrument to be judged as having excellent content validity are shown in table 11.3.

Table 11.3 Recommended criteria for an instrument's acceptability

	3–5 SMEs	6–10 SMEs
All items' CVRs	1.00	≥ 0.78
Overall CVI	≥ 0.90	≥ 0.90

Source of content: Polit and Beck 2006, 496.

Construct Validity

Constructs are abstractions of theoretical, non-observable concepts. Being non-observable, constructs are "constructed" in language and graphics. Classic examples of constructs are psychological concepts, such as intelligence, motivation, and anxiety. For example, although intelligence itself is not visible, its effects are. Similarly, although satisfaction itself is not visible, its effects are. *Construct validity* is the degree to which an instrument measures the constructs that it claims to measure. Therefore, if an instrument is intended to measure users' satisfaction, it should include measurable aspects associated with users' satisfaction.

Construct validity is assessed by evaluating the degree of correlation between the instrument and the variables it supposedly measures. The three components of construct validity are convergent validity, discriminant (divergent) validity, and concurrent validity.

- Convergent validity is the degree of correlation between the instrument and other instruments designed to measure similar constructs, or the degree of correlation among items measuring the same construct. For example, the degree of convergent validity is high when the results of two instruments measuring self-efficacy have a high positive correlation.

- **Discriminant (divergent) validity** is the degree to which the instrument does *not* positively correlate to instruments measuring dissimilar constructs or the degree to which items measuring dissimilar constructs are uncorrelated. For example, discriminate validity is high when the results of an instrument measuring self-efficacy and another instrument measuring locus of control (people's feelings whether they control the situation or others are in control) have a strong negative correlation.
- **Concurrent validity** is the instrument's ability to discriminate between groups it should differentiate. For example, an instrument with concurrent validity would be able to discriminate between expert users and novice users of an alert system.

Factor analysis is a statistical technique that analyzes the correlations and is used to assess construct validity. Factor analysis identifies the underlying set of relationships (factors) in an instrument. These factors comprise variables that are highly correlated among themselves, but minimally correlated with other variables (Carter 2016, 732–733). In addition to identifying the underlying factors, factor analysis is used to reduce the factors to the fewest number. (See discussion in chapter 2.) The relationships are reported as eigenvalues and factor loadings, which are terms for the output of factor analysis. Minimum values are typically 1 for eigenvalues and 0.40 for factor loadings (Huck 2012, 491–494). Numerous studies build evidence of the instrument's construct validity when the studies show high degrees of correlation between the instrument and the variables it supposedly measures and when the studies identify the same common factors.

Criterion Validity

Criterion validity (also called criterion-related validity, discussed in chapter 2) is the assessment of an instrument against a *criterion*—an established instrument for which the validity and reliability are known and accepted. For example, researchers compared the calorie-burning and step-counting estimates of an armband activity monitor to two gold standards. One gold standard was a calorimetry of energy (calorie) expenditure, and the other was a manual count of the study participants' steps in a video recording of their activities. The armband monitor's results were strongly correlated to the calorimetry's readings, but the correlation with step counts was poor. Interpreting these results in terms of criterion validity, the armband monitor was a valid tool to estimate energy expenditure; however, it was not a valid tool to estimate the number of steps (Tierney et al. 2013, 889).

Reliability of Instruments

Reliability is the extent to which a procedure or an instrument yields similar results over repeated trials, over time, across similar groups, within individuals, and across raters. Reliability means that, over time, a test or observation is dependable and consistent in its measurement. Consistency, dependability, and reproducibility characterize reliable instruments. Reliability was discussed in chapter 2; this section builds upon that discussion.

Three aspects of reliability are interrater reliability and intrarater reliability, test-retest reliability, and internal consistency reliability. While these characteristics are related, they assess reliability from different perspectives. Interrater reliability and intrarater reliability assess the instrument's standardization. Test-retest reliability assesses the stability of an instrument in different situations. Internal consistency reliability assesses whether all the instrument's items are related to the same concept.

Interrater Reliability and Intrarater Reliability

Interrater reliability and intrarater reliability involve the degree of agreement in the results among repeated administrations of an instrument or test. The results of instruments or tests, by one rater or multiple raters, should be consistent. This consistency, known as **rater reliability** indicates the extent to which subjectivity has been eliminated. Inconsistency and variability should be minimal.

Interrater reliability means that different persons completing the instrument or test have reasonably similar results. For example, chapter 8 describes the steps in conducting a systematic review, and, in step 6, two or more independent reviewers decided whether the identified articles were relevant to their topic and should be included in their systematic review. As part of this process, the reviewers' consistency—their interrater reliability—in their decisions, yes-include or no-exclude, was assessed.

Intrarater reliability means that the same person completing the instrument or test at different times will have reasonably similar results. For example, researchers could assess intrarater reliability by having the same coding professional who originally coded a patient record recode that same record at a later date and then compare the similarity of the codes.

Two common statistical tests to assess rater reliability are the intraclass correlation coefficient (ICC) and the Cohen's kappa (κ) coefficient. Each will be described here.

Intraclass Correlation Coefficient The ICC is a versatile test of interrater reliability and intrarater reliability for continuous data that can be used for a variety of purposes (Huck 2012, 70). It evaluates the consistency of measurements by multiple raters and is used when data are organized as groups, rather than as paired observations. The ICC describes the strength of the resemblance among data in the same group and is applied to assess the consistency or reproducibility of quantitative measurements made by different raters measuring the same quantity. The ICC detects both interrater and intrarater consistency (or, conversely, variability). Therefore, in terms of interrater inconsistency, the ICC would detect systematic differences (variability) among raters. For example, one rater's scores are routinely higher or lower than the scores of the other raters. However, in terms of intrarater inconsistency, the ICC would also detect one rater's unusual deviation (outlier) from his or her past patterns of measurements.

Generally, the ICC is the ratio of between-groups variance to total variance. There are several models of ICC based on its original derivation from Pearson product-moment correlation coefficient and its evolution based on analysis of variance (ANOVA) (Lee et al. 2012, 150). The ICC is preferred to Pearson product-moment correlation coefficient when the sample size is small (≤15). Data are organized in tables with the measured object in the rows and each rater's measurements in a column. The ICC assesses the interrater (raters in the column) effect in relation to the grouping (row) effect, using two-way ANOVA. To interpret the ICC, the ICC will approach 1.0 when there is no variance within the raters' scores.

Cohen's Kappa Coefficient The Cohen's kappa (κ) coefficient (also sometimes called *Cohen's kappa,* the *kappa statistic,* and the *kappa coefficient*; the Greek letter "κ" means kappa) is used to assess interrater reliability and intrarater reliability of nominal data (Huck 2012, 71). As described in chapter 8's discussion of interrater reliability between the independent reviewers screening articles for the systematic review, kappa coefficient is used when there are two raters and their ratings, such as agree or disagree, are dichotomous. The formula to calculate the kappa coefficient and an example are provided in chapter 8. The kappa coefficient measures the strength of agreement or homogeneity—the consensus—among raters. Like the ICC, the kappa coefficient establishes the extent of reliability. The kappa coefficient is also similar to the ICC, in that data are organized in a table in which the raters are the columns and measured attributes (variables) are the rows. Table 11.4 provides general rubrics to interpret the kappa coefficient.

Table 11.4 Interpretation of Cohen's kappa (κ) coefficient

Kappa Statistic	Strength of Agreement
< 0.00	Poor
0.00–0.20	Slight
0.21–0.40	Fair
0.41–0.60	Moderate
0.61–0.80	Substantial
0.81–1.00	Almost perfect

Source: Landis and Koch 1977, 165.

Test-Retest Reliability

Test-retest reliability, as explained in chapter 2, determines whether the instrument is consistent over time or when used multiple times. Test-retest reliability measures how stable and reproducible an instrument's results are (Huck 2012, 69). Repeated administrations of instruments that have test-retest reliability will result in reasonably similar findings. The measure is capable of giving consistent results independent of the situation or the state of the test taker. If changes occur in the intervening period between tests, the results may be different (threat to internal validity of study design). The following are two statistical techniques to assess test-retest reliability (Hopkins 2014, 22):

- Pearson product-moment correlation coefficient (sample size > 15)
- ICC (sample size ≤ 15)

A perfect correlation is 1.0; no correlation is 0 (negative correlations are reported as 0). The minimally acceptable correlation coefficient is ≥ 0.70 for groups and 0.90 to 0.95 for individuals (Scientific Advisory Committee of the Medical Outcomes Trust 2002, 199). Pearson product-moment correlation coefficient is further described in chapter 9; ICC was addressed in the previous section.

Internal Consistency Reliability

Internal consistency reliability is the homogeneity of an instrument's items. An instrument with internal consistency reliability measures a single construct, a single characteristic, a single skill, or a single quality. The items "hang together" (Huck 2012, 71). The following three statistical techniques are commonly used to assess internal consistency (Huck 2012, 71–74):

- Split-half reliability coefficient—two halves of the test, such as even items and odd items, are correlated and then the Spearman-Brown correction formula applied.
- Kuder-Richardson formula—this is an improvement on split-half reliability coefficient because it is not affected by items' order.
- Cronbach's alpha—this is an improvement on both split-half reliability coefficient and Kuder-Richardson formula because it evaluates more complex scoring, such as partial credit.

Cronbach's alpha test is common in health informatics and HIM investigative studies (sometimes seen with the Greek letter "α" that means alpha). Chapter 2 provides examples of researchers assessing the reliability of their instruments using Cronbach's alpha. The minimum level of acceptability varies by the type of instrument and the number of test takers. For most instruments in health informatics and HIM, an acceptable Cronbach's alpha is ≥ 0.70 for groups and 0.90 to 0.95 for individuals (Scientific Advisory Committee of the Medical Outcomes Trust 2002, 199).

Factors in Selecting an Instrument

Researchers consider multiple factors when determining which instrument to use in their studies. These factors include the researchers' purpose, the instrument's validity and reliability, its format, attributes, and feasibility. These factors are discussed in the following subsections.

Purpose of the Research

The most important factor in selecting an instrument is the purpose of the research—the data collected must be relevant to the research question. Researchers should match their study's purpose to the instrument's purpose. Reading the description and critique of an instrument in a reference book or database, such as the Health IT Survey Compendium (AHRQ 2017), is just the first step. Researchers then obtain a sample of the instrument itself (often for free or at nominal cost) and read it in its entirety to be sure that the instrument exactly matches their purpose. Researchers pay special attention to the instrument's theoretical underpinning and the operational definitions of terms. These aspects are also discussed in the following paragraphs.

Theoretical Underpinning Researchers develop instruments as they work with a theory. Thus, the instrument reflects the theory's assumptions about knowledge and reality. For example, the decision to use an instrument that evolved from existential psychology in a study using Skinner's behaviorism would be problematic because these two theoretical bases are entirely different.

Operational Definitions Operational definitions represent concepts in observable and measurable terms (see discussion in chapter 10). Developers of instruments operationalize concepts based on the theory with which they are working; if different developers use different theories, their concepts will also be defined differently. For example, research on decision support systems may investigate aspects of expertise. Cognitive theories and knowledge engineering theories have different operational definitions of expertise (Herling 2000, 11–12). (See table 1.1 in chapter 1 for examples of publications on information processing and cognitive learning theories and knowledge engineering theories.) Cognitive theories provide the following definition: Expertise is the ability to rapidly organize and process "small bits of information" into "meaningful and creative ways to solve problems and comprehend solutions" (Kuchinke 1997, 81, 82). In contrast, knowledge engineering theories provide the following definition: Expertise is the compiled task knowledge that an expert has gained while in the practice of domain-specific behaviors in an ongoing search for better ways of doing things, including problem solving (Herling 2000, 12). Thus, the cognitive theories operationalize expertise in terms of characteristics, such as organizing ability and processing ability, whereas the knowledge engineering theories operationalize expertise in terms of what is needed to replicate it, as in artificial intelligence, such as types of knowledge, practice, and behaviors.

Researchers need to verify that the instrument operationalizes concepts the same way that they do. For example, researchers studying workplace social support would want to ensure that the instrument collects data about social support in the workplace from colleagues, rather than social support in the home from family members. If researchers select an instrument that operationalizes terms differently than they do, this choice will undermine the research study by collecting data unrelated to the research question.

Satisfactory Ratings for Validity and Reliability

An instrument's validity and reliability are key considerations when making a selection. Acceptable levels of validity and reliability vary by the type of instrument and the type of research. Instruments measuring attitudes, perceptions, and personality traits tend to have lower levels than standardized aptitude tests. Moreover, newer instruments initially tend to have lower reliability than older instruments. As the instruments are further developed, tested, and refined, their levels of validity and reliability increase. If at all possible, researchers select instruments that other researchers have already developed and refined. The validity and reliability of such existing instruments are established. Researchers who are using an existing instrument should state the instrument's content validity, construct validity, and reliability in their report.

Construction of a valid and reliable instrument is a research project in and of itself. Researchers should undertake the difficult task of developing an instrument only after they have investigated and verified that an appropriate instrument does not already exist.

As discussed in chapter 2, the development of a survey questionnaire includes deciding on its content, checking its validity, pilot testing it, and other tasks. The following example further illustrates this process. To conduct a statewide assessment of health information technology (HIT) workforce needs, a team of health informatics and HIM researchers developed a quantitative employer needs assessment survey (Fenton et al. 2013, 1–2). First, the researchers conducted 12 focus groups with employers to obtain qualitative data from which to develop the survey's content. The researchers then constructed the survey through multiple cycles, during which they analyzed transcripts of the focus groups' discussions and content of facilitators' whiteboards, reviewed the survey, checked its validity, and tested it. Drafting the written survey took the research team five to six weeks of intensive work. After the paper version of the survey was completed, it was loaded into an online survey tool for which additional testing was required. For the online survey, the research team also spent time considering web design features, such as a progress completion bar and navigational buttons (Fenton et al. 2013, 3).

Researchers also check whether the instrument's validity and reliability have been established for their study's setting (patient's home, academic health center, and such), population (socioeconomic, race, veteran, rural, educational level, so forth), or both. An instrument's validity and reliability may vary when used in settings or with populations different from the setting or population in which or with which it was developed. Therefore, prior to using an instrument, researchers confirm that its validity and reliability have been established in the setting and for the population of their study.

Style and Format of the Instrument

The instrument should be written in a style that is clear and direct. Clearly worded instruments are more likely to collect accurate data than vague or imprecise instruments. Confused respondents may simply quit and leave the instrument incomplete, or they may misinterpret the instrument and thereby provide erroneous information. Brevity, directness, and an attractive format also increase the response rate (discussed later in the chapter).

Instruments are available in various formats, such as paper-based or web-based, and in multiple languages (English, Spanish, Korean, and others). Formats can also target certain age groups, such as a pediatric format and another matched version for the parents of pediatric patients. These other formats have their own validities and reliabilities. Therefore, prior to using an instrument, researchers should confirm that its validity and reliability have been established for the format that they intend to use.

Attributes of Items

Items within an instrument can have different attributes, such as type, level, scales, and the use of standardized categories. *Type* involves how the items are constructed. *Level* refers to whether the items collect data at the numerical or categorical level. *Scales* are a form of categorical item. Standardized categories are grouping for subpopulations that come from the literature or authoritative sources. This subsection addresses these attributes.

Structured, Unstructured, and Semistructured Types Three types of structures for questions are structured, unstructured, and semistructured. (See also the discussion of this topic in chapter 2.)

- **Structured questions**, also known as *closed-ended questions*, are those questions in which the participant can choose a particular response from a finite list of possible responses. The advantages of structured questions are that they are easier for the participant to complete and for the researcher to tabulate and analyze than unstructured questions. An example of a structured question is: What is your gender? ___Male ___Female
- **Unstructured questions**, also known as *open-ended questions*, are those questions that do not have a specific choice of answers and the participants can provide free-form responses in oral or written form. The advantages of unstructured questions are that they allow in-depth questions and may uncover aspects of a problem unknown to the researcher. The real-world case at the beginning of the chapter highlights the value of this second advantage. In the case, unstructured data are called "hidden gems and associations" and are considered essential to improve the health of populations. An example of an unstructured question is: What barriers prevent you from routinely exercising?
- **Semistructured questions** begin with structured questions and then follow with open-ended questions to clarify. Semistructured questions have the advantages of obtaining comparable data for analysis and potentially providing insights. An example of a semistructured question is: Would you consider yourself physically fit? ___Yes ___No. Why or why not?

Structured questions are often used in quantitative research. Unstructured questions and semistructured questions are often used in exploratory and qualitative research. Sometimes researchers use a combination of all three types. The purpose of the research determines which type or types of questions the researchers use.

Numerical and Categorical Levels Structured questions may be formatted at the numerical level or at the categorical level. Table 11.5 shows examples of numerical and categorical levels. For more details, see the discussion of data levels in chapter 9. When feasible, items at the numerical level are preferable to items at the categorical level (Alreck and Settle 2004, 113). Researchers need to collect the data at the level, numerical or categorical, that matches their proposed statistical analyses.

Table 11.5 Example of numerical and categorical levels

Numerical	Categorical
_____Indicate the number of hours that you work per week (whole numbers).	Mark the number of hours that you work per week: ☐ 19 or fewer hours per week ☐ 20 to 29 hours per week ☐ 30 to 39 hours per week ☐ 40 to 49 hours per week ☐ 50 to 59 hours per week ☐ 60 or greater hours per week

Numerical items request that the respondent enter a number. Numerical items result in metric data (interval or ratio, see chapter 9). Statistical analysis of metric data has fewer limitations than statistical analysis of categorical items. However, in writing a numerical item, researchers are careful to explicitly specify the unit of measure. For example, the question, "How long ago was your last visit to the dentist?" does not give the respondent an explicit unit of measure. The respondent may write, for example, 365 days, 52 weeks, or 1 year.

Categorical items require the respondent to select the appropriate category or grouping. Categorical items result in nominal or ordinal data, which are discussed in chapter 9. Statistical analysis of nominal and ordinal data has greater limitations than statistical analysis of numerical data. Composing good categorical items requires attention to detail. The categories must be collectively all-inclusive, mutually exclusive, and sufficiently broad or narrow, and they must form meaningful clusters. These concepts are explained as follows:

- **All-inclusive:** All respondents must fit into a category, even if it is "other." Typically, there are unusual or exceptional cases that warrant the category "other." Moreover, the lack of a matching category, even if it is "other," frustrates the respondents.

- **Mutually exclusive:** Categories should not overlap, which could confuse the respondents.
- **Form meaningful clusters:** Categories should make sense and be meaningfully distinct. The set of categories under the column "Poor Clusters," in figure 11.2 does not form a reasonable progression because 13 years of schooling are grouped in one category and then there are four categories for the years it takes to earn a baccalaureate degree (college freshman, college sophomore, college junior, and college senior). The other column in figure 11.2, "Meaningful Clusters" shows of a set of categories that form a reasonable, balanced progression.
- **Sufficiently narrow or broad:** The number of categories for a question must be at least two (for example, yes or no; true or false) and generally should not exceed eight. Respondents have difficulty seeing shades of meaning beyond eight categories. It is recommended that, when in doubt, use the narrower (greater number) categories because categories can always be combined; however, broad categories cannot be disaggregated into fine-grained categories, if the detailed data were not collected in the first place (Aleck and Settle 2004, 112–113). On the other hand, requesting that participants respond to many categories and unnecessarily narrow categories may lower the response rate and introduce inaccuracy.

Figure 11.2 Examples of poor and meaningful clusters for categorical items about levels of education

Poor Clusters	Meaningful Clusters
Kindergarten to 12th grade	High school education
College freshman	Associate's degree
College sophomore	Baccalaureate degree
College junior	Graduate degree
College senior	
Graduate school	

Scales Scales are a form of categorical item that uses progressive categories, such as size, amount, importance, rank, or agreement. (See table 11.6 and the discussion of scales in chapter 2.) Each category is also called a *point;* a scale with five categories is a five-point scale. Reliability increases steadily from a two-point scale to a seven-point scale. However, after seven points, the improvement is trivial and insignificant. Thus, if the literature provides researchers with no information on the appropriate number of scale points, they should choose a seven-point scale. HIM researchers used a scale on a survey that allowed respondents to categorize their competence, from very weak to very strong, in educational subdomains related to HIM (Sandefer and Karl 2015, 26). (See figure 11.3.)

Table 11.6 Common scales

Scale	Purpose	Example
Two-point	Dichotomous question	Yes, no Favor, oppose True, false
Three-point	Importance, interest, or satisfaction Satisfaction with amounts	Very, fairly, not at all Too much (many), just (about) right, not enough (too few)
Four-point	Generic Measurement of amounts	Excellent, good, fair, poor Very much, quite a bit, some, very little
Likert (five-point)	Indication of agreement or disagreement	Strongly agree, agree, neutral, disagree, strongly disagree
Verbal frequency (five-point)	Frequency	Always, often, sometimes, rarely (seldom), never
Expanded Likert (seven-point)	Extra discrimination desirable	Very strongly agree, strongly agree, agree, neutral, disagree, strongly disagree, very strongly disagree

Source: Forrestal 2016, p. 591.

Figure 11.3 Excerpt from survey illustrating use of scale in health informatics and HIM research

Survey on Competence
Rate your level of competence in the following educational subdomains:

	Very Weak	Weak	Neutral	Strong	Very Strong
Classification systems					
Health record content and documentation					
Data governance					
Data management					
Secondary data sources					

Source: Content derived from Sandefer and Karl 2015.

A commonly used scale is the **Likert scale** (named for its developer, Rensis Likert), which allows respondents to record their level of agreement or disagreement along a range of five categories (see table 11.6). The categories along the scale's range are "strongly agree, agree, neutral, disagree, strongly disagree."

Researchers, marketers, and others use semantic differential scales to discover consumers' perspectives or organizations' public relations images. **Semantic differential scales** allow respondents to rate products, healthcare organizations, or other services using adjectives that are polar opposites on the ends of a continuum. Figure 11.4 shows how a semantic differential scale allows respondents to select ratings between polar opposites. Up to 20 adjective pairs may be used. Half the items should begin with the positive adjective of the pair and the other half with the negative adjective. This type of scale is difficult to construct because it is challenging to identify polar-opposite adjectives that capture the major attributes of a product, an organization's image, or services. However, a well-constructed semantic differential scale can provide a valuable profile of a product's, organization's, or program's image (Alreck and Settle 2004, 132–134).

Figure 11.4 Example of a semantic differential scale

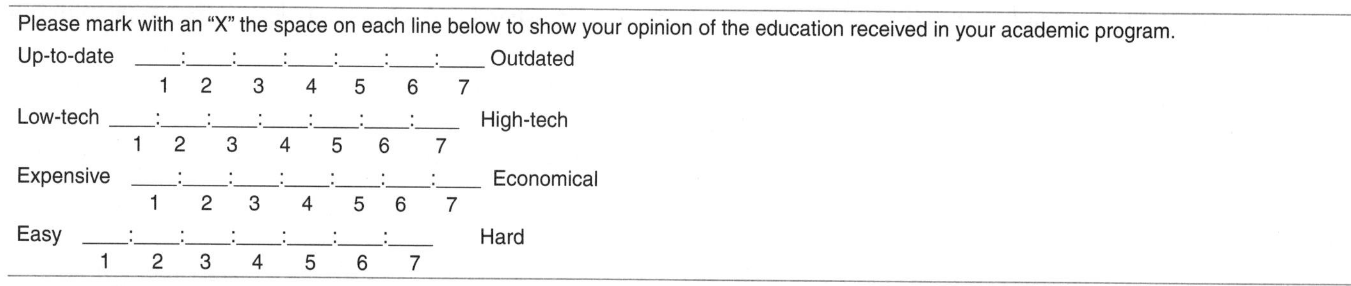
Please mark with an "X" the space on each line below to show your opinion of the education received in your academic program.

Up-to-date ____:____:____:____:____:____:____ Outdated
1 2 3 4 5 6 7

Low-tech ____:____:____:____:____:____:____ High-tech
1 2 3 4 5 6 7

Expensive ____:____:____:____:____:____:____ Economical
1 2 3 4 5 6 7

Easy ____:____:____:____:____:____:____ Hard
1 2 3 4 5 6 7

Source: Forrestal 2016, 592.

Standardized Categories If at all possible, researchers use standardized categories for groups, such as races, age groups, and other subpopulations (also called *subgroups*). Using standardized categories allows researchers to compare and contrast their results with the results of other researchers as reported in the literature. Researchers find these standardized categories during their literature review or in the resources of authoritative organizations, such as the Centers for Disease Control and Prevention (CDC), CMS, AHRQ, and other agencies and organizations. In figure 11.5, the example of standardized categories for age groups comes from the CDC (Xu et al. 2016, 4) and the example of races or ethnicities come from the National Institutes of Health (NIH 2015). Chapter 12 explains how subgroups are involved in statistical analysis.

Figure 11.5 Examples of standardized categories: age groups and races or ethnicities

Age Groups by Years[1]
Under 1 year
1–4
5–14
15–24
25–34
35–44

(Continued)

Figure 11.5 (*Continued*)

Age Groups by Years[1]
45–54
55–64
65–74
75–84
85 and over
Races[2]
American Indian or Alaska Native
Asian
Black or African American
Native Hawaiian or Other Pacific Islander
White
Ethnicities[2]
Hispanic or Latino
Not Hispanic or Latino

Sources of content: [1]Xu et al. 2016, 4; [2]NIH 2015.

Feasible Logistics

Instruments may be in the public domain or proprietary. Public domain means that the creator of a literary work, musical composition, invention, or other material can no longer restrict or receive a royalty for the use of the material. Works and materials in the public domain are not protected by copyright, patent, trademark, or other laws. While it may seem that materials on the Internet are public domain, often, they are not. When the copyright status is not clearly stated, it is best to contact the content owner to request permission for use of the content.

Instruments in the public domain can be copied and used freely. Instruments that are proprietary must be purchased and cannot be copied. When purchasing an instrument, researchers should be aware of hidden costs. For example, some instruments must be scored by the institute or researcher holding the instrument's copyright. The cost of scoring can significantly increase the cost of the study. Other hidden costs include having to purchase the user's manual or the scoring guide. However, a free instrument that collects inaccurate data only tangentially related to the researcher's topic would be unsuitable. Therefore, while cost is a factor, the overall quality of the study should be the priority.

Examples of Instruments Used in Health Informatics and HIM

Health informatics and HIM researchers use a variety of instruments. One of the commonly referenced instruments is the System Usability Scale (SUS) (Brooke 1986). The SUS is a 10-item instrument for evaluating hardware, software, mobile devices, websites, applications, and other products and services (HHS 2016). SUS has been referenced in over 1,300 articles and publications and is considered an engineering and computer industry standard. It is discussed in chapter 6 and shown in figure 6.2. The SUS is in the public domain (Brooke 2013, 29). Another instrument, the Software Usability Measurement Inventory (SUMI) assesses software quality from the user's point of view (Kirakowski and Corbett 1993). In the software engineering and computer industries, the SUMI is the de facto standard for analyzing the users' experience of Internet and desktop software applications (Kirakowski 2017). The SUMI is proprietary and must be purchased. A third instrument, the Questionnaire for User Interaction Satisfaction (QUIS) was created by a multidisciplinary team. QUIS assesses users' satisfaction with specific factors of computer interfaces, such as the screen, multimedia, online tutorials, and other factors (University of Maryland 2015). To use this proprietary instrument, researchers must purchase a license.

Techniques and Tools of Data Collection

Techniques and tools to collect data vary by the method of the research. For example, observations may use different instruments than surveys. The following section reviews various techniques and tools in surveys, observations, elicitation, and data mining.

Surveys

Surveys systematically collect data about a population (entire group) to determine its current status regarding certain factors. *Census surveys* collect data from all the members of the population. A **sample survey** collects data from representative members of the population. Surveys are a form of self-report research in which the individuals themselves are the source of data. Two survey formats are interviews (oral) and questionnaires (written or electronic).

In an interview survey, researchers orally question the members of the population. Researchers can question members of the population as individuals or as a group. Examples of interview surveys are telephone surveys and focused interviews (explained in chapter 3). Focused interviews and collection of data through interview guides are described in chapter 3. Typically, interviews are recorded and transcribed for later analyses. Questionnaire surveys query members of a population by providing participants a means to record and submit their responses electronically or in print form. Questionnaire surveys are described in detail in chapter 2.

Observations

Observation includes many ways of collecting data by noting and recording. Data collection tools used to document researchers' observations include activity lists, audiotapes, case notes, check sheets, clinical data (such as laboratory values or weight), logs, observation forms, questionnaires, surveys, videotapes, and other tools. These tools *must* be developed and tested prior to their use. Observations reflect the approach that the researchers are taking, quantitative or qualitative.

In a quantitative study, researchers use tools to collect categorical or numerical data. For example, in an evaluation study investigating users' ability to navigate a computer application, the researchers can collect data on keystrokes, time spent viewing a screen, and audit trails. In one instance, a research team investigated whether sending adolescent patients text-message reminders could improve their adherence in taking their medications. Self-reported data were collected via online or telephone surveys, depending on the patients' and their parents' preference (Johnson et al. 2016, 450).

In the qualitative approach, the researchers code all the recorded observations so that the observations can be analyzed later. Audiotapes and videotapes must undergo the additional step of transcription, prior to coding and analysis. Moreover, qualitative studies emphasize triangulation (obtaining data from multiple data sources; see chapter 3). Observation results in vast volumes of data, often called rich data. *Rich data* are thick descriptions and layers of extensive details from multiple sources. For example, if the phenomenon of interest was the exchange of health information during patient transfers, rich data would describe the scene; the participants' words, actions, and intentions; social relationships around the phenomenon; and many more details (Schultze and Avital 2011, 3). Data collection continues to **saturation**, a point of closure when there is repetition and convergence of information and no new themes, ideas, or concepts are emerging. Collecting data via observation is resource-intensive in terms of time, energy, and cost.

Elicitation

Elicitation is a technique of data collection that evokes, brings out, or draws out knowledge, ideas, perceptions, beliefs, memories, needs, and other, often hidden, phenomena. The purpose—obtaining unarticulated or tacit knowledge—is what classifies a technique as elicitation.

Elicitation includes many of the data collection techniques that have been discussed in previous chapters and sections, such as interviews, questionnaires, and observations. Other techniques of elicitation that have not been previously discussed include reviewing and analyzing documents, storytelling, brainstorming, role playing, and many others (Gavrilova and Andreeva 2012, 528).

The goal of elicitation is to uncover informants' unarticulated knowledge (Johnson and Weller 2001, 491). Examples of unarticulated knowledge include tacit understandings, which are difficult to verbalize, and assumptions. Elicitation techniques can be systematic (structured) or free-flowing (open-ended or unstructured), and there is a broad range of types, including audio, expert, graphic, interview, knowledge, photo, and video. Elicitation is used in wide variety of fields including anthropology, computer science, economics, health-related fields, and many other fields.

Decision support systems (DSS) are often based upon knowledge elicited from experts. In the development of the DSS, system developers could arrange individual sessions with experts and explain to the experts that they will be presented with a problem and that their solution of the problem using the DSS will be observed and recorded. The developers might also question the experts in the process of the solution to find out why the experts took their chosen approach or made a particular action. The developers would record all the actions and answers, usually with video recordings (Gavrilova and Andreeva 2012, 530). The information from the video recordings can then be used to improve the DSS.

In another healthcare example investigators used photo elicitation to prompt hospital informants about their views of sources of waste (Goff et al. 2013, 826–827). A purposive sample of 20 personnel at an academic health center were asked to take up to 10 photos of waste in a two-week period. Then, shortly after the end of the photo-taking period, the researchers conducted semistructured interviews with the participants. During the audiotaped interviews, the participants showed the researchers each photo and described the waste it depicted. While in this study the participants took the photos, photo elicitation can also involve the researchers having photos and showing them to the participants. In both versions, this technique is used to encourage in-depth discussions.

In health informatics and HIM, investigators could use elicitation techniques to obtain information from users and experts, such as users' system requirements and experts' opinions during the development of health information technologies. The complex questions and problems that are faced by investigators in health informatics and HIM are well suited to the techniques of elicitation.

Data Mining

Data mining is the use of various analytic tools to discover new facts, valid patterns, and relevant relationships in large databases (Naidu and Tiwari 2014, 109). Data mining is considered secondary data analysis because data miners use databases created by others, often for purposes unrelated to research and data mining. The process of performing data mining is covered in detail in chapter 7.

Data Sources

Researchers have many sources of data available to mine. These sources include both primary sources and secondary sources, such as those listed in table 1.3 in chapter 1.

Primary sources, also called *primary data,* are firsthand sources, as discussed in chapter 1. In this case, *firsthand* means that they are either the original data obtained by researchers who conducted the research study or data that were collected to serve a specific purpose. For example, researchers collect primary data to answer a specific research question whereas patient records are created for a specific purpose, to provide care for a specific patient (documentation in patient records also supports billing and legal issues).

Secondary sources, also called *secondary data,* are secondhand sources. As described in chapter 1, secondary sources are primary sources that have been aggregated, summarized, critiqued, analyzed, or manipulated. For example, secondary sources derived from health records include registries, indexes, and administrative records. Secondary sources also include manipulated data. Sources of manipulated data include public-domain databases compiled by governmental agencies as well as other researchers' data or databases.

Data Access

Access to data is critical for researchers who conduct secondary analyses or combine their primary research with data from public databases. When seeking access to data, researchers must consider whether they need approval or permission to gain access, the types of data available (individual or aggregate, public-domain or proprietary), and the location of the data. In addition, researchers must arrange a secured way to collect their data, in accordance applicable rules and regulations, such as the Health Insurance Portability and Accountability Act (HIPAA) of 1996 for patient data, and the organization's policies.

- **Approval or permission:** Researchers need to obtain approval or permission from relevant oversight entities and, in the case of individually identifiable data, additional approval may be required. Data can range from totally uncontrolled to highly protected. For example, data from the US government or companies' annual reports are often easily accessed online by anyone, whereas healthcare organizations' proprietary financial data are much more difficult to obtain. Researchers need to allow sufficient time to obtain the approvals or permissions.
- **Individual or aggregate data:** Data that identify specific individuals are less accessible and more heavily protected than aggregate data. To use identifiable data, researchers must obtain approvals from all involved institutional review boards (IRBs) (discussed later in this chapter and in detail in chapter 14). For example, researchers may need to obtain the approval of the IRB of the university where they work and from the IRB of the healthcare organization

from which they received the identifiable data. Some organizations may require informed consent from subjects to review data. In addition, accessing personally identifiable data has become more complex with the implementation of the provisions of HIPAA, the Health Information Technology for Economic and Clinical Health (HITECH) Act of 2009, and the federal Common Rule. (See chapter 14.)

- **Public-domain or proprietary data:** US government data are often accessible under the Freedom of Information Act; some have been posted on the Internet. State registry data also are often accessible. Access to and use of proprietary data require permission from the owner of the database. An example of proprietary data is the data held by Internet companies. These data come from the Internet companies' tracking of consumers' movements, transactions, demographics, and other activities. Profiles from these data include consumers' preferences and health status. These data are stored or created outside of HIPAA protection (Glenn and Monteith 2014, 1).
- **Location of data:** The ease of access to data varies widely by the data's location. For example, researchers can easily access data in anonymized (deidentified) public databases that can be transferred over the Internet, but data in historical paper records can be difficult to access, as the investigator may need to physically go to the site of storage within the organization's hours of operation and in accordance with its security rules.

Sampling and Samples

In sampling, researchers select a set of subjects or units to represent a larger population. The sample is the set of units that the researchers select. Accurate identification of the target population and its sample is essential to the success of research studies. This section discusses target populations and samples, data sampling methods and types of samples, sample sizes and their calculation, and response rates. This section builds on chapter 2's discussion of sampling in survey research, because sampling techniques are also used in other research methods.

Target Population and Sample

The *target population* is the set of individuals (or objects) of interest to the researchers and the focus of their research study. Determining the exact characteristics of the study's target population is important because the research's results and conclusions are only applicable to this population. Target populations can be health informatics and HIM professionals, patients, clinicians, healthcare organizations, websites, blogs, and many other groups of individuals or objects. In research studies, populations are shown as "N" (letter in upper case).

A *sample* is a set of units, such as portion of a target population. Researchers often use samples because studies involving entire populations can be impractical, impossible, or too expensive. For example, very few researchers would have enough funding to poll all US citizens about their opinions on storing their health data on the Internet. Researchers, however, might be able to identify a sample group of citizens who are representative of the entire population and poll them. Individual humans are one type of units. In other studies, the units could be bacteria, mice, families, schools, television shows, historical documents, websites, and so on. In research studies, samples are represented as "n."

Data Sampling Methods and Types of Samples

Data sampling methods and types of samples differ between the quantitative and qualitative approaches. Quantitative researchers try to obtain large unbiased samples that they have *randomly* identified. Their goal is that the sample is representative of the target population. Qualitative researchers focus on small sample sizes that they have *purposefully* identified to provide them with rich data. Their goal is that the sample explains the research question through either unusual cases or typical cases.

Sampling is the process of selecting the units to represent the target population. The **sampling frame** is the list of subjects from which the sample is drawn (Dillman et al. 2014, 3). Quantitative researchers should ensure that the list is representative of all the elements of the target population. Coverage errors and sampling errors are two types of errors that may occur in sampling.

A **coverage error** occurs when elements of the population are missing from the sampling frame, creating a systematic (nonrandom) discrepancy between the target population and the sampling frame (Dillman et al. 2014, 3). For example, in a quantitative study of a healthcare organization's patients' interest in using an electronic personal health record, a coverage error could occur if the researchers only surveyed patients who accessed the healthcare organization's patient portal while excluding patients who had *not* accessed the patient portal, but who *are* part of the healthcare organization's patient population. To avoid a coverage error, quantitative researchers may want to examine other researchers' published studies to learn how those researchers successfully determined their sampling frame.

A **sampling error** is a difference between the population and sample due to pure chance. If several samples are drawn from the same population, there are random variations. These variations are sampling error. A sampling error reduces the reliability of the study (Alreck and Settle 2004, 59–60). One way to avoid a sampling error is to use a larger sample.

The two major methods of sampling reflect the differing goals of quantitative and qualitative researchers. Quantitative researchers use random sampling (except when they use a convenience sample); qualitative researchers use nonrandom sampling. The two types are described as follows:

- *Random sampling* is the unbiased selection of subjects from the population of interest. More specifically, random sampling is a method of selecting a sample from a target population in which all its members have an equal and independent chance of being selected for the research study. This method underpins many statistical tests that health informatics and HIM professionals encounter. To generate random samples, researchers can use either a feature of spreadsheet applications called the *random number generator,* an option of statistical packages called *select cases,* or a table of random numbers from a basic statistics textbook. Four common types of random sampling are *simple random sampling*, *stratified random sampling, systematic sampling*, and *cluster sampling.* Table 11.7 provides descriptions of these types of random sampling. Researchers using these methods attempt to make the random sample as representative of the population as possible. Researchers document their sample selection procedures so that they be explained in the methods section of their study in such detail that other researchers can replicate their procedures.
- **Nonrandom (nonprobability) sampling** does not use statistical methods of probability to select samples, and all members of the target population do *not* have an equal and independent chance of being selected for the research study. Five common types of nonrandom sampling are *convenience sampling,* **purposive sampling**, **snowball sampling**, **quota sampling**, and **theoretical sampling**. Table 11.7 provides descriptions of these types of nonrandom sampling. Qualitative researchers record, describe, and justify their procedures and decisions in selecting their nonrandom samples because other researchers should be able to replicate their process.

Table 11.7 Types of random and nonrandom sampling

Type of Sampling	Description
Random sampling	
Simple	The selection of units from a population gives every unit exactly the same chance of being included in the sample. When a unit has been selected, it is returned to the population so that the other units' chances remain identical (for example, in population of 500, each unit has a 1 in 500 chance of being selected).
Stratified	The selection of units from a population proportionally mirrors characteristics that divide the population. For example, the human population includes males and females. The male and female subgroups are called *strata* (singular, *stratum*). The percentage of the stratum in the sample should equal the percentage of the stratum in the population. Therefore, if the population were equally divided among the genders, the sample should be 50 percent male and 50 percent female. Other percentages would cast doubt on the results.
Systematic	Units of the sample are selected from a list by drawing every *n*th unit. For example, health informatics and HIM professionals could choose every fourth surgery on the surgical schedule for surgical case review.
Cluster	The sample is clusters of units. The population is first divided into clusters of units, such as family, school, or community, and then clusters are randomly sampled.
Nonrandom sampling	
Convenience	The sample is opportunistically selected from easily recruited and accessible subjects. Also known as an *accidental sample,* its use diminishes the generalizability and credibility of the research.
Purposive	Qualitative researchers use their expertise to select both representative units and unrepresentative units of the population.
Snowball	Initial contacts (units) suggest additional contacts who also could be informative. Snowball sampling is also called *chain* or *nominated sampling*.

(*Continued*)

Table 11.7 (*Continued*)

Type of Sampling	Description
Quota	Subjects are selected to ensure proportionate representation of various strata present in the population. This method increases the study's representativeness.
Theoretical	Subjects are selected as topics emerge to ensure representation of those topics and to build theory.

Source: Adapted from Forrestal 2016, 593.

Sample Size

Sample size is the number of subjects the researcher determines should be included in the study in order to represent the population. If statistical tests are planned, the sample size must be large enough to support them and detect statistical significance (Farrokhyar et al. 2013, 207, 209) (see chapter 9 about statistical tests and chapter 12 about statistical significance). This section builds upon the discussion in chapter 2 of sample size in survey research, because sample size is also a concern in other research methods.

Sample Size Calculation

Sample size calculation refers to the quantitative and qualitative procedures used to estimate the appropriate sample size (Hayat 2013, 945–946). Prior to estimating the appropriate sample size, researchers collect and consider the available quantitative and qualitative information about the study's purpose, the statistical tests to be used, and the target population and make initial decisions. It must be emphasized that sample size calculation is a "best guess" and never an absolute rule (Farrokhyar et al. 2013, 210).

First, the researchers review their purpose. If a researcher's purpose is to explore clinicians' views of a proposed minor change in an application's graphic user interface, 30 randomly selected clinicians at a one academic health center may be sufficient. However, a study comparing the efficacy of various treatment protocols for breast cancer warrants a sample size in the thousands. Moreover, research that involves many variables also needs larger sample sizes. Generally, the higher the stakes, such as misdiagnosis or potential harms to users, the larger the sample should be.

Researchers also take into account the relationships among their desired level of significance, power, effect size (degree of change), statistical test, and sample size (Hayat 2013, 944). The seriousness of committing a type I or type II error is also considered. These concepts are explained in chapter 12.

Researchers obtain demographic information or a profile of the target population. If subgroups exist in the target population, the proportions of the subgroups are obtained. For example, in a survey of administrative leaders about the use of a health information system, some members of the target population may be chief information officers (CIOs) and other members may be chief financial officers (CFOs). The proportion of each subgroup is determined so that the sample for each subgroup is adequate and proportionally correct.

Other information that researchers consider includes the population's heterogeneity and its typical response and attrition rates (Brink et al. 2006, 137). **Heterogeneity** means variation or diversity. The more heterogeneous a population, the larger the sample needs to be to ensure that it includes all the diverse units in the population. Similarly, the sample size increases as the response rate declines or the attrition rate rises. Researchers also consider ethics. It is unethical to expose more participants to potential risks than is necessary. On the other hand, it is also unethical to expose *any* participants to risk if the study has too few participants to attain results with practical and statistical significance (Hayat 2013, 945). Finally, the size of the sample should be economical, providing the level of detail needed to answer the question, but not wasting time, money, and resources through excessive numbers of participants (Noordzij et al. 2010, 1388; Brink et al. 2006, 137).

Statistical formulas are used to calculate adequate sample sizes. Formulas depend on the sampling method used, such as simple random sampling or stratified random sample, and on the amount of information the researcher has about the population. Software packages and online calculators available to assist researchers include OpenEpi (2013), PASS (NCSS Statistical Software 2015), PowerandSampleSize.com (HyLown Consulting LLC 2016), RAT-STATS (OIG 2015), and PS: Power and Size Calculation (DuPont and Plummer 2014).

One commonly used formula for determining optimal sample size requires that the researcher know or decide on the size of the population, the proportion of subjects needed, and an acceptable amount of error. The formula results in the necessary number of responses from or observations of the sample. This number must be adjusted by the target audience's typical response rate or attrition rate to arrive at the number of instruments to be distributed or observations made.

The following example illustrates use of this formula for arriving at the sample size for a simple random sample. Figure 11.6 shows each calculation for the example. (Refer to chapter 2 for the calculation for arriving at the sample size for a stratified random sample.) Suppose a research team at a health center wants to determine the sample size for a study on clinicians' opinions of a feature of the center's clinical decision support system. The investigative team knows that the number of clinicians is 800 but has little other information about the population's characteristics. Having no other specific data, the general convention is to select p = 0.5 (where p is the proportion of subjects needed) and B = 0.05 (where B is the acceptable amount of error). Using the basic formula, the team members calculate that in this situation a sample of 267 is needed if they are willing to accept 5 percent error due to variability in the sampling. Finally, the team determines the number of surveys to distribute by multiplying the sample size by the typical response rate. Thus, if 50 percent of the clinicians typically respond to surveys, the team must double the sample and distribute 534 surveys for the opinion study.

Figure 11.6 Basic example of sample size calculation

Elements of the formula
Sample size = n
Size of population = N
Proportion of subjects needed = p
Acceptable amount of error = B

Data from the case
N = 800
p = 0.5
B = 0.05

Formula

$$n = \frac{Np(1-p)}{(N-1)\frac{(B2)}{4} + (p)(1-p)}$$

Calculations

$$n = \frac{(800)(0.5)(1.0-0.5)}{(800-1)\frac{(0.52)}{4} + (0.5)(1.0-0.5)}$$

$$n = \frac{200}{(799)(0.000625) + 0.25}$$

$$n = \frac{200}{0.75}$$

n = 267

Source: Forrestal 2016, p. 594.

Response Rate

Response rate is a critical issue for surveys and interviews. *Response rate* is the number of people who complete the survey or are interviewed divided by the total number of people in the sample. (See chapter 2 for more information on response rate.) There are two considerations related to response rate: overall numbers and response bias (also known as *nonresponse bias*). Low response rates and biased responses are threats to internal validity.

Ensuring an adequate response rate is of particular concern for surveys. Researchers review the literature for the response rates of their intended audience, factors affecting response rates, and successful strategies. To maximize the response rate, it is recommended that researchers use a mixed-mode approach that contacts participants in multiple ways (for example, postal paper questionnaires, telephone interviews, web-based surveys, and other contact mechanisms) and allows them to respond in the mode of their choice (Dillman et al. 2014, 14). In one study, researchers used an approach for a survey that combined postal letters and e-mails, provided paper and web-based questionnaires, and offered a $2.00 incentive, and achieved a 63 percent response rate within 10 days and a 77 percent response rate within 2 months when data collection ended (Dillman et al. 2014, 22–23).

Researchers also are on guard for bias in response. **Response bias** is when there is a systematic difference, such as computer-savviness or age, between the responders (participants) and nonresponders (nonparticipants). The characteristics of volunteers for a study may also differ from those of nonvolunteers. To prevent response bias, researchers seek to establish the similarity of both responders and nonresponders to the population (see chapter 2 for more information).

Data Collection Procedures

As has been discussed, data collection procedures differ between quantitative and qualitative studies, but the two types have some procedures in common. This section discusses procedures related to data collection that are common to both quantitative and qualitative researchers.

Approvals of Oversight Committees

In the United States, federal regulations govern research on human subjects. The purpose of the regulations is to protect humans from researchers' abuses. To comply with federal regulations, organizations have IRBs (also referred to as *human subjects committees*), which are administrative bodies established to protect the rights and welfare of human subjects recruited to participate in an institution's research activities. IRBs provide oversight for the research studies conducted within their institutions. As specified by both federal regulations and institutional policies, IRBs have the authority to review and approve or reject research studies within their jurisdictions. They also may require modifications to the research protocols.

Prior to conducting studies, researchers must obtain written approvals from the IRB and other oversight entities of their organizations. To obtain approvals, researchers complete the organization's documentation, providing descriptions of their research plan and copies of their informed consent forms. (See chapter 14 for a complete discussion of IRBs.) Researchers must allow sufficient time in their plan for the IRB to review the intended research, meet, and respond.

Training and Testing

Training of investigators and testing of research instruments help ensure that reliable data are collected. Researchers and their assistants (if any) may require special training. For example, publishers of some psychological tests require verification that the researchers and their assistants have had the specialized training on the tests in order to administer the tests. The researchers must obtain this verification (or select another instrument). To effectively conduct interviews or to observe vignettes, researchers and their assistants also need training. If the research requires that instruments be scored, training on scoring also should occur.

Researchers and their assistants also test the data collection instruments before collecting real data. Such tests identify ambiguous instructions and inconsistent definitions. Also, if the scoring for the instrument is done by a computerized scoring algorithm, the algorithm is checked to ensure that it is functioning properly.

Pilot Study

A *pilot study* is a trial run of the data collection and scoring procedures (chapter 2 provides more information about pilot studies for surveys). Pilot studies obtain valuable information for researchers as follows:

- *Confirmation of details*—for example, volumes of materials or numbers of study assistants needed, costs, and likely response rates
- *Detection of potential problems*—for example, biases in sample selection; flawed performance of equipment, hardware, software, or the website; poorly worded instructions, unclear questionnaire items, and leading questions in interviews; log jams (gridlock) in the distribution method; errors in the scoring key; and discrepancies between the order of items on the data collection instrument and the order on the data entry screen

Conducting a pilot study allows researchers to work out the logistical details of their data collection plan and enhances the likelihood of the research's successful completion.

Assembling and Storing Data

Researchers include a mechanism in the research plan for assembling their data and preparing them for analysis. Depending upon the research method used, procedures should be in place for transcribing interviews, data entry, scoring, and quality checks on data entry. The plan also addresses how the researchers will safeguard the confidentiality of their data. If videotapes are involved, where will they be stored? Because sensitive data may be on personality tests, where will these documents be stored and how will they be secured? How will the confidentiality of data on computer hard drives, laptops, external storage devices, and websites be ensured? In accordance with the rules of applicable oversight entities, the plan also must include a mechanism for disposition of the data (storage, archiving, and destruction) after the termination of the research.

Review Questions

1. Review the research designs and research methods in chapters 1 through 8. Which research design would a researcher select if the researcher wanted to identify and describe factors associated with high patient engagement and use of a healthcare organization's patient portals? Explain your rationale.
2. A health center implemented a new concierge service that offered assistance in parking and transportation and information on nonclinical issues. The health center had reviewed concierge service models from other organizations, but it had not specifically explored its own patients' views on this type of service prior to implementation. With so little information, which data collection technique would researchers choose to investigate patients' views of this new service?
3. A student research team wants to work with the university's librarians on a quantitative project that investigates users' satisfaction with a library interface. What should be the team's first step in the data collection process? What does this step involve and why is it important?
4. What are at least three instruments that researchers could use to investigate patients' views of a healthcare organization's patient portal?
5. What are the types of validity related to instruments? Provide a definition for each type.
6. What are the aspects of instrument reliability and how are they assessed?
7. What type of question do researchers use when they conduct a focus group and allow the participants to engage in a free-flowing conversation? What is an advantage of this type of question?
8. Two members of a student research team want to skip the pilot study and "just get to it." They explain that team is already running behind in its timeline for this research project and skipping the pilot study will get the team back on schedule. How should you and the other team members respond?
9. What is the difference between a coverage error and a sampling error?
10. What are four types of random sampling and five types of nonrandom sampling? How are all the types defined? Which type of sampling and sampling type would a quantitative researcher choose when the population is characterized by three subgroups?

Application Exercises

1. Patient-reported outcome measures (PROMs or PROs), also known as patient-reported experience measures (PREMs) are becoming increasingly important in healthcare. PROMs can be collected in symptom and quality of life information (SQLI) systems.

   In the past, most information collected about patient outcomes reflected the providers' views of their patients' outcomes. Today, CMS and other payers are also interested in their beneficiaries' or members' perspectives. For example, the CMS has implemented a Health Outcomes Survey (HOS), the first patient-reported outcome measure used in Medicare managed care. The purpose of the HOS is "to gather valid, reliable, and clinically meaningful health status data from the Medicare Advantage (MA) program to use in quality improvement activities, pay for performance, program oversight, public reporting, and to improve health" (CMS 2016b).

   Health informatics researchers and clinicians have developed online tools to collect PROM data. Obtain the article "Patient-reported outcome measures: An on-line system empowering patient choice" (Wilson et al. 2014).

What operational definition of PROMs do the article's authors use? What is the source of this operational definition? What is the Oxford shoulder scale (OSS), and why did the researchers use it?

2. This application exercise gives you the opportunity to apply terms related to survey research. Obtain the articles "Effect of tele-emergency services on recruitment and retention of US rural physicians" (Potter et al. 2014) and "Perceptions of the benefits of telemedicine in rural communities" (Potter et al. 2016).
   a. Review the Tele-emergency Survey Instrument in the Appendix 1 of the 2014 article. What type of questions are items numbers 3 through 7? How many points does the scale have?
   b. Per the 2016 article, when was the survey administered? In total, how many staff members responded to the survey? In total, how many hospitals did the staff-member respondents represent?
   c. Read the 2014 article. What is the research question? How many respondents were there, and how many hospitals did the respondents represent? How many surveys did Potter and colleagues conduct?
   d. Consider the following statement in the 2016 article: "This study employed mixed methods to identify ways communities may change when a rural hospital adopts telemedicine services." What does "mixed methods" mean? Who would you expect to be interviewed or surveyed based on the statement? What recommendation related to the community do the researchers make?
3. Obtain the article "Use of electronic health record documentation by healthcare workers in an acute care hospital system" (Penoyer et al. 2014) through your university's library (it is only available through a library license): After reading the article, answer the following questions:
   a. How was the survey administered?
   b. What type of sample did the researchers use?
   c. What is face validity and how did the researchers assess it? What other aspects of the instrument did they have their evaluators assess?
   d. What limitations of the study did the researchers report? Does the study have external validity? Why or why not?
   e. The researchers used a convenience sample and face validity. Considering those two aspects of the study, how could the researchers increase the rigor of their research in a subsequent study?

References

Agency for Healthcare Research and Quality (AHRQ). 2017. Health IT Survey Compendium. Accessed January 10, 2017. https://healthit.ahrq.gov/health-it-tools-and-resources/health-it-survey-compendium.

Alreck, P.L., and R.B. Settle. 2004. *The Survey Research Handbook,* 3rd ed. New York: McGraw-Hill/Irwin.

Behavioral Measurement Database Services (BMDS). 2015. HaPI (Health and Psychosocial Instruments). http://bmdshapi.com/.

Brink, H., C. van der Walt, and G.van Rensburg. 2006. *Fundamentals of Research Methodology for Health Care Professionals*, 2nd ed. Cape Town, South Africa: Juta Press.

Brooke, J. 2013. SUS: A retrospective. *Journal of Usability Studies* 8(2):29–40.

Brooke, J. 1986. SUS: A quick and dirty usability scale. Available for download in references for Usability.gov. System Usability Scale. http://www.usability.gov/how-to-and-tools/methods/system-usability-scale.html.

Buros Center for Testing. 2016. Test Reviews and Information. http://buros.org.

Carter, S.R. 2016. Using confirmatory factor analysis to manage discriminant validity issues in social pharmacy research. *International Journal of Clinical Pharmacy* 38(3):731–737.

Centers for Medicare and Medicaid Services (CMS). 2016a. CMS Quality Strategy 2016. https://www.cms.gov/medicare/quality-initiatives-patient-assessment-instruments/qualityinitiativesgeninfo/downloads/cms-quality-strategy.pdf

Centers for Medicare and Medicaid Services (CMS). 2016b (June 27). Health Outcomes Survey (HOS). https://www.cms.gov/Research-Statistics-Data-and-Systems/Research/HOS/index.html?redirect=/hos.

Dillman, D.A., J.D. Smyth, and L.M. Christian. 2014. *Internet, Phone, Mail, and Mixed-Mode Surveys: The Tailored Design Method, 4th* ed. Hoboken, NJ: John Wiley & Sons.

Dowding, M. 2016 (February 10). The role of IT in population health management. *Leadership* +. Healthcare Financial Management Association. http://www.hfma.org/Leadership/PopulationHealthIT.

DuPont, W.D. and WD. Plummer, Jr. 2014. PS: Power and Sample Size Calculation version 3.1.2. Department of Biostatistics, Vanderbilt University. http://biostat.mc.vanderbilt.edu/wiki/Main/PowerSampleSize.

Farrokhyar, F., D. Reddy, R.W. Poolman, and M. Bhandari. 2013. Why perform a priori sample size calculation? *Canadian Journal of Surgery* 56(3):207–213.

Federal Aviation Administration (FAA). 2017. Human Factors: Workbench Tools. Accessed January 10, 2017. http://www.hf.faa.gov/workbenchtools/default.aspx.

Fenton, S.H., E. Joost, J. Gongora, D.G. Patterson, C.H.A. Andrilla, and S.M. Skillman. 2013. Health information technology employer needs survey: An assessment instrument for HIT workforce planning. *Educational Perspectives in Health Informatics and Information Management*: 1–36.

Forrestal, E. 2016. Research methods. Chapter 19 in *Health Information Management: Concepts, Principles, and Practice*, 5th ed. Edited by P.K. Oachs and A.L. Watters. Chicago: AHIMA Press.

Gavrilova, T., and T. Andreeva. 2012. Knowledge elicitation techniques in a knowledge management context. *Journal of Knowledge Management* 16(4):523–537.

Glenn, T. and S. Monteith. 2014. Privacy in the digital world: Medical and health data outside of HIPAA protections. *Current Psychiatry Rep*orts 16(11):1–11.

Goff, S.L., R. Kleppel, P.K. Lindenauer, and M.B. Rothberg. 2013. Hospital workers; perceptions of waste: A qualitative study involving photo-elicitation. *BMJ Quality and Safety* 22(10):826–835.

Hayat, M.J. 2013. Understanding sample size determination in nursing research. *Western Journal of Nursing Research* 35(7):943–956.

Health Research and Educational Trust (HRET). 2015 (August). Approaches to Population Health in 2015: A National Survey of Hospitals. Chicago, IL: Health Research & Educational Trust. www.hpoe.org/pophealthsurvey.

Herling, R.W. 2000. Operational definitions of expertise and competence. *Advances in Developing Human Resources* 2(1):8–21.

HIMSS Analytics. 2015 (December 10). Essentials Brief: 2015 Population Health Study. http://www.himssanalytics.org/research/essentials-brief-2015-population-health-study.

Hopkins, W. 2014. A New View of Statistics. http://complementarytraining.net/wp-content/uploads/2013/10/Will-Hopkins-A-New-View-of-Statistics.pdf.

Huck, S.W. 2012. *Reading Statistics and Research,* 6th ed. Boston: Pearson.

HyLown Consulting LLC. 2016. Power and Sample Size.Com. http://powerandsamplesize.com.

Johnson, J.C. and S.C. Weller. 2001. Elicitation techniques for interviewing. Chapter 24 in *Handbook for Interview Research: Context and Method*. Edited by J.F. Gubrium and J.A. Holstein. Thousand Oaks, CA: Sage: 491–514.

Johnson, K.B., B.L. Patterson, Y.X. Ho, Q. Chen, H. Nian, C.L. Davison, J. Slagle, and S.A. Mulvaney. 2016. The feasibility of text reminders to improve medication adherence in adolescents with asthma. *Journal of the American Medical Informatics Association* 23(3):449–455.

Kaplan, R.M. M.L. Spittel, and D.H. David, eds. 2015. *Population Health: Behavioral and Social Science Insights.* Rockville, MD: Agency for Healthcare Research and Quality. http://www.ahrq.gov/professionals/education/curriculum-tools/population-health/index.html.

Kirakowski, J. 2017. What Is SUMI? Accessed January 10, 2017. http://sumi.uxp.ie/about/whatis.html.

Kirakowski, J. and M. Corbett. 1993. SUMI: The Software Usability Measurement Inventory. *British Journal of Educational Technology* 24(3):210–212.

Kuchinke, K.P. 1997. Employee expertise: The status of the theory and the literature. *Performance Improvement Quarterly* 10(4):72–86.

Landis, J.R. and G.G. Koch. 1977. The measurement of observer agreement for categorical data. *Biometrics* 33(1):159–174.

Lawshe, C.H. 1975. A quantitative approach to content validity. *Personnel Psychology* 28(4):563–575.

Lee, K.M., J. Lee, C.Y. Chung, S. Ahn, K.H. Sung, T.W. Kim, H. J. Lee, and M.S. Park. 2012. Pitfalls and important issues in testing reliability using intraclass correlation coefficients in orthopedic research. *Clinics in Orthopedic Surgery* 4(2):149–155.

Miles, M.B., A.M. Huberman, and J. Saldaña. 2014. *Qualitative Data Analysis: A Methods Sourcebook,* 3rd ed. Thousand Oaks, CA: Sage Publications.

Naidu, H. and A. Tiwari. 2014. Data mining and data warehousing. *International Journal of Engineering Sciences and Research Technology* 3(11):109–111.

National Institutes of Health (NIH). 2015 (April 8). Racial and Ethnic Categories and Definitions for NIH Diversity Programs and for Other Reporting Purposes. Notice Number: NOT-OD-15-089. http://grants.nih.gov/grants/guide/notice-files/NOT-OD-15-089.html.

NCSS Statistical Software. PASS [Power Analysis and Sample Size software]: Overview. 2015. http://www.ncss.com/software/pass.

Noordzij, M., G. Tripepi, F.W. Dekker, C. Zoccali, M.W. Tanck, and K.J. Jager. 2010. Sample size calculations: Basic principles and common pitfalls. *Nephrology Dialysis Transplantation* 25(10):1388–1393.

Office of Inspector General (OIG). 2015. RAT-STATS-Statistical Software. https://oig.hhs.gov/compliance/rat-stats.

OpenEpi. 2013 (April 6). http://www.openepi.com/Menu/OE_Menu.htm.

Polit, D.F. and C.T. Beck. 2006. The content validity index: Are you sure you know what's being reported? Critique and recommendations. *Research in Nursing and Health* 29(5):489–497.

Sandefer, R. and E.S. Karl. 2015. Ready or not: HIM is changing—results of the new HIM competencies survey show skill gaps between education levels, students, and working professionals. *Journal of the American Health Information Management Association* 86(3):24–27.

Schultze, U., and M. Avital. 2011. Designing interviews to generate rich data for information systems research. *Information and Organization* 21(1):1–16.

Scientific Advisory Committee of the Medical Outcomes Trust. 2002. Assessing health status and quality-of-life instruments: Attributes and review criteria. *Quality of Life Research* 11(3):193–205.

Tierney, M., A. Fraser, H. Purtill, and N. Kennedy. 2013. Study to determine the criterion validity of the SenseWear Armband as a measure of physical activity in people with rheumatoid arthritis. *Arthritis Care and Research* 65(6):888–895.

University of Maryland Laboratory for Automation Psychology and Decision Processes. 2015. Questionnaire for User Interaction Satisfaction (QUIS). http://www.lap.umd.edu/quis/.

US Department of Health and Human Services (HHS). 2016. System Usability Scale (SUS). https://www.usability.gov/how-to-and-tools/methods/system-usability-scale.html.

Wilson, F.R., W. Pan, and D.A. Schumsky. 2012(July). Recalculation of the critical values for Lawshe's content validity ratio. *Measurement and Evaluation in Counseling and Development* 45(3):197–210.

Xu, J., S.L. Murphy, K.D. Kochanek, and B.A. Bastian. 2016. Deaths: Final data for 2013. *National Vital Statistics Reports* 64(2): 1–16. http://www.cdc.gov/nchs/data/nvsr/nvsr64/nvsr64_02.pdf.

Resources

Carlson, K.D., and A.O. Herdman. 2012. Understanding the impact of convergent validity on research results. *Organizational Research Methods* 15(1):17–32.

Coiera, E. 2014. Communication spaces. *Journal of the American Medical Informatics Association* 21(3):414–422.

Gentles, S.J., C. Charles, J. Ploeg, and K.A. McKibbon. 2015. Sampling in qualitative research: Insights from an overview of the methods literature. *Qualitative Report* 20(11):1772–1789.

Grigore, B., J. Peters, C. Hyde, and K. Stein. 2013. Methods to elicit probability distributions from experts: A systematic review of reported practice in health technology assessment. *PharmacoEconomics* 31(11):355–369.

Knol, A.B., P. Slottje, J.P. van der Sluijs, and E. Lebret. 2010. The use of expert elicitation in environmental health impact assessment: A seven step procedure. *Environmental Health* 9(19):1–16.

Landers, R.N. 2015. Computing intraclass correlations (ICC) as estimates of interrater reliability in SPSS. *Winnower3*:e143518.81744. doi: 10.15200/winn.143518.81744. http://neoacademic.com/2011/11/16/computing-intraclass-correlations-icc-as-estimates-of-interrater-reliability-in-spss.

Maruyama, G. and C.S. Ryan. 2014. *Research Methods in Social Relations,* 8th ed. Chichester, UK: John Wiley & Sons.

McHugh, M.L. 2012. Interrater reliability: The kappa statistic. *Biochemia Medica* 22(3):276–282.

Penoyer, D.A., K.H. Cortelyou-Ward, A.M. Noblin, T. Bullard, S. Talbert, J. Wilson, B. Schafhauser, and J.G. Briscoe. 2014. Use of electronic health record documentation by healthcare workers in an acute care hospital system. *Journal of Healthcare Management* 59(2):130–144.

Polit, D.F. 2014. Getting serious about test-retest reliability: A critique of retest research and some recommendations. *Quality of Life Research* 23(6):1713–1720.

Potter, A.J., M.M. Ward, N. Natafgi, F. Ullrich, A.C. MacKinney, A.L. Bell, and K.J. Mueller. 2016 (Summer). Perceptions of the benefits of telemedicine in rural communities. *Perspectives in Health Information Management*:1-13. http://perspectives.ahima.org/perceptions-of-the-benefits-of-telemedicine-in-rural-communities.

Potter, A.J., K.J. Mueller, A.C MacKinney, and M.M. Ward. 2014. Effect of tele-emergency services on recruitment and retention of US rural physicians. *Rural and Remote Health* 14:2787. http://www.rrh.org.au/articles/subviewnew.asp?ArticleID=2787.

Shrout, P.E. and J.L. Fleiss. 1979. Intraclass correlations: Uses in assessing rater reliability. *Psychological Bulletin* 86(2):420–428.

Strauss, M.E. and G.T. Smith. 2009. Construct validity: Advances in theory and methodology. *Annual Review of Clinical Psychology* 5(1):1–25.

Wilson, J., F. Arshad, N. Nnamoko, A. Whiteman, J. Ring, and B. Roy. 2014. Patient-reported outcome measures: An on-line system empowering patient choice. *Journal of the American Medical Informatics Association* 21(4):725–729.

Wolpin, S.E., B. Halpenny, G. Whitman, J. McReynolds, M. Stewart, W.B. Lober, and D.L. Berry. 2015. Development and usability testing of a web-based cancer symptom and quality-of-life support intervention. *Health Informatics Journal* 21(1):10–23.

Zamanzadeh, V., A. Ghahramanian, M. Rassouli, A. Abbaszadeh, H. Alavi-Majd, and A. Nikanfar. 2015. Design and implementation content validity study: Development of an instrument for measuring patient-centered communication. *Journal of Caring Sciences* 4(2):165–178.

12 Analyzing Data and Presenting Results

Elizabeth J. Forrestal, PhD, RHIA, CCS, FAHIMA

Learning Objectives

- Analyze statistical data for decision making.
- Interpret descriptive and inferential statistics.
- Describe the use of quantitative and qualitative data in decision making.
- Present research results in formats consistent with recognized standards.
- Use key terms associated with analyzing data and presenting results appropriately.

Key Terms

Absolute risk (AR)
Absolute risk reduction (ARR)
Alpha level (α)
Area under the curve (AUC)
Beta (B)
Claim
Conclusion validity
Confidence interval (CI)
Confidence level
Data cleaning
Effect size
Imputation
Intention-to-treat (ITT) analysis
Likelihood ratio (LR)
Negative predictive value (NPV)
Null hypothesis significance testing (NHST)
Number needed to treat (NNT)
P value
Positive predictive value (PPV)
Power
Precision
Primary analysis
Primary data
Qualitative data analysis
Quantitative data analysis
Receiver operating characteristic (ROC) curve
Relative risk reduction (RRR)
Secondary analysis
Secondary data
Sensitivity
Significance level
Specificity
Statistical analysis plan (SAP)
Statistical conclusion validity
Supervised learning
Type I error
Type II error
Unit of analysis
Unsupervised learning
Warrant

Researchers inspect, dissect, and explore their data during data analysis. Through analysis, researchers transform their data into results. **Quantitative data analysis** examines, probes, and transforms large amounts of numerical data into understandable information through the application of descriptive statistics and inferential statistics. **Qualitative data analysis** is a systematic process of working with data to create coherent descriptions and explanations of phenomena (Miles et. al 2014, 10).

This chapter completes part II's exploration and study of the research process by presenting the fifth component, analyze data, and the sixth component, present results. Chapter 9 presented applied statistics that are found in general statistics books and are typically covered in freshman- or sophomore-year statistics courses. This chapter builds upon that foundation. It presents additional information about working with quantitative data and addresses specialized statistical techniques and terms often found in the health and health informatics and HIM literature.

The chapter begins with quantitative data analysis, then moves into qualitative data analysis. The chapter concludes with how to present and discuss results. For statistical formulas and computations or in-depth qualitative analytic practices, readers are advised to seek books specializing in those topics, some of which are listed in the resources section at the end of this chapter.

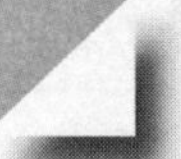

Real-World Case

Researchers at a consulting and analytic firm developed an approach for analyzing data from healthcare organizations (Korenda et al. 2015, 2). The researchers have suggested that this approach could eventually help healthcare organizations identify ways to improve care and to lower costs. This approach could be especially helpful to healthcare organizations that serve high-risk patient populations, such as dual-eligible beneficiaries.

Dual-eligible beneficiaries are Medicare beneficiaries whose low income also qualifies them for Medicaid. Dual-eligible beneficiaries often have multiple chronic conditions, significant disabilities, or both. They are among "the sickest and poorest individuals covered by either Medicare or Medicaid" (Musumeci 2015, 3). Consequently, their costs are higher than the costs of other patient populations. On average, Medicare fee-for-service per-capita spending is more than twice as high for dual-eligible beneficiaries than for non-dual-eligible beneficiaries (MEDPAC 2016, 35).

In their analysis, Korenda and colleagues combined claims data (medical and pharmacy data), sociodemographic data, and lifestyle data. The researchers

> *used data from the Medicare Current Beneficiary Survey (MCBS), an annual nationally representative survey of Medicare beneficiaries administered by the Center[s] for Medicare and Medicaid Services. This survey provides detailed information on healthcare insurance coverage, spending by payment source (Medicare, Medicaid, private insurance, and out-of-pocket spending), and the use of prescription drugs and long-term care services, as well as information on a rich set of socioeconomic and demographic characteristics, such as marital status, living arrangements, education, and income level. It also provides information on survey participants' Medicare claims. (Korenda et al. 2015, 4)*

The data set included MCBS records for 15,573 individuals, with 19 percent of the sample identified as dual-eligible beneficiaries.

Using cluster analysis, the researchers segmented the data set into five groups based on similarities and differences in demographics (age, marital status) and health status (body mass index, depression, year-over-year change in health status). These five groups were "Older and likely to be widowed," "Young and disabled," "Older and overweight," "Older and healthy weight," and "The survivors." The researchers presented descriptive statistics on each segment. For each segment, the table displayed percentages for sociodemographics, lifestyle variables, health conditions, and healthcare costs. Each segment contained about 20 percent dual-eligible beneficiaries, except for the "young and disabled" segment that had 71 percent dual-eligible beneficiaries. (Note: Some people younger than 65 years, the usual eligibility age for Medicare, are eligible for Medicare; for example, patients of any age with end-stage renal disease may be eligible.)

Using logistic regression, the researchers identified variables that differentiated dual-eligible beneficiaries from non-dual-eligible beneficiaries. Separate regressions were performed on the entire data set and on each of the five segments. The regression results were given as odds ratios. For example, in the segment "Older and likely to be widowed," the odds ratios for "has difficulty eating solid foods because of dental problems" and "tooth loss" were 4.02 and 3.26, respectively. In contrast, no variables related to dental issues were identified for the segment "older and overweight."

Based on their analysis, the researchers stated three take-aways for healthcare organizations:

- Segmenting a data set is helpful because conducting separate regressions on the five segments identified variables associated with dual eligibility that were masked when the entire data set was analyzed. Over half of the variables associated with dual eligibility would have been missed had the researchers only analyzed the entire data set.
- Analyzing claims data only is insufficient because many variables associated with dual eligibility came from the MCBS and are not contained in claims data.
- Creating segments of a patient population gives healthcare organizations accurate, actionable information about subpopulations such as dual-eligible beneficiaries. Having knowledge of these segments of patient populations and the variables associated with those segments allows healthcare organizations to identify high-risk groups or other groups of interest and to design interventions specific to their needs.

The optimal interventions identified in this research have the potential to improve health and reduce costs (Sanky et al. 2012, 221). For example, consider the segment "Older and likely to be widowed" that has dental issues. These dental issues may result in poorer health because of poor nutrition that results from not being able to eat properly. Toward this segment, a healthcare organization could target a dental health initiative. The "Older and overweight" subpopulation could be omitted from this initiative because dental health was not identified as associated with dual eligibility for this segment. For both segments, however, healthy eating is an issue; therefore, both segments could be targeted for a healthy eating initiative.

Quantitative Data Analysis

Research data can be subjected to more than one statistical test or technique. Descriptive statistics and tabular and graphical displays explore and describe the data. Inferential statistics are performed to make predictions and test hypotheses. Researchers maximize the use of their data by using a variety of statistical tests and techniques to analyze different aspects of their data. Quantitative data analysis is a broad topic and encompasses many concepts, including the statistical analysis plan, statistical significance versus practical significance, null hypothesis testing and significance level, power, type I and type II errors, preparing data for analysis, descriptive statistics, inferential statistics, data analysis in data mining, statistical conclusion validity, and quantitative analytic software programs.

Statistical Analysis Plan

A **statistical analysis plan (SAP)** is a document that contains technical and detailed descriptions of the statistical analyses that will be performed on a research study's variables and other data (FDA 1998, 43). Quantitative researchers develop their SAP as part of their overall plan for the research study. The purpose of the SAP is to determine whether the data collection strategies will obtain all the necessary data for the planned statistical tests. Additionally, in the study's overall planning, the SAP is important because the types of statistical tests affect decisions about the sample size and about the specific data to be collected. The plan should also take into account that data analysis is time-intensive and ensure that sufficient time is allocated to analyze the data. This section describes the listings of all the planned statistical tests and data elements.

Listing of Statistical Tests

In the SAP, researchers determine which statistical tests they will perform on their data. Researchers decide these tests based on their research question, hypotheses, and the literature. The literature presents accepted statistical tests that other researchers have used to analyze similar data. The literature also includes critiques of analytic approaches. Researchers should inspect these critiques for ways to use the criticisms to improve their own study. In the plan, the researchers also establish the criteria to determine significance. *Significance* is the conclusion that the effect was *not* just a random chance or a fluke but is something that is real. The criteria are values, typically 0.05 or 0.01. The statistical tests and the criteria for significance are determined *before* any data collection. Researchers may also want to have a statistician review the SAP to check for any oversights.

Researchers describe the statistical tests in the methods section of scholarly papers. The descriptions of the tests and decisions should be precise and clear so that other researchers can replicate the procedures using similar data.

Listing of Data Elements

The SAP lists each data element required for each planned statistical test for each hypothesis. A table is a useful tool for this part of the analytic plan. One column is the hypothesis; each row in this column is a hypothesis (alternative and null). The next column is the relevant variables or factors; each row in this column is the variables or factors relating to that row's hypothesis (immediately to the left). The third column is the statistical tests; the row is the specific statistical test which will use the variables or factors immediately to the left to test that row's hypothesis (Thompson 2009, 56). Other tactics are to conduct mock statistical analyses on fabricated data and create empty shells for the manuscript's tables and figures early in the planning of the research (Thomas and Peterson 2012, 774). This planning process attempts to ensure that the researcher collects all necessary data during data collection and avoids discovering during analysis that critical data items are missing.

In addition to the data directly relevant to their research question, researchers typically collect sociodemographic data, such as sex, age, race, and income level, about the participants. Also collected are data that allow the researchers to compare their participants (subjects or responders) to known characteristics of the entire population of interest. These known characteristics could be credentials, professional titles, work settings, geographic locations, and other relevant factors.

This comparison attempts to verify that the study's participants are representative of the target population; thus, supporting the general soundness of inferences and conclusions about the population. Researchers also include the study's unit of analysis and their plan for data preparation in the SAP.

Statistical Significance Versus Practical Significance

Researchers use the word *significance* in two ways. First, there is *statistical significance,* which is related to significance testing determined from statistical tests. This meaning indicates that the association or difference is actual, and not a random chance. Statistical significance is based on calculations. The size of the sample is an element in the calculation. A very large sample can create statistical significance just by its sheer size. Conversely, a very small sample can mask statistical significance just because the numbers are so small.

Second, there is *significance* that relates to the importance of the finding and whether the association or difference can or should affect decisions, practices, or policies. This *practical significance* may be signified by the use of the word *significance* alone or by the phrase, *clinical significance*. The word significance alone is the common, dictionary definition of the word as importance or meaningfulness. To show practical significance, researchers include the effect size which is the magnitude of the difference or relationship between the variables (effect size is discussed later in this chapter).

Researchers are careful in their use of these terms because statistical significance does *not* guarantee practical or clinical significance. Statistically significant findings can be trivial. For example, researchers studying a managerial decision support system could find that an improved algorithm increased the speed of calculating staffing needs by a statistically significant 0.5 second. While statistically significant, managers are not likely to purchase a new decision support system for staffing based on half a second. However, in research on collision avoidance systems, 1 second can make the difference between a near-crash and a crash; 0.5 second would be both statistically significant and practically significant.

Null Hypothesis Significance Testing and Significance Level

The purpose of **null hypothesis significance testing (NHST)** is to determine the likelihood that the research study's findings are *not* the result of random chance or a biased sample. NHST is also known as *statistical significance testing (SST), hypothesis testing, null hypothesis testing,* and *significance testing*. Many statistical tests are used in NHST, including the *Z*-test as well as many of the statistical tests described in chapter 9, such as the independent one-sample *t*-test, the independent-measures *t*-test, the chi-square test, and the analysis of variance (ANOVA). As discussed in chapter 9, selection of the specific statistical test depends on various factors, such as the purpose of the research, the level of the data, the nature of the target population, and other factors.

Typically, NHST is applied to the null hypothesis, as its name implies. NHST analyzes the study's data to obtain the probability value and then compares that probability to a pre-established significance level (Barry 2013, 140–141). This comparison establishes whether the study's findings are statistically significant. With NHST, researchers determine whether results are due solely to random chance. If results are not due solely to random chance, the null hypothesis is rejected in favor of the alternative hypothesis. (See chapter 9 for more information on null and alternative hypotheses.)

A **significance level** is a pre-established threshold that determines whether the null hypothesis is rejected. The significance level is also known as the **alpha level** (α). The significance level is established prior to conducting any statistical tests. The alpha level is set at a probability level, such as 0.001, 0.01, or 0.05. A probability of 0.001 is more stringent (lower) than a probability of 0.01. Common alpha levels are 0.05 and 0.01. Researchers set the lower alpha level when they want to minimize the chance that they might erroneously reject the null hypothesis when it is actually true (see discussion of type I error later in this chapter). Moreover, the more severe the consequences of being wrong about the findings, the more stringent (lower) the probability is set. For example, in studies related to detecting differences between students' test performance, the probability may be set at 0.05. However, in studies analyzing results on HIV, the probability is set more stringently at 0.001.

Statistical tests for significance result in a *P* value. A ***P* value** is a statistical summary of the compatibility between the observed data and what would be predicted or expected if all the assumptions, such as normal distribution, used to compute the *P* value were correct. The *P* value, then, is the probability that the chosen test statistic will fall within a range of specific values (Greenland et al. 2016, 339). Therefore, if the calculated *P* value is 0.05 or less, the null hypothesis is rejected and if the calculated *P* value is 0.051 or more, the null hypothesis cannot be rejected.

P values are often misunderstood and misused (Greenland et al. 2016, 338). As a result, research methodologists and biostatisticians recommend that researchers examine confidence intervals and effect sizes (discussed later in the chapter), as well as providing the exact *P* value, not just whether it was above or below the threshold. Additionally, these experts recommend that researchers examine assumptions they have made. These assumptions include statistical assumptions and assumptions in the research protocol and data collection (Greenland et al. 2016, 340). Generally, in using *P* values, researchers need to be aware that *P* values do *not* measure whether a hypothesis is true or the importance of a study's results. Moreover, practitioners and policymakers reading *P* values in a published study need to be aware that *P* values should not be the *sole* basis of business decisions or policies (Wasserstein and Lazar 2016, 131–132).

Power

Power is the probability of identifying real differences or relationships between groups. Specifically, power is the likelihood of failing to reject a false null hypothesis. When researchers fail to reject a false null hypothesis, the researchers have wrongly determined that there is no difference or relationship when, in fact, there is. Power is usually set at 0.80 or higher (Barry 2013, 242). If power is set at 0.80, there is a 20 percent chance that the researcher will wrongly determine that no difference or relationship exists in the results, when there actually is a difference or relationship. For example, the researcher could falsely state that a training workshop made no difference in the use of the decision support system, when in fact the training workshop *did* make a difference. The cutoff set for power depends on the research. Power is less stringent than significance level because failing to assert a difference or relationship has fewer ramifications for researchers and the general public than falsely asserting a difference or relationship when none really exists.

Type I Error and Type II Error

Researchers can make two types of errors associated with null hypothesis significance testing. A **type I error** occurs when the researcher erroneously rejects the null hypothesis when it is true; in actuality, there is no difference or relationship. A **type II error** occurs when the researcher erroneously fails to reject the null hypothesis when it is false; in actuality, there is a difference. For example, let us consider the following hypotheses:

- Null hypothesis: There is no difference in the mean times to triage health maintenance organization (HMO) patients on the medical help line between the nurses who participate in a three-hour workshop on the clinical diagnostic decision support system and the nurses who do not participate in the workshop.
- Alternative hypothesis (one-tailed): The mean time to triage HMO patients on the medical help line will be less for nurses who participate in a three-hour workshop on the clinical diagnostic decision support system than for nurses who do not participate in the workshop.

A researcher committing a type I error would reject the null hypothesis when the null hypothesis is true—there is no difference or relationship. This error is a false positive because the researcher incorrectly reports that there is a difference in the performance of the two groups. Continuing in the error, he or she would report that the workshop reduced the nurses' triage time. However, there is no difference between the two groups' performance; the three-hour workshop does not affect performance. Alpha levels are associated with type I errors. Researchers who set the alpha level at 0.05 have a 5 percent chance of making this error, whereas those who set the alpha level at 0.01 have a 1 percent chance of making the error.

Power is associated with type II errors. In the previous example, the researcher would make a type II error if he or she failed to reject the null hypothesis and it was indeed false. This error is a false negative because the researcher erroneously reports that there was no difference between the performance of the nurses who participated in the workshop and the nurses who did not participate. In fact, there was a difference, and the workshop did reduce the triage time, as predicted. **Beta (B)** designates the probability of making a type II error because power is 1.0 – B. For a power of 0.80, B is set at 0.20; the researcher has a 20 percent chance of failing to reject the null hypothesis when an association or difference actually exists.

Researchers use prescribed language when reporting the results of NHST. Researchers may only state "reject the null" or "fail to reject the null." Researchers cannot write "accept the alternate hypothesis" or "accept the null hypothesis." The reasoning of NHST is similar to the courtroom. In the courtroom, there are only two choices: "guilty" or "not guilty." A verdict is announced as "not guilty" because there was insufficient evidence to prove guilt beyond a reasonable doubt. There is no verdict of "innocent" because the only choices are "guilty" or "not guilty" (Motulsky 2014, 137–138).

Preparation of Data

"Garbage in, garbage out," a commonly used phrase on how computers work, also applies to research. The quality of study results depends upon the quality of its data. Data must be prepared prior to analysis because many different types of errors may occur during data collection and data entry. Preparation minimizes the effects of these errors on their studies' results.

Data preparation begins with the data collection plan. The data collection plan could, for example, include procedures that validate data as they are collected or are being entered into the study's database. Electronic systems can place limits on data types, such as requiring numerical characters. These limits prevent the entry of alphabetical characters and symbols. Logic checks that verify the validity of dates, such as no future dates or dates before the year 1880, could also be in place.

Data preparation continues when data are assembled. Depending on the research method, procedures should be in place for transcribing interviews, data entry, scoring, and quality checks on data entry. Other activities that are performed as part of data preparation and that are discussed in this section are selecting a unit of analysis, intention-to-treat analysis, addressing missing values, and data cleaning.

Selecting the Unit of Analysis

A **unit of analysis** is the group, object, or phenomenon for which the researchers have collected data to analyze. The unit of analysis is the focus of the study. The unit of analysis should match the unit of randomization. If individual patients from several group-physician practices were randomly assigned to arms of a study, then the individual patients' responses should be analyzed. If the group-physician practices were randomly assigned to arms of a study, then the practices' scores are analyzed. Selecting the correct unit of analysis increases the likelihood that the study's results will be accurate. Explicitly stating the unit of analysis in the research plan may help researchers avoid a unit of analysis error.

The unit of analysis is often confused in research papers. As discussed in chapter 9, a unit of analysis error is a misuse of statistics. Consequences of unit of analysis errors include type I errors and misleading conclusions (Sedgwick 2014, 1).

Intention-to-Treat Analysis

Intention-to-treat (ITT) analysis is defined as the principle in which subjects of a randomized controlled trial (RCT) are analyzed within the group to which they were originally allocated with no regard to noncompliance or deviations from the protocol (Alshurafa et al. 2012, 1). The purpose of ITT analysis is to minimize bias, maintain the effects of randomization, and reliably indicate the effects of treatments. For example, ITT analysis continues to count subjects in the groups to which they were originally assigned even if they drop out, are lost to follow-up, or switch groups. ITT analysis results in an accurate, although potentially conservative, reflection of the effectiveness of treatment. ITT analysis is recommended by research methodologists, statisticians, and the US Food and Drug Administration (FDA) (Alshurafa et al. 2012, 1). ITT analysis is reported in the results section of a scholarly paper, often in conjunction with a flow diagram showing the number of subjects in each of the groups at each phase of the trial (enrollment into trial, intervention, follow-up, and data analysis) (Schulz 2010, 3).

Addressing Missing Values

Missing values are a common problem in health research, including health informatics and health information management (HIM) research that investigates e-health, electronic health records (EHRs), and big databases (Montez-Rath et al. 2014, 1328; Haneuse et al. 2016, 82). A systematic review of articles in leading medical journals found that 95 percent of the articles on RCTs had missing outcome data (Bell et al. 2014, 3). It is important to address missing values and to address them properly to reduce the risk of bias and to validate the study's conclusions.

When values are missing, the data are incomplete; variables do not contain data values for some subjects or cases. Missing values can occur because of attrition, such as subjects who withdraw or "drop out" of a study prematurely or are lost to follow-up (see chapter 4). In other cases of missing values, the subjects fail to complete items on a survey or the entire survey, are unavailable for some sessions, or in some other way omit data or are omitted. These variables are *missing* values.

Researchers can proactively minimize missing values. For example, if respondents in a pilot study omitted or skipped items in an instrument, the instrument could be improved to reduce these omissions. The SAP can also be written so that available data are used rather than lost. For example, in longitudinal studies, persons (patients) may be lost to follow-up. The SAP could specify that person-years (number of years that the patient was in the study) rather than the number of persons are to be used in the statistical tests.

Despite efforts to gather and enter complete data, missing values may still occur. Experts categorize missing values into three patterns, described as follows:

- **Missing completely at random (MCAR):** Missing data are determined to be missing completely at random. For example, a portion of questionnaire data was accidentally lost—so, truly at random.

- **Missing at random (MAR):** MAR is a confusing misnomer because the missing data are not randomly missing; they are selectively missing based on some characteristic, factor, or other variable (Cummings 2013, 656). An analysis would solely depend on the available data and ignore the missing data. For example, a researcher is studying a decision support system's ability to predict an outcome based on the patients' adherence to the treatment protocol. The data on the patients who drop out (are nonadherent) are not calculated into the system's prediction. Therefore, we cannot rely on the system's prediction.
- **Missing not at random (MNAR):** A missing value is unknown or is unobserved data; whether its absence is random cannot be determined (Blankers et al. 2010, 3).

Until proven otherwise, the missing values are considered systematically biased and different from the present data in ways that affect statistical tests.

Researchers who fail to resolve missing values face several risks. Their study's randomization may be compromised because subjects may drop out disproportionately from groups, thereby introducing a selection bias (Haneuse et al. 2016, 83). Missing values can also jeopardize the assumptions that underpin statistical tests, reducing the study's power and invalidating their conclusions (Bell et al. 2014, 1). More generally missing values jeopardize the management of the data (Dziura et al. 2013, 356).

Several statistical techniques can be used to address missing data (Montez-Rath et al. 2014, 1328). Two common rudimentary techniques to resolve missing values are case deletion and single imputation. In *case deletion,* a case with missing values is entirely deleted from the study. In a modified form of case deletion, a case is only excluded from calculations for which it has missing data. **Imputation** is the substitution of values for the missing values. A common form of single imputation is the substitution of the mean of the available values for the missing data. Both case deletion and single imputation have the advantage of simplicity. The disadvantages of both techniques are the loss of cases and the potential for bias because the missing data may not be random.

Instead of these rudimentary techniques, experts recommend approaches that use the power of computers and statistical software programs, such as maximum likelihood estimation (MLE)—which is also known as *full-information likelihood (FIML)*—and multiple imputation (MI), to handle missing values (Little et al. 2014, 12). MLE uses the existing values to infer the missing values. As an example, people who read "mnagment" can infer that the intended word is "management"; they infer the "a" and the "e" that are missing. MLE uses a similar modeling process (Little et al. 2014, 153–154). MI provides substitutes for missing values; the substitutes are predicted by producing multiple data sets using existing values, performing statistical tests on each of these data sets, and combining the results into an overall value. Researchers should always fully describe the techniques that they used to address their missing data.

Cleaning Data

Data cleaning (also called *data cleansing* and *data scrubbing*) is the "process of detecting, diagnosing, and editing faulty data" (Van den Broeck et al. 2005, 0966). It is used to validate the accuracy of data. Researchers clean their data prior to data analysis because data errors occur despite researchers' efforts to prevent them. The purposes of data cleaning are to find and correct these errors and to minimize their impact on the research study's results. Data cleaning includes finding duplications (such as two questionnaires were returned by the same subject), checking internal consistency (for example, a mismatch between city and Zip code), and identifying outliers (values outside the expected range, such as age 42 years in a study on infant mortality). Data cleaning may be lengthy, requiring many hours of detailed work. Researchers should report the number and types of errors and how they cleaned them.

Descriptive Statistics

This chapter builds upon chapter 9 by adding several more descriptive statistics. This section covers sensitivity, specificity, and predictive values; receiver operating characteristic (ROC) curve analysis; and measures of effect.

Sensitivity, Specificity, and Predictive Values

Sensitivity, specificity, and predictive values are used in epidemiological studies about disease and risk for disease (refer to chapter 5 for further discussion of epidemiological methods). These measures are also used in evaluation studies of decision support systems and of data mining algorithms (refer to chapter 6 for more information on evaluation studies).

Sensitivity and Specificity Sensitivity and specificity are gauges of performance. Prior to discussing sensitivity and specificity, it is helpful to recap and build upon the information from table 5.3 in chapter 5 as follows:

- **True positive (TP),** correct labeling of an individual as having the disease or outcome
- **False negative (FN),** incorrect labeling of an individual as *not* having the disease or outcome when he or she *does*; false negatives are associated with type II errors
- **True negative (TN),** correct labeling of an individual as *not* having the disease or outcome when he or she *does not*
- **False positive (FP),** incorrect labeling of an individual as *having* the disease or outcome when he or she does *not*; false positives are associated with type I errors

Sensitivity is the ability of a measure to detect a characteristic (such as disease) when the characteristic exists. In a population with a characteristic, sensitivity indicates the proportion of people with the characteristic that will have a *positive* result. In other words, sensitivity expresses the ability of a test to maximize true positives (Chang et al. 2012, A-1). For this reason, sensitivity is also known as the *true positive rate*. Sensitivity is reported as a percentage. A 100 percent sensitive measure would identify everyone who has the disease or other characteristic that the measure seeks to detect. In health informatics, a sensitive decision support rule would be able to correctly identify a prescription error (the true positive in this example). Sensitivity is calculated by dividing the number of true positives (TP) by the number of true positives (TP) and false negatives (FN). The formula is as follows:

$$\text{Sensitivity} = \frac{\text{TP}}{\text{TP} + \text{FN}}$$

Specificity is the ability of a measure to detect the absence of a characteristic (again, such as disease) when the characteristic is absent. Specificity is also known as the *true negative rate*. In a population *without* a characteristic, specificity is the proportion of people without a characteristic that will have a *negative* result, known as a *true negative*. Specificity expresses the ability of a test to minimize false positives (Chang et al. 2012, A-1). Like sensitivity, specificity is reported as a percentage. A 100 percent specific measure would identify everyone *without* the disease or other characteristic being measured. In health informatics, a specific decision support rule would be able to correctly identify nonprescription errors (avoiding alert overload). Specificity is calculated by dividing the number of true negatives (TN) by the number of false positives (FP) and true negatives (TN). The formula is as follows:

$$\text{Specificity} = \frac{\text{TN}}{\text{FP} + \text{TN}}$$

Sensitivity is related to type II errors. A highly sensitive measure results in few false negatives (type II errors). In a false negative, a few subjects who *have* the disease (or other characteristic) are identified as *not* having the disease (characteristic). For example, a screening examination, such as a Papanicolaou (Pap) test, might falsely show that the specimen is negative, when, in fact, it is cancerous. However, a highly sensitive measure may result in many false positives. In that case, many subjects are identified as having the characteristic when, in fact, they do not.

On the other hand, specificity is related to type I errors. A highly specific measure results in few false positives (type I errors). Therefore, in a population without the characteristic, highly specific measures identify all the persons *without* the characteristic as *not* having the characteristic. For instance, a highly specific measure identifies all healthy people as being without disease. However, a highly specific measures may result in many false negatives, indicating that individuals do not have the condition (the illness or other characteristic being studied) even though they actually have it.

In the real world, a trade-off exists between sensitivity and specificity because tests are rarely 100 percent sensitive and 100 percent specific. Performance measures attempt to strike a reasonable balance. This reasonable balance is often based on whether false positives or false negatives are more consequential or detrimental. Erring on the side of generating excess false positives makes it is more likely that *all* possible cases are identified. However, patients who are falsely identified as potentially having a disease may be harmed by anxiety, additional diagnostic tests, and healthcare costs. False-positives may also lead to alert-overload for clinicians, who then might ignore potentially accurate alerts (Woods et al. 2014, 569). Erring on the side of generating excess false negatives makes it more likely that all healthy people are identified, but some people with the condition could be missed, thus delaying or omitting their treatment.

Sensitivity and specificity can be merged into one number, called the **likelihood ratio (LR)**. Likelihood ratios quantify the change in the certainty of the diagnosis conferred by test results (Chang et al. 2012, A-2). Likelihood ratios can be positive (LR+) or negative (LR–).

- A positive likelihood ratio (LR+) is calculated by dividing sensitivity by 1 – specificity (specificity/1–specificity). The formula is:

$$\frac{[TP/(TP+FN)]}{[1-(TN/(FP+TN))]}$$

- A negative likelihood ratio (LR–) is calculated by dividing 1–sensitivity by specificity (1–sensitivity/specificity). The formula is:

$$\frac{[1-(TP/(TP+FN))]}{[TN/(FP+TN)]}$$

Likelihood ratios convert the pretest odds of a diagnosis (positive or negative) to the posttest odds.

The next subsection describes a predictive values that are more useful than sensitivity and specificity because predictive values allow clinicians to state what a negative or positive test result means for an individual patient.

Positive Predictive Value and Negative Predictive Value Predictive values are useful because they put the results of positive and negative indicators into context. Predictive values provide an indicator of the likelihood of a disease or event following the results of a positive or negative measure. For example, after a positive screening test for cancer, how likely is it that the patient has cancer (LaMorte 2016)?

The **positive predictive value (PPV)** is the probability that a person has the characteristic when the measure is positive. The PPV is also known as the *precision rate* (particularly in information retrieval) or *posttest probability of disease*. For example, the PPV provides the likelihood of a patient having a disease when the laboratory test result is positive. A positive predictive value is calculated by first multiplying sensitivity by the prevalence of the disease or item of interest. The prevalence of a characteristic in the population affects the PPV (Lalkhen and McCluskey 2008, 222). As discussed in chapter 5, prevalence is the proportion of people (or objects) in a population that has a particular characteristic at a specific point in time or over a specific period of time. Prevalence can be obtained from the literature. The PPV calculation is completed as follows:

$$PPV = \frac{\frac{TP}{TP+FN}\times \text{Prevalence}}{\left(\frac{TP}{TP+FN}\times \text{Prevalence}\right)+(1-\text{Prevalence})\times\left(1-\frac{TN}{FP+TN}\right)}$$

The **negative predictive value (NPV)** is the probability that a person does *not* have a characteristic when the measure is *negative*. The NPV provides the likelihood of a patient *not* having a disease when the laboratory test result is *negative*. The formula for NPV also adjusts for prevalence and is calculated as follows:

$$NPV = \frac{\frac{TN}{FP+TN}\times(1-\text{Prevalence})}{\left[\frac{TN}{FP+TN}\times(1-\text{Prevalence})\right]+\left[\text{Prevalence}\times\left(1-\frac{TP}{TP+FN}\right)\right]}$$

Practitioners can use positive predictive value (PPV) and negative predictive value (NPV) to estimate individuals' probability of disease or other characteristics of interest. The inclusion of sensitivity and specificity in the formulas shows that the PPV and NPV are related to sensitivity and specificity.

Receiver Operating Characteristic Curve Analysis

Receiver operating characteristic (ROC) curves plot sensitivity versus specificity at different thresholds and graphically show a measure's ability to predict an outcome. ROC curve analysis measures performance. Commonly, ROC analysis is used to measure the performance of predictive algorithms (such as in decision support systems), diagnostic tests (such as sputum tests), screening examinations (such as mammograms), and other detection technologies.

ROC curves visualize the trade-off between sensitivity and specificity. They graph all different possible cut points between sensitivity (true positive rate) and the false positive rate (1 –Specificity). In terms of the graph, the *y*-axis is the sensitivity (true positive rate) and the *x*-axis is the false positive rate (1 – Specificity).

In interpreting ROC curves, the **area under the curve (AUC)** is the performance of the predictive algorithm or other detection technology. Perfect performance yields 100 percent (1.0) of the AUC and is seen as a point at upper left corner (perfect classification) of figure 12.1. The size of the AUC indicates how predictive the algorithm or test is (the larger the AUC, the more predictive the algorithm or test is). On the other hand, totally random guessing yields 50 percent (0.5) and a diagonal line from the bottom left corner to the top right corner (line of no discrimination). Figure 12.2 shows random guessing.

Figure 12.1 Generic ROC curve showing sensitivity and specificity

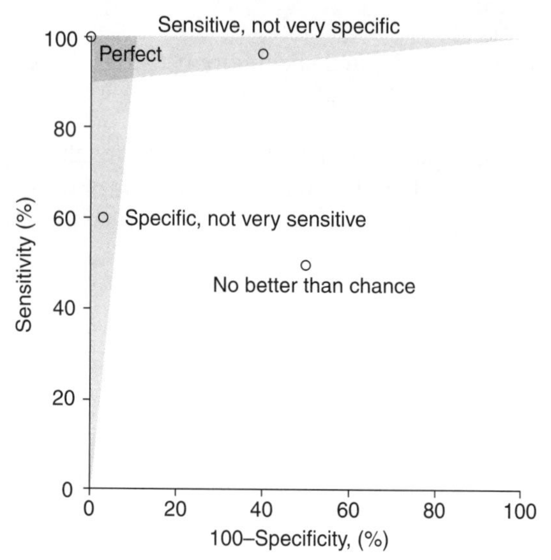

Source: Chang et al. 2012, A-2. Reprinted with permission of the Agency for Healthcare Research and Quality.

Figure 12.2 ROC curve showing random guessing

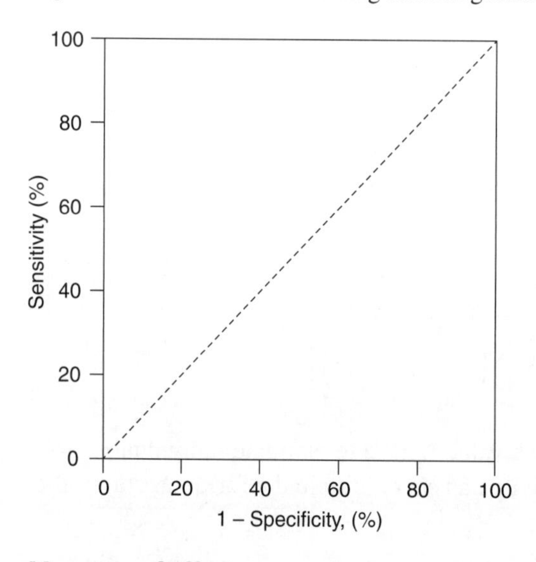

Measures of Effect

Measures of effect put a study's results in context for practitioners by providing information about the magnitude of the association or difference. Measures of effect can also be used to determine statistical significance. In NHST, the *effect size* is the extent to which the null hypothesis is false and represents the degree to which the sample's results differ from the null hypothesis. Measures of effect show the practical significance of a study's findings. This section will discuss confidence intervals, odds ratios (ORs), risk reduction statistics, and other indexes of effect.

Confidence Intervals A **confidence interval (CI)** is a range of values for a sample's characteristic, such as the mean, within which it is estimated that the population's characteristic lies (Ravid 2011, 39). CIs indicate the **precision** (the degree of certainty) of the estimate. Confidence limits, an upper limit and a lower limit, are on each end of the CI range. Using different formulas, CIs can be calculated for means, proportions, risk ratios, ORs, and other statistics.

Confidence levels are the probability that the CI includes the population's value. Researchers set their confidence levels to represent their desired level of certainty. Desired certainty can be set at any percentage, but common percentages are 90 percent confidence level (10 percent significance level), 95 percent confidence level (5 percent significance level), and 99 percent confidence level (1 percent significance level). (For information on significance levels, see the previous discussion of alpha levels). If the confidence level is set at 95 percent, researchers would be confident that the true results will be in the CI's range 95 percent of the time.

Confidence intervals provide a way to measure the precision of the estimate. Narrower CIs have greater precision than wider CIs. The width of calculated CIs is affected by various factors, including heterogeneity of the sample, sample size, and the selected confidence level, described as follows:

- Greater heterogeneity (more variance) of the sample's measurements or scores results in wider CIs. Greater homogeneity (less variance) in the measurements or scores of the sample results in narrower CIs.
- Smaller sample sizes result in wider CIs than larger sample sizes. Researchers can increase the precision of their study by increasing their sample size.
- Higher confidence levels, such as 95 percent, have wider CIs than lower confidence levels, such as 90 percent. The interval needs to be wider to support the claim that the population's parameter is included (Schünemann et al. 2011, 12.4.1).

In reporting CIs, researchers provide the sample's statistic, such as mean, the confidence level, and the upper and lower confidence limits. For example, researchers conducted a study investigating youth's exposure to Internet-based tobacco advertising (Dunlop et al. 2016). One aspect of the study was to measure exposure to tobacco branding on social media. When comparing exposures between 2010 and 2013, the researchers found that youths participating in the study in 2010 were statistically significantly less likely to report exposure to tobacco branding on social media than youths interviewed in 2013. This finding is based on the OR that the researchers calculated as one of the statistical tests in the analysis of their data (*ORs* are discussed in the next section and in chapter 5). The researchers set their CI at 95 percent. The calculated OR between 2010 and 2013 is 0.26. The lower limit of the CI is 0.20 and the upper limit was 0.33. The calculated *P* value is < 0.001. The OR is reported as a lower likelihood because the calculated statistic is less than 1.0. This information is presented as follows in the article: (odds ratio [OR] 0.26, 95% CI 0.20–0.33, $P < 0.001$). The 0.26 OR is for this sample of youths. With the CI of 95 percent, the researchers are 95 percent confident that the OR for the youth population is between 0.20 and 0.33. Interpretation of CIs depends on information on the study, such as sample size, familiarity with the field's literature, such as typical confidence levels, and professional knowledge, such as understanding of the practical significance of the reported findings.

Odds Ratio The OR is the chance of an event occurring in one group compared to the chance of it occurring in another group. In studies using a control group, the OR compares the probability of the outcome under study occurring in the experimental group that received the intervention versus the control group that did not. In other words, the OR is the ratio of the odds of the treatment group to the odds of the control group. Therefore, the individual odds of both groups are calculated. Consequently, an OR can be thought of as a ratio of ratios. The OR is also known as *relative odds* and the *cross-product ratio*.

As described in chapter 5, ORs are often calculated in case-control studies. In these epidemiological studies, the OR is explained as a measure that quantifies the relationship between an exposure (intervention) and an outcome (CDC 2012, 3-45). The step-by-step procedure for calculating ORs is provided in chapter 5 and recapped in table 12.1. Researchers adhere to the organization of the data into the columns and rows shown in table 12.1 because it is the standardized notation (CDC 2012, 6-42).

ORs are interpreted for decision making in terms of whether they equal or are greater or less than 1. Table 12.2 shows that odds greater than 1 increase the likelihood of an outcome while odds less than 1 decrease the likelihood of an outcome.

Table 12.1 Sample calculations for odds ratios, relative risk ratios, absolute risk reduction, relative risk reduction, and number needed to treat

	Disease or Intervention	No Disease or No Intervention	Total	Ratios
Exposed	100 (A)	1900 (B)	A + B = 2000	Risk rate = A/(A + B) = 5%
Not exposed	80 (C)	7920 (D)	C + D = 8000	Risk rate = C/(C + D) = 1%
Total	A + C = 180	B + D = 9820	A + B + C + D = 10,000	
	A/C = 1.25	B/D = 0.24		Odds ratio = (A/C)/(B/D) = 5.21
				Relative risk = [A/(A + B)]/[C/(C + D)] = 5
				Absolute risk reduction = [A/(A + B)] − [C/(C + D)] = 4%
				Relative risk reduction = {[A/(A + B)] − [C/(C + D)]}/[C/(C + D)] = 4%
				Number needed to treat = 1/[A/(A + B)] − [C/(C + D)] = 25

A = number of people with both the disease and exposure
B = number of people with the exposure but not the disease
C = number of people with the disease but not the exposure
D = number of people with neither the disease nor the exposure
A + C = total number of persons with disease (case-patients)
B + D = total number of persons without disease (controls)
A + B = total number of people exposed
C + D = total number of people not exposed
Source: CDC 2012, 3-45, 6-41.

Table 12.2 Interpreting odds ratios and relative risks for decision making

Result	Odds Ratio	Relative Risk
1	No relationship or equal likelihood (intervention or exposure makes no difference)	No difference in risk between exposed group and unexposed group
> 1	Positive relationship; exposed (experimental) group has greater likelihood	Greater risk of bad outcome in exposed group
< 1	Negative (inverse) relationship; exposed (experimental) group has lesser likelihood	Less of risk of bad outcome in exposed group

Source: Adapted from Szumilas 2010, 227; Irwig et al. 2008, 214.

Risk Reduction Statistics Risk reduction statistics allow researchers and practitioners to know the probability of success for an intervention or exposure and each outcome's expected probability. Analyses are conducted related to exposures to interventions or to risks, such as health hazards. Risk reduction statistics include absolute risk, absolute risk reduction, relative risk, relative risk reduction, and number needed to treat.

Absolute risk (AR) (often known simply as *risk rate*) is the probability of an occurrence of an event in an entire population of subjects (experimental group and control group). The event is usually adverse, but it could be beneficial. For an adverse event, AR is a measure of the size of the risk. The AR is calculated by taking the number of events in a group and dividing that number by the total number of subjects in that group. Refer to table 12.1, which shows risk rates (ARs) of 5 percent and 1 percent.

Absolute risk reduction (ARR) is the arithmetic difference between the event rate of two groups. The ARR is also known as the *risk difference*. In the example in table 12.1, the ARR (4 percent) is the difference between the two groups' ARs (5 percent minus 1 percent). The ARR is interpreted as the control (unexposed) group having a 4 percent reduced risk of the outcome.

Relative risk (RR) compares the rate of risk of an outcome in exposed subjects (or experimental group) to the rate of risk of an outcome in unexposed subjects (or control group). Thus, RR provides different perspective on an occurrence's risk than AR because RR views an occurrence's risk as *relative* to another group's risk. RR also measures the magnitude of the association between an exposure, such as food item or intervention, and an outcome, such as disease or improved performance. RR is also known as the *risk ratio* (CDC 2012, 6-40).

RR is used in experimental and epidemiological studies. In an experimental study, the experimental group is exposed to an intervention, and the control group is not. In epidemiological studies, the disease (attack) rate in the exposed group is compared to the disease (attack) rate in the unexposed group (refer to chapter 5). The individual risks of both groups, the experimental (exposed) group and the control (unexposed group), are calculated. The ratio of these two risks is then calculated. Consequently, RR can be thought of as a ratio of ratios. As described in chapter 5, RRs are often calculated in cohort (prospective or incidence) studies. The step-by-step procedure for calculating RR is provided in chapter 5 and recapped in table 12.1. Relative risks are interpreted for decision making in terms of whether they equal or are greater or less than 1 (refer to table 12.2).

Occasionally, OR is used interchangeably with RR, in retrospective case-control studies. In table 12.1, the OR of 5.21 is similar to the RR of 5.0 (CDC 2012, 3-46).

Relative risk reduction (RRR) is the percentage that an intervention reduces risk in the experimental group compared to the control group. Generally, RRR is the reduction in terms of percentage that an intervention will produce in the probability of occurrence of the characteristic of interest. Relative risk reduction is also known as the *relative difference*. The calculation of the RRR is the ratio between the absolute risk reduction (ARR) and the risk rate (C/C+D) in the *unexposed group* (control group). In table 12.1, RRR is 4 percent.

Number needed to treat (NNT) is the number of people who need to receive the intervention for one person to benefit from the intervention (Sedgwick 2015, 1). The NNT is viewed as a user-friendly statistic because it is fairly straightforward to understand. The NNT is reciprocal to the ARR and is calculated as 1 divided by the absolute risk reduction (1/ARR). In table 12.1, the NTT is calculated as 1 divided by 4 percent (0.04) and shows that 25 people would need to receive the intervention in order for 1 person to benefit.

Other Indexes of Effect Size **Effect sizes** are indexes that quantify the degree to which a study's results should be considered important or unimportant. The larger the value of the effect size, the greater the presence of the phenomenon under study. Effect sizes are valuable statistical tests because, unlike NHST, they are unaffected by sample size. For researchers and readers, the effect size is the practical significance of the study's findings.

There are several indexes of effect size, including Cohen's *d*, Hedges's *g*, Glass's delta (Δ), and R^2. Research methodologists write about "families" of indexes because some indexes are related to statistical tests for differences, others to statistical tests for relationships, and others to differences in ratios.

Thresholds have been suggested for interpreting measures of effect in terms of practical significance. The practical significance of effect sizes varies by the statistical test. The thresholds of practical significance for the effect sizes of the commonly encountered statistical tests discussed in chapter 9 are as follows (Cohen 1992, 157):

- One-way analysis of variance (ANOVA): Small = 0.20, medium = 0.50, and large = 0.80
- Pearson product-moment correlation coefficient: Small = 0.10, medium = 0.30, and large = 0.50
- Multiple regression: Small = 0.02, medium = 0.15, and large = 0.35

Research methodologists caution that these are only suggested thresholds and interpretation of the effect size must be put into the context of the research question and practical significance in the field (Kelley and Preacher 2012, 146). Finally, effect sizes only reflect the magnitude of the result; they do *not* establish cause-and-effect relationships.

Inferential Statistics

Inferential statistics allow the researchers to make inferences about a population's parameters (characteristics) from the sample's statistics (characteristics). Multiple statistical tests can be applied to research data. To see different aspects of their data, researchers often analyze their data using more than one test.

Two major dimensions that determine the selection of the appropriate statistical test are the purpose of the research and the assumptions of parametric tests. Statistical tests vary by the purpose of the research—to infer differences or to infer associations. Data that meet the assumptions can have *parametric tests* applied to them (refer to the assumptions for parametric tests in chapter 9). If the data do not meet the assumptions, then *nonparametric tests* must be applied. Consequently, statistical tests can be organized into four divisions, as follows:

- Difference and parametric: Independent one-sample *t*-test, independent measures *t*-test, paired *t*-test, one-way analysis of variance (ANOVA), two-way ANOVA, one-way repeated measures ANOVA, multivariate ANOVA (MANOVA), and analysis of covariance (ANCOVA)
- Difference and nonparametric: One-sample median test, chi-square goodness of fit, Mann-Whitney *U* test, chi-square test of independence, Fisher exact test, Wilcoxon signed-rank test, Kruskal-Wallis test, and Friedman test
- Association and parametric: Pearson product-moment correlation coefficient, simple regression, and multiple regression
- Association and nonparametric: Spearman rank order correlation

Table 9.1 in chapter 9 reflects these four divisions. In chapter 9, these statistical tests are described with examples of their application and with some of the other names by which they are known.

Once purpose and parametric assumptions are considered, other factors then affect the selection of statistical test, as follows:

- Level of data affects classification as parametric or nonparametric. Nominal and ordinal data must have nonparametric tests applied to them. Continuous data have parametric tests applied to them. Continuous data that have been grouped also have nonparametric tests applied to them. For example, blood pressure readings categorized as "low" "medium/normal," and "high" are continuous data that have been grouped and can have nonparametric tests applied to them.
- When the size of the sample is less than 30, nonparametric statistical tests are applied; a sample greater than 30 in size has parametric statistical tests applied (provided the parametric assumptions are met).
- The number of variables affects the selection. For example, a simple regression has one independent variable and one dependent variable. However, multiple regression, a family of statistical tests may have one or more independent variables and one or more dependent variables, depending upon the specific regression model.
- The independence of the samples affects the selection. Dependent samples require certain statistical tests, such as the paired *t*-test or one-way repeated measures ANOVA. Terms associated with dependent samples include *matched, paired, clustered,* or *repeated measures*.
- Randomness of the sample underpins parametric statistical tests. Nonrandom samples require nonparametric statistical tests.
- Linearity of associations between data is common in research. Linearity is an assumption of parametric statistical tests. Nonlinear associations require nonparametric tests. However, as chapter 9 points out, many statistical tests, such as ANOVA, are robust enough to withstand some deviations. *Robust* means resistant to errors.

These other factors may require a statistical test not listed in the previous bullets or in table 9.1. Researchers should consult with a statistician about other appropriate statistical tests for their study design and data.

Sensitivity analysis is the investigation of a study's results to see whether results differ as decisions on handling the data are changed or whether results differ for subgroups within the data (refer to the discussion in chapter 9). Sensitivity analysis is not the same as sensitivity and specificity. For example, in the discussion of the results of the hypothetical decision support system for predicting sepsis located in chapter 9, the results varied by sex. The researchers would have been unaware of this difference had they not investigated male and female subgroups (refer to table 9.5).

One purpose of sensitivity analysis is to check the robustness of the study's results. A study's results are robust when the results remain fairly consistent, despite variations in the handling of the data (such as how missing data were addressed). Another purpose of sensitivity analysis is to put actionable information into the hands of decision makers. For this purpose, researchers conduct subgroup analyses. Often, decision makers want to know whether all groups respond in the same way to an intervention or whether certain groups respond differently. Examples of subgroups include races, age groups, geographic areas, and types of professionals. If subgroup analysis is planned, the subgroups must first contain sufficient numbers of cases to make statistical analysis feasible. Second, the subgroups should be operationally defined as they are in the literature. For example, refer to figure 11.5 in chapter 11 for the subgroups of ages and races and ethnicities used by the Centers for Disease Control and Prevention (CDC) (Xu et al. 2016, 4) and the National Institutes of Health (NIH).

Data Analysis in Data Mining

Data mining is the use of semiautomated and automated processes for exploring large databases and detecting relevant patterns and relationships (Tufféry 2011, 4). It analyzes data to generate descriptive or predictive models. Conducting studies using data mining is described in chapter 7. This chapter builds on the processes described in chapter 7 by adding information on data analysis in data mining.

Data mining is secondary analysis of data. Researchers make a distinction between primary analysis and secondary analysis. **Primary analysis** is the analysis of original research data by the researchers who collected the data for a specific study. Similarly, **primary data** are the data researchers collect to answer their own specific research question.

Secondary analysis is any research in which researchers use data for purposes not defined nor predicted in the original study's design (Yardley et al. 2014, 102). The secondary data analysis could reuse the data to answer a different question than the original study asked, combine the data set from the original study with another data set, or apply different statistical tests to the original study's data. These data that were originally collected for another specific purpose are called **secondary data**.

Data mining differs from other types of quantitative analysis. First, data mining can begin *without* a precise, preestablished hypothesis, as researchers explore the data in the database to generate hypotheses. Second, data mining projects are secondary analysis, because the data used in data mining, such as claims data, were not collected for the new analysis. Third, data mining differs from statistics because data mining must deal with heterogeneous data fields, such as images (positron-emission tomography scans), signals (electrocardiograms and electroencephalograms), laboratory data (glycated hemoglobin [HbA1c] and cholesterol levels), clinicians' interpretation of the data, patients' impressions, and other medical data.

The next subsections address general methods of data mining and influential methods of data mining.

General Data Mining Methods

Data mining methods are algorithms that are used on databases, after initial data preparation, to find patterns in data or build models (Cios et al. 2000, 17). In this definition, the terms *algorithm*, *pattern*, and *model* have specific meanings, as follows:

- **Algorithm:** An iterative, computational sequence of steps or rules that transform inputs to outputs (Kotu and Deshpande 2015, 4).
- **Pattern:** Event or combination of events in a database that occurs more often than expected, such that its occurrence is statistically significant and is not random chance (Berson et al. 2000, 110–111). Patterns are differentiated from models because patterns reflect the data in the database whereas models reflect a predefined purpose.
- **Model:** "A data mining model is a description of a specific aspect of a dataset. It produces output values for an assigned set of input values" (Ray 2011, 517). A model describes the original, historical database upon which it was built and can be applied to new data to make predictions (Berson et al. 2000, 110). Modeling can be unsupervised (undirected) learning or supervised (directed) learning. In **unsupervised learning**, modeling is exploratory in that there is no dependent variable of interest (target) and the algorithm searches through the database to discover potentially significant relationships or patterns among fields in the database (Ahlemeyer-Stubbe and Coleman 2014, 16–18). In **supervised learning**, the model is built on a training database when the values or other attributes of the independent variables are *known* and the target is *known*. During the model's training phase, the algorithms learn the relationship (dependency) and, then, during subsequent deployment in other databases, can predict the target (Ahlemeyer-Stubbe and Coleman 2014, 16–18).

The steps of the algorithm create the model by identifying and analyzing the patterns in a subset of the data set. The algorithm runs many times, iteratively, to create the best model. This model can then be applied to the entire data set to identify patterns or trends that can inform decision making.

Dozens of data mining methods exist, and several methods can be valid choices in mining a database (McCormick et al. 2014, 404–405). Moreover, different methods can be used iteratively, with each method providing a different insight into the data. Factors in choosing a method include the type of data available and the amount of preparation needed prior to applying the software. Table 12.3 presents examples of several general types of data mining methods: rough sets, fuzzy sets, Bayesian models, evolutionary computation, machine learning, artificial neural networks, and clustering (Cios et al. 2000, 19).

Table 12.3 Selected general data mining methods

Method	Description
Rough sets	Patterns from imprecise or incomplete data sets are extracted and analyzed to define approximate boundaries between regions and thereby categorize objects into classifications. Rough sets can be usefully applied to medical data in EHRs to classify patients by diseases because the boundaries between diseases are often vague, with overlapping signs and symptoms (Gardiner and Gillett 2015, 1782).
Fuzzy sets	Structural relationships in imprecise or incomplete data sets are identified, and the potential degree of membership or nonmembership of an object in a class is quantitatively described (value between 0 and 1). Fuzzy sets can represent and summarize qualitative (nonnumeric) data into membership classifications, such as young and old or short and tall (Zeng et al. 2012, 36).
Bayesian models (probabilistic graphical dependency models, Bayes networks, belief networks)	Classification is expressed as probabilities based upon subject matter experts' degrees of belief in propositions' truth or falsity. Two estimates, expressed as probabilities between zero and one, are used to weigh and infer the truth of hypotheses. The two estimates represent (1) commonsensical experience prior to observing data (prior probability), and (2) informed expectation that the observed data are true (likelihood). Probabilities of relationships can be represented graphically, such as the relationships between signs, symptoms, and various diseases (Perfors et al. 2011, 302–304, 313).
Evolutionary computation	Search and optimization algorithms are based on Darwin's theory of evolution (survival of the fittest). Variation operators, called *crossovers* and *mutations,* are randomly applied to data objects in a population of candidate solutions (data models), and the iteration with the greatest fit to an organizational objective, such as accuracy, is selected. Four major evolutionary algorithms are genetic algorithm, genetic programming, evolutionary strategies, and evolutionary programming (Li et al. 2014, 2).
Machine learning	In this type of artificial intelligence, computer programs learn from their previous experiences and perform tasks in ways similar to intelligent agents (humans). Computer algorithms automatically (without online human guidance) extract information and reveal and summarize relationships in data in the form of decision trees or production rules (Carbonell et al. 1983, 69–70).
Artificial neural networks (ANNs)	Descriptive and predictive models that, mimicking the functioning of the human brain, are organized in interconnected units, known as *neurons*. ANNs are a form of artificial intelligence that processes numerical data and produces complicated nonlinear models relating the independent variables (inputs) to the dependent predictive variables (outputs) (Mobley et al. 2000, 188; Tufféry 2011, 217).
Clustering	Natural groups within data are revealed by unsupervised learning. Objects within a group are similar to each other and are dissimilar from objects data outside the group (Tufféry 2011, 235).

Influential Data Mining Methods

Derived from the general types of methods are hundreds of specific and hybrid methods and many with multiple variations (Vleugel et al. 2012, 244–245). Researchers identified the 10 most widely-used and well-known data mining methods (Wu et al. 2008, 3–27). These most influential specific methods are described in table 12.4.

Table 12.4 Influential data mining methods

Name	Description
C.5 (successor of C4.5)	Classifier that predicts into which category (class) new data belong. Supervised learning (Quinlan 1966, 7).
k-Means	Method to cluster or partition a database into user-identified groups (clusters) of similar data (k = number of user-specified clusters). Often used to explore data. Semisupervised learning (Morissette and Chartier 2013, 15–16).
SVM (support vector machines)	Classifier that categorizes data into two classes and determines the dividing line (hyperplane). Often used to identify hypotheses. Supervised and semisupervised learning (Vapnik 1999, 996–999).
Apriori	Approach to find frequent item sets in a transaction database and derive association rules. Item sets are variables (items) that are often connected, such as groups of purchases in a grocery store (for example, bread, peanut butter, and jelly). Association rules represent the various correlations and relations among

(*Continued*)

Table 12.4 (*Continued*)

Name	Description
	the attributes of variables. In healthcare, variables could be medical data (patient characteristics, disease stage, and other clinical factors) that are often associated with a certain disease. Often used to detect previously unrecognized relationships. Unsupervised learning (Kosters et al. 2003, 284–285).
EM (expectation-maximization)	Method of clustering and modeling by using the statistical technique of maximum likelihood estimation. This technique finds the population that is the most likely to produce the recorded (observed) data. EM is a two-step method in which two sets of variables, recorded (labeled) and missing values (absent or hidden), are used to estimate a population parameters. The resulting model can be used to estimate missing values or outcomes from a set of parameters. Semisupervised learning (McLachlan and Krishnan 2008, 1–2).
PageRank	Method that explores links (associations, such as hyperlinks) in a network of objects (such as web pages) and determines their relative importance (rank). The search engine Google uses PageRank as one of its techniques to rank web pages by their importance. The method has applications beyond ranking the importance of webpages, such as determining which species are critical for sustaining ecosystems. Supervised learning (Brin and Page 1998, 109).
AdaBoost	Method of creating a classifier that takes multiple weak algorithms and combines ("boosts") them into a single strong ensemble algorithm. The accuracy of weak algorithms' results is barely above random chance, whereas strong algorithms have high accuracy. Supervised and semisupervised learning (Freund and Schapire 1997, 124–126).
*k*NN (k-Nearest Neighbor)	Supervised classifier that stores the labeled training data from a historical database and categorizes new (unlabeled) data based on the classes of the closest labeled data (nearest neighbors); considered a *lazy learner* because it builds no models during training. Supervised learning (because the algorithm is provided a labeled training data set) (Jiang et al. 2014, 194–195).
Naive Bayes	Family of classifers that share the assumption that every feature of the data being classified is independent of (has no effect on) all other features given in the category. Supervised learning (Friedman et al. 1997, 131–132).
CART (Classification and Regression Trees)	Classifier that creates classification trees and decision trees. The procedure is capable of handling both continuous and nominal data, both independent variables (predictors) and dependent variables (targets, outcomes), and missing values. Classification trees put data into binary classes (survive, not survive). Regression trees predict numerical or continuous values (costs, additional years of life). Supervised learning (Breiman et al. 1984, 1–5).

Statistical Conclusion Validity

Statistical conclusion validity is the extent to which the statistical conclusions about the relationships in the data are reasonable. Statistical conclusion validity judges the soundness of conclusions that the researchers derived from their study's findings. The following threats to statistical conclusion validity exist:

- *Lack of power*: Power is related to type II errors. A difference or relationship existed, but the study did not detect it. Small sample sizes can mask effects of interventions.
- *Lack of reliability:* Reliability is the ability to consistently reproduce similar findings. Reliability can be compromised when researchers use faulty instruments or procedures to collect data.
- *Extreme heterogeneity of the subjects:* The random diversity of the respondents or phenomenon makes the difference or association undetectable.
- *Use of an inappropriate statistical test:* The researchers' conclusions cannot be trusted if a statistical test is used when the underlying assumptions of parametric tests are violated.
- *Fishing:* Researchers' conclusions are questionable if they run many statistical tests just to find a statistically significant result without an a priori hypothesis. Fishing is also known as *data dredging, hunting, snooping,* and p-*hacking*.

Researchers' decisions in selecting their research design, collecting data, and analyzing their data can affect statistical conclusion validity. Figure 12.3 shows the types of validity across research design, data collection (instrument), and data analysis.

Figure 12.3 Three prongs of statistical conclusion validity: Research design, data collection, and data analysis

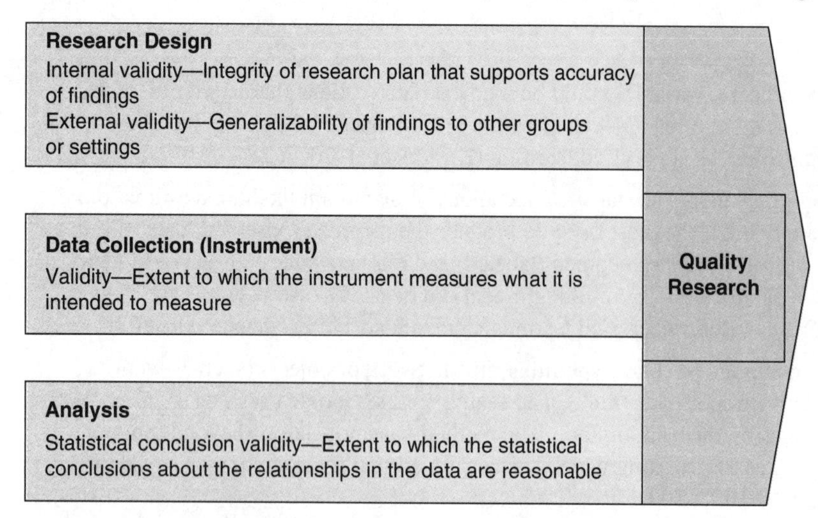

Quantitative Analytic Software Programs

Quantitative analytic software programs assist researchers in analyzing their data by performing the computations and providing tables and graphs. However, the researchers, not the software program, are analyzing the data. The researchers select the statistical test and enter various parameters, such as confidence levels.

Researchers conducting quantitative studies can select from dozens of software packages for the analysis of their data. Many free general and proprietary data analysis software packages and free data-mining software packages are available.

For basic descriptive statistics, researchers can use spreadsheet software, such as Microsoft Excel. However, most researchers choose to use dedicated statistical packages because these packages require less manipulation of the data than spreadsheets, and because they perform many more statistical procedures. Other factors that influence the choice of software are level of data, planned analytic techniques, and cost. Statistical data analysis software packages often offer free trials and tutorials. Researchers should explore the capabilities of various packages before selecting one. Descriptions of commonly used analytic software programs are provided in table 12.5.

Table 12.5 Quantitative analytic software packages

Software Package	Description
Epi Info	Public domain suite of interoperable software tools from the CDC. The software supports data analyses with epidemiological statistics, maps, and graphs for public health professionals who may lack an information technology background.
IBM SPSS Statistics	Integrated family of more than a dozen modules that addresses the entire statistical analysis process of planning, data collection, analysis, and reporting.
JMP	Family of integrative and visual statistical tools that link data, statistics, and graphics.
LISREL	Set of statistical applications for data manipulation, basic statistical analyses, regression analyses, structural equation modeling, and linear and nonlinear modeling.
Minitab	Comprehensive set of statistical tools for exploring, analyzing, graphing, and interpreting data.
SAS/STATS	Comprehensive set of tools from traditional statistics to Bayesian inference and modeling tools for massive data.
STATISTICA	Comprehensive array of analytic software products for data analysis, data management, data visualization, and data-mining procedures that includes techniques for predictive modeling, clustering, classification, and exploration.

Qualitative Data Analysis

In *qualitative data analysis,* researchers systematically use techniques to understand, explain, and interpret their data. Qualitative analysis is applied to nonnumerical observations, such as gestures, activities, space, and perceptions.

Qualitative researchers collect data through open-ended items on questionnaires, unstructured interviews, examination of photographs, and many other methods. Relevant data may also be collected from health records, such as free-form clinician progress notes or from other free texts, such as blogs.

Qualitative researchers interpret their data, seeking patterns and connections, to make sense and understandings (Merriam 2009, 175–176). Analysis of qualitative data is a cyclical and iterative process. Data collection, data analysis, and generation of hypotheses and theories are concurrent, intertwined activities. Qualitative researchers collect data, pose hypotheses, find gaps, collect more data, refine hypotheses, and conclude their analyses when the theory accounts for both confirming and disconfirming data. These data are progressively reduced into fewer and fewer categories and, eventually, into themes. A general framework describes this cyclical and iterative process of data analysis in terms of three major activities: data condensation, data display, and conclusion drawing and verification (Miles et al. 2014, 10–14). Table 12.6 describes each of these activities.

Table 12.6 Major activities in qualitative analysis process

Activity	Description
Data condensation	Organizing and condensing data by selecting, focusing, simplifying, distilling, abstracting, and transforming data into meaningful categories
Data display	Assemblage of categories into extended text, diagram, matrix, chart, or other array that promotes systematic thinking, extrapolation, detection of interrelationships, discernment of patterns, and discovery of higher order categories or themes
Conclusion drawing and verification	Interpreting higher order categories and themes in terms of the study's question and establishing the validity of the conclusions by checking and rechecking the data until all data are accounted for or explained

Source: Miles et al. 2014, 10–14.

Over 25 years ago, a researcher identified more than 20 types of qualitative analytic techniques (Tesch 1990, 77–99). Many techniques were similar and represented differences in the researchers' philosophies or academic backgrounds. Moreover, qualitative researchers may use a variety of overlapping techniques, rather than just one technique (Holloway and Wheeler 2010, 285).

This section addresses grounded theory and content analysis, two commonly used techniques of qualitative analysis. The section also discusses conclusion validity and qualitative analytic software programs.

Grounded Theory

The purpose of grounded theory is to discover or generate theories through the analysis of data. Consequently, *grounded theory* refers both to the theories that the technique generates and the technique itself. The theories are called *grounded* theories because they closely fit their data, including diverse data. With regard to the technique, the name emphasizes that the data generate the theories through coding, categorization, and comparison. Grounded theory is also known as the *constant comparative method*. (Refer to the example of the constant comparative method in chapter 3.)

One of grounded theory's developers, Dr. Barney Glaser, explained that the theory emerged as he and his fellow researchers analyzed their data on the interactions between hospital staff members and dying patients (Glaser 1965, 436). Conceptualization is the core of grounded theory. Conceptualization results in the identification of latent (hidden) patterns; enduring relevance and meaning; and abstractions of time, place, and people. These conceptualizations form the generalizations of theories (Glaser 2002, 787).

In grounded theory, data collection, data analysis, and generation of hypotheses and theories are concurrent, intertwined activities. In data collection, qualitative researchers observe the phenomena. They record and code these observations as incidents. The unit of analysis is the incident. Each incident is coded. The coded incidents are the data of qualitative researchers. Often, qualitative researchers represent the data by selecting illustrative or characteristic quotes.

Grounded theory is an iterative process. The stages of the process as shown in table 12.7. Researchers develop conceptual categories inductively to fit the coded data. Some researchers may use pre-established categories that apply to the small group under observation. Redesign, collection, and recoding of additional data occur constantly as subsequent observations reveal gaps or discrepancies in the categories that need additional observations (this is why the method is referred to as the *constant comparative method*). Data collection, coding, and analysis continue until all the data fit or are accounted for in the discovered or generated theory.

Table 12.7 Stages of grounded theory

Stage		Activities
1	Comparing incidents applicable to each category	✧ Code incidents to all applicable categories (laughter, coughing, inflection, and body-language are included as well as statements) (known as *open coding* or *level 1 coding*). ✧ Compare current incident with coding of past incidents. ✧ Compare categories' relationships. ✧ Record "memos" (reflective notes to oneself) and diagrams of ideas, relationships, noted discrepancies, notions about emerging theory, and other reflections.
2	Integrating categories and their properties	✧ Compare, constantly, properties of categories. ✧ Create framework by integrating categories (known as *axial coding* or *level 2 coding*). ✧ Integrate diverse properties. ✧ Make sense of theory expressing relationships as paradigm, model, or conditional matrix.
3	Delimiting the theory	✧ Solidify theory to core categories as fewer changes are made to integrate incidents (selective coding). ✧ Modify theory to increase logical clarity. ✧ Discover underlying uniformities and reduce categories. ✧ Account for differences with higher level concepts ("dimensionalization"). ✧ Achieve parsimony of variables and formulation. ✧ Attain "dense" categories and theoretical "saturation." ✧ Generalize to other relevant contexts. ✧ Delimit list of categories.
4	Writing theory	✧ Summarize memos on each category. ✧ Validate theory by pinpointing coded data behind it. ✧ Write theory using categories as major sections (themes).

Source: Glaser 1965, 439–443.

Gee and colleagues reported on their use of grounded theory to analyze data on patients' use of personal health records (PHRs) through various provider portals (Gee et al. 2015, 231). PHRs have been promoted as a way for chronically ill patients to take a greater role in managing their care themselves (self-management) and meaningfully communicate with their healthcare providers. Eighteen patients were purposively selected to participate in a qualitative study. The researchers selected these patients because they were PHR users between the ages 50 and 65 years, spoke English, had at least one chronic condition, and had been identified by their providers as frequent, engaged, and experienced users of the PHR for self-management support and for provider-patient communication. The researchers wanted to learn how these patients were using the PHRs for self-management and communication.

The researchers conducted semistructured interviews, which were digitally recorded and transcribed verbatim. In addition to the recordings and transcriptions, data included demographic data, field notes collected during each encounter with the participant, and memos (spontaneously written thoughts on analysis). The researchers primarily analyzed the data using the grounded theory approach of constant comparative analysis. They identified four major thematic categories that captured the perceptions of the chronically ill users of PHRs: (1) patient engagement and health self-management, (2) access to and control over personal health data, (3) promotion of productive communication, and (4) opportunities for training and education. The researchers learned that the participants did not always find the PHR easy to use. However, all the participants in the study found that the PHR was useful for the self-management of their illness and for productive interactions with their provider. The information learned from the participants suggested that making improvements to the portal and providing education to both patients and providers may increase the usefulness of the system for experienced users and may encourage new users to adopt it.

Content Analysis

Content analysis is the systematic analysis of communication. It is a "technique for making replicable and valid inferences from texts (or other meaningful matter) to the contexts of their use" (Krippendorff 2013, 24). (See also the discussion of content analysis in chapter 3.) Most often, researchers use content analysis to study written documentation. However, they may analyze other modes of communication, such as speech, body language, images and photographs, music, television shows, commercials, movies, and other symbolic matter (such as office layout).

The purposes of content analysis are to (1) identify dominant findings and make generalizations, and (2) study and predict behaviors. Content analysis may be quantitative or qualitative. In quantitative content analysis, the researchers count and tabulate the number of times a unit of analysis (text or other communication) is used. In qualitative content analysis, the researchers progressively reducing the units of analysis into fewer and fewer categories and, eventually, into themes.

Content analysis is characterized as essentially being a coding operation (Babbie 2016, 328). The coded texts (or communications) are the data. Researchers iteratively cycle through the following process:

- Identify a unit of analysis (text or other means of communication). A *unit of analysis* is a single, meaningful, undivided whole (Chenail 2012, 266). The units of analysis may be words, images, sentences, times, settings, or other elements.
- Code the unit of analysis. Coding is the labeling of words or word groups (segments) with annotations or scales. These labels are characteristics of the segments.
- Assess reliability of the coding by checking the agreement between and among coders (researchers, their assistants, or both).
- Identify key terms, characteristics, or other attributes from the coding.
- Categorize the data by classifying groups of coded data with similar meanings. Categorization is a major step in the analysis. These categories must include, without exception, all the meanings transmitted by the original communication. The categories must be mutually exclusive and have both internal integrity (homogeneity within each category) and external integrity (heterogeneity between and among categories). Additionally, the process of developing the categories should be transparent.
- Abstract the categories into overarching themes.

Content analysis can be either deductive or inductive. In deductive content analysis, the researchers are testing an existing theory or model in a fairly established body of knowledge. Thus, the analysis moves from the generalization (theory or model) to the data. In inductive content analysis, little is known about a topic. Inductive content analysis builds theory and the body of knowledge by moving from limited data on specific observations to generalization.

Alpert and associates used content analysis in a case study that evaluated how well portals convey information to patients (Alpert et al. 2016, 2). They conducted interviews with 31 patients using critical incident technique, a qualitative technique in which the researchers asked the participants to identify their best and worst experiences with the object being studied (in this case, the portal). The interviews, on average lasting 14 minutes, were audio recorded and transcribed. The researchers also conducted two clinician focus group sessions, again using critical incident technique. The first focus group had eight physicians. The second focus group had five clinicians (four nurses and one emergency medical technician). The average length of both focus group sessions was 51 minutes.

The researchers gathered over 140 critical incidents, with 71.8 percent being negative and 28.2 percent being positive (Alpert et al. 2016, 1). Three positive incident categories were instant medical information access, clear health information, and patient vigilance. Four negative incident categories were standardized content, desire for direct communication, website functionality, and difficulty interpreting laboratory data (Alpert et al. 2016, 1). The research showed two general ways to refine the portal: improve communication by being direct and interactive and increase patients' engagement by greater "perceived personalization" (Alpert et al. 2016, 1). The researchers concluded that "simple modifications [to portals] such as increased interactivity and personalized messages, can make portals...easily accessible, and trusted information sources" (Alpert et al. 2016, 1).

Conclusion Validity

Conclusion validity is the extent to which observations, patterns, and inferences are reasonable. Conclusion validity is the qualitative counterpart of quantitative research's statistical conclusion validity. Conclusion validity may be judged by the following criteria:

- Clarity of the logic in assigning categories
- Exhaustiveness of search for confirming and disconfirming data

- Ability of final interpretation to encompass evidence and patterns
- Inclusion of critical examinations of researchers' perspectives and their potential to bias interpretations
- Convincing warrant for the researchers' claims

The terms *warrant* and *claim* have specialized meaning in qualitative research. **Warrant** means justification, and **claim** means interpretation. Credibility, transferability, dependability, and confirmability are the characteristics of high-quality qualitative research (Guba and Lincoln 1989, 236–243). Refer to table 1.3 for the specialized definitions of these characteristics. These characteristics support qualitative researchers' conclusion validity. Conclusion validity is the justified reasonableness of the final interpretation to fit the data.

Qualitative Analytic Software Programs

Qualitative analytic software does *not* conduct analysis—qualitative researchers do. The researchers perform the actual analysis and interpretation of their data (Humble 2012, 125). However, software can *assist* researchers in analyzing their data. For example, the programs facilitate manual tasks, such as retrieving specific coded excerpts from transcripts of interviews. Software packages can also assist qualitative researchers throughout the research process in organizing, managing, collecting, coding, and analyzing their volumes of data.

The software used in qualitative research is known as *CAQDAS (computer-aided qualitative data analysis software).* Many qualitative analytic software packages are available (Predictive Analytics Today 2016a; Predictive Analytics Today 2016b.). Experts advise, however, that researchers carefully explore software to ensure a fit between the program's features and the researchers' question, design, and methods (Humble 2012, 129; Cope 2014, 323). Some software is freeware; other types are proprietary (see table 12.8 for examples). Free trials and tutorials are often available.

Table 12.8 Free and proprietary qualitative analytic software programs

Name	Description
ATLAS.ti	Set of tools that can code and analyze text-based data from open-ended surveys, transcriptions of focus groups, or other sources. ATLAS.ti can also be used to code non-text-based types of qualitative data, such as photographs. It allows the retrieval of specific information based on search criteria and has the ability to export data as an IBM SPSS data set.
CDC EZ-Text	Free software program from the CDC that helps investigators create, manage, and analyze semistructured qualitative databases. Investigators can use the software to enter data, create online codebooks, apply codes to specific response passages, develop case studies, conduct database searches to identify text passages, and export data in a wide array of formats for further analysis with other analytic software programs.
HyperRESEARCH and HyperTRANSCRIBE	HyperRESEARCH is a cross-platform software for qualitative analysis that assists in coding and retrieving data, building theories, and conducting analyses of data. The software has multimedia capabilities that allow work with text, graphics, audio, and video sources. HyperTRANSCRIBE assists with the transcription of audio or video data from its source to a text file by giving keyboard control over the looping and playback of audio or video files.
NVivo	Software for collecting, organizing, and analyzing data from almost any source. NVivo is used to code and analyze unstructured, text-based data from open-ended surveys, transcriptions of focus groups, or other sources. It allows investigators to retrieve specific quotes based on search criteria and can create tabular data representing the counts of specific codes. The data can be exported to quantitative statistical packages.

(*Continued*)

Table 12.8 (*Continued*)

Name	Description
QDA Miner	Software package for coding, annotating, retrieving, and analyzing small and large collections of documents, such as interview transcripts and journal articles, and images, such as photographs and drawings. QDA Miner integrates with a statistical data analysis tool and a content analysis tool so that data can be related to numerical and categorical data.
Qiqqa	Research management software that can manage thousands of PDFs and scans. Qiqqa has optical character recognition so PDFs can be searched, and it can tag and report text annotations.

Presentation of Results and Discussion

Researchers present the results of their study in the results and discussion sections of their reports or scholarly papers. The results section includes both tabular and graphical displays and narrative. The discussion section expands upon the results section by interpreting the results and putting them in context.

Tabular and Graphical Display

Researchers generate tabular and graphical displays to present their results (see chapter 9 for more details on tables and graphical displays). Creation and refinement of the tables and graphs occur throughout the processes of analysis of data and presentation of results. The researchers' choice of table versus graph depends on the information that the researchers are communicating. Tables are used when exact numerical values are being presented and the reader will be comparing a few values at a time. Graphs are selected when visual comparisons are needed, such as in the presentation of trend data. This subsection builds upon the information on tables and graphical displays in chapter 9.

The purpose of tables and graphs is to support the readers' understanding of the research's results. Points to remember when constructing tables and graphs include the following:

- Tables, graphs, and figures have titles.
- Tables have stub heads, spanner heads, and column heads for clarification.
- Sources are cited.
- Time frames and dates are noted.
- Multiple tables, charts, graphs, and figures are numbered.
- Both axes of graphs are labeled with bar titles, legends, and scale captions as necessary.
- Keys show the meaning of shadings and colors.
- Scales start at zero.
- Graphics are for emphasis; they should not dilute the effect with clutter.
- Tables and graphics should be able to stand on their own, being understandable even without reading the narrative text.

One rule of thumb is that data should be presented in only one way or mode (Day and Gastel 2012, 92). A particular data element may be presented in narrative text, in a table, or in a graph or other figure, but not repeated in multiple modes. Researchers select the mode that most clearly communicates information about the particular data element.

Narrative

Researchers follow a two-step process when presenting their results (also called *findings*). The first step is writing the section of the manuscript called *the results*. In the results section, the researchers report their results with no commentary, explanation, or interpretation. The second step is writing the section of the manuscript called *the discussion*. In the discussion, the researchers comment on, explain, and interpret their results. Also included in the discussion are conclusions and recommendations for future research. The style of language, the content of the results and discussion, and interpretation are described in the follow subsections.

Style of Language in Narrative

Researchers describe their results in the past tense; general truths, such as well-known theories, are stated in the present tense. The style of writing for scientific manuscripts is objective, precise, and factual. Researchers avoid subjective interjections and emotional hyperbole as well as jargon. In the research results, researchers are careful to maintain a neutral tone. They are merely recording their results in a narrative form.

Results

In the results, the researchers present the results for each hypothesis. Restating the hypothesis aids the readers. The researchers state whether the results support the hypotheses. They also document characteristics about the sample and describe the results of the statistical tests that investigated whether the sample resembled or differed from the target population. Supplemental statistical tests also are described. Attention is paid to the appropriate use of the term *statistical significance* as previously discussed in the chapter's section on Statistical Significance Versus Practical Significance.

Discussion

In the discussion section of the manuscript, the researchers focus on their study's important results, highlighting their practical significance. It is in this section of the manuscript that researchers add to the field's body of knowledge by describing their study's results in terms of the existing literature and the field's theories or models. For example, the researchers compare their results to the results of the studies that they had singled out as key contributions to the field in their literature review. The researchers explain why their findings were similar to or differed from those of other researchers. Additionally, the researchers explicitly return to their research question and aims, explaining whether they answered their question and fulfilled their aims, or why they did not. Finally, of particular importance is the researchers' explanation of how their results expand or advance the theory or model underpinning their study.

The researchers also state their assumptions and the limitations of their research. For example, researchers describing a questionnaire study might state that one assumption is that people are honest and that one limitation is the study's cross-sectional time frame. Concluding their discussion, the researchers suggest implications for practice. The results of a research study usually raise new questions. These new questions become the recommendations for further research.

Interpretation

In the discussion section, the researchers are interpreting their study's results by relating them to the theory underpinning their study, to the literature, and to practice. In making this interpretation, the following questions may be helpful:

- What theoretical significance do the results have?
- What practical significance do the results have?
- How do the results explicitly link to the larger body of knowledge?
- How have the results improved the field's research model?
- How have the results expanded the body of knowledge?
- What new definitions have the researchers added to the field's area of practice?
- How do the results support practitioners in the workplace?
- What problems do the results solve?
- What valid conclusions can the researchers and the readers draw?
- What subsequent research studies need to be conducted to answer questions that this study raised or to address problems that this study faced?

Answers to these questions result in new information. For example, the results might have expanded existing theory by clarifying ambiguities or closing gaps. Additionally, actionable information may have been placed into the hands of practitioners in the workplace. Finally, the field's scholarship may have been advanced because the study presents new information and avenues for continued research.

Review Questions

1. What do the abbreviations ITT and NTT mean? For what purpose would a researcher use each of these acronyms?
2. The following ROC curve was presented in a research article on detecting fraud and shows how the researchers' model was functioning to detect fraud. Inspect the ROC curve in figure 12.4. Is the model predictive of fraud? Based on the AUC, why or why not?

Figure 12.4 ROC curve optimized toward sensitivity

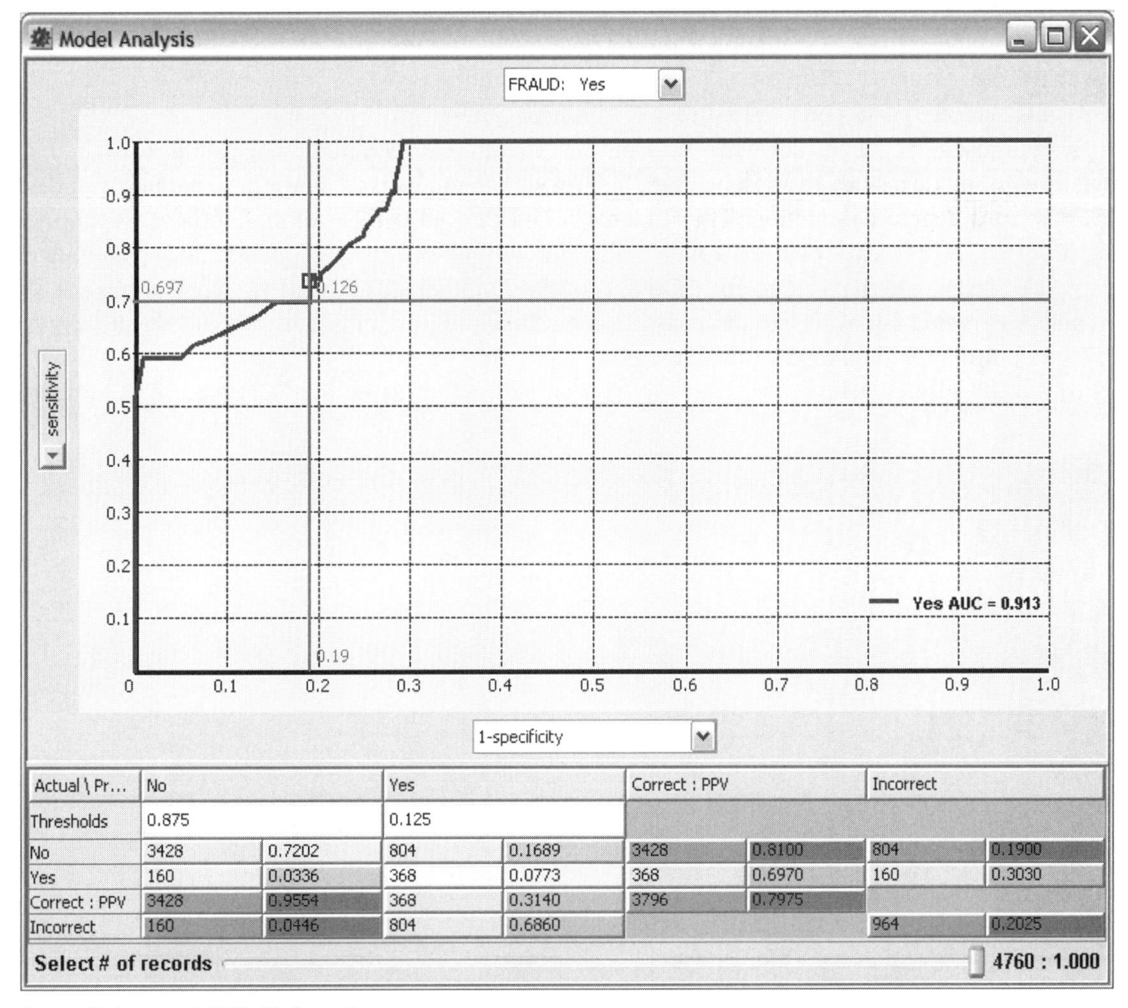

Source: Rudman et al. 2009, 20, figure 6.

3. Your subordinate, Hannah, created an application to enhance the organization's clinician dashboard. This application captured data from the patients' electronic health records (EHRs) and presented the clinicians with a line graph of the data. Hannah selected a convenience sample of 18 clinicians (3 cardiologists, 5 neurologists, 3 nephrologists, and 7 dermatologists). When a clinician logged into the patient's EHR, line graphs of the following data were presented: weight for the past 5 years, height for the past 5 years, and hematocrit and hemoglobin levels. The application also included red stars if the body mass index, which is calculated from weight and height, categorized the patient as overweight or obese or underweight or if the hematocrit or hemoglobin level indicated anemia.

   Hannah created her own questionnaire in which she asked the clinicians to indicate their agreement with the following statement: "This application for the dashboard is very helpful to my treatment of my patients." The clinician indicated whether he or she strongly disagreed (rating of 1) to strongly agreed (rating of 5). Hannah performed a one-sample *t*-test on her data. Hannah told you that she decided to scrap her application because the result of statistical test was not significant. You told her that she should *not* to base her decision on the statistical test. Why would you make that statement?

4. What is statistical conclusion validity and why does it matter?
5. What is content analysis and when is it used?
6. What is conclusion validity and how is it assessed?
7. A large, multispecialty group practice installed kiosks in its gastroenterology clinic, its dermatology clinic, and its cardiology clinic. The purpose of the kiosks was to allow patients to enter data into or update their Internet-based personal health records (PHRs). Prior to installing the kiosks, the organizational leaders had analyzed the data on PHR usage and had found that few patients had used the portal to access the online PHR. The leaders decided that the cause of the low usage was the patients' lack of Internet access. Therefore, the leaders decided to address this problem by making Internet access available right at the clinics. Three months after installing the kiosks, the usage was the same as it had been prior to the installation. Could a qualitative research study have improved the leaders' decision? Why or why not?
8. Explain how the results and the discussion sections of a manuscript differ.
9. What two factors should researchers consider when determining how to present a particular data element?
10. A team of students is working on a study of students' satisfaction with the university's program that helps students track their progress toward degree completion. The students found that 36 percent of students were extremely satisfied with the program, 35 percent of students were satisfied with the program, 15 percent of students were neutral, 8 percent were dissatisfied, and 6 percent were extremely dissatisfied. The team is working on the first draft of its report and has created figure 12.5 to insert as a way to show their findings. How should the team revise figure 12.5 prior to submitting the final report to the instructor?

Figure 12.5

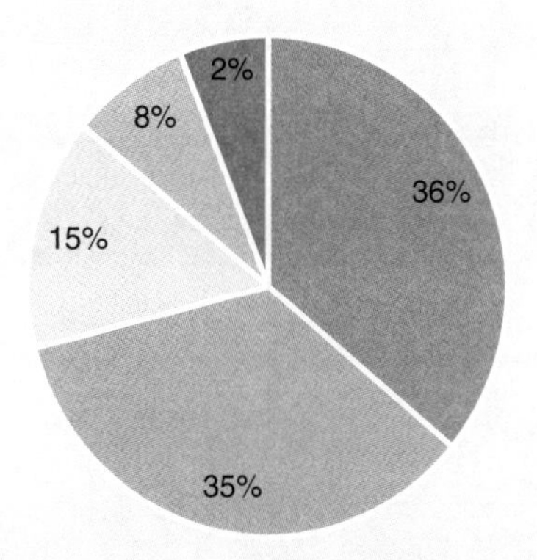

Application Exercises

1. The real-world case in this chapter described a research study in which researchers presented an analytic approach that could identify dual-eligible beneficiaries, an especially costly patient population for healthcare organizations. The researchers segmented a very large data set into five groups. Conducting regressions, the researchers identified variables that differentiated dual-eligible beneficiaries from the nondual-eligible beneficiaries. The regressions' results were given as ORs. Certain variables increased a Medicare beneficiary's odds of being a dual-eligible beneficiary. For example, in the segment "Older and likely to be widowed," having "tooth loss" made the beneficiary 3.26 times more likely of being a dual-eligible beneficiary. The researchers presented all the statistically significant ORs in a table. Interpret the following information and explain its meaning in a sentence:
In the segment "The survivors," a statistically significant OR was 0.24 for the variable of "Respondent's home: one-family detached."
2. A team of college students completed a quantitative research project on the perceptions of college students and college professors of activity trackers. The team members wrote in the first draft of their paper that their results, based on their statistical analysis, showed a significant difference between the perspectives of college students and college professors of activity trackers. The caption of their table showing their results contained the following

note: *Significant at $P > 0.05$. Can you identify the errors in the team's first draft and suggest how the paper should be corrected?

3. The chapter discusses the problem of missing data in health research. The chapter briefly noted that a systematic review of articles in leading medical journals found that 95 percent of the articles on RCTs had missing outcome data (Bell et al. 2014, 3). The chapter has discussed many terms used in this article on missing data. In this application, you see how the terms are used in context.
   One of the authors' purposes in conducting this research was to evaluate the extent, handling, and sensitivity analysis of missing data from RCTs reported in "top tier medical journals" (*BMJ*, *Journal of the American Medical Association*, *Lancet*, and the *New England Journal of Medicine*). The RCTs had been published between July and December 2013. The researchers reported the following results: "Of the 77 identified eligible articles, 73 (95%) reported some missing outcome data. … The most commonly used method to handle missing data in the primary analysis was complete case analysis (33, 45%), while 20 (27%) performed simple imputation, 15 (19%) used model based methods, and 6 (8%) used multiple imputation. … Reports of ITT or modified ITT were found in 52 (85%) trials, with 21 (40%) of them including all randomized participants" (Bell et al. 2014, 1).
   a. Why does it matter if missing data are addressed?
   b. "Complete case analysis" is the same as "case deletion." Why do you think so many studies reported case deletion and simple imputation as the method of addressing missing data?
   c. What is imputation and what is a possible reason why multiple imputation was the least likely technique to be used?
   d. What is sensitivity analysis and why does it matter?

References

Ahlemeyer-Stubbe, A. and S. Coleman. 2014. *A Practical Guide to Data Mining for Business and Industry*. Chichester, UK: Wiley.

Alpert, J.M., A.H. Krist, R.A. Aycock, and G.L. Kreps. 2016. Applying multiple methods to comprehensively evaluate a patient portal's effectiveness to convey information to patients. *Journal of Medical Internet Research* 18(5):e112.

Alshurafa, M., M. Briel, E.A. Akl, T. Haines, P. Moayyedi, S.J. Gentles, L. Rios, C. Tran, N. Bhatnagar, F. Lamontagne, S.D. Walter, and G.H. Guyat. 2012. Inconsistent definitions for intention-to-treat in relation to missing outcome data: Systematic review of the methods literature. *PLoS ONE* 7(11):e49163.

Babbie, E. 2016. *The Practice of Social Research,* 14th ed. Boston: Cengage Learning.

Barry, B.H. 2013. *Explaining Psychological Statistics,* 4th ed. Hoboken, NJ: Wiley.

Bell, M.L., M. Fiero, N.J. Horton, and C.H. Hsu. 2014. Handling missing data in RCTs: A review of the top medical journals. *BMC Medical Research Methodology* 14(118): 1–8.

Berson, A., S. Smith, and K. Thearling. 2000. *Building Data Mining Applications for CRM*. New York: McGraw Hill.

Blankers, M., M.W.J. Koeter, and G.M. Schippers. 2010. Missing data approaches for ehealth research: Simulation study and a tutorial for nonmathematically inclined researchers. *Journal of Medical Internet Research* 12(5):e54.

Breiman, L., J. Friedman, R.A. Olshen, and C.J. Stone. 1984. *Classification and Regression Trees*. Boca Raton, FL: CRC Press.

Brin, S. and L. Page. 1998. The anatomy of a large-scale hypertextual Web search engine. *Computer Networks and ISDN Systems* 30(1–7):107–117.

Carbonell, J.G., R.S. Michalski, and T. Mitchell. 1983. Machine learning: A historical and methodological analysis. *AI Magazine* 4(3):69–79.

Centers for Disease Control and Prevention (CDC). 2012. *Principles of Epidemiology in Public Health Practice: An Introduction to Applied Epidemiology and Biostatistics*, 3rd ed. Atlanta, GA: Centers for Disease Control and Prevention. Self-study course SS1978. https://www.cdc.gov/ophss/csels/dsepd/ss1978/ss1978.pdf.

Chang, S.M., D.B. Matchar, G.W. Smetana, and C.A. Umscheid. 2012. *Methods Guide for Medical Test Reviews*. AHRQ publication no. 12-EC017. Rockville, MD: Agency for Healthcare Research and Quality. https://effectivehealthcare.ahrq.gov/search-for-guides-reviews-and-reports/?pageaction=displayProduct&productID=558.

Chenail, R.J. 2012. Conducting qualitative data analysis: Reading line-by-line, but analyzing meaningful qualitative units. *Qualitative Report* 17(1):266–269.

Cios, K.J., A. Teresinska, S. Konieczna, J. Potocka, and S. Sharma. 2000. A knowledge discovery approach to diagnosing myocardial perfusion. *IEEE Engineering in Medicine and Biology Magazine* 19(4):17–25.

Cohen, J. 1992. A power primer. *Psychological Bulletin* 112(1):155–159.

Cope, D.G. 2014. Computer-assisted qualitative data analysis software. *Oncology Nursing Forum* 41(3):322–323.

Cummings, P. 2013. Missing data and multiple imputation. *JAMA Pediatrics* 167(7):656–661.

Day, R.A. and B. Gastel. 2012. *How to Write and Publish a Scientific Paper*, 7th ed. Cambridge, UK: Cambridge University Press.

Dunlop, S., B. Freeman, and D. Perez. 2016. Exposure to Internet-based tobacco advertising and branding: Results from population surveys of Australian youth 2010–2013. *Journal of Medical Internet Research* 18(6):e104.

Food and Drug Administration (FDA) Center for Drug Evaluation and Research and Center for Biologics Evaluation and Research. 1998(September). *Guidance for Industry: E9 Statistical Principles for Clinical Trials*. http://www.fda.gov/downloads/drugs/guidancecomplianceregulatoryinformation/guidances/ucm073137.pdf.

Freund, Y. and R.E. Schapire. 1997. A decision-theoretic generalization of on-line learning and an application to boosting. *Journal of Computer and System Sciences* 55(1):119–139.

Friedman, N., D. Geiger, and M. Goldszmidt. 1997. Bayesian network classifiers. *Machine Learning* 29(2):131–163.

Gardiner, E.J., and V.J. Gillet VJ. 2015. Perspectives on knowledge discovery algorithms recently introduced in chemoinformatics: Rough set theory, association rule mining, emerging patterns, and formal concept analysis. *Journal of Chemical Information and Modeling* 55(9):1781–1803.

Gee, P.M., D.A. Paterniti, D. Ward, and L.M. Soederberg Miller. 2015. e-Patients perceptions of using personal health records for self-management support of chronic illness. *CIN: Computers, Informatics, Nursing* 33(6):229–237.

Glaser, B.G. 2002. Grounded theory and gender relevance. *Health Care for Women International* 23(8):786–793.

Glaser, B.G. 1965. The constant comparative method of qualitative analysis. *Social Problems* 12(4):436–445.

Greenland, S., S.J. Senn, K.J. Rothman, J.B. Carlin, C. Poole, S.N. Goodman, and D.G. Altman. 2016. Statistical tests, *P* values, confidence intervals, and power: A guide to misinterpretations. *European Journal of Epidemiology* 31(4):337–350.

Guba, E. and Y. Lincoln. 1989. *Fourth Generation Evaluation*. Newbury Park, CA: Sage.

Haneuse, S., A. Bogart, I. Jazic, E.O. Westbrook, D. Boudreau, M.K. Theis, G.E. Simon, and D. Arterburn. 2016. Learning about missing data mechanisms in electronic health records-based research: A survey-based approach. *Epidemiology* 27(1):82–90.

Holloway, I. and S. Wheeler. 2010. *Qualitative Research in Nursing and Healthcare*, 3rd ed. Ames, IA: Wiley-Blackwell.

Humble, A.M. 2012. Qualitative data analysis software: A call for understanding, detail, intentionality, and thoughtfulness. *Journal of Family Theory and Review* 4(2):122–137.

Irwig, L., J. Irwig, L. Trevena, and M. Sweet. 2008. *Smart Health Choices: Making Sense of Health Advice*. London, UK: Hammersmith Press.

Jiang, L., Z. Cai, D. Wang, and H. Zhang. 2014. Bayesian citation-KNN with distance weighting. *International Journal of Machine Learning and Cybernetics* 5(2):193–199.

Kelley, K. and K.J Preacher. 2012. On effect size. *Psychological Methods* 17(2):137–152.

Korenda, L., D. Byler, K. Bingham, T. Schiltgen, and G. Scott. 2015 (December). Drilling Down on Dual Eligibles. Deloitte Center for Health Solutions. http://dupress.com/articles/dual-eligibles-quality-of-health-care-analytics.

Kosters, W.A., W. Pijls, and V. Popova. 2003 (July). Complexity analysis of Depth First and FP-growth implementations of APRIORI. In *Machine Learning and Data Mining in Pattern Recognition: Third International Conference, MLDM 2003. Leipzig, Germany, July 5–7, 2003, Proceedings*. Edited by P. Perner and A. Rosenfeld. Berlin, Germany: Springer-Verlag: 284–292.

Kotu, V. and B. Deshpande. 2015. *Predictive Analytics and Data Mining: Concepts and Practice with RapidMiner*. Waltham, MA: Morgan Kaufmann.

Lalkhen, A.G. and A. McCluskey. 2008. Clinical tests: Sensitivity and specificity. *Continuing Education in Anaesthesia, Critical Care and Pain* 8(6):221–223.

LaMorte, W.W. 2016 (June 15). Screening for Disease: Positive and Negative Predictive Value. Boston University School of Public Health. http://sphweb.bumc.bu.edu/otlt/MPH-Modules/EP/EP713_Screening/EP713_Screening5.html.

Li, S., L. Kang, and X.M. Zhao. 2014 (January). A survey on evolutionary algorithm based hybrid intelligence in bioinformatics. *BioMed Research International.* doi: 10.1155/2014/362738.

Little, T.D., T.D. Jorgensen, K.M. Lang, and E.W.G. Moore. 2014. On the joys of missing data. *Journal of Pediatric Psychology* 39(2):151–162.

McLachlan, G.J. and T. Krishnan. 2008. *The EM Algorithm and Extensions*, 2nd ed. Hoboken, NJ: John Wiley and Sons.

Medicare Payment Advisory Committee (MEDPAC). 2016 (June). *Data Book: Health Care Spending and the Medicare Program.* http://www.medpac.gov/-documents-/data-book.

Merriam, S.B. 2009. *Qualitative Research: A Guide to Design and Implementation.* San Francisco, CA: Jossey-Bass.

McCormick, T.H., R. Ferrell, A.F Karr, and P.B. Ryan. 2014. Big data, big results: Knowledge discovery in output from large-scale analytics. *Statistical Analysis and Data Mining* 7(5):404–412.

Mobley, B.A., E. Schechter, W.E. Moore, P.A. McKee, and J.E. Eichner. 2000. Predictions of coronary artery stenosis by artificial neural network. *Artificial Intelligence in Medicine* 18(3):187–203.

Montez-Rath, M.E., W.C. Winkelmayer, and M. Desai. 2014. Addressing missing data in clinical studies of kidney diseases. *Clinical Journal of the American Society of Nephrology* 9(7):1328–1335.

Morissette, L. and S. Chartier. 2013. The *k*-means clustering technique: General considerations and implementation in *Mathematica. Tutorials in Quantitative Methods for Psychology* 9(1):15–24.

Motulsky, H. 2014. *Intuitive Biostatistics: A Nonmathematical Guide to Statistical Thinking*. New York, NY: Oxford University Press.

Musumeci, M. 2015 (December). Financial and Administrative Alignment Demonstrations for Dual Eligible Beneficiaries Compared: States with Memoranda of Understanding Approved by CMS. Kaiser Family Foundation Issue Brief. https://kaiserfamilyfoundation.files.wordpress.com/2015/12/8426-07-financial-alignment-demonstrations-for-dual-eligible-beneficiaries-compared-dec-2015.pdf.

Perfors, A., J.B. Tenenbaum, T.L. Griffiths, and F. Xu. 2011. A tutorial introduction to Bayesian models of cognitive development. *Cognition*. 120(3):302–321.

Predictive Analytics Today. 2016a. Top 17 Free Qualitative Data Analysis Software. http://www.predictiveanalyticstoday.com/top-free-qualitative-data-analysis-software./

Predictive Analytics Today. 2016b. Top 15 Qualitative Data Analysis Software. http://www.predictiveanalyticstoday.com/top-qualitative-data-analysis-software./

Quinlan, J.R. 1996 (March). Improved use of continuous attributes in C4.5. *Journal of Artificial Intelligence Research* 4:77–90

Ravid, R. 2011. *Practical Statistics for Educators*. 4th ed. Lanham, MD: Rowman and Littlefield.

Ray, R. 2011. *Enterprise Resource Planning*. New Delhi, India: Tata McGraw Hill Education.

Rudman, W.J., J.S. Eberhardt, W. Pierce, and S. Hart-Hester. 2009 (Fall). Healthcare fraud and abuse. *Perspectives in Health Information Management* 6:1–24.

Sanky, M., P.D. Berger, and B.D. Weinberg. 2012. A segmentation approach to patient health intervention. *Journal of Medical Marketing* 12(4):221–228.

Schulz, K.F., D.G. Altman, D. Moher, for the CONSORT Group. 2010. CONSORT 2010 statement: Updated guidelines for reporting parallel group randomized trials. *Annals of Internal Medicine* 152(11):1–7.

Schünemann, H.J., A.D. Oxman, G.E. Vist, J.P.T Higgins, J.J. Deeks, P. Glasziou, and G.H. Guyatt. 2011 (March). Confidence intervals. Section 12.4.1 in *Cochrane Handbook for Systematic Reviews of Interventions Version 5.1.0.* Edited by Higgins, J.P.T. and S. Green. http://handbook.cochrane.org/chapter_12/12_4_1_confidence_intervals.htm.

Sedgwick, P. 2015. Measuring the benefit of treatment: Number needed to treat. *BMJ* 350:h2206. doi: 10.1136/bmj.h2206.

Sedgwick, P. 2014. Unit of observation versus unit of analysis. *BMJ* 348:g3840. doi: 10.1136/bmj.g3840. Errata published in *BMJ* 2015;351:h5534. doi: 10.1136/bmj.h553.

Szumilas, M. 2010 (August). Explaining odds ratios. *Journal of the Canadian Academy of Child and Adolescent* 19(3):227–229.

Tesch, R. 1990. *Qualitative Research: Analysis Types and Software Tools.* New York, NY: Falmer Press.

Thomas, L. and E.D. Peterson. 2012. The value of statistical analysis plans in observational research: Defining high-quality research from the start. *Journal of the American Medical Association* 308(8):773–774.

Thompson, B.G. 2009. Descriptive data analysis. *Air Medical Journal* 28(2):56–59.

Tufféry, S. 2011. *Data Mining and Statistics for Decision Making.* Chichester, UK: John Wiley and Sons.

Van den Broeck, J., S.A. Cunningham, R. Eeckels, and K. Herbst. 2005. Data cleaning: Detecting, diagnosing, and editing data abnormalities. *PLoS Medicine* 2(10): e267. doi: 10.1371/journal.pmed.0020267.

Vapnik, V.N. 1999. An overview of statistical learning theory. *IEEE Transactions on Neural Networks* 10(5):988–999.

Vleugel, A., M. Spruit, and A. van Daal. 2012. Historical Data Analysis Through Data Mining from an Outsourcing Perspective: The Three-Phases Model. Chapter 17 in *Organizational Applications of Business Intelligence Management: Emergency Trends*. Edited by Herschel, R.T. Hershey, PA: IGI Global: 236–260.

Wasserstein, R.L., and N. A. Lazar. 2016. The ASA's statement on *P*-values: Context, process, and purpose. *American Statistician* 70(2):129–133.

Woods, A.D., D.P. Mulherin, A.J. Flynn, J.G. Stevenson, C.R. Zimmerman, and B.W. Chaffee. 2014. Clinical decision support for atypical orders: Detection and warning of atypical medication orders submitted to a computerized provider order entry system. *Journal of the American Medical Informatics Association* 21(3):569–573.

Wu, X., V. Kumar, J.R. Quinlan, J. Ghosh, Q. Yang, H. Motoda, G.L. McLachlan, A. Ng, B. Liu, P.S. Yu, Z. Zhou, M. Steinbach, D.J. Hand, and D. Steinberg. 2008. Top 10 algorithms in data mining. *Knowledge and Information Systems* 14(1):1–37.

Xu, J., S.L. Murphy, K.D. Kochanek, and B.A. Bastian. 2016. Deaths: Final data for 2013. *National Vital Statistics Reports* 64(2):1–16. http://www.cdc.gov/nchs/data/nvsr/nvsr64/nvsr64_02.pdf.

Yardley, S.J., K.M. Watts, J. Pearson, and J.C Richardson. 2014. Ethical issues in the reuse of qualitative data: Perspectives from literature, practice, and participants. *Qualitative Health Research* 24(1):102–113.

Zeng, A., T. Li, J. Zhang, and D. Liu. 2012. An Incremental Approach for Updating Approximations of Rough Fuzzy Sets Under the Variation of the Object Set. In *Rough Sets and Current Trends in Computing: 8th International Conference, RSCTC 2012, Chengdu, China, August 17–20, 2012: Proceedings,* vol. 7413. Edited by Yao, J., Y. Yang, R. Slowinsky, S. Greco, H. Li, S. Mitra, and L. Polkowski. New York: Springer: 36–45.

Resources

Cohen, D. and B. Crabtree. 2006 (July). Evaluative Criteria. In *Qualitative Research Guidelines Project*. Robert Wood Johnson Foundation. http://www.qualres.org/HomeEval-3664.html.

Cohen, J. 1988. *Statistical Power Analysis for the Behavioral Sciences,* 2nd ed. Hillsdale, NJ: Lawrence Erlbaum Associates.

Creswell, J.W. 2014. *Research Design: Qualitative, Quantitative, and Mixed Methods Approaches*, 4th ed. Thousand Oaks, CA: Sage.

Indrayan, A. 2013. *Medical Biostatistics*, 3rd ed. Boca Raton, FL: Chapman and Hall/CRC Press.

Maxwell, J.A. 2013. *Qualitative Research Design: An Interactive Approach*, 3rd ed. Thousand Oaks, CA: Sage.

Miles, M.B., A.M. Huberman, and J. Saldaña. 2014. *Qualitative Data Analysis: A Methods Sourcebook*. 3rd ed. Thousand Oaks, CA: Sage.

Niazkhani, Z., P. Habibollah, J. Aarts, S. Adams, and R. Bal. 2010 (December). Reporting qualitative research in health informatics: REQ-HI recommendations. *Studies in Health Technology and Informatics* 169:877–881.

Selya, A.S., J.S. Rose, L.C. Dierker, D. Hedeker, and R.J. Mermelstein. 2012. A practical guide to calculating Cohen's f(2), a measure of local effect size, from PROC MIXED. *Frontiers in Psychology* 3(111):1–6.

Silverman, D. 2016. *Qualitative Research,* 4th ed. Thousand Oaks, CA: Sage.

Silverman, D. 2013. *Doing Qualitative Research,* 4th ed. Thousand Oaks, CA: Sage.

Stang, A. and C. Poole. 2013. The researcher and the consultant: A dialogue on null hypothesis significance testing. *European Journal of Epidemiology* 28(12):939–944.

Wassertheil-Smoller, S. and J. Smoller. 2015. *Biostatistics and Epidemiology: A Primer for Health and Biomedical Professionals,* 4th ed. New York: Springer.

White, S. 2016. *A Practical Approach to Analyzing Healthcare Data*, 3rd ed. Chicago: American Health Information Management Association.

PART III

Information to Knowledge

13 The Grant Process and Proposal Writing

14 Research and Ethics

15 Disseminating Information

13 The Grant Process and Proposal Writing

Valerie Watzlaf, PhD, MPH, RHIA, FAHIMA

Learning Objectives

- Evaluate the grant writing process, aspects of the grant proposal, and methods used to obtain grant funding.
- Compare and contrast the types of funding agencies and application guidelines and how grants can be used to fund health informatics research.
- Apply knowledge of the peer review process, general review criteria, scoring and ranking of the proposal, and the entire panel review process when deciding which grants to fund.
- Assess whether a proposal meets the requirements of the content section and application.
- Determine why a grant may not be accepted and funded.
- Summarize how grant writing can be used effectively in health informatics research to seek funds to conduct the research.

Key Terms

Approach
Biographical sketch
Budget
Centers for Scientific Review (CSR)
Confidentiality form
Conflict of interest form
Cost sharing
Eligibility criteria
Face page
Grant
Grantee
Indirect costs
Innovation
Investigators
Key personnel
Letter of intent
Matching requirements
National Institutes of Health (NIH)
National Library of Medicine (NLM)
Panel of reviewers
Peer-reviewed research
Principal investigator (PI)
Program officer
Proposal reviewer
Request for application (RFA)
Scientific review group (SRG)
Scientific review officer (SRO)
Seed money
Significance
Streamlining

Researchers in health informatics may wish to seek grants to fund the research process. A **grant** in healthcare research is a financial assistance award for peer-reviewed research that extends health and decreases illness and disability (NIH 2016a). Grant writing, or proposal writing, takes a great deal of time and effort, but it is doable and should be pursued by health informatics professionals. This chapter explains the steps in the grant-writing process and provides examples specific to health informatics. Health informatics professionals may choose to be the primary investigator (PI) in a research project, or they can serve as co-investigators, consultants, grant writers, or key staff members for intervention studies such as clinical and community trials. Whatever roles they play, it is important for health informatics researchers to immerse themselves in current research projects. Their expertise is vital to the success of health informatics research. This chapter covers the process of writing a grant proposal, including preparation, finding a granting agency, writing the proposal, the granting agency staff and volunteers who will review the grant proposal, the grant proposal review process, and revising and resubmitting a proposal.

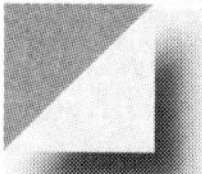

Real-World Case

There are many opportunities for funding in the health informatics field. Many are found in **requests for applications (RFAs)**, which are sometimes called *requests for proposals (RFPs)* or *funding opportunity announcements (FOAs)*, issued by grant-giving entities. For example, the US Department of Health and Human Services (HHS) through the Agency for Healthcare Research and Quality (AHRQ) has created a funding opportunity titled "Exploratory and Developmental Grant to Improve Health Care Quality through Health Information Technology (IT) (R21)." This FOA invites researchers to submit grant proposals for research in which they will use health information technology (HIT)—such as electronic health records (EHRs), computerized provider order entry (CPOE) systems, telemedicine, clinical decision support, mobile apps, and health kiosks—to improve healthcare quality outcomes, manage HIT workflow and workload, and reduce the costs of adopting HIT (HHS 2013). The funding announcement outlines the following sections that must be included in the grant proposal:

- *Background and significance:* Demonstrate gaps in the literature and show how the results of the research will help to inform future health informatics research.
- *Theoretical framework:* Reflect on the ability of the study to generate awareness into HIT applications by using traditional healthcare analytic theories as well as other innovative theories related to human factors and industrial and systems engineering.
- *Research design and methods:* Use a wide range of quantitative and qualitative methods with a well-thought-out study design and statistical analysis plan (SAP).
- *HIT intervention:* If the proposed study uses an HIT intervention (such as a new EHR system), describe the new or revised HIT intervention and demonstrate a need for it.
- *Secondary data analysis or economic analysis:* If secondary data analyses are used, explain how the proposed research project is different from the study that collected the data, and describe the data sets used as well as completeness, reliability, and accuracy of the data.
- *Dissemination:* Describe how research results will be disseminated to those who can benefit from future HIT research.
- *Privacy and security protections of the HIT:* Include a plan for privacy and security protections in the development and implementation of HIT systems.
- *Project administration:* Identify who will oversee the project and include a project timeline.
- *Appendix:* Add any additional information relevant to the grant proposal.

Preparing to Write a Grant

Grant writing is the process in which an individual or team of researchers explain their research plan in hopes that a grant-seeking entity will give (grant) them monies to conduct the research explained in the grant proposal. Grant proposal writing is an art. To be successful, the grant writer should be creative, immersed in the scientific area at hand, and fully aware of the granting agency's requirements and recommendations. Grant writing can be a tedious, arduous task, but it can provide great rewards if the grant proposal is accepted and the research is funded. With a grant, the researcher can complete a study in an area that may not have been explored before, making the researcher a pioneer in a scientific area.

Specific researchers write the grant proposal; however, if the grant is awarded, the **grantee** (recipient of the grant money) is a university, healthcare center, or other organization that the researchers are affiliated with, not the individual researchers. Therefore, once the grant is awarded, the organization must abide by the terms and requirements of the grant. A program officer or grants management specialist, employed by the granting agency, will work with the grantees to assist them in managing the award. Before writing a grant proposal, researchers must understand research trends and problems in the proposed area of study and establish their credibility as **investigators**, personnel who carry out research.

Monitor Research Trends and Problems in Areas of Expertise

To be successful in securing a funded grant, the researchers must monitor research trends and be experts in the area in which they are seeking funding. For example, if the investigators are interested in securing a grant award in the area of International Classification of Diseases, 10th Revision, Clinical Modification (ICD-10-CM) and International Classification of Diseases, 10th Revision, Procedure Classification System (ICD-10-PCS), they should know a great deal about ICD-10-CM and ICD-10-PCS and its strengths and weaknesses, methods of improvement, other research on ICD-10-CM and ICD-10-PCS, and the gaps in that research. Additionally, they should have a fundamental knowledge base about classification systems in general. Providing this evidence to the funding agency will illustrate the need for the proposed research and why it should be funded by the agency.

Build Credibility in Area of Expertise Through Publication

Granting agencies take a calculated risk by providing monies to carry out the proposed research, and they therefore seek evidence in the grant proposal that the investigators are worth that risk. One way for grant seekers to build credibility as an expert in a specific area is to provide as many examples of scholarly work as possible, such as publications, presentations, and collaborations with other experts in the field of study. A history of scholarly work demonstrates to the granting agency that the researchers are well known in their research area. **Peer-reviewed research** is research that is examined and evaluated by experts in the same or a related research field or scientific area (see chapter 15). Most scholarly publications, such as journal articles, are peer-reviewed and therefore demonstrate that experts in that same field acknowledge the expertise of the author. This recognition is something that granting agencies value. For example, for a grant proposal to research ICD-10-CM and ICD-10-PCS, the investigators should list their publications and presentations in areas related to classification systems and clinical terminologies, including ICD-10-CM and ICD-10-PCS. The investigators could also strengthen their proposal by noting any relevant collaborations, such as serving on a taskforce that examines clinical terminologies and classification systems, or serving on committees that examine the effectiveness of ICD-10-CM and ICD-10-PCS. In addition, documenting in the proposal any preliminary research or previous grant awards in the same or similar area can aid the grantee in securing the grant.

Sources of Grants

An important part of grant writing is identifying potential funding entities. Investigators often begin this process by approaching entities that fund preliminary research, such as their employer's or university's funding agency or a foundation. Once this research is complete, investigators can continue to the local, state, or federal levels for additional funding sources.

Internal Sources and Foundations

New investigators with little prior experience in grant writing and investigators in a pioneering research area may initially look for "seed" money to start exploring the research topic. **Seed money** is funding, often from an internal source or a foundation, that enables an investigator to begin research in a new area of interest. For example, most universities and even some healthcare centers have research monies available for new investigators within their university or healthcare center. These monies may include research and development funds available from specific university schools or foundations established within the healthcare facility. At the University of Pittsburgh School of Health and Rehabilitation Sciences (SHRS), the SHRS Research and Development Fund is available to students and faculty interested in pursuing research. Similarly, the University of Minnesota's Clinical and Translational Science Institute and the Institute for Health Informatics sponsors the Informatics Seed Grants Program, whose goal is to support junior faculty in researching health informatics so that they can then go on to apply for larger funding at the state or federal level. There are several topic areas of interest, such as designing an informatics intervention to increase vaccination rates or creating new informatics systems to increase medication compliance (University of Minnesota 2015).

Internal entities have specific granting requirements that investigators must follow to get seed money. Such requirements may include administrative restrictions on the types of research funded, limits on travel costs, and rules about the number of graduate student assistants that can be hired.

Several foundations provide seed money or other funding for health informatics research. Investigators should search for funding foundations specific to their area of inquiry. Grant databases are available to aid in the search for funding from foundations, but use of these databases can sometimes be costly. In many cases, a web search of the funding available from foundations is equally reliable and effective.

The AHIMA Foundation is one example of a foundation that funds certain types of research. For example, it provides the Dissertation Assistance Award program, which supports research undertaken by doctoral candidates as part of an academic program in areas relevant to health information management (HIM). To qualify for an award from this program, the student acting as the principal investigator must be enrolled in an accredited doctoral degree program in an area related to HIM (computer science, business management, education, public health, and so forth) and must be an active or student member of the American Health Information Management Association (AHIMA). The student must complete all requirements for the doctoral degree, other than the dissertation, by the award date. (The **principal investigator [PI]** is the leader of the research project for which the grant proposal is being written. The PI's role in the grant is to carry out all aspects of the grant procedures, hire appropriate staff to conduct the research, manage the budget and report all progress to the granting agency.)

Local and State Entities

Once the preliminary research is complete, investigators may continue to seek larger sources of funding, such as grants from local and state funding agencies. These agencies usually fund research only if it is relevant to the state or local residents served by the agency. For example, state and local agencies may fund health informatics research that benefits a local healthcare facility, individuals within a community, or a local school. Therefore, when applying for state or local grants, investigators should emphasize in the grant proposal how the proposed research will benefit the community or state. For example, a state agency in Pennsylvania provided funding to the University of Pittsburgh Department of Health Information Management for the purpose of enhancing HIT and systems within the department. The funding was used to help develop seminars for students, faculty, and clinical instructors in the areas of HIT, privacy, and security, and to stage recruitment fairs to attract the best and brightest students into HIM and HIT. This project was helpful to the community, and ultimately the state of Pennsylvania, because it expanded the potential HIT workforce. It is vital to search for all appropriate funding entities that relate to the research idea.

Federal Entities

Federal funding is probably the most sought-after and therefore the most competitive source of monies for research. A federal grant can be more prestigious and lucrative than any other type of funding. When seeking federal funding for health informatics research, investigators should search opportunities offered by all relevant federal entities. The AHRQ and Health Resources and Services Administration (HRSA) fund health informatics research projects. Furthermore, the **National Library of Medicine (NLM)** and other agencies that are part of the **National Institutes of Health (NIH)** may fund health informatics research topics that focus on a specific group of individuals, such as older adults, or a specific disease or condition, such as kidney or heart disease or cancer. For example, a researcher who is interested in determining whether smartphones can be effectively used by elderly Americans to record their dietary intake might seek funding from the National Institute of Aging (NIA), which falls under the jurisdiction of the NIH. Another federal funding agency that may support certain health informatics research projects is the National Institute on Disability, Independent Living, and Rehabilitation Research (NIDILRR). For example, investigators might seek funding through NIDILRR to develop a web-based disability research registry that includes healthcare services appropriate to the specific disability as well as community and social services. Many federal agencies will send e-mails to prospective grantees when an RFA is posted. Similarly, many universities send faculty a monthly list of prospective links from potential funding agencies so researchers can decide which grants to pursue. Some entities, such as NIH, provide automatic notification of RFAs to investigators on request.

Writing the Grant Proposal

Grant-funding organizations evaluate grant proposals from several perspectives. The scientific merit of the proposal is measured by many components, such as the **significance** or importance of the research area, the methodological **approach** for carrying out the research, the innovativeness of the research or technologies that are being tested, and the qualifications of the investigators. Other aspects of the grant proposal that are equally important include the programmatic, financial, and administrative requirements. Therefore, to construct an effective grant proposal, the investigator or researcher must closely adhere to the application guidelines, paying particular attention to the following:

- *Application criteria:* The investigator must make sure that the grant is submitted on time, meets eligibility requirements, meets format requirements, and stays within the budget allocated.
- *The mission and rules of the funding agency:* The investigator should align project objectives with the agency's mission and focus on its funding priorities, timelines, and matching requirements.
- *The proposal content:* Several months before the proposal due date, the investigator should write a draft of the proposal and form a mock review committee to review it before submission. This mock committee can provide constructive feedback to strengthen the proposal before actual submission. It is also recommended that a professional editor review the entire manuscript for grammar, spelling, and punctuation, as well as to identify phrasing that does not make sense or could be improved.

Excellent examples of federal grant proposals are available online from the National Cancer Institute (NCI 2016). Also, online appendix 13A provides a sample of a grant proposal that received funding from the AHIMA Foundation. That example provides a general view of how a small grant may be written for content and format.

Other areas of granting agencies that are important to be familiar with include their application criteria and performance requirements as specified in the application.

Basic Application Criteria

Each granting agency will have its own application criteria, and the investigator should know the specific criteria well before beginning the grant-writing process. A grant-writing workshop may prove beneficial to the investigator, especially if he or she is writing a grant for the first time. Grant-writing workshops are offered by several universities, healthcare centers, and the NIH. The following sections on eligibility, timeliness, format, budget limits, and submission procedures describe application criteria of relevance to most, if not all, grants.

Eligibility

Eligibility criteria specify the types of facilities eligible to apply for funding. The investigator must examine these criteria carefully to make sure that the facility meets them. For example, a grant may only be available to health centers as defined under Section 330 of the Public Health Service Act that are applying on behalf of a managed care network or plan that has received federal grants for two subsequent years. If the investigator has questions regarding eligibility, he or she should contact the program officer or grant representative to be certain that all eligibility criteria are met.

Timeliness

Meeting deadline dates is an important part of the grant process. RFAs list the dates when the application is available and completed applications can be submitted, the date and time that application is due, the date when the letter of intent is due (if required), and the dates when the funding can start and end. The application due date is probably the most important date. If the application due date is not met, the granting agency may reject the application.

Letter of intent deadlines are also very important. A **letter of intent** describes the focus and goal of the research project and enables the granting agency to determine whether a full application is of interest. Some, but not all, RFAs require a letter of intent. Some make it an optional component. After the letter of intent is received, the applicant receives feedback regarding the research topic without having to submit a full grant proposal. A one- to two-page letter of intent can save the grant writer precious time and effort if the granting agency determines that the focus of the research project is not in accord with its mission. If, however, the granting agency determines that the research area is one of great interest to them, the feedback received will guide the investigator in framing a better research proposal.

Format

RFAs state the maximum number of pages to include in the proposal, how to format and submit documents, and what to include in required attachments. It is imperative that researchers comply with these specific directions. For example, if the application states that the methodology section should not exceed 20 pages, the investigator must abide by these rules. Failure to meet the page limitations may disqualify the proposal. Similarly, if the application requires the use of 10-point Times New Roman font, then all parts of the grant proposal must be in this format.

Additionally, the sections of the grant must be labeled as outlined in the application guidelines, and all required attachments must be provided in the requested format. For example, if the grant guidelines state that a one-page curriculum vitae (CV) be included for all personnel listed in the grant as attachments to the application, then it is imperative that the applicant abide by this rule and truncate existing CVs to meet the one-page limit. The application may also require that financial documentation supporting the grant project, such as letters of support or Internal Revenue Service (IRS) determination letters of tax-exempt status, be attached.

Budget Limits

The proposal must include a budget, which must not exceed the maximum limits stated in the application guidelines. Granting agencies are unlikely to examine a proposal if it exceeds the budget limits in the RFA. Sometimes, the RFA lists the budget as an estimated amount. If this is the case, it is best to stay close to or less than the estimate when framing the budget section.

Submission Procedures

The application will explain how investigators can submit their grant proposals. Many granting entities, including the NIH, require that proposals be submitted electronically. Because of this, it is important to work with an administrative assistant or grant writer to formulate the steps needed to successfully submit the grant application online. Online submission procedures may be complicated, and the submission process can take more time than anticipated. The investigator should be prepared and allot time to this process, especially if it is the first time an investigator is submitting a grant electronically.

Minimum Performance Requirements as Specified in Applications

The minimum requirements for grant applications are typically specified in an RFA. Always follow the instructions in the specific RFA, as different RFAs will have different performance requirements. These instructions include the project or proposal objectives, timelines, in-kind contributions, the agencies funding priorities, and the content of the application.

Project Objectives

Investigators should list all objectives of the research project and describe in detail how the project will meet each objective. Start and end dates for completing each activity are necessary, as is listing the personnel who will complete each activity.

Timelines

A grant proposal may include multiple project timelines, such as one for each objective, so the proposal reviewers can see how every part of the project is planned. Some grant applications require that quarterly timelines be developed to show all project activities and grant expenditures for each quarter. Others require that timelines be developed for the entire project period, specifying activities, personnel, and outcomes. Online appendix 13A, figure 1 displays an example of a timeline for a research proposal that examines effective and efficient public health reporting using ICD-10-CM and ICD-10-PCS.

Matching Requirements or Cost Sharing (In-Kind Contributions)

Some grant applications have **matching requirements** or **cost-sharing** rules, which are any costs of the specific research project that are not going to be funded by the granting agency and therefore can be shared or matched with the entity submitting the grant, who in turn can seek these funds through their own entity or other funding agencies. Therefore, the applicant for this type of grant must discuss how in-kind contributions will be used and the portion of the project costs that would be funded by an entity other than the agency sponsoring the grant. For example, a granting entity might state that the matching requirement is 25 percent of the total project costs and allow the investigator to seek monies to cover this cost from state, local, or private funds.

Entity Funding Priorities

As noted earlier, different granting entities have different funding priorities, and they will not fund projects that do not fit with those priorities. Therefore, the PI should pay special attention to explaining how the project's objectives serve the target population, geographical region, or specific community. Some granting entities will consider only those projects that provide intervention to human subjects, so clinical and community trials may be given priority. Examples of funding priorities are provided in the following sections.

Target Population A *target population* relates to a specific group of individuals on which the granting agency would like the research to focus. For example, NIA targets individuals older than 65 years, and NIDILRR targets individuals with disabilities. Other granting entities will focus only on children or individuals with behavioral health issues. Investigators should explain in their proposal the target population or population under study, including who will be in the study, how they will become a part of the study, why these specific subjects will be a part of the study, whether a sample will be used, and why and how the sample will be selected.

Geography Some funding entities focus on a certain geographic area. For example, many of the foundations will only fund those projects that will make a difference in a specific community, city, town, or borough. State funding entities may focus on a particular region of the state. Some funding entities may focus on a specific population *and* geographic area. For example, a state department of health may focus on children in need of vaccinations in a low-income region of the state. The applicant must read the funding announcement carefully to make sure his or her proposal will meet any geographical requirements. The applicant should explain where the study will be conducted and if it will include one facility or multiple facilities and why.

Intervention RFAs may include intervention requirements. Under this type of requirement, the applicant must introduce a health-related intervention of some kind within the target population to qualify for funding. For example, the University of Minnesota Informatics Seed Grant described earlier in the chapter specified that interventions related to health informatics were needed.

Content

Once all of the program announcement criteria have been scrupulously reviewed and the applicant believes that the criteria are met, the content of the grant proposal can be written. It is important to start by developing an outline of the proposal. The outline should contain a timeline that lists what must be done to produce the content of the grant proposal within the funder's required time frame.

The applicant should assess the potential competition in the field and determine the resources needed to compete. In addition, an organizational assessment should be developed and other investigators sought as collaborators. Many granting agencies favor proposals from multi-entity collaborations when innovative research projects are planned. A mentor who has expertise in the subject matter should be chosen to evaluate the grant proposal and provide constructive criticism.

Proper training and experience is vital for the PI and co-investigators seeking to respond to a specific grant announcement. They should peruse grant applications from successful grantees that are sometimes available through NIH and web searches, read the instructions for the grant application several times, and refrain from rushing into the grant writing process. It should take at least two to three months to write the grant proposal, and the specific aims should be developed early and reviewed with colleagues, contact persons within the granting agency, and other individuals knowledgeable about the topic of interest (NIH 2016b).

The content of the grant usually includes the following parts (NIH 2016b):

- **Section I:** Face page, description/abstract, key personnel, budget, biographical sketch, and other support
- **Section II:** Specific aims; background, significance, and preliminary studies; research design and methods; approach; results; human subjects; vertebrate animals; literature cited; contractual agreements and consultant agreements
- **Section III:** Appendixes

These parts are described in more detail in the next sections.

Section I: Introductory Materials The introductory materials consist of five main parts: face page, description or abstract, listing of key personnel, budget, biographical sketch, and other support.

The **face page** is very similar to a title page. It typically includes the following, although the specific items included in the face page vary based on the specific grant announcement and funding entity:

- The title of the project
- Whether the grant is in response to an RFA

- The name, degrees, position title, and mailing address of the PI
- Dates of the proposed project
- Costs requested for the proposed project
- Performance sites
- Congressional district of applicant and/or other districts that benefit financially from the application
- Applicant organization, type of organization, and official signing for the applicant organization
- Signature of PI

The *abstract* serves as a succinct description of the proposed work that can stand alone, separate from the application. It states the hypothesis, objectives, why the objectives are important and innovative, and how the proposed methods will accomplish the established goals. It should be written carefully because it will determine which peer reviewers will review the application. Most NIH abstracts have a strict 200-word limit. It can be challenging to include relevant information while staying within this limit. It is recommended that the abstract be written after the major content of the research methods is completed, so all pertinent data are included.

The **key personnel** are all staff, professional and non-professional, who are working on a study. This section lists the name, position title, department, organization, and role in the project for the PI or PIs, co-investigators, collaborators, consultants, statisticians, and any other personnel who have important roles in the research project, such as research assistants. Sometimes, a summary of key personnel, their role in the project, and percentage of time per person per year are requested in the application guidelines.

The **budget** is money allowed for a research project. It can be specific or broad-based, depending on the requirements of the grant application. Most grant applications have a format for the budget. The budget normally includes salary and fringe benefits for personnel, as well as expenses for equipment, supplies, travel, patient care costs, contractual costs, consulting costs, telephone calls, paper, computer usage, and equipment maintenance. The budget must be realistic in relation to the research plan. As with the abstract, the budget should be prepared after the research plan is completed so all costs are included. Over- or underestimated expenses in the budget may alert the proposal reviewers that the investigator does not truly understand the research project. Each budget line item must be justified; for example, the specific functions of the personnel, consultants, statisticians, and collaborators must be explained so the granting entity can understand their value. Grants that cover multiple years should contain budgets that reflect each year and include changes in costs (such as salaries and fringe benefits) over time.

Applications usually provide a standard form for the **biographical sketch**, which typically includes the name and title of each key personnel, along with that person's educational background, relevant publications, roles in research, and professional experience (including employment history). Although there is some overlap with the key personnel section, the biographical sketch includes more detail. All staff, professional and nonprofessional, should be listed, even if their salaries are not part of the budget. Reviewers look for a ranking of personnel by the percentage of time each will spend on the project.

Other supportive documentation included in a grant application may include endorsement letters, other applications or proposals pending review or funding, and applications planned or being prepared for submission. Each item should mention the source of support, project title, percentage of time devoted to the project, project period dates, project description, and whether it overlaps, duplicates or is being replaced, or supplemented by the present application.

Additional resources allocated to the project should be described. These could include laboratory, clinical, computer, office, and other facilities and resources.

Section II: Research Plan The research plan comprises specific aims; background, significance, and preliminary studies; research design and methods; approach; results; human subjects; vertebrate animals; literature cited; and contractual agreements and consultants.

As discussed in chapter 5, the *specific aims* are the research objectives and goals for the project. Specific aims should be clearly defined and relate directly to the hypothesis to be tested. The first step in writing the content of the grant proposal is to state the research problem clearly and succinctly. The problem must coincide with the project hypothesis and specific aims.

Grant applications may ask that objectives or specific aims be listed with outcomes or performance indicators that relate to each objective. Each outcome should be measurable and focus on the problem.

The section on background, significance, and preliminary studies details the importance of or need for the research project. Some granting entities label this section *Impact, Need,* or *Rationale*. It states why the research must be done, how the project is different from previous research studies, and whom the research will benefit. This section also demonstrates the knowledge of the researcher by citing reviews of existing research and showing the gaps and flaws in that research. Once these deficiencies are explained, the applicant should state how the proposed research would address them. The key to this section is to be succinct and organized. If preliminary research can be briefly summarized, include the summary in this section, particularly if it illustrates the importance of the study. If preliminary research was extensive, it is described in a separate section on preliminary studies.

In the section on research design and methods, the applicant should describe the study design and methods in detail and provide support for their use. This section should be organized so each experiment or research method relates to a specific aim of the study. If the methods are not innovative, the applicant should describe how established they are and why each method is necessary for this research project. If the methods are innovative, then the applicant should explain how the new methods hold promise in moving the field forward and establish that the methods are sound and effective. If graphics of any kind are used in this section, they should be included in the body of the proposal and also in the appendix. This is recommended because the research plan may be separated from the rest of the application, and it should contain all relevant information to stand on its own. The methods should be described in logical order, and in relation to the following:

- Time—when the study will be conducted and for how long
- Place—facilities involved
- Persons—the population under study

The data collection process is also included in this section. It describes the following:

- How the data will be collected (for example, by questionnaire, interview, or abstracting)
- What data will be collected and why
- How the data will be categorized and why
- Who will collect the data
- Training techniques
- Where the data will be stored
- How patient identifiers will be handled
- How the data will be accessed
- How confidentiality of the data will be protected

The reasons why an approach is chosen should be explained and its methods specified. For example, it is not appropriate to state, "Many different health information technologies in different health information networks across several healthcare facilities will be used to assess differences in the outcomes of care." Reviewers want to know *which* health information technologies, across *what* networks, and in *what* type of healthcare facilities. The more specific the information, the more confident the reviewers will be that the applicant understands the research and can successfully carry out the project.

The results section should show how the data will be analyzed by describing the type of statistical tests that will be performed and why they are needed. Dummy tables that demonstrate how the data will be displayed may effectively demonstrate an understanding of the project's statistical analyses. A statistician should be consulted to help write this section. The applicant should show the limits and the benefits to the kind of results expected, and he or she should define criteria for success or failure of a specific test. Specific statistical tests such as frequency distributions, chi-square tests, confidence intervals, sensitivity and specificity, and other validity and reliability tests should be listed, when applicable, for each procedure described.

The human subjects section includes a demographic description of the study population, how informed consent will be obtained, how confidentiality will be safeguarded, and how human subjects will be protected during the research process. Institutional review board (IRB) approval letters are included in this section to demonstrate that the facility where the research will be conducted has approved the study protocol. (Sometimes, applications do not require IRB approval for the proposal but the applicant must promise to seek it before research is conducted.)

If vertebrate animals will be used, methods of protection should be described, and IRB letters of approval should be included.

All literature cited, discussed, or reviewed in any section of the grant proposal should be referenced in its own section and also cited at the end of the grant.

Finally, section II of the proposal should explain any contractual agreements pertinent to the grant proposal, and any consultants that may be used. Letters of support from these individuals or companies should be included. For example, a coding consultant may be needed to assign ICD-10-CM and ICD-10-PCS codes.

Section III: Appendixes The appendixes include tables, figures, criteria, a summary of laboratory tests or techniques, the data collection forms or survey instruments, and other items that are important and relevant to the grant proposal. Appendixes serve to clarify the topic described in the grant proposal. Any information not pertinent to the current research project should be excluded.

Grant Proposal Review Criteria

Granting agencies do not give funds to grantees based solely on their individual scholarship or expertise. To the contrary, the most important criteria used when reviewing proposals are the scientific merit and scholarship of the actual grant proposal, as determined by peer review; the alignment of the proposal with the funder's mission and priorities; and whether financial and administrative requirements identified in the application are met.

Peer Review

Peer reviewers (experts in the scientific area of the proposed project) evaluate the grant proposal based on specific review criteria. The general review criteria that peer reviewers use for investigator-initiated grant proposals for NIH include the following five items (NIH 2016c):

- **Significance:** Does the study address an important area of research and how will this area be advanced or moved forward if the research is completed?
- **Approach:** Are the conceptual framework, design, methods, and analyses sound and well developed, and integrated in relation to the specific aims or goals of the project? Do the PIs acknowledge potential problems with the proposal and discuss methods to address these problems?
- **Innovation:** Is the current proposal unique, original, and innovative? Does it challenge existing clinical practice and use novel concepts, approaches, and technologies?
- **Investigators:** Are the PIs and co-PIs well trained to carry out this research? Is the research appropriate to the experience of the personnel listed in the grant proposal?
- **Environment:** Does the scientific environment and physical environment contribute to success of the research proposed? Are collaborative arrangements effective in carrying out the research proposed, and is there institutional support?

Other granting agencies use similar types of criteria, but NIH is emphasized here because it is considered the standard for grant proposal review criteria.

Other areas that peer reviewers assess in determining scientific merit include the following:

- **Protection of human subjects as required by federal law:** Reviewers assess whether the grant proposal addresses the risk to subjects, the adequacy of protections against risk, benefits of the research to subjects and others, the importance of the knowledge to be gained, and for clinical trials, a data and safety monitoring plan (see chapter 14 for more information on the protection of human subjects).
- **Inclusion of women, minorities, and children as required by federal law:** Reviewers evaluate whether the grant proposal addresses the inclusion (or exclusion) of individuals on the basis of sex/gender, race, and ethnicity, as well as the inclusion (or exclusion) of children to determine if the exclusions and inclusions are justified in terms of the scientific goals and research strategy proposed.
- **Use of vertebrate animals:** If the grant proposal includes the use of animals, reviewers consider whether the proposal justifies their use and includes a plan for the care of those animals.
- **Biohazards:** Reviewers assess whether materials or procedures proposed to be used in the grant proposal are potentially hazardous to research personnel and/or the environment, and, if needed, determine whether adequate protection is included in the research plan.

Programmatic Requirements for Grant Recipients

As has been noted, grant-funding entities only award grants to fund research that serve their mission and meet their programmatic requirements. For example, NIH's mission is to lead the way toward important medical discoveries that improve people's health and save lives. Priority is given to healthcare for children, minorities, women, and seniors, and to efforts that advance healthy lifestyles. Therefore, it is usually in the investigator's best interest to include women and minorities in NIH proposals. Other requirements can be specific to a program within the granting agency. For example, the NLM and the National Heart, Lung, and Blood Institute (NHLBI) are both parts of NIH, but they have distinct programmatic requirements based on their distinct missions.

Financial Requirements

Even if a proposal aligns with the grant-giving entity's mission and meets the programmatic requirements, the grant request may not be funded because it fails financial review. Each RFA includes the financial requirements, and most state the maximum amount to be awarded and the time period for the award. For example, some grant announcements state that the maximum amount is $500,000 per year for a period of three years and encourage the grantee to apply for renewal of the grant at the end of the three-year period, whereas other grants provide funding of $500,000 for a one-year period with no opportunity for renewal. Because the financial requirements may pose some limitations on how the proposal is written, the requirements should be reviewed before writing of the project proposal begins.

Most granting agencies state the total funding amount in the RFA and indicate whether it includes indirect costs. Direct costs are all costs that coincide with the research project. **Indirect costs**, or *facilities and administration costs,* cover such items as office space, use of library resources, electricity, and so forth. Indirect costs can be a large part of the total budget, so it is imperative that grant applicants carefully read the RFA regarding financial requirements to determine whether indirect costs are included in or excluded from the total funding amount for the grant. Although the indirect costs are not specifically charged to a research project, they represent real costs and expenditures for the grantee's employer or the sponsoring facility. Some granting agencies allow no indirect costs. Granting agencies within the federal government allow indirect costs of approximately 50 percent to 60 percent of the total award, or they allow the indirect rate that has been established for a facility or university. The research office at the organization that will be awarded the grant can help prepare the proposed budget and assist in meeting the essential financial requirements outlined in the RFA. A research office representative can also answer questions from the funding agency regarding the budget for a research project.

Administrative Requirements

The granting agency will assess whether a proposal meets various administrative requirements before awarding a grant. At NIH, administrative review may include evaluation of the project's alignment with NIH's funding principles, review of the project budget, assessment of the applicant's management systems, determination of applicant eligibility, and determination of public policy requirements. Before the award is granted, NIH administrators may also request additional information about the proposal, such as information regarding other grant support (to demonstrate no overlap with other funding sources in regard to budget and commitment by investigators), as well as IRB approvals for human subjects, animals, and education on the protection of human research participants requirements (see chapter 14). The continued eligibility of the PI for the time period in which grant funds are awarded may need to be verified; a cost analysis to determine the validity of the budget as proposed in the grant proposal may be requested; and compliance with other public policy requirements related to financial conflict of interest and age and sex discrimination may be reviewed.

Key Individuals in the Granting Agency Process

Every granting agency has key individuals who work toward achieving the goals of specific RFPs. It will benefit the PI to become acquainted with the key individuals in the RFA because they can answer questions about the application process and requirements, the mission and purpose of the granting agency, whether the research project is a good fit for their agency, and what areas the PI should focus on to have a higher level of success in funding.

Program Officer

The **program officer** leads a specific RFA and is the primary person who will address any questions that investigators may have while developing the proposal. It is recommended that applicants call or e-mail program officers with questions early in the grant proposal development process so that the officers can steer researchers in the proper direction. For example, an investigator may be interested in designing a patient safety education tool that encourages patients to use HIT to communicate directly with their healthcare providers. However, after contacting the program officer and explaining their ideas regarding the development of the tool, the researchers may decide to change some of their objectives to better meet the goals of the RFA. In this way, the program officer reminds the researchers to revisit the grant announcement and pay greater attention to the program goals.

Proposal Reviewers

A **proposal reviewer** (or *peer reviewer*) is an individual with an extensive background or experience in a research area who reviews the grant proposals and provides comments. In some circumstances, individuals with a minimal background in the subject area still may be suitable reviewers if they supplement their expertise with additional reading in that grant proposal's subject area, and demonstrate interest in that area. Proposal reviewers are asked to review a specific proposal based on their background. They are normally required to supply the granting agency with their CV and other application information in order to become proposal reviewers. Most reviewers are volunteers, but sometimes payment can be provided for their work on the review process.

Grant Proposal Review Process

The granting agency is responsible for several steps of the review process. It is the agency's responsibility to select appropriate proposal reviewers, to provide appropriate evaluation criteria that the proposal reviewers use to evaluate the grant proposal, and to organize an effective overall assessment of the proposal. This overall assessment includes initial reviews, meetings, and final recommendations. For investigator-initiated grants, the NIH peer review process consists of having one or more of the **Centers for Scientific Review (CSR)** referral officers review the initial application (NIH 2016c). The CSR referral officers determine the most appropriate **scientific review group (SRG)** to assess the proposal's scientific and technical merit. The application is then assigned to a study section. NIH has many different study sections that consist of many peer reviewers. If an application may fit into more than one study section, it will be assigned to each of those sections for review. The grantee may state in a cover letter which study sections they prefer to review their application, and these requests are seriously considered within NIH. However, if the grant proposal is in response to a specific RFA, then the study section is listed within the announcement and the application would be reviewed by that group. Steps within the peer review process at NIH include the following (NIH 2016c):

- The application is received and assigned to a study group.
- The **scientific review officer (SRO)** reviews the application for completeness and content, and assigns the most appropriate proposal reviewer.
- The application is assigned to reviewers, and they provide written critiques and lead the discussion at the meeting.
- The proposal reviewers submit critiques and scores to CSR.
- The reviewers are given a list of proposals that fall in the lower half of the scoring. These proposals will not be discussed at the meeting. This process, **streamlining**, does not mean that the proposal has been disapproved, but grantees are encouraged to resubmit after receiving the critique.
- The members of the study sections meet for about two days, during which time reviewers present and discuss their critiques. Priority scores are marked on the scoring sheet, which is then tabulated by CSR. Scoring is done privately.
- After approximately two days, the priority score and percentile ranking is available online to the grantee and via e-mail. Summary statements typically are available in approximately one month and include the full critique, the SRG's summary of the meeting discussion, study section recommendations, and other pertinent information.

Details of the review process are discussed in the sections that follow and include the role of the proposal reviewers, assessment and ranking of the grant proposal, the final decision of the funding agency and reasons why a grant proposal may not get funded.

Role of Proposal Reviewers

Steps that the proposal reviewers must follow and items they should submit in order to partake in the review of grant proposals vary among granting agencies, but for the most part, these steps include:

- Submitting a CV or a resume with experience listed in specific clinical or science areas

- Reviewing the list of proposal applications to determine which are appropriate for review based on their area of expertise and focus of the proposal application
- Receiving and completing a confidentiality and conflict of interest form
- Receiving the proposal, evaluation form, and instructions for review via e-mail

Other areas that proposal reviewers may be required to submit to include confidentiality and disclosure of conflict of interests and the scores and comments on each proposal reviewed.

Confidentiality and Disclosure of Conflict of Interest

The **confidentiality form** states that the reviewer will keep all information in the proposal application confidential. It must be signed and dated by the proposal reviewer to attest to his or her commitment to not disseminate confidential information about the proposal before, during, or after the review. When evaluating proposals, reviewers gain insight into all aspects of scientific research conducted or planned by many different individuals. Reviewers should take utmost care to maintain confidentiality of the information shared during this process because the ideas within the grant proposals are novel creations of the specific PI and research entity—if reviewers do not keep those ideas confidential, others may unfairly claim them to be their own. Proposal reviewers should delete electronic copies and shred paper copies of grant proposals after review, and not share the information with anyone outside of the granting agency.

The **conflict of interest form** asks the reviewer to inform the program officer of any conflicts of interest based on the area of focus for the grant application. Conflicts of interest may occur if the proposal reviewer is a consultant to the same organization that is requesting funds, or to one of its competitors; if the proposal reviewer has employed individuals who are listed on the grant application; if the PI or co-investigator were students of the proposal reviewer; or if the reviewer has a financial interest in the outcomes of the proposed study. By completing and signing conflict-of-interest forms, proposal reviewers attest to the fact that they have disclosed any potential conflicts of interest with the grant application before them. The granting agency determines whether the disclosures are grounds for disqualifying the reviewer from scoring and commenting on the proposal.

Scoring and Commenting on Proposals

After the confidentiality and conflict of interest forms are signed and accepted by the granting agency, the proposal reviewer evaluates the grant proposal. Typically, two or three reviewers evaluate each grant proposal. The reviewers individually score the research project's potential for funding and offer detailed comments on the scientific merits and weaknesses of the grant proposal. Usually, a score of 1 is given to the highest-ranking proposals, and 9 is given to those that rank the lowest. A score of 5 is considered average. Some granting agencies use more specific numbers, such as 2.5 or 3.3, to score reviews. Some evaluation forms ask the proposal reviewer to rank their reviewer expertise in relation to the subject matter of the proposal. This ranking assists in the final decision, especially if two very different rankings are provided by two different reviewers.

Proposal reviewers should thoroughly read the entire grant proposal, but they are asked to focus their evaluation on the practicality, feasibility, relevance, and cost-effectiveness of the proposed project. One of the major areas of focus for reviewers is whether the hypotheses are unambiguous and scientifically plausible. For example, if a researcher's hypothesis is to evaluate the effectiveness of HIT in improving the quality of care, the first question a reviewer may have is "How is this feasible or practical when assessing the quality of care is such a broad area?" The reviewer will begin to look within the grant proposal for other hypotheses or specific aims that narrow the focus of the research. Also, proposal reviewers will focus on the relevance of the grant proposal in relation to the granting agency's goals. If the proposal is not relevant to the granting agency's mission, then it will be quite difficult to receive a favorable score.

The budget is another major area of focus for the proposal reviewer. As has been noted, the budget should be fair in relation to the expected accomplishments and should not approach the maximum amount that can be allocated unless the researchers can show that the maximum amount is needed to meet the project objectives. Also, the researchers should seek from their organization some services in-kind or matching funds. This demonstrates to the proposal reviewer that the researcher's employer may sustain the project after the grant monies are depleted. For example, in-kind services may include providing a computer laboratory or health information systems network so that additional grant monies need not be requested for additional computers or HIT services.

Once evaluation forms from the reviewers are submitted with their final scores and specific comments, a panel of reviewers meets to discuss all the grant applications received and make final recommendations.

Panel Assessment and Ranking

The panel of reviewers may include the proposal reviewers, or it may include a second level of reviewers different from the proposal reviewers. This choice depends on the granting agency and their specific requirements. In any event, the panel uses their collective expertise to evaluate the grant proposal and compile a score. The ranking informs the funding entity's decision whether to fund the grant proposal. At NIH, each application is discussed and then assigned a single overall score based on the five criteria listed earlier in this chapter (significance, approach, innovation, investigator, and environment). The weight given to each criterion varies depending on the nature of the grant application. For example, in some HIT grants innovation may be weighted more heavily than the other areas if the focus of that RFA is on innovative technology practices. Also, the appropriate use and explanation of human subjects, animals, and safeguards against biohazards are taken into account in the priority score, as previously described. At NIH, the best possible score a panelist can give is 1 and the worst is 9. The scores of the panelists are averaged and multiplied by 100 to arrive at an overall score (NIH 2016c).

Funding Entity's Decision

After the scoring is complete, the funding entity takes the panel critique, scoring, and recommendations under consideration. It then decides whether to fund the proposal, decline to fund it, or seek more information from the potential grantee. If the decision is made to seek further information, then the proposal is deferred and the panel may make a site visit to the potential grantee. If the decision is to not fund the grant and not seek further information, then a priority score is not assigned to the proposal and the proposed budget is not discussed.

The panel's assessment of the proposal is just one factor in the decision-making process of the funding entity. Other factors, which include the entity's purpose, emphasis, or funding priorities, past performance, and available funds, are discussed in the following sections.

Entity's Purpose, Emphasis, or Funding Priorities

As has been noted in this chapter, before a funding entity awards funds, it must be confident that the proposal reflects the entity's purpose, focus, and funding priorities. For example, if researchers propose to examine the effects of stroke on family members by developing a web-based tool that collects the subjects' experiences while caring for a family member who has had a stroke, the funding entity must decide whether this research is in accordance with its purpose and funding priorities. Even if a proposal received an excellent review and recommendation from the panel of reviewers, it may not reflect the mission of the granting agency.

Principal Investigator's or Institution's Past Performance

Another important aspect in the determination of providing the grant award is the previous performance of the PI or grantee with the same granting agency. If the PI had a prior award and demonstrated that he or she has good leadership, budgeting, and organizational skills and promptly provides reports and updates regarding the research progression, the grant-giving entity will feel more confident that the PI will demonstrate these same behaviors in subsequent research and, therefore, the entity may be more inclined to offer the PI another grant.

When considering a grantee's past performance, grant-funding entities scrutinize how budgets were used. It is imperative that the PI use the budget appropriately. In some cases, investigators do not complete the grant project as written with the funds provided because they did not budget the funds appropriately. Therefore, the PI may need to curtail the progression of the grant because the monies are depleted. This outcome does not demonstrate effective management skills. If a PI or grantee has a reputation of poor budget management of previous awards, the funding agency may reconsider providing funds again, even if the proposal received a favorable priority score.

Funds Available

Obviously, a funding entity's decision about a proposal will depend on the funds available. Sometimes, however, the grant-giving entity allocates more or less funds than what was originally stated in the RFA. For example, a proposal submitted to the Centers for Disease Control and Prevention (CDC) to examine the use of the EHR in physician offices and its impact in improving infectious diseases in the elderly might receive more funds than requested if the CDC believes the proposal truly reflects the mission of the agency and does not think that the research can be carried out completely with the amount requested.

Reasons Why a Proposal May Not Get Funded

Agencies usually limit the number of grantees that can be selected for each RFA and have a limited amount of money to distribute. Therefore, most grant applicants will not get funded.

However, the following increase the odds of rejection:

- The proposal includes objectives that are not specific enough to be measurable.
- The project is overly ambitious with a large amount of activities proposed.
- The methodology is not detailed enough, does not relate to the objectives cited, and does not convince the reviewers that the investigator knows what he or she is doing.
- The proposal does not have alternative methodological approaches to try if the first approach is not successful.
- The proposal lacks a thorough review of the literature, which causes the reviewers to think that the researchers do not know the subject area.
- The proposal does not indicate which data were obtained by the investigator and which data are from other authors reported in the literature or other reports.
- The hypothesis and goals of the study are not related to the funding agency's priorities and preferred target population.
- The qualifications of investigators are not clearly stated.
- The evaluation plan is inappropriate or absent.
- The proposal does not have an itemized budget, or the funding limits are exceeded. (NIMH 2016)

Rejection of a proposal is not a closed door on funding for the research project. If the proposal was not rejected because it is not aligned with the funding agency's priorities and target population, the proposal can be revised and resubmitted.

Revising Grant Proposals

When a proposal is not funded, applicants receive comments and criticisms from the reviewers. PIs should use this information to determine whether to resubmit the application. If the reviewers thought the idea was needed and interesting, the proposal may be worth revising. If revision is deemed worthwhile, the applicant or investigator should reevaluate, redesign and resubmit the proposal. It is not unusual for an investigator to submit a grant proposal several times before it is accepted and funded.

The PI should meet with their research team and determine whether the comments received fall into the challenging category or the fixable problem category. Even if the proposal is not revised, the PI can learn many things from a rejected proposal, especially if the comments received are detailed and provide suggestions for improvements. The PI may learn that he or she needs to hire a grant writer to assist in the editing and overall organization of the grant, or the PI may decide to do more preliminary research work before submitting a new or revised proposal. In some cases, investigators may find that they need to sit down with their research team and assess the problems they are having with their current innovation and think about a novel way to attack the problem. The program officer for the granting entity can be a great resource and can also help in the review of changes that are made to a revised proposal to determine whether it is improved enough for resubmission.

Review Questions

1. The author states that "grant writing is an art." Why must a grant writer be creative, immersed in the scientific area at hand, and fully aware of the granting agency requirements and recommendations? Include information to support your answer.
2. Why is peer reviewed research an important part of the grant writing process?
3. Investigators should be experts in the research trends and problems within their area of study. If investigators are interested in securing a grant in the area of privacy and security in health information when using telemedicine, where should their expertise lie?
4. How do the general review criteria that peer reviewers use for investigator-initiated grant proposals for NIH help evaluate the scientific merit of those proposals?

5. Why might the PI reach out to the program officer when thinking about resubmitting a previously rejected grant proposal?
6. What are the differences between direct and indirect costs?
7. What are some reasons why a grant proposal may not be accepted and funded?
8. What are the basic steps that a researcher should follow when completing an effective grant proposal?
9. What are the steps within the peer review process at NIH?
10. When should the abstract of the grant proposal be written, and why might the abstract be a particularly challenging part of the grant proposal to write?

Application Exercises

1. Visit the NIH's Grants and Funding website (NIH 2017) and click the Funding tab. Near the top of the page, search for a funding opportunity in health informatics, and select a funding opportunity from the search results. Briefly describe the research that they are seeking and discuss whether it meets the grant criteria discussed in this chapter.
2. Read the grant proposal application in online appendix 13A. Take the role of a proposal reviewer and assign it a score from 0 (poor) to 100 (excellent) using the following criteria:
   I. Impact: Introduction, purpose statement of need, objectives or specific aims (20 points)
   II. Methodology: Research design, research methods, statistical analysis (40 points)
   III. Feasibility: Organization/management plan, personnel, and timetable (20 points)
   IV. Evaluation: Measurement for success, intended distribution (20 points)
3. Find a foundation that funds health informatics research. Describe why you think this foundation would be a good place to apply for a health informatics grant.

References

National Cancer Institute (NCI). 2016 (March). Epidemiology and Genomics Research Program. Sample Cancer Epidemiology Grant Applications. http://epi.grants.cancer.gov/funding/grantsmanship/sample-grants.html#orientation.

National Institutes of Health (NIH). 2016a (May 24). What Does NIH Look For? https://grants.nih.gov/grants/what-does-nih-look-for.htm.

National Institutes of Health (NIH) Office of Extramural Research. 2016b (January 28). Grants and Funding: Write Your Application. https://grants.nih.gov/grants/how-to-apply-application-guide/format-and-write/write-your-application.htm.

National Institutes of Health (NIH) Office of Extramural Research. 2016c (September 12). Grants and Funding: Peer Review. http://grants.nih.gov/grants/peer_review_process.htm.

National Institute of Mental Health (NIMH). 2016. Common Mistakes in Writing Applications. https://www.nimh.nih.gov/funding/grant-writing-and-application-process/common-mistakes-in-writing-applications.shtml.

University of Minnesota. 2015. Informatics Seed Grants, Request for Proposals. https://healthinformatics.umn.edu/research/funding-opportunities/informatics-seed-grants.

US Department of Health and Human Services (HHS). 2013. Funding Opportunity Announcement (FOA) Number PA-14-001: Exploratory and Developmental Grant to Improve Health Care Quality through Health Information Technology (IT) (R21). http://grants.nih.gov/grants/guide/pa-files/PA-14-001.html.

Resources

National Institutes of Health (NIH). 2017. Grants and Funding. http://grants.nih.gov/grants/oer.htm.

14 Research and Ethics

Laurinda B. Harman, PhD, RHIA, FAHIMA

Learning Objectives

- Assess ethical issues related to research involving human subjects based on a review of unethical clinical research projects.
- Determine how governments and institutions act to protect human subjects at international, national, and local levels.
- Assess the ongoing value of the Belmont Report to the protection of human subjects.
- Determine adherence to the processes and policies of institutional review boards.
- Construct the elements of and process for informed consent.
- Defend why a researcher should know the aspects of research misconduct.

Key Terms

Autonomy
Belmont Report
Beneficence
Bioethics committees
Biomedical research
Caring
Civil monetary penalties
Code of ethics
Common Rule
Declaration of Helsinki
Ethics
Exempt from review
Expedited review
Federal Policy for the Protection of Human Subjects
Federal-wide assurance of compliance (FWA)
Fidelity
Full review
Gelsinger case
Health Information Technology for Economic and Clinical Health (HITECH) Act
Health Research Extension Act
Holmesburg Prison studies
Honesty
Human Genome Project (HGP)
Human radiation experiments
Informed consent
Jewish Chronic Disease Hospital study
Justice
National Research Act
Nonmaleficence
Nuremberg Code
Office for Civil Rights (OCR)
Office for Human Research Protections (OHRP)
Office of Research Integrity (ORI)
Policy and Procedure Order 129
Privacy Rule
Research misconduct
Respect for persons
Sanctity
Security Rule
Tearoom Trade study
Tuskegee Study of Untreated Syphilis in the Negro Male
Utility
Vioxx case
Vulnerable population
Willowbrook hepatitis studies

International ethics guidelines, national laws and regulations, and institutional oversight activities all aim to protect human subjects in research. However, ethical challenges persist despite these efforts. This chapter discusses commonly encountered ethical principles and examines research projects that violated them. The chapter also explains the US laws and regulations that provide a framework for the protection of human subjects in research projects and describes federal efforts to promote research integrity. It concludes with a discussion of an ethical climate for research.

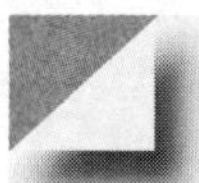

Real-World Case

The **Jewish Chronic Disease Hospital study** was an experiment conducted in 1963 in which live cancer cells were injected into 22 weak and chronically ill patients. The purpose of the research was to measure the ability of the patients to reject foreign cells (Langer 1966, 663). The patients were told that the injections were a test of their resistance to disease, to which they gave their oral consent. The researchers intentionally avoided the word *cancer* because the word's emotional impact might have deterred patients from giving their consent (Langer 1966, 663–664). Thus, the patients were *not* told that they would receive cancer cells, the injection was a part of a research study, and the injection was unrelated to any treatment for them. Withholding this information was an ethical breach that left the patients unaware that the injections were part of an experiment unrelated to the treatment of their disease (Katz 1992, 248).

Biomedical Research and Ethics

Biomedical research is "the broad area of science that looks for ways to prevent and treat diseases that cause illness and death in people and in animals" (NJABR 2016). This research encompasses the life sciences, such as biology and physiology, and the physical sciences, such as chemistry. Teams that conduct biomedical research include physicians, health informaticists, engineers, and other professionals. **Ethics** is commonly defined as the "norms for conduct that distinguish between acceptable and unacceptable behavior" (Resnick 2015). This section begins by explaining why ethics is important in biomedical research and then describes how two sets of researchers took divergent approaches in their consideration of the ethical implications of their work. This section also discusses several ethical principles and provides notorious examples of biomedical research studies that breached these principles. Finally, ethical codes applicable to researchers in health informatics and health information management (HIM) are discussed.

What Is Ethics in Research and Why Is It Important?

A preeminent ethical principle in research is to protect human research subjects from harm. This protection requires that researchers ensure voluntary participation, get informed consent (voluntary agreement with full knowledge of risks and benefits, as discussed in detail later in the chapter), balance the risks and benefits of the research for its participants, and respect privacy and confidentiality.

Researchers must be particularly sensitive to ethical challenges when the participants are members of a vulnerable population. **Vulnerable populations** are those people who "are likely to be vulnerable to coercion or undue influence, such as children, prisoners, pregnant women, mentally disabled persons, or economically or educationally disadvantaged persons" (45 CFR 46.111(b)). Other examples of people who may be vulnerable to undue influence include patients, employees, students, and people with disabilities or chronic diseases.

Two Approaches to Ethics in Research

Two famous research studies illustrate very different approaches to ethics in research. The **Tuskegee Study of Untreated Syphilis in the Negro Male**, also known as the US Public Health Service Syphilis Study, was conducted by the US Public Health Service (PHS) between 1932 and 1972 in rural counties around Tuskegee, AL. The researchers did not tell 399 African-American men participating in the study that they had syphilis and, moreover, after the discovery of penicillin (definitive treatment) in the 1940s, the investigators blocked the men from being treated (Reverby 2001, 24). In contrast, the **Human Genome Project (HGP)**, an "international, collaborative research program whose goal was the complete mapping and understanding of all the genes of human beings," prioritized the ethical implications of its investigations

(NHGRI 2016). The following sections describe the Tuskegee Study and the Human Genome Project so that one can see how different they are in relation to ethics in research. The Human Genome Project considered ethical and other implications from the very beginning of their study whereas the Tuskegee Study did not.

The Tuskegee Study

In 1932, the Tuskegee Study of Untreated Syphilis in the Negro Male began with the purpose of obtaining information about the course of untreated syphilis. As a part of the Tuskegee study, PHS researchers tested 4,400 African-American male residents of Macon County, AL. The investigators found a 22 percent rate of syphilis in the men and identified 399 African-American men who had never received treatment for this disease (Pence 2003, 397). The study initially involved 600 African-American men: the 399 men with untreated syphilis as well as 201 men who did not have the disease. The men were poor and mostly illiterate sharecroppers (farmers who rent the land) (Brandt 1978, 23). The PHS researchers did not tell the men with syphilis that they had the disease. Instead, the researchers led the men to believe that they were receiving special treatment from the PHS for their "bad blood" (Brandt 1978, 24). In fact, the men did not receive the period's conventional treatments for syphilis (such as mercury and arsenic); instead, the men received tonics and aspirins, which the researchers used to deceive them into thinking that they were receiving meaningful treatments (Reverby 2001, 2, 24). Every few years, the PHS researchers visited Macon County to evaluate the study's progress (Pence 2003, 398). The researchers acted to prevent the men from receiving treatments by tracking them to other public health departments and by intervening with local physicians (Reverby 2001, 24). In the 1940s, when penicillin became available as a definitive treatment for syphilis, the PHS researchers prevented the men in the study from being drafted into military service during World War II because drafted soldiers were routinely treated for the disease (Katz 1992, 249).

During the 1930s and 1940s, a few PHS researchers were critical of the study's scientific methods, with the result being some minor modifications, such as adding a control group and performing autopsies (Reverby 2009, 48). In 1956, the first external criticism occurred. Dr. Count Gibson heard Dr. Sidney Olansky, a PHS leader and researcher, speak about the study. After reading articles published on the study, Gibson wrote Olansky to question the study's ethics. Olansky replied to Gibson's letter with "bits of the information" and avoided the issue of denying treatment (Reverby 2009, 72). Moreover, Gibson was convinced by his colleagues that questioning the PHS was inadvisable if he wanted a successful career (Reverby 2009, 72). In 1957, the 25th year of the study, the PHS held a meeting about the study's future. PHS decided to continue the study and to give the subjects fake treatments of iron tonics and aspirin, "special certificates of participation" signed by the US Surgeon General, and one dollar for every year of "service" (Reverby, 2009, 73). In 1965, PHS researchers met again about the study, and they decided it still served a purpose (Brandt 1978, 26). In 1966, the US Surgeon General issued Policy and Procedure Order Number 129 (discussed later in the chapter), which required institutions receiving PHS research grants have mechanisms to protect human subjects (Jones 2008, 94). Technically, the order did not apply to research studies conducted by PHS; however, ethically, the PHS researchers should have upheld the spirit of the order's requirements.

Upon learning about the study, Peter Buxton, a PHS psychiatric social worker, questioned the morality of the Tuskegee Study in multiple letters and when meeting with officials (Jones 2008, 94). In 1969, the Centers for Disease Control and Prevention (CDC) responded to his complaints by convening a blue-ribbon panel of experts to consider whether the Tuskegee study should be continued. The sole panelist unfamiliar with the study insisted that it be terminated and that the men receive treatment for their condition (Lederer 2005, 21). That panel member was outvoted. In 1972, Buxton showed copies of the research articles published about the study and his correspondence with PHS officials to an Associated Press reporter (Jones 2008, 94–95). The reporter forwarded the materials to her superiors at the Associated Press, who gave the story to Jean Heller, another of its reporters. Heller conducted telephone interviews with CDC officials, who confirmed the study's existence (Jones 2008, 95). On July 25, 1972, Heller broke the story, "Syphilis Victims in U.S. Study Went Untreated for 40 Years" (Heller 1972). A public outcry ensued, and, in August 1972, the CDC convened another blue-ribbon panel, the Tuskegee Syphilis Study Ad Hoc Advisory Panel. Based on the advisory panel's recommendation, the Assistant Secretary of Health, Dr. Merlin K. DuVal of the US Department of Health, Education, and Welfare (now the US Department of Health and Human Services [HHS]) terminated the Tuskegee study on November 16, 1972 (DuVal 1972). The outrage over the Tuskegee study also led to the National Research Act of 1974, which set the stage for today's federal protections of human research subjects.

Ethical breaches that occurred during the study included lying to people, preventing people from getting medical treatment, and taking advantage of poor people with limited educations. The PHS researchers had multiple opportunities to consider the ethics of the Tuskegee study. As early as the 1930s and 1940s, internal experts questioned the study's scientific methods. Questionable scientific methods should have been a flag that the study was not being properly conducted. Dr. Gibson specifically questioned the ethics of the study, but his concerns were discounted. In 1957, the PHS could have decided to end the study instead of deciding to give fake treatments, certificates, and money to the subjects. Again, after Buxton raised concerns, the study could have been terminated. Only the outrage of the public ended the study. For almost 40 years, the PHS researchers involved in the Tuskegee study were blind to its ethical implications.

The Human Genome Project

Three decades after James Watson and Francis Crick discovered the structure of DNA in 1953, the HGP, which sought to map and sequence human DNA, was launched in the mid-1980s and was completed as a formal research project in 2003 (Collins et al. 2003, 286). Unlike the Tuskegee study, leaders of the HGP considered ethical and other implications from the very beginning of the project. The HGP was "the first large-scale research project to include a component dedicated to examining broader societal issues, such as how to protect people's privacy and prevent discrimination" (Green et al. 2015, 31). Between 3 percent and 5 percent of the HGP budget was set aside to investigate these societal issues through its Ethical, Legal, Social Implications (ELSI) program (Collins et al. 2003, 289).

The ELSI program began receiving funding in 1988 (Seltzer et al. 2011, 17). An early ELSI working group identified the following ethics-related topics for research:

- Fairness in the use of genetic information
- Impact of knowledge of genetic variation on the individual
- Privacy and confidentiality of genetic information
- Impact of the HGP on genetic counseling
- Reproductive decisions influenced by genetic information
- Issues raised by the introduction of increased genetic information into mainstream medical practice
- Uses and misuses of genetics in the past and their relevance to the present
- Commercialization of the products of the HGP
- Conceptual and philosophical implications of the HGP (HHS and DOE 1990, 67–69)

ELSI research has informed public policy. For example, the federal Genetic Information Nondiscrimination Act (GINA) of 2008 (Public Law 110–233) prohibits genetic discrimination by most health insurers and employers (NHGRI 2015).

Ethical Principles and Examples of Breaches of Ethical Principles

Ethical principles in biomedical research include autonomy, beneficence, care, fidelity, honesty, justice, nonmaleficence, sanctity, and utility. Unfortunately, these ethical principles are sometimes violated. Several notorious cases are presented in this section in relation to the relevant principles.

Autonomy

In the research context, **autonomy** (self-determination) refers to the ability of research participants to understand what their participation in a research study involves and to give their informed consent. **Informed consent** signifies that the subject was given a complete and understandable explanation of the experiment and its risks and based his or her decision to participate or not to participate on that information, without being coerced or unduly influenced (45 CFR 46.116). Autonomy does not mean that the participant can control the outcomes of the research or what might happen to the participant; rather, it means that the participant understands the potential risks and benefits of the research and chooses to be participate without coercion or fear of the consequences of refusing to participate.

Research participants did not have autonomy in the **Tearoom Trade study**, a research project to examine the sexual behavior of men in public restrooms conducted by Laud Humphreys in St. Louis, MO, in the late 1960s, a time when engaging in homosexual sex was illegal (Humphreys 1970, 15; Galliher et al. 2004, 27–28). ("Tearoom" was slang for a place where homosexual encounters occurred.) To gain trust of the subjects, Humphreys pretended to the men that he was gay and that he was a lookout to prevent them from being caught by the police (Galliher et al. 2004, 28).

After confirming (by watching through windows) that the men had engaged in a homosexual act, he then recorded their license plates when they left the restroom. Based on this information, he acquired data on the men from city and county directories (Humphreys 1970, 15). He subsequently disguised himself and interviewed the men in their homes while pretending that he was conducting a social health survey. Some of these men were socially prominent and had families, and they could have been harmed had their identities become known; however, Humphreys completely and carefully protected their identities (Lenza 2004, 25). Nevertheless, the research project violated the subjects' autonomy because Humphreys deceived them (Lenza 2004, 23). The research project has been controversial since it was first published (Nardi 1995, 1). In research methods textbooks, the study is presented as "an example of covert and deceptive research methods that endangered subjects without their consent" (Lenza 2004, 20).

Beneficence

Beneficence means doing good for others. In biomedical research, a study demonstrates beneficence when it intends to build on the body of knowledge in a manner that will help the research participants or future patients. A person dying of cancer may not benefit from research on a new medication but may decide to participate in the hope that determining a drug's effectiveness may help others.

In 1994, President Bill Clinton appointed the Advisory Committee on Human Radiation Experiments to investigate reports of possible unethical **human radiation experiments** sponsored by the several federal agencies and conducted by researchers affiliated with government agencies, universities, hospitals and other research institutions between 1944 and 1974 (Faden 1996, 5, 777). Examples of the cases compiled by the Advisory Committee involved plutonium injections and total-body irradiation; experimentation on sick hospital patients, prisoners, and children; intentional environmental releases of radiation; and radiation exposures of uranium miners and atomic veterans (US military personnel potentially exposed to radioactivity during testing or use of atomic weapons or devices or during other service-related activities in the Marshall Islands, other Pacific islands, New Mexico, Nevada, Japan, and other locations) (Faden 1996, 7).

These experiments violated the ethical principle of beneficence because the experiments "offered no prospect of medical benefit to human subjects" (Advisory Committee 1995, 803). For example, many atomic bomb tests were conducted to investigate the effectiveness and the effects of nuclear weapons. "More than 200,000 people, including soldiers, sailors, air crews, and civilian test personnel, were engaged to staff the tests, to participate as trainees or observers, and to gather data on the effects of the weapons" (Advisory Committee 1995, 455). In one case, on July 1, 1946, the United States exploded an atomic bomb at the Bikini Atoll in the Marshall Islands (located near the equator in the Pacific Ocean) and the atoll's 167 inhabitants were relocated (Guyer 2001, 1371–1374). Atomic bomb tests continued in the Marshall Islands between 1946 and 1958, and, consequently, "Bikini and other islands in the Marshall Island chain remain hazardous for living organisms" (Guyer 2001, 1371).

The Advisory Committee's extensive investigation resulted in 23 findings and 18 recommendations (Advisory Committee 1995, 777–799, 801–839). Recommendations 1 and 3 are illustrative of the committee's conclusions:

- *Recommendation 1:* "The Advisory Committee recommends … that the government deliver a personal, individualized apology and provide financial compensation to the subjects (or their next of kin) of human radiation experiments in which efforts were made by the government to keep information secret from these individuals or their families, or from the public, for the purpose of avoiding embarrassment or potential legal liability, or both, and where this secrecy had the effect of denying individuals the opportunity to pursue potential grievances" (Advisory Committee 1995, 803).
- *Recommendation 3:* "The Advisory Committee recommends … that for subjects who were used in experiments for which there was no prospect of medical benefit to them and there is evidence specific to the experiment in which the subjects were involved that (1) no consent, or inadequate consent, was obtained, or (2) their selection as subjects constituted an injustice, or both, the government should offer a personal, individualized apology to each subject" (Advisory Committee 1995, 805).

Caring and Fidelity

The ethical principle of **caring** focuses on the importance of relationships and on the connections between oneself and others (Noddings 1990, 124). It "can best be understood as a positive emotional and supportive response" to a person or people who need care, with the aim of affirming the caregivers' "commitment to their well-being, our willingness to identify with them in their pain and suffering, and our desire to do what we can to relieve their situation" (Callahan 1990, 144). Caring is also understood to extend beyond the relationship between caregiver and care recipient to a broad array of personal, professional, and societal relationships (Pettersen 2011, 51–52).

Fidelity is related to loyalty and good faith. It means being faithful—keeping promises and honoring contracts and agreements. Good faith includes avoiding conflicts of interest. Thus, researchers state any conflicts of interest that they may have when conducting research, such as having a financial interest in a medical device, technology, or drug that they are investigating. Research professionals also have a duty to honor their words and actions.

The **Gelsinger case** represents a violation of the ethical principles of caring and fidelity. Jesse Gelsinger was an 18-year-old with an inherited genetic disorder that affected his ability to metabolize nitrogen (a component of proteins) and eliminate the resulting ammonia from his body (Savulescu 2001, 148). He was relatively fit, having controlled his disorder with a special low-protein diet and drugs, but he had had episodic crises when he went off his diet and ammonia toxicity built up in his body (Wilson 2010, 298). In 1999, he participated in a gene therapy trial at the University of Pennsylvania that involved having an adenovirus vector carrying the corrected gene infused directly into his liver through a catheter (Savulescu 2001, 148). In September 1999, four days after Gelsinger received the highest dose of the vector given in the 18-subject trial (Marshall 1999, 2244), he died of multisystem organ failure (Scully 2000, S56).

The principle of fidelity was violated in this case because one of the researchers conducting the trial and the University of Pennsylvania had a conflict of interest. They were primary stakeholders in a biogenetics company that would profit from the gene technology (Nelson and Weiss 2000). Other ethical violations, related to caring, also occurred. The researchers had not adequately evaluated Gelsinger before the trial and therefore did not realize that pre-erythroblast cells (immature red blood cells) in his bone marrow were depressed, possibly because of another genetic disorder or a viral infection (Savulescu 2001, 148). Moreover, the researchers deviated from their protocol as approved by the Food and Drug Administration (FDA). Gelsinger's ammonia levels were 30 percent to 60 percent higher than the protocol's criterion of eligibility (Savulescu 2001, 148). Additionally, the researchers failed to report that, prior to Gelsinger receiving the infusion, two subjects in earlier trials had experienced serious adverse effects (Smith and Byers 2002, 107). Per FDA requirements, the trial should have been halted at that point. Also, the consent form that Gelsinger signed did not disclose that monkeys given a similar treatment in a previous study had died of ammonia toxicity (Savulescu 2001, 149).

Gelsinger's death resulted in two lawsuits, one filed by his family and another by the federal government. The family's suit was settled out of court for an undisclosed amount of money and with a promise from the University of Pennsylvania to improve its oversight of research (Sibbald 2001, 1612). In 2005, the US Department of Justice reached a settlement with the university and the researchers. The university paid $517,496 in fines, and the researchers' clinical investigations were restricted (Couzin and Kaiser 2005, 1028).

Honesty

In the context of a research study, **honesty** is a complete, truthful accounting for all parts of the research study. Failure to be honest can involve *lies of commission* (intentional lying) or *lies of omission* (failure to tell the truth when it is known). Lies of commission could involve intentionally reporting inaccurate results, whereas lies of omission could involve failing to fully disclose results, such as potential harm to patients, or suppression of unfavorable results.

The **Willowbrook hepatitis studies** were a series of experiments on institutionalized children with severe intellectual disabilities at Willowbrook State School, a state-sponsored institution for children with intellectual disabilities located in New York City. Between the 1940s and the 1960s, the Willowbrook State School population increased from about 3,000 residents to over 6,000 residents, and hepatitis was widespread in the overcrowded facility (Krugman 1986, 158). Between the mid-1950s and 1976, researchers intentionally exposed newly admitted children to the hepatitis virus. The researchers' purpose was to learn more about the natural course of the disease (Krugman 1986, 159–160). These studies represent a violation of honesty because the researchers intentionally misled the parents to believe that their children were being vaccinated *against* hepatitis; instead the children were being infected with the virus (Rothman 1982, 7). Moreover, as happened in the Tuskegee study, the research was continued after a treatment for the disease had been found and the studies' ethics had been questioned (Rothman 1982, 7).

The **Vioxx case** involves a pharmaceutical company that violated the principle of honesty by marketing a drug while knowingly suppressing information about its serious adverse side-effects (Krumholz et al. 2007, 121). The case began in 1999, when Merck and Co. launched the painkiller rofecoxib under the brand name Vioxx. This medication became one of the company's five most profitable drugs, with $2.5 billion in sales per year (Cavusgil 2007, 452). However, within a year of the product's launch, practicing physicians observed cardiovascular problems in their patients taking Vioxx (Lyon and Mirivel 2011, 57). Moreover, in 2000, researchers published an article about the comparative gastrointestinal side effects, such as ulcers and bleeding, of Vioxx and naproxen (an older, established painkiller) (Bombardier et al. 2000, 1520). During the study, researchers also monitored any cardiovascular events, such as myocardial infarctions (heart attacks), that the subjects had. The subjects taking Vioxx had more myocardial infarctions than subjects taking naproxen; however, this result was explained away by suggesting that naproxen may have a "protective effect" against myocardial infarctions (Bombardier et al. 2000, 1526; Smith 2006, 380). Merck did not specifically investigate these adverse cardiovascular effects.

Other research also suggested problems with Vioxx. For example, in April 2001, Merck conducted an intention-to-treat analysis (ITT, refer to chapter 12) of data from two research trials that had investigated whether the use of Vioxx affected the development or progression of Alzheimer's disease (Fielder 2008, 106). External researchers who inspected documents from a Vioxx lawsuit reported that the company's internal ITT analysis had shown a significant increase in mortality among the Vioxx patients (Psaty and Kronmal 2008, 1813). In 2000, another trial began to investigate whether Vioxx could prevent the recurrence of colon polyps. Minutes from an internal May 2003 safety meeting regarding this trial showed that subjects in the Vioxx group had a 20 percent higher risk of heart attack or stroke than subjects receiving the placebo. The reported risk continued to increase until September 2004, when it was 120 percent higher than the risk with placebo (Cavusgil 2007, 454). Based on this conclusive evidence, the company withdrew Vioxx from the market; however, in the years between 1999 and 2004, up to 38,000 patients had died from cardiovascular complications with a total of 160,000 injured (Drugwatch 2016).

Despite the initial warnings, Merck aggressively marketed Vioxx between 2001 and 2004. The marketing campaign began with a press release titled "Merck Reconfirms Favorable Cardiovascular Safety of Vioxx" on May 22, 2001 (Topol 2004, 1707). The campaign continued with numerous publications in scholarly journals and presentations at national meetings. Whenever other researchers published reports showing the adverse cardiovascular effects of Vioxx, the company claimed that the study designs were flawed (Topol 2004, 1707). In conclusion, the company's marketing campaign and other communications "systematically distorted communication involving its drug Vioxx … in ways that hindered patients and physicians from making an informed choice about using and prescribing the drug" (Lyon 2007, 377).

Merck has paid at least $6 billion to settle lawsuits resulting from the drug's use (Loftus 2016). For example, in 2007, Merck agreed to pay $4.85 billion to settle 27,000 lawsuits from patients claiming the drug caused their heart attacks and strokes, although the company admitted no wrongdoing (Wadman 2007, 324). Additionally, after pleading guilty to a misdemeanor, Merck agreed in 2011 to pay $950 million to settle the US Department of Justice's allegations that the company had misbranded Vioxx as a treatment for diseases that were not covered when the FDA approved the drug (Loftus and Kendall 2011). In 2016, Merck further agreed, while admitting no wrongdoing, to pay $830 million to settle a suit brought by shareholders who alleged that they had paid inflated prices for the company's shares because its executives made misleading statements about Vioxx's safety (Loftus 2016).

Justice

In research, **justice** means individuals are treated fairly during enrollment and when they participate in a study. Justice requires that researchers do not provide preferential treatment to specific individuals or groups. It also requires that no undue burden for participation is placed on any group, such as prisoners or other vulnerable populations. For example, individuals who lack access to or cannot afford healthcare should *not* be offered temporary healthcare as an incentive to enroll in a clinical trial, because they may conclude that they do not have any other alternatives and because the healthcare services would end when the study ends. Moreover, participants cannot be enrolled as a convenience to the researcher.

The **Holmesburg Prison studies** refer to unjust experiments conducted with prisoners as subjects at Holmesburg Prison in Philadelphia, PA, from the early 1950s through the mid-1970s (Hornblum 1999, 383). The lead researcher in many of these experiments was Albert Kligman, a dermatologist at the University of Pennsylvania (Hornblum 1998, xix), who used the prisoners to test pharmaceutical companies' consumer products, such as deodorants, detergents, hair dyes, diet beverages, toothpaste, eye drops, shampoos, and suntan lotions (Hornblum 2000, 421). In other experiments, researchers infected the prisoners with skin wart viruses, such as herpes simplex virus and human papillomavirus (Hornblum 1999, 384). At Holmesburg Prison, the prisoners' incentive for participating was money (Hornblum 2000, 422); one prisoner estimated that he made between $400 and $600 in one year (Hornblum 1998, 22). Between 1964 and 1968, Kligman conducted research for the U.S. Army using 320 prisoners to test the effects of mind-altering drugs (Perper and Cina 2010, 92). For Dow Chemical, Kligman and his team of researchers applied dioxin (the carcinogenic toxin in Agent Orange) and other herbicides to the prisoners' skin because the company wanted to know whether its workers had developed an acne-like condition as a result of handling the chemical compounds (Perper and Cina 2010, 92–93). For many of these experiments, the prisoners were unaware of experiments' purposes and the chemicals used (Hornblum 1998, xxi). The researchers' careers flourished, but "the prisoners were left with physical scars, horrible memories, and a fear of scientists and physicians" (Hornblum 2000, 425).

Nonmaleficence, Sanctity, and Utility

Other ethical principles include nonmaleficence, sanctity, and utility; these principles can be applied to the studies already discussed.

The ethical principle of **nonmaleficence** means doing no harm. The principles of beneficence and nonmaleficence can be traced back to the Greek physician Hippocrates who, in 400 BCE wrote, the "physician must … have two special objects in view with regard to disease, namely, to do good or to do no harm" (Hippocrates 340 BCE, Book I, Section II. 5). A research study's intervention should not knowingly harm a participant. For example, in the Willowbrook Hepatitis Study, nonmaleficence was the ethical principle that was violated because the researchers deliberately infected the children with hepatitis, making them sick.

Sanctity is the principle that humans are valued and have rights just because they exist. Humans deserve to be treated well and with respect because they are human (Novak 2007, xi–xiii). In other words, humans do not need to serve a purpose. Under this principle, researchers should not use people as a means to an end. This principle was violated in several of the studies discussed previously, such as the Tuskegee Study.

Utility involves considering the usefulness of an act, which is evaluated by its effects, including its benefits and costs. The principle of utility is engaged when a researcher considers several alternative methodological paths or weighs participation options for a study's subjects. Researchers are obligated to assess or predict the consequences of the research, even though those consequences are not guaranteed. Utility helps researchers determine whether the study will lend itself to the greatest benefit and the least harm. The principle of utility was violated during the Jewish Chronic Disease Study because the subjects were not provided any alternative methodological pathways other than to receive live cancer cells, nor were they told that the cells were cancerous.

Codes of Ethics for Researchers

A **code of ethics** incorporates principles discussed in the previous section to express a profession's core values and promote ethical behavior of the profession's members (Spielthenner 2015, 195). The code provides both a statement for the public and a level of expectation that guides practice, but it does not provide a set of rules about how to act in all situations. Although a code of ethics cannot guarantee ethical behavior, resolve all ethical issues, or fully capture the richness and complexity involved in making responsible ethical choices, it sets forth values and ethical principles and offers ethical guidelines to which professionals can aspire and by which their actions can be judged. Codes of ethics for health informatics and HIM professionals, such as those listed below, have been issued:

- A Code of Professional Ethical Conduct for AMIA (AMIA 2016)
- Code of Ethics for Health Information Professionals (IMIA 2016)
- AHIMA Code of Ethics (AHIMA 2016)

These codes have provisions that specifically apply to researchers. For example, principle IV of the AMIA code provides ethical guidelines regarding society and research (AMIA 2016). In the IMIA code, rule of conduct D.2.a. states that health information professionals have a duty to ensure that only data relevant to legitimate research are collected, and rule of conduct D.4 states that such professionals "refuse to participate in or support practices that violate human rights" (IMIA 2016). Principle V in the AHIMA code of ethics details the HIM profession's expectations regarding research, as follows.

V. Advance health information management knowledge and practice through continuing education, research, publications, and presentations. A health information management professional shall:

5.1. Develop and enhance continually professional expertise, knowledge, and skills (including appropriate education, research, training, consultation, and supervision). Contribute to the knowledge base of health information management and share one's knowledge related to practice, research, and ethics.
5.2. Base practice decisions on recognized knowledge, including empirically based knowledge relevant to health information management and health information management ethics.
5.3. Contribute time and professional expertise to activities that promote respect for the value, integrity, and competence of the health information management profession. These activities may include teaching, research, consultation, service, legislative testimony, advocacy, presentations in the community, and participation in professional organizations.
5.4. Engage in evaluation and research that ensures the confidentiality of participants and of the data obtained from them by following guidelines developed for the participants in consultation with appropriate institutional review boards.
5.5. Report evaluation and research findings accurately and take steps to correct any errors later found in published data using standard publication methods.
5.6. Design or conduct evaluation or research that is in conformance with applicable federal or state laws.
5.7. Take reasonable steps to provide or arrange for continuing education and staff development, addressing current knowledge and emerging developments related to health information management practice and ethics. (AHIMA 2016)

It is useful to review professional codes of ethics to ground one's thinking on ways to behave and think about potential issues that may arise when conducting research or assisting researchers. In the next section, ethical guidelines, laws, and regulations that exist to protect human subjects are discussed.

International Protection of Human Research Subjects

Multiple guidelines, laws, and regulations contribute to the protection of human research subjects. These protections exist internationally, nationally, and at the local level. For the international level, this section describes the Nuremburg Code and the Declaration of Helsinki.

The Nuremburg Code

At the international level, the **Nuremberg Code**, dating to 1947, is a set of 10 ethical principles that guide human experimentation (NIH 2009). The code emerged from the US military tribunal known as the Doctors' Trial, in which Nazi doctors were tried in Nuremberg for war crimes because they performed medical experiments on civilian prisoners (Shuster 1997, 1437). These experiments subjected individuals to hypothermia (excessively low body temperature), castration by x-rays, intrauterine injections, exposure to high-altitude conditions through decompression chambers, bone transplantation, forced ingestion of saltwater, and injection with typhus and malaria (Bassiouni et al. 1981, 1639–1640). In response to these horrific acts, the first principle of the Nuremberg Code is a precise statement on the requirements for voluntary informed consent "whenever human beings are asked to make sacrifices for the sake of others" (Katz 1996, 1665).

Declaration of Helsinki

The **Declaration of Helsinki** is an international statement of ethical principles for biomedical research involving humans (WMA 2016). The declaration was first adopted in 1964 and has been routinely updated. The current version dates to 2013. While the declaration primarily guides physicians, the World Medical Association (WMA) encourages everyone who conducts biomedical research involving humans to adopt its principles. The declaration states that the goal of generating new knowledge through research can never take precedence of the rights of individual subjects. Moreover, the declaration addresses other issues, such as risks and benefits, vulnerable groups and individuals, privacy and confidentiality, informed consent, and other issues.

Federal Laws and Regulations

In the United States, human research subjects are protected by numerous federal laws and regulations related to research, including Policy and Procedure Order 129, the National Research Act of 1974, the Belmont Report, the Federal Policy for the Protection of Human Subjects ("Common Rule"), HIPAA, HITECH, and the Health Research Extension Act of 1985.

Policy and Procedure Order 129

In 1966, the US Surgeon General issued Policy and Procedure Order 129, which contained directives concerning research and investigations involving human subjects in institutions receiving PHS grant money (Stewart 1966). The order was the result of years of study by PHS staff and advisory groups, and it required that an institutional committee review researchers' proposals to "assure an independent determination: (1) of the rights and welfare of the individual or individuals involved, (2) of the appropriateness of the methods used to secure informed consent, and (3) of the risks and potential medical benefits of the investigation" (Stewart 1966, 351). The order was the origin of *institutional review boards (IRBs)*, the administrative bodies established to protect the rights and welfare of human research subjects recruited to participate in research activities associated with healthcare organizations and other institutions. As previously noted in the section on the Tuskegee study, the order did not apply to PHS-run research programs (Jones 2008, 94).

National Research Act of 1974

Public outcry over the ethical lapses in the Tuskegee study led to the passage in 1974 of the National Research Act (Public Law 93-348), which provides a framework for the protection of human subjects in biomedical and behavioral research. The law created the National Commission for the Protection of Human Subjects of Biomedical and Behavioral Research, which was charged with developing guidelines for the use of human subjects in biomedical and behavioral research. The legislation directed the commission to consider the following:

- The boundaries between biomedical and behavioral research and the accepted and routine practice of medicine
- The role of assessment of risk-benefit criteria in the determination of the appropriateness of research involving human subjects
- Appropriate guidelines for the selection of human subjects for participation in such research
- The nature and definition of informed consent in various research settings (National Commission for the Protection of Human Subjects of Biomedical and Behavioral Research 1979, 1)

The National Research Act requires that human subjects in research must be protected. It set the stage for the issuance of another important set of principles, detailed in the Belmont Report.

Belmont Report

The Belmont Report is the ethical and regulatory foundation for biomedical and behavioral research on human subjects in the United States. Written following the National Research Act and published in 1979 as the *Ethical Principles for the Protection of Human Subjects of Research,* the report focuses on the following three basic ethical principles:

- Respect for persons involves recognition of the personal dignity and autonomy of individuals and special protection of those persons with diminished autonomy. Its application is in informed consent. This principle requires that subjects, to the degree that they are capable, be given the opportunity to choose what shall or shall not happen to them. The process contains three elements: information, comprehension, and voluntariness.
- Beneficence entails an obligation to protect persons from harm by maximizing anticipated benefits and minimizing possible risks of harm. Its application is the assessment of risks and benefits of the research. This principle requires that the nature and scope of the risks and benefits are carefully and systematically assessed.
- Justice requires that the benefits and burdens of research be distributed fairly. This principle is applied in the selection of subjects for a research project. The principle requires that the procedures and outcomes in the selection of research subjects must be fair. (National Commission for the Protection of Human Subjects of Biomedical and Behavioral Research 1979, 4–10)

The Belmont Report also includes the concept of ethics review boards, such as those required by the previously discussed Policy and Procedure Order 129. These review boards came to be known as IRBs.

Federal Policy for the Protection of Human Subjects and the "Common Rule"

In 1981, in response to the Belmont Report, HHS and the FDA created the **Federal Policy for the Protection of Human Subjects** (45 CFR 46) by revising the following existing regulations (Federman et al. 2001, 24–26; HHS 2016a):

- Basic 1974 regulations governing the protection of human subjects in research supported or conducted by HHS (then known as the Department of Health, Education and Welfare) (HHS 2016a)
- Kefauver-Harris Amendments (Public Law 87-781) to the Federal Food, Drug, and Cosmetic Act, which authorized the FDA to evaluate the safety of drugs and included a provision requiring the informed consent of participants in the testing of new drugs (Federman 2001, 24–25).

The revised policy includes the federal regulations that protect the rights, welfare, and well-being of subjects involved in research (at first, only that conducted or supported by the HHS), and gives the **Office for Human Research Protections (OHRP)** oversight of compliance with the federal regulations. Moreover, the federal policy incorporates major portions of the Belmont Report. HHS continues to revise and expand the protections in 45 CFR 46, generally clarifying language, addressing emerging issues, and adding protections for specific vulnerable populations (OHRP 2012). The policy currently encompasses the following five subparts (HHS 2016b):

- Subpart A, known as the **Common Rule**, offers a basic set of protections for all human subjects of research conducted or supported by HHS; this subpart was revised in 1981 and 1991, with technical amendments made in 2005. Currently, 18 federal departments and agencies have adopted Subpart A (HHS 2016c).
- Subpart B identifies additional protections for pregnant women, human fetuses, and neonates involved in research. Fetuses and neonates are vulnerable populations because they cannot consent to research; pregnant women are given additional protection because their participation in research may affect the health of the fetus.
- Subpart C provides protections for prisoners participating in biomedical and behavioral research. As noted earlier in the chapter, prisoners may not be able to make a truly voluntary and uncoerced decision to participate in research (45 CFR 46.302).
- Subpart D gives additional protections to children involved as subjects in research. Children have not reached their full intellectual and emotional development and may be vulnerable to coercion or undue influence.
- Subpart E covers registration of IRBs that conduct review of human research studies conducted or supported by HHS.

In 2015, HHS and several other federal departments and agencies proposed revisions to modernize, strengthen, and make the Common Rule more effective (HHS 2015, 53933). At the time of the publication of this book, no final rule has been issued.

The Common Rule contains three general provisions for the protection of human subjects (45 CFR 46):

- Institutional assurance of compliance—in other words, researchers' institutions, such as universities or other organizations, must agree to comply with the federal regulations
- Obtainment of IRB approval before research begins
- Acquisition of informed consent from all human subjects in the research project

These three general provisions are discussed in the next sections.

Institutional Assurance of Compliance

Federal-wide assurance of compliance (FWA) is a formal, written, and binding commitment in which an institution promises to comply with applicable regulations governing research with human subjects and stipulates the procedures through which compliance will be achieved, "regardless of whether the research is subject to federal regulation" (45 CFR 46.103(b)(1)). To ensure compliance, the OHRP conducts (a) compliance ("not-for-cause") audits, which are general surveillance visits to evaluate an institution's overall compliance, and (b) complaint ("for-cause") investigations, which occur because the OHRP has received specific allegations of investigators' misconduct or reports of a serious incident, such as the death of a healthy subject (OHRP 2016).

In addition to its investigative responsibilities, the OHRP also promotes regulatory compliance and ethical research practices by providing educational programs and materials on ethics and producing guidelines and interpretations of specific regulatory provisions.

Institutional Review Boards

IRBs provide mandatory review, oversight, guidance, and approval for research projects conducted at an institution that involve human subjects or data sources about human subjects (for example, medical records, a tumor registry or Medicare data). The regulations define research as "a systematic investigation, including research development, testing and evaluation, designed to develop or contribute to generalizable knowledge. Activities which meet this definition constitute research for purposes of this policy, whether or not they are conducted or supported under a program which is considered research for other purposes" (45 CFR 46.102(d)). This definition excludes investigations that are not intended to develop or contribute to generalizable knowledge, such as internal organizational activities to improve operations and quality.

The regulation describes the membership of IRBs (45 CFR 46.107). The IRB board must have at least five diverse members, with a minimum of one member having a scientific background, one member having a nonscientific background, and one member being unaffiliated with the institution. Most IRBs have 10 to 14 members, including members with expertise in vulnerable subjects and in various research designs and methods. IRBs may also use consultants with specialized expertise in research or the area of proposed experiments. An IRB member may not participate in reviews of proposals or continuing reviews of any project in which he or she has an interest. The IRB's meetings are scheduled per the needs of the institution.

Researchers submit their proposals to conduct research to their institution's IRB. Institutions have specific forms for these proposals, which researchers must complete and submit, usually electronically. When studies involve multiple organizations, such as projects with researchers from different organizations or subjects from different organizations, the researchers must submit proposals and obtain approval from the IRBs at all involved institutions. IRBs review and have the authority to approve, require modifications in (to secure approval), or disapprove all research activities covered by 45 CFR 46 (45 CFR 46.109(a)). This review and authority includes initial reviews of proposals and continuing reviews of studies.

There are three categories of reviews: exempt, expedited, and full. The IRB determines the appropriate category of review. However, the researcher can indicate a possible category on the proposal form.

Exempt from review is a category of review for research projects that do not collect identifiable information and do not pose a risk to subjects. The requirements for informed consent and yearly IRB renewal do not apply to projects deemed exempt from review. To help researchers assess whether their research project might be exempt, the HHS regulations describe the following examples of exempt research projects (45 CFR 46.101(b)(1–6)):

1. Research conducted in educational settings, involving normal educational practices (such as comparisons of online learning and face-to-face learning)
2. Research involving the use of educational tests (cognitive, diagnostic, aptitude, achievement), survey procedures, interview procedures, or observation of public behavior, unless the data are collected in a way that allows identification of the subjects
3. Research involving the use of educational tests (cognitive, diagnostic, aptitude, achievement), survey procedures, interview procedures, or observation of public behavior, unless the data are collected in a way that allows identification of the subjects if the subjects are elected or appointed public officials or candidates for public office or if federal statute requires without exception that the confidentiality of the personally identifiable information will be maintained throughout the research and thereafter
4. Research involving the collection or study of existing data, documents, records, pathological specimens, or diagnostic specimens, if these sources are publicly available or if the information is recorded by the investigator in such a manner that subjects cannot be identified directly or through identifiers linked to the subjects
5. Research and demonstration projects that are conducted by or subject to the approval of [federal] department or agency heads, and which are designed to study, evaluate, or otherwise examine: (i) public benefit or service programs; (ii) procedures for obtaining benefits or services under those programs; (iii) possible changes in or alternatives to those programs or procedures; or (iv) possible changes in methods or levels of payment for benefits or services under those programs
6. Taste and food quality evaluation and consumer acceptance studies approved by the FDA or the Environmental Protection Agency or the Food Safety and Inspection Service of the US Department of Agriculture

IRB exemptions usually are determined by the IRB chair or a designated IRB member.

Expedited review is a category of review for minor changes in previously approved research during the period (of one year or less) for which approval is authorized, and research projects that involve no more than minimal risk for subjects and are in one of the following authorized categories (45 CFR 46.110):

1. Clinical studies of drugs and medical devices *if* an investigational new FDA drug application or an FDA investigational device exemption application is not required or the medical device is cleared or approved for marketing and the medical device is being used in accordance with its cleared or approved labeling
2. Collection of blood samples by finger stick, heel stick, ear stick, or venipuncture
3. Prospective collection of biological specimens for research purposes by noninvasive means, such as hair and nail clippings
4. Collection of data through noninvasive procedures (not involving general anesthesia or sedation and excluding x-rays or microwaves) routinely employed in clinical practice, such as magnetic resonance imaging, electrocardiography, strength testing, and so forth
5. Research involving materials (data, documents, records, or specimens) that have been collected, or will be collected solely for nonresearch purposes (such as medical treatment or diagnosis)
6. Collection of data from voice, video, digital, or image recordings made for research purposes
7. Research on individual or group characteristics or behavior (including, but not limited to, research on perception, cognition, motivation, identity, language, communication, cultural beliefs or practices, and social behavior) or research employing survey, interview, oral history, focus group, program evaluation, human factors evaluation, or quality assurance methodologies
8. Continuing review of research previously approved by the convened IRB as follows: (a) where (i) the research is permanently closed to the enrollment of new subjects; (ii) all subjects have completed all research-related interventions; and (iii) the research remains active only for long-term follow-up of subjects; (b) where no subjects have been enrolled and no additional risks have been identified; or (c) where the remaining research activities are limited to data analysis
9. Continuing review of research, not conducted under an investigational new drug application or investigational device exemption, where categories 2 through 8 do not apply but the IRB has determined and documented at a convened meeting that the research involves no greater than minimal risk and no additional risks have been identified (45 CFR 46.110)

Expedited review is often considered a quick review, and it may mean that the researcher does not have to wait for an IRB meeting. Expedited reviews are conducted by the IRB chair or a designated IRB member and are not conducted during an IRB meeting. In reviewing the research, the reviewers may exercise all the authorities of the IRB except that the reviewers may not disapprove the research. A research activity may be disapproved only after review in accordance with the nonexpedited procedure (full review).

Full review is a category of review for research projects that represent more than minimal risk for the subjects and, therefore, are presented to a quorum of IRB members, who may discuss the proposal at length. The IRB pays special attention to the proposed study's research methods, risks and benefits to subjects, the process of informed consent, and selection and enrollment of subjects. Some IRBs may use a primary reviewer system, designating two persons to do a full analysis of the project. The primary reviewer encourages all board members to participate in the discussion.

After the review of the proposal, the IRB notifies the researchers and the institution in writing of its decision to approve or disapprove the proposed research, or of modifications required to secure IRB approval of the research activity. If the IRB decides to disapprove a research study, it includes in its written notification a statement of the reasons for its decision and gives the researchers an opportunity to respond in person or in writing.

IRBs conduct continuing review of research at intervals appropriate to the degree of risk, but not less than once per year, and have authority to observe or have a third-party observe the consent process and the research. In continuing reviews, the researcher completes and submits a form on the conduct and progress of the research project. IRBs also must approve any changes to an approved study protocol, except corrections of an administrative nature, such as typographical or spelling errors. IRBs also have the authority to suspend or terminate research that is not being conducted in accordance with their requirements or that has been associated with unexpected serious harm to subjects (45 CFR 46.113).

The regulations require that IRBs have meeting space and sufficient staff to support their reviews and record-keeping duties (46.103(b)(2)). The federal regulations also describe requirements for the documentation that must be maintained regarding activities of the IRB. The documentation includes the following:

- Copies of all reviewed research proposals, any accompanying scientific evaluations, approved sample consent documents, progress reports submitted by researchers, and reports of injuries to subjects, as applicable
- Minutes of IRB meetings, which shall be in sufficient detail to show attendance at the meetings; actions taken by the IRB; the vote on these actions, including the number of members voting for, against, and abstaining; the basis for requiring changes in or disapproving research; and a written summary of the discussion of controverted issues and their resolution
- Records of continuing review activities
- Copies of all correspondence between the IRB and the investigators
- A list of IRB members that identifies them by name with earned degrees and other information sufficient to describe each member's chief anticipated contributions to IRB deliberations
- Written procedures the IRB will follow for conducting its initial and continuing review of research and for reporting its findings and actions to the researcher and the institution; for determining which projects require review more often than annually; for ensuring researchers' prompt reporting to the IRB and other appropriate officials any unanticipated problems involving risks to subjects or others or any serious or continuing noncompliance with this policy or the requirements or determinations of the IRB; for any suspensions or terminations of IRB approval; and other procedural details (45 CFR 46.115)

The records must be retained for at least three years, and records relating to research that is conducted is to be retained for at least three years after completion of the research. All records must be accessible for inspection and copying by authorized representatives of the federal department or agency at reasonable times and in a reasonable manner.

IRBs also receive any reports of unanticipated problems involving risks to human subjects and others (such as the researchers themselves or staff members) and adverse events (OHRP 2007). *Unanticipated problems* are defined as issues that are unexpected; are related or possibly related to the research study; and suggest that the research places subjects or others at a greater risk of harm (including physical, psychological, economic, or social) than was previously known or recognized. *Adverse events* are untoward or unfavorable medical occurrences. Upon becoming aware of the unanticipated problem or adverse event, the researchers must promptly report it within one to two weeks, depending upon its severity.

The OHRP recommends that investigators include the following information when reporting an adverse event, or any other incident, experience, or outcome as an unanticipated problem to the IRB:

- Appropriate identifying information for the research protocol, such as the title, and investigator's name
- Detailed description of the adverse event, incident, experience, or outcome
- Explanation of the basis for determining that the adverse event, incident, experience, or outcome represents an unanticipated problem
- Description of any changes to the protocol or other corrective actions that have been taken or are proposed in response to the unanticipated problem (OHRP 2007)

The OHRP's recommendations are intended to help ensure that the review and reporting of unanticipated problems and adverse events occur in a timely, meaningful way so that human subjects and others are protected from avoidable harms.

Informed Consent

Informed consent predates the Belmont Report. For medical care, such as surgeries, the concept dates to the early 20th century (Faden and Beauchamp 1986, 120). However, in this period, patients' informed consent for medical experimentation generally was not obtained, although healthy subjects were "informed of the nature and consequences of their participation and then asked to give their consent" (Katz 1996, 1663). By the mid-1960s, some physicians, such as Henry K. Beecher and Maurice H. Pappworth, questioned the ethics of not obtaining patients' informed consent for experimentation on them (Gaw 2012, 150).

Today, *informed consent* is used to refer to both a process and a signed form. Investigators must obtain informed consent from potential research participants before conducting the research. An IRB's scope of authority includes the process of and forms for obtaining informed consent. To comply with federal regulations, IRBs usually have specific requirements for consent forms regarding the format, content, and reading level, and they may reject proposals noncompliant with the requirements. Federal regulations require that the basic elements of informed consent provide the following information to each subject:

- A statement that the study involves research, an explanation of the purposes of the research and the expected duration of the subject's participation, a description of the procedures to be followed, and identification of any procedures that are experimental
- A description of any reasonably foreseeable risks or discomforts to the subject
- A description of any benefits to the subject or to others that may reasonably be expected from the research
- A disclosure of appropriate alternative procedures or courses of treatment, if any, that might be advantageous to the subject
- A statement describing the extent, if any, to which confidentiality of records identifying the subject will be maintained
- For research involving more than minimal risk, an explanation as to whether any compensation will be given and an explanation as to whether any medical treatments are available if injury occurs and, if so, what the compensation and treatments consist of, or where further information may be obtained
- An explanation of whom to contact for answers to pertinent questions about the research and research subjects' rights, and whom to contact in the event of a research-related injury to the subject
- A statement that participation is voluntary, refusal to participate will involve no penalty or loss of benefits to which the subject is otherwise entitled, and the subject may discontinue participation at any time without penalty or loss of benefits to which the subject is otherwise entitled (45 CFR 46.116(1–8))

When applicable, additional elements of informed consent may also be provided to subjects, such as additional costs that may result from the subject's participation, consequences of a subject's decision to withdraw from the research, and other elements. The information that is given to the subject must be in language understandable to the subject. Informed consent, whether oral or written, cannot include any exculpatory (tending to clear from guilt) language through which the subject is made to waive or appear to waive any of his or her legal rights; the language in the informed consent also cannot release or appear to release the researcher, sponsor, institution, or its agents from liability for negligence.

As a general guide, everyone involved in the process of informed consent should grasp the concepts of understanding, voluntariness, disclosure, and comprehension.

Understanding means that a consent form must be presented and written in language understandable to the prospective subject. "For example, presenting information in a disorganized and rapid fashion, allowing too little time for consideration or curtailing opportunities for questioning, all may adversely affect a subject's ability to make an informed choice" (National Commission for the Protection of Human Subjects of Biomedical and Behavioral Research 1979, 7). Additionally, presenting information using medical and legal jargon may limit a subject's ability to make an informed choice. For non-English-speaking subjects, the consent form must be translated into their native language. For illiterate subjects, the investigator in charge of informed consent must explain the study in terms they can understand and answer the subjects' questions. To assess participants' understanding, the researcher should ask and answer the following questions:

- What do the study participants understand about the research?
- Do the study participants understand the potential risks and benefits?
- Do the patients know what their rights are?
- Do they know that they can withdraw from the research study at any time?
- Do they know they can withdraw data or tissue samples?
- Do the participants understand their responsibilities in participating in the trial?

To judge understanding, the authors of the Belmont Report offer the following standard: "Persons, knowing that the procedure is neither necessary for their care nor perhaps fully understood, can decide whether they wish to participate in the furthering of knowledge. Even when some direct benefit to them is anticipated, the subjects should understand clearly the range of risk and the voluntary nature of participation" (National Commission for the Protection of Human Subjects of Biomedical and Behavioral Research 1979, 7).

Voluntariness means that an agreement to participate in research is only valid if the participant voluntarily gives consent, without coercion and undue influence (National Commission for the Protection of Human Subjects of Biomedical and Behavioral Research 1979, 7–8). Moreover, participants may feel "unjustifiable pressures" to agree when persons in positions of authority or influence, such as physicians, teachers, and employers, and other influential persons, "urge a course of action for a subject" (National Commission for the Protection of Human Subjects of Biomedical and Behavioral Research 1979, 8).

Researchers can support the voluntary nature of consent by providing sufficient time for subjects to review the consent form, highlighting the sections of the consent form that describe risk, and encouraging the participant to ask questions. During the experiment, the subject should be able to withdraw for any reason.

Disclosure, under the Common Rule, means that informed consent must describe the potential risks and benefits of a research study. For example, a clinical trial must include the potential risks and benefits of the medication, procedure, or device, and a nonmedical research study must identify the risks and benefits of tools and methods used in its interventions, such as social media or group interactions. Plus, the process of informed consent must include disclosure of appropriate alternative procedures or courses of treatment, if any, that might be advantageous to the subject.

Another set of federal regulations requires researchers to disclose any financial conflicts of interest (42 CFR 50, Subpart F). Financial conflicts may result if the researchers receive anything of monetary value, such as consulting fees, stocks, patents, and other payments or rights. In addition to supporting informed consent, the disclosure requirement promotes objectivity in research by establishing standards to ensure there is no reasonable expectation that the design, conduct, or reporting of research funded under PHS grants or cooperative agreements will be biased by any conflicting financial interest of a researcher (42 CFR 50.601).

Comprehension involves the capability of a subject to make decisions about whether to enroll in a research study. It is a function of intelligence, rationality, and maturity, and the researcher is obligated to adapt the presentation of the information to the subject's capacities in those areas. Each subject should be considered on his or her own terms because the principle of respect for persons requires giving each subject the opportunity to choose, to the extent he or she is able, whether to participate in research (National Commission for the Protection of Human Subjects of Biomedical and Behavioral Research 1979, 7). For example, a person who is marginally literate may not have adequate literacy skills or knowledge to make informed decisions about enrolling in a clinical trial. A person with mild dementia may not remember from one day to the next what decisions have been made. When a potential subject is incompetent, incapacitated, or a minor, federal regulations allow a legally authorized representative to give informed consent (45 CFR 46.102(b)). Subjects with diminished capacities who cannot give consent on their own include infants and young children, some individuals with intellectual disabilities, and comatose patients.

Researchers are responsible for obtaining informed consent. The process of informed consent is complete only when all the information relevant to the study has been explained to the potential subject, the subject's understanding of the experiment and its risks and benefits has been determined, and the form has been signed by the subject or legally authorized representative. The next sections will consider other laws and regulations applicable to research.

HIPAA and HITECH Act

The **Office for Civil Rights (OCR)** is the agency within the HHS that enforces federal civil rights laws and HIPAA of 1996 (Public Law 104-191). The OCR investigates allegations of violations of HIPAA. If the OCR finds evidence that supports the complaint, it requires the noncompliant institution to voluntarily comply or take corrective action. If the institution does not take satisfactory action to resolve the matter, the OCR may impose fines known as **civil monetary penalties**. If the complaint could be a violation of the criminal provision of HIPAA, the OCR may refer the case to the Department of Justice for investigation (OCR 2016).

One important element of HIPAA related to research ethics is the **Privacy Rule**, which establishes minimum standards to protect the privacy of health information that identifies individuals who are living or deceased. The Privacy Rule "balances an individual's interest in keeping his or her health information confidential with other social benefits, including health care research" (NIH 2004, i.). Where research is concerned, the Privacy Rule protects the privacy of individually identifiable health information, while at the same time ensuring that researchers continue to have access to health information necessary to conduct research.

Individually identifiable health information, including demographic information collected from an individual, is information created or received by a healthcare provider, health plan, employer, or healthcare clearinghouse that identifies the individual, or reasonably could be used to identify the individual (such as name, address, birth date, and Social Security number) and that relates to the past, present, or future physical or mental health or condition (such as medical records and claims data); provision of healthcare to the individual; or past, present or future payment for the provision of healthcare to the individual (NIH 2004, 4). The Privacy Rule creates a subset of individually identifiable health information known as *protected health information* (PHI). "PHI is individually identifiable health information transmitted by electronic media, maintained in electronic media, or transmitted or maintained in any other form or medium" (NIH 2004, 2). It also includes identifiable health information about subjects of clinical research.

The Privacy Rule works with the Common Rule. The HIPAA Privacy Rule establishes the conditions under which PHI may be used or disclosed for research purposes by covered entities (health plans, health care clearinghouses, and healthcare providers that electronically transmit any health information associated with transactions). The Privacy Rule also defines how individuals will be informed of uses and disclosures of their medical information for research purposes, and their rights to access information about them held by covered entities.

An individual's PHI may be used and disclosed for research if that individual provides written permission in the form of an authorization. Researchers must obtain a signed authorization before using or disclosing PHI for research. An authorization differs from an informed consent in that an authorization focuses on privacy risks and states how, why, and to whom the PHI will be used, disclosed, or both for research. The authorization must be written in plain language that is understandable to a layperson. Moreover, the Privacy Rule specifies that a valid research authorization must include six core elements and three required statements. The six core elements generally are as follows:

- Description of PHI information to be used or disclosed, such as a medical record or laboratory result
- Persons or entities permitted to use or disclose the PHI, such as the investigator or the research team
- Persons or groups that may have access to or receive the PHI, such as the research team's staff members or research institute
- Title of the study and its purpose
- Date or event upon which the authorization expires
- Signature and date of the subject or legally authorized representative (NIH 2004, 12)

The general content of the three required statements is as follows:

- Explanation of how the participant can revoke (take back) his or her authorization
- Explanation that the participant has right to refuse and information about the consequences of refusal
- Explanation that once the PHI is released, the PHI may no longer be protected by the Privacy Rule (NIH 2004, 12)

The authorization pertains *only* to the research study described in it; the authorization does not cover nonspecific research or future, unspecified projects. The authorization need not have a fixed expiration date or state a specific expiration event; the form can list "none" (that is, no expiration date) or "the end of the research project." An authorization can be combined with an informed consent document or other permission to participate in research. Whether combined with an informed consent or separate, the authorization must contain the six core elements and three required statements.

De-identified health information is not PHI. Therefore, it is not protected by the Privacy Rule (NIH 2004, 9). However, the Privacy Rule only allows two methods to de-identify health information. The first method is statistical verification. The second method is the removal of 18 types of identifiers (NIH 2004, 9–10).

The Privacy Rule allows use and disclosure of PHI without authorization in the following circumstances: under a waiver of the authorization requirement, as part of a limited data set with a data use agreement, preparatory to research, and to research decedents' information (NIH 2004, 13–17).

The Privacy Rule added another layer of documentation, forms, and procedures that must be completed before research begins. Some institutions have created privacy boards, whereas other institutions have added the responsibility for compliance with the Privacy Rule to the role of IRBs. If a privacy board exists, it focuses on authorizations, waivers, and other requirements of the Privacy Rule. If a privacy board does not exist, the IRB handles review and approval of HIPAA requirements as part of the IRB initial review. In some instances, IRBs added Privacy Rule requirements to the informed consent form. In other instances, a separate set of forms was created. Researchers can usually find guidance on their institution's website about institutional procedures for compliance with the Privacy Rule.

Currently, research data are collected, transmitted, stored, and shared electronically. Federal regulations require the protection of these data. The HIPAA Security Rule (45 CFR 160 and 45 CFR 164 Subparts A and C) protects the security of electronically stored PHI that is created, received, used, or maintained by a covered entity. The Security Rule requires appropriate administrative, physical, and technical safeguards to ensure the confidentiality, integrity, and security of electronic PHI:

- *Administrative safeguards* are administrative actions, policies and procedures to manage the selection, development, implementation, and maintenance of security measures to protect electronic PHI and manage the conduct of the covered entity's or business associate's workforce in relation to the protection of that information.

- *Physical safeguards* are physical measures, policies, and procedures to protect a covered entity's or business associate's electronic information systems and related buildings and equipment from natural and environmental hazards, and unauthorized intrusion.
- *Technical safeguards* include the technology and the policy and procedures for its use that protect electronic PHI and control access to it. (45 CFR 164.304)

The American Recovery and Reinvestment Act (ARRA) of 2009 (Public Law 111-5) provided stimulus opportunities for health information technology, including the **Health Information Technology for Economic and Clinical Health (HITECH) Act**. The HITECH Act strengthened existing privacy and protections for individuals' health information (HHS 2013, 5566).

Health Research Extension Act of 1985

In 1985, Congress passed the **Health Research Extension Act** (Public Law 99-158) (42 CFR 493). The act mandated the secretary of HHS to issue a regulation requiring institutions receiving research awards to establish an administrative process to review reports of scientific misconduct and report to the federal government their investigations into the misconduct (ORI 2016). Congress passed this law following several publicized cases of research misconduct at leading universities in the late 1970s and early 1980s. For example, a researcher fabricated data during his medical residency and cardiology fellowship at Emory University, and at Brigham and Women's Hospital, a teaching affiliate of Harvard University (Culliton 1983, 31). In another case, a researcher falsely claimed that he successfully transplanted skin without immunosuppression in a mouse experiment. Instead, he faked the transplantation by using a pen to color a square patch of skin on the mice. A laboratory assistant discovered the fake transplants by washing off the ink with alcohol (Weissmann 2006, 587).

The **Office of Research Integrity (ORI)** is the agency in the HHS that monitors compliance with the Health Research Extension Act. The ORI is charged with promoting research integrity and preventing research misconduct. **Research misconduct** includes falsifying data, fabricating data and results, and plagiarizing (HHS 2005, 28386). Research misconduct does *not* include honest error or differences of opinion.

Consequences of research misconduct include debarment from receiving federal research grants for a period of time, such as three years or more, depending on the seriousness of the research misconduct; however, they may still participate in nonfederal research. Being barred from participating on PHS advisory committees; being required to have superiors certify the study's activities and supervise the research; and retracting articles, correcting articles, or both (HHS 2005, 28393).

Support and Training for Researchers

Institutions that have research programs and receive external funding usually have research administration departments. These departments, often known as grants and sponsored programs offices, assist in identifying funding opportunities, interpreting the funding agency's regulations, and preparing proposals for submission. Once the funding is received, these offices assist researchers in understanding the terms of the grant award, monitoring expenses, and reporting. At the research project's completion, they assist in "grant closeout," which is the final determination that all work required by the grant has been accomplished.

The National Institutes of Health (NIH) requires education on the protection of human research participants for all individuals who will be involved in the design or conduct of NIH-funded human subjects research (NIH 2008). Therefore, most institutions require all researchers, staff, and administrators associated with research to participate in educational programs about the responsible conduct of research. Some institutions have designed their own programs, and others participate in a collaborative institutional training initiative. Topics covered by the programs include the history of human subject protections, current regulatory information, protections for vulnerable populations, and ethical issues. Other topics include publication and authorship, intellectual property, conflict of interest, plagiarism, data fabrication, reporting of misconduct, and privacy and security of research data. In addition, many institutions involved in research have extensive websites explaining the rules for researchers and answering frequently asked questions.

Local-Level Ethical Research Guidelines and Procedures

At the local level, there are also guidelines and procedures that must be followed when dealing with ethics in research. These include bioethics committees that can assist institutions in handling ethical issues related to research and other executive level commitments in meeting the regulations that oversee ethics in research.

Bioethics Committees

Bioethics committees, also known as *institutional ethics committees,* provide guidance on ethical issues related to patient care (Annas and Grodin 2016, 556–557). Bioethics committees began in hospitals and date to the mid-1970s, when their members advised physicians in end-of-life decisions (Jonsen 2003, 362–363). Members of these committees can include researchers, ethicists, physicians and other healthcare providers, clergy, administrators, patients, and patient advocacy representatives.

Bioethics committees have three purposes:

- To advise clinicians, administrators, other institutional members, and patients and their family members as they address ethical conflicts, issues, and problems that affect the care and treatment of patients or that involve other aspects of the organization or its stakeholders.
- To educate institutional members about ethics, ethical problems, and ethical decision making.
- To assist in the development of policy. For example, the bioethics committees may provide policies related to clinical ethical issues, such as advanced directives, the withdrawal of life support, and end-of-life decisions. (Mercurio 2011, 2)

Thus, although bioethics committees and IRBs focus on different issues (patient care versus human research in accordance with federal regulations), bioethics committees may assist IRBs and researchers in considering ethical issues of research.

Ethical Climate for Research

In an ethical climate for research, all members of an institution's research community uphold the ethical guidance outlined in the professional codes, laws, and regulations. The response of executive-level management to federal laws and regulations promoting research integrity and protecting human subjects and their data is crucial. It sets the tone for the entire institution and affects the attitude of the institutions' researchers. Researchers who must complete complex documents and time-consuming procedures need to feel that the institution supports their efforts. The establishment of a supportive, ethical climate for research involves the following four institutional activities:

- Interdisciplinary proactive identification and discussion of emerging ethical issues in the community of researchers
- Ongoing, open dialogue about personal roles and responsibilities
- Widely disseminated messages and the integration of ethics into institutional policies and procedures to make ethics visible and evident throughout the institution
- Use of responsible conduct of research issues to identify areas needing attention (Ferguson et al. 2007, 196)

An ethical climate for research encourages ethical behavior that adheres to legal and professional guidelines and discourages unethical behavior that can result in negative publicity for the institution.

Review Questions

1. Which ethical principles were violated in the Jewish Chronic Disease Hospital study? How were they violated? Would the study meet today's standards for informed consent? Why or why not?
2. The chapter states that the Willowbrook hepatitis studies violated the ethical principle of honesty. Were any other ethical principles violated in this study? If so, how were they violated? Would this study meet today's standards for informed consent? Why or why not?
3. The chapter states that the Holmesburg Prison studies violated the ethical principle of justice. Were any other ethical principles violated in this study? If so, how were they violated? Would this study meet today's standards for informed consent? Why or why not?
4. Consider the following statement: In the United States, human subjects are protected by federal regulations; however, human subjects in other countries do not have similar protections. Do you agree with the statement and what are your reasons for agreeing or disagreeing?
5. Consider the following statement: The Belmont Report, while valuable when it was written in 1979, no longer contributes to the protection of human subjects because federal regulations have replaced it. Do you agree with the statement and what are your reasons for agreeing or disagreeing?

6. You are on a research team that is studying students' views about learning medical terminology by comparing responses from students based on their majors in the health professions, such as clinical laboratory science, health informatics, occupational therapy, physical therapy, and so forth. Your team had planned to "code" the data collection forms so that you could track respondents and nonrespondents and send follow-up requests only to the nonrespondents. Two of your team members come to the team's meeting and announce that they have found a way to finish the project ahead of schedule. They have read the regulatory clause suggesting that "research conducted in educational settings involving normal educational practices" is exempt from IRB review. They reason that students' views about medical terminology would be a "normal educational practice," and the team could therefore skip completing and submitting a proposal to the IRB. How should you respond to your fellow team members?
7. What is the composition of an institutional review board?
8. Your research team has discovered an unanticipated problem in its research project and has taken a corrective action, changing the study's protocol, in response to this discovery. Must your team report this change to the IRB?
9. What are the eight basic requirements of informed consent per 45 CFR 46.116?
10. A researcher's manuscript has been accepted for publication. As the researcher was reading the galley proofs (final typeset version prior to publication), she realized that she had inadvertently submitted an early draft version of her manuscript that did not include all the study's results. This draft version omitted responses from seven participants. The inclusion of these responses did not change the study's overall results. The results were still statistically significant; however, the measure of effect was less in the final calculations than in the preliminary calculations. The researcher decides to make no changes in the accepted manuscript because the overall findings were unchanged. Has the researcher committed research misconduct? Explain your reasoning.

Application Exercises

1. To familiarize yourself with the types and extent of research misconduct, go to the Office of Research Integrity website (ORI 2016a) and review the Misconduct Case Summaries and the PHS Administrative Action Bulletin Board.
   a. Based on your review, did the researchers in these cases tend to make a single mistake of misconduct or did they repeat their misconduct?
   b. What are some of the time frames for debarment and supervision?
   c. What ethical principles discussed in the chapter does research misconduct violate? How does research misconduct violate these principles?
2. Publishing articles that include falsified data or fabricated data or plagiarized content is a form of research misconduct. Such articles could be retracted, corrected, or both. Complete the following activities to enhance your understanding of research misconduct and its consequences.
   a. In 1988, Stephen E. Breuning was prosecuted and convicted of research misconduct (Garfield and Welljams-Dorof 1990, 1424). Use PubMed's Single Citation Matcher (NCBI 2016) to search the author Breuning, SE. Note that PubMed lists the retraction date of some of the author's articles. Click one of the retracted titles and see the retraction notice.
   b. Go to the PHS Administrative Action Bulletin Board (ORI 2016b). Find a researcher whose articles must be retracted or corrected. Go to PubMed (NCBI 2016) to check whether the retraction or correction has occurred.
3. The OHRP oversees the federal-wide assurance application process, conducts site visits, and receives and reviews complaints regarding research studies. Review information on the OHRP's webpage for Compliance and Reporting (OHRP 2016).
   a. In the category Determination Letters, the OHRP describes findings of the review, which may include findings of noncompliance and a listing of corrective steps to be taken. Read three recent determination letters posted on the OHRP website. What were the topics of the research and what was the complaint?
   b. Review the types of determinations listed in Determination Letters. List at least five types of determinations.

References

42 CFR 50 Subpart F: Promoting objectivity in research. 2011.
42 CFR 50.601: Purpose. 2011.
45 CFR 46.101(b): Basic HHS policy for protection of human research subjects. 2005.
45 CFR 46.102(b): Definitions. 1991.
45 CFR 46.103(b)(1): Assuring compliance with this policy—research conducted or supported by any federal department or agency. 2005.
45 CFR 46.107: IRB membership. 1991.
45 CFR 46.109(a): IRB review of research. 2005.
45 CFR 46.110: Categories of research that may be reviewed through an expedited review procedure. 2005.
45 CFR 46.111(b): Criteria for IRB approval of research. 1991.
45 CFR 46.113: Suspension or termination of IRB approval of research. 2005.
45 CFR 46.116: General requirements for informed consent. 2005.
45 CFR 46.302: Purpose. 1978.
45 CFR 160: General administrative requirements. 2000.
45 CFR 164 Subpart A: General provisions. 2013
45 CFR 164 Subpart C: Security standards for the protection of electronic protected health information. 2003.
45 CFR 164.304: Definitions. 2013.
American Health Information Management Association (AHIMA). 2016. Code of Ethics. http://bok.ahima.org/doc?oid=105098.
American Medical Informatics Association (AMIA). 2016. Ethics. https://www.amia.org/about-amia/ethics.
Annas, G. and M. Grodin. 2016. Second thoughts: Hospital ethics committees, consultants, and courts. *AMA Journal of Ethics* 18(5):554–559.
Bassiouni, M.C., T.G. Baffes, and J.T. Evrard. 1981. An appraisal of human experimentation in international law and practice: The need for international regulation of human experimentation. *Journal of Criminal Law and Criminology* 72(4):1597–1666.
Bombardier, C., L. Laine, A. Reicin, D. Shapiro, R. Burgos-Vargas, B. Davis, R. Day, M.B. Ferraz, C.J. Hawkey, M.C. Hochberg, T.K. Kvien, and T.J. Schnitzer. 2000. Comparison of upper gastrointestinal toxicity of rofecoxib and naproxen in patients with rheumatoid arthritis. *New England Journal of Medicine* 33(21):1520–1528.
Brandt, A.M. 1978. Racism and research: The case of the Tuskegee Syphilis Study. *Hastings Center Report* 8(6):21–29.
Callahan, D. 1990. *What Kind of Life? The Limits of Medical Progress*. Washington, DC: Georgetown University Press.
Cavusgil, E. 2007. Merck and Vioxx: An examination of an ethical decision-making model. *Journal of Business Ethics* 76(4):451–461.
Collins, F.S., M. Morgan, and A. Patrinos. 2003. The Human Genome Project: Lessons from large-scale biology. *Science* 300 (5617):286–290.
Couzin, J. and J. Kaiser. 2005. As Gelsinger case ends, gene therapy suffers another blow. *Science* 307(5712):1028.
Culliton, B.J. 1983. Coping with fraud: The Darsee case. *Science* 220(4592):31–35.
Drugwatch. 2016 (May 26). Vioxx Lawsuit. https://www.drugwatch.com/vioxx/lawsuit.
DuVal, M.K. 1972. Memorandum terminating the Tuskegee syphilis study, 11/16/1972. National Archives Catalog. http://research.archives.gov/description/650716.
Faden, R.R. and T.L. Beauchamp. 1986. *A History and Theory of Informed Consent*. New York: Oxford University Press.
Faden, R.R. 1996. The Advisory Committee on Human Radiation Experiments: Reflections on a presidential commission. *Hastings Center Report* 26(5):5–10.
Federman, D.D. and the Committee on Assessing the System for Protecting Human Research Subjects, Board on Health Sciences Policy, Institute of Medicine. 2001. *Preserving Public Trust: Accreditation and Human Research Participant Protection Programs*. Washington, DC: National Academies Press.
Ferguson, K., S. Masur, L. Olson, J. Ramirez, E. Robyn, and K. Schmaling. 2007. Enhancing the culture of research ethics on university campuses. *Journal of Academic Ethics* 5(3):189–198.

Fielder, J.H. 2008. The Vioxx debacle revisited. *IEEE Engineering in Medicine and Biology Magazine* 27(4):106–109.

Galliher, J.F., W.H. Brekhus, and D.P. Keys. 2004. *Laud Humphreys: Prophet of Homosexuality and Sociology*. Madison: University of Wisconsin Press.

Garfield, E. and A. Welljams-Dorof. 1990. The impact of fraudulent research on the scientific literature: The Stephen E. Breuning case. *Journal of the American Medical Association* 263(10):1424–1426.

Gaw, A. 2012. Exposing unethical human research: The transatlantic correspondence of Beecher and Pappworth. *Annals of Internal Medicine* 156(2):150–155.

Green, E.D., J.D. Watson, and F.S. Collins. 2015. Twenty-five years of big biology. *Nature* 526(7571):29–31.

Guyer, R.L. 2001. Radioactivity and rights: Clashes at Bikini Atoll. *American Journal of Public Health* 91(9):1371–1376.

Heller, J. 1972 (July 26). Syphilis victims in the U.S. study went untreated for 40 years. *New York Times*: 1, 8.

Hippocrates. 400 BCE. Book I, Section II, Second Constitution 5 in *Of the Epidemics*. Translated by Francis Adams. Internet Classics Archive. http://classics.mit.edu//Hippocrates/epidemics.html.

Hornblum, A.M. 2000. Subjected to medical experimentation: Pennsylvania's contribution to "science" in prisons. *Pennsylvania History: A Journal of Mid-Atlantic Studies* 67(3):415–426.

Hornblum, A.M. 1999. Ethical lapses in dermatologic "research." *Archives of Dermatology* 135(4):383–385.

Hornblum, A.M. 1998. *Acres of Skin: Human Experiments at Holmesburg Prison: A True Story of Abuse and Exploitation in the Name of Medical Science*. New York: Routledge.

Humphreys, L. 1970. Tearoom trade: Impersonal sex in public places. *Trans-action* 7(3):10–25.

International Medical Informatics Association (IMIA). 2016. IMIA code of ethics—updated version 2016. http://imia-medinfo.org/wp/imia-code-of-ethics.

Jones, J.H. 2008. The Tuskegee syphilis experiment. In *The Oxford Textbook of Clinical Research Ethics*. Edited by Emanuel, E.J., C. Grady, R.A. Crouch, R.K. Lie, F.G. Miller, and D. Wendler. New York: Oxford University Press: 89–96.

Jonsen, A.R. 2003. *The Birth of Bioethics*. New York: Oxford University Press.

Katz, J. 1992. Abuse of human beings for the sake of science. In *When Medicine Went Mad: Bioethics and the Holocaust*. Edited by Caplan, A.L. Totowa, NJ: Humana Press: 233–270.

Katz, J.D. 1996. The Nuremberg Code and the Nuremberg Trial: A reappraisal. *Journal of the American Medical Association* 276(20):1662–1666.

Krugman, S. 1986. The Willowbrook hepatitis studies revisited: Ethical aspects. *Clinical Infectious Disease* 8(1):157–162.

Krumholz, H.M., J.S. Ross, A.H. Presler, and D.S. Egilman. 2007. What have we learnt from Vioxx? *BMJ* 334 (7585):120–123.

Langer, E. 1966. Human experimentation: New York verdict affirms patient's rights. *Science* 151(3711):663–666.

Lederer, S.E. 2005. Experimentation on human beings. *OAH [Organization of American Historians] Magazine of History* 19(5):20–22.

Lenza, M. 2004. Controversies surrounding Laud Humphreys' tearoom trade: An unsettling example of politics and power in methodological critiques. *International Journal of Sociology and Social Policy* 24(3–5): 20–31.

Loftus, P. 2016 (January 15). Merck to pay $830 million to settle Vioxx shareholder suit. *Wall Street Journal*. http://www.wsj.com/articles/merck-to-pay-830-million-to-settle-vioxx-shareholder-suit-1452866882.

Loftus, P., and B. Kendall. 2011 (November 23). Merck to pay $950 million in Vioxx settlement. *Wall Street Journal (Online)*. http://www.wsj.com/articles/SB10001424052970204531404577054472253737682.

Lyon, A. 2007. "Putting patients first": Systematically distorted communication and Merck's marketing of Vioxx. *Journal of Applied Communication Research* 35(4):376–398.

Lyon, A. and J.C. Mirivel. 2011. Reconstructing Merck's practical theory of communication: The ethics of pharmaceutical sales representative-physician encounters. *Communication Monographs* 78(1):53–72.

Marshall, E. 1999. Gene therapy death prompts review of adenovirus vector. *Science* 286(5448):2244–2245.

Mercurio, M.R. 2011. The role of a pediatric ethics committee in the newborn intensive care unit. *Journal of Perinatology* 31(1):1–9.

Nardi, P.M. "The breastplate of righteousness": Twenty-five years after Laud Humphreys' *Tearoom Trade: Impersonal Sex in Public Places*. *Journal of Homosexuality* 30(2):1–10.

National Commission for the Protection of Human Subjects of Biomedical and Behavioral Research. 1979 (April 18). *The Belmont Report: Ethical Principles and Guidelines for the Protection of Human Subjects of Research*. Bethesda, MD: US Department of Health Education and Welfare. https://www.hhs.gov/ohrp/regulations-and-policy/belmont-report.

National Human Genome Research Institute (NHGRI). 2016. What was the Human Genome Project? https://www.genome.gov/12011238/an-overview-of-the-human-genome-project/.

National Human Genome Research Institute (NHGRI). 2015. The Ethical, Legal, and Social Implications Research Program, overview. https://www.genome.gov/10002329/elsi-research-program-fact-sheet/.

National Institutes of Health (NIH). 2009. Laws Related to the Protection of Human Subjects: The Nuremberg Code. https://history.nih.gov/about/timelines/nuremberg.html.

National Institutes of Health (NIH). 2008. Guidance on NIH Office of Extramural Research (OER) on-line tutorial Protecting Human Research Participants (PHRP), Notice number: NOT-OD-08-054. https://grants.nih.gov/grants/guide/notice-files/NOT-OD-08-054.html.

National Institutes of Health (NIH). 2004. Protecting personal health information in research: Understanding the HIPAA Privacy Rule. https://privacyruleandresearch.nih.gov/pdf/HIPAA_Booklet_4-14-2003.pdf.

Nelson, D. and R. Weiss. 2000 (September 19). Penn researchers sued in gene therapy death; teen's parents also named ethicist as defendant. *Washington Post*.

New Jersey Association for Biomedical Research (NJABR). 2016. What is biomedical research? http://njabr.com/education/general-background-on-biomedical-research/what-is-biomedical-research.

Noddings, N. 1990. A response. *Hypatia* 5(1):120–126.

Novak, D. 2007. *Sanctity of Human Life*. Washington, DC: Georgetown University Press.

Office for Civil Rights (OCR). 2016. How OCR enforces the HIPAA Privacy & Security Rules. https://www.hhs.gov/hipaa/for-professionals/compliance-enforcement/examples/how-OCR-enforces-the-HIPAA-privacy-and-security-rules/index.html.

Office for Human Research Protections (OHRP). 2016. Compliance and reporting. http://www.hhs.gov/ohrp/compliance/index.html.

Office for Human Research Protections (OHRP). 2012. Archive of policy documents no longer in effect. http://wayback.archive-it.org/4657/20150930181808/http://www.hhs.gov/ohrp/archive/policy/archive.html.

Office for Human Research Protections (OHRP). 2007. Unanticipated problems involving risks & adverse events guidance (2007). https://www.hhs.gov/ohrp/regulations-and-policy/guidance/reviewing-unanticipated-problems.

Pence, G.E. 2003. The Tuskegee Study. In *Contemporary Issues in Bioethics*, 6th ed. Edited by Beauchamp, T.L. and L. Walters. Belmont, CA: Wadsworth:394–401.

Perper, J.A. and S.J. Cina. 2010. *When Doctors Kill: Who, Why, and How*. New York: Springer.

Pettersen, T. 2011. The ethics of care: Normative structures and empirical implications. *Health Care Analysis* 19(1):51–64.

Psaty, B.M. and R.A. Kronmal. 2008. Reporting mortality findings in trials of rofecoxib for Alzheimer disease or cognitive impairment: A case study based on documents from rofecoxib litigation. *Journal of the American Medical Association* 299(15):1813–1817.

Reverby, S.M. 2009. *Examining the Tuskegee Study: The Infamous Syphilis Study and Its Legacy*. Chapel Hill: University of North Carolina Press.

Reverby, S.M. 2001. More than fact and fiction: Cultural memory and the Tuskegee Syphilis Study. *Hastings Center Report* 31(5):22–28.

Rothman, D.J. 1982. Were Tuskegee and Willowbrook "studies in nature"? *Hastings Center Report* 12(2):5–7.

Savulescu, J. 2001. Harm, ethics committees and the gene therapy death. *Journal of Medical Ethics* 27(3):148–150.

Scully, S.P. 2000. Gene therapy: clinical considerations. *Clinical Orthopaedics and Related Research* 379(Suppl):S55–S58.

Seltzer, D., L. Zoloth, C.L.H. Traina, and L. Kiesling. 2011. Paved with good intentions: Rethinking the ethics of ELSI research. *Journal of Research Administration* 42(2):15–24.

Shuster, E. 1997. Fifty years later: The significance of the Nuremberg Code. *New England Journal of Medicine* 337(20):1436–1440.

Sibbald, B. 2001. Death but one unintended consequence of gene-therapy trial. *Canadian Medical Association Journal* 164(11):1612.

Smith, L. and J.F. Byers. 2002. Gene-therapy in the post-Gelsinger era. *JONA's [Journal of Nursing Administration] Healthcare Law, Ethics, and Regulation* 4(4):104–110.

Smith, R. 2006. Lapses at the *New England Journal of Medicine*. *Journal of the Royal Society of Medicine* 99(8):380–382.

Spielthenner, G. 2015. Why comply with a code of ethics? *Medicine, Health Care, and Philosophy* 18(2):195–202.

Stewart, W.H.. 1966. Surgeon General's Directives on Human Experimentation—Policy and Procedure Order 129. https://history.nih.gov/research/downloads/Surgeongeneraldirective1966.pdf.

Topol, E.J. 2004. Failing the public health—rofecoxib, Merck, and the FDA. *New England Journal of Medicine* 351(17):1707–1710.

US Department of Health and Human Services (HHS). 2016a. 45 CFR 46 FAQs: What is the historical basis for the current human research regulations 45 CFR Part 46? https://www.hhs.gov/ohrp/regulations-and-policy/guidance/faq/45-cfr-46.

US Department of Health and Human Services (HHS). 2016b. 45 CFR 46. https://www.hhs.gov/ohrp/regulations-and-policy/regulations /45-cfr-46/index.html.

US Department of Health and Human Services (HHS). 2016c. Federal policy for the Protection of Human Subjects ("common rule"). https://www.hhs.gov/ohrp/regulations-and-policy/regulations/common-rule/index.html.

US Department of Health and Human Services (HHS). 2015. Federal Policy for the Protection of Human Subjects; proposed rules. *Federal Register* 80(173):53933–54061.

US Department of Health and Human Services (HHS). 2013. Modifications to the HIPAA Privacy, Security, Enforcement, and Breach Notification Rules under the Health Information Technology for Economic and Clinical Health Act and the Genetic Information Nondiscrimination Act; other modifications to the HIPAA rules; final rule. *Federal Register* 78(17):5566–5702.

US Department of Health and Human Services (HHS). 2005. Public health service policies on research misconduct [42 CFR Parts 50 and 93]; final rule. *Federal Register* 70(94):28370–28400.

US Department of Health and Human Services (HHS) and US Department of Energy (DOE). 1990. *Understanding Our Genetic Inheritance: The U.S. Human Genome Project: The First Five Years, FY 1991–1995*. NIH publication no. 90-1580. http://web.ornl.gov/sci/techresources/Human_Genome/project/5yrplan/firstfiveyears.pdf.

Wadman, M. 2007. Merck settles Vioxx lawsuits for $4.85 billion. *Nature* 450(7168):324–325.

Weissmann, G. 2006. Science fraud: From patchwork mouse to patchwork data. *Federation of American Societies for Experimental Biology Journal* 20(6):587–590.

Wilson, R.F. 2010. The death of Jesse Gelsinger: New evidence of the influence of money and prestige in human research. *American Journal of Law and Medicine* 36(2–3): 295–325.

World Medical Association (WMA). 2016. WMA Declaration of Helsinki—Ethical principles for medical research involving human subjects. http://www.wma.net/en/30publications/10policies/b3.

Resources

Alliance for Human Research Protection. 2016. Ethical violations/investigations today. http://ahrp.org/ethical-violations-and-investigations-today.

Alliance for Human Research Protection. 2005. Pharma ethics: Merck CEO resigns—Vioxx deceptive marketing/AIDS drug experiments foster kids. http://ahrp.org/pharma-ethics-merck-ceo-resigns-vioxx-deceptive-marketing-aids-drug-experiments-foster-kids.

Association of Clinical Research Professionals. 2013. The process of informed consent. http://www.acrpnet.org/pdf/ACRPWhitePaperTheProcessofInformedConsent.pdf.

Beecher, H.K. 1966. Ethics and clinical research. *New England Journal of Medicine* 274(24):1354–1360.

Branzke, H. 2012. Sanctity-of-life: A bioethical principle for a right to life? *Ethical Theory and Moral Practice* 15(3):295–308.

Citro, C.F., D.R. Ilgen, and C.B. Marrett, eds. 2003. *Protecting Participants and Facilitating Social and Behavioral Sciences Research*. Washington, DC: National Academies Press.

Curfman, G.D., S. Morrissey, and J.M. Drazen. 2005. Expression of concern: Bombardier et al., "Comparison of upper gastrointestinal toxicity of rofecoxib and naproxen in patients with rheumatoid arthritis," *N Engl J Med* 2000;343:1520–8. *New England Journal of Medicine* 353(26):2813–2814.

Goodman, H. 1998 (July 21). Studying prison experiments research: For 20 years, a dermatologist used the inmates of a Philadelphia prison as the willing subjects of tests on shampoo, foot powder, deodorant, and later, mind-altering drugs and dioxin. *Baltimore Sun*. http://articles.baltimoresun.com/1998-07-21/news/1998202099_1_holmesburg-prison-kligman-philadelphia.

Hanna, K.E. 1995. The Ethical, Legal, and Social Implications Program of the National Center for Human Genome Research: A missed opportunity? In *Society's Choices: Social and Ethical Decision Making in Biomedicine*. Edited by Bulger, R.E., E.M. Bobby, H.V. Fineberg, and Committee on the Social and Ethical Impacts of Developments in Biomedicine, Institute of Medicine. Washington, DC: National Academies Press: 432–457.
Harman, L.B. and F.H. Cornelius, eds. 2017. *Ethical Health Informatics: Challenges and Opportunities*, 3rd ed. Burlington, MA: Jones & Bartlett Learning.
3rd ed. Burlington, MA: Jones & Bartlett Learning.
Hornblum, A.M. 2013 (December 28). NYC's forgotten cancer scandal. New York Post. http://nypost.com/2013/12/28/nycs-forgotten-cancer-scandal.
Humphreys, L. 1970. Tearoom Trade: Impersonal Sex in Public Places. London: Duckworth.
Humphreys, L. 1975. Tearoom Trade: Impersonal Sex in Public Places, 2nd ed. New York: Aldine Publishing.
National Academy of Sciences; National Academy of Engineering; Institute of Medicine; Committee on Science, Engineering, and Public Policy. 2009. On Being a Scientist: A Guide to Responsible Conduct in Research, 3rd ed. Washington, DC: National Academies Press. http://www.nap.edu/catalog/12192/on-being-a-scientist-a-guide-to-responsible-conduct-in.
National Center for Biotechnology Information (NCBI). 2016. PubMed Single Citation Matcher. https://www.ncbi.nlm.nih.gov/pubmed/citmatch.
Office for Civil Rights. 2007. Frequently Asked Questions: HIPAA Privacy Rule for researchers. https://privacyruleandresearch.nih.gov/faq.asp.
Office of Research Integrity (ORI). 2016a. Office of Research Integrity home page. http://ori.hhs.gov.
Office of Research Integrity (ORI). 2016b. PHS Administrative Action Bulletin Board. https://ori.hhs.gov/ORI_PHS_alert.html?d=update.
Office of Research Integrity (ORI). 2016c. About ORI. https://ori.hhs.gov/about-ori.
Pappworth, M.H. 1962. Human guinea pigs: A warning. Twentieth Century 171:66–75.
Shivayogi, P. 2013. Vulnerable population and methods for their safeguard. Perspectives in Clinical Research 4(1):53–57.

15 Disseminating Information

Elizabeth J. Forrestal, PhD, RHIA, CCS, FAHIMA

Learning Objectives

- Select a format for disseminating research results consistent with the researcher's purpose.
- Explain the processes of poster presentations and oral presentations.
- Determine the appropriate content for an effective oral presentation.
- Demonstrate the appropriate organization, content, and format of a journal publication.
- Apply criteria in the review of a research article.
- Discuss the means and purpose of alternative dissemination formats.
- Use key terms associated with disseminating information through presentations, publications, and research project websites appropriately.

Key Terms

Article
Claim of primacy
Dissemination
Impact factor
IMRAD
Manuscript
Oral paper presentation
Paper
Peer review
Poster presentation
Proceedings
Research project website
Submission guidelines
White paper

Dissemination is the planned, strategic distribution of information to a targeted audience. For researchers, dissemination is sharing the results and other information from their research study. Target audiences include practitioners, other researchers, policy makers, patients, and other individuals or groups. The planned strategies used by researchers include articles, books, brochures, newsletters, presentations, press releases, policy briefs, postings on websites, social media, white papers, and many others. This chapter discusses processes related to poster presentations, oral paper presentations at conferences and meetings, journal publications, white papers, and research project websites.

Researchers disseminate information from their research because this information is the evidence on which practitioners, policy makers, and others base decisions and take actions. Dissemination also adds the researchers' information to the field's body of knowledge and can inform future research projects.

Dissemination of information is essential to the accessibility, availability, and eventual use of that information. Health informatics and HIM researchers disseminate their research results for three purposes. First, researchers disseminate their research results to advance the fields of health informatics and HIM because new knowledge builds and expands the scientific bases of these fields. Second, researchers disseminate this new information so it can be implemented in the workplace and thereby move forward the practices of health informatics and HIM. Finally, researchers disseminate their research results to advance their own careers in academia, the private and public sectors, and other professional arenas.

This chapter has two aims. The first is to prepare readers to clearly and appropriately present the results of their own research studies in ways that provide information to practitioners, other researchers, and other interested individuals and groups. The second aim is to help readers learn to assess the information presented in research articles and determine whether the articles' results and conclusions are applicable to their own work environments.

Real-World Case

Cartoons are everywhere around us—in newspapers' cartoon and editorial pages, magazines, online humor, greeting cards, educational materials and textbooks, and other print and electronic sources (Bartlett 2013, 215–216). In figure 10.3 in chapter 10, cartoons are listed as an information source; however, cartoons may also be an innovative way to disseminate research results.

Two research studies investigated how cartoons could be used in disseminating results. A qualitative study that investigated the social activism of people with mild dementia used cartoons as a way to report its results (Bartlett 2013, 215). The cartoons were then exhibited and viewers were allowed to comment on the cartoons. Based on the commentary, the researcher recommended that cartoons be used judiciously because not everyone finds cartoons funny and some people prefer written text (Bartlett 2013, 224). Moreover, cartoons must be used ethically. The cartoons should do no harm, such as stereotyping the participants or marginalizing important questions (Bartlett 2013, 223). A mixed methods study investigated how cartoons could be used as a knowledge dissemination intervention (KDI) (Lafrenière et al. 2014, 104). The KDI study's researchers sent an e-mail with a link to four webpages to the target audience's members who were researchers and ethicists in nutrition and genetics and institutional review board members. The webpages combined text and cartoons about gaps in the nutrition and genetics literature. Respondents completed a survey that assessed the effectiveness of the KDI. A large majority of the respondents reported that combining text and cartoons effectively communicated information, and some respondents even noted that the cartoon-based KDI was "entertaining and stimulating" (Lafrenière et al. 2014, 111). Thus, used correctly and for the right audience, cartoons could be an effective way to make research results available and accessible.

Formats for Disseminating Research

To achieve the purposes of dissemination described above, health informatics and HIM researchers must select a way to disseminate their research that best suits their target audience (Cleary et al. 2007, 225). Depending on their target audience, researchers decide whether to present, publish, or use a multipronged approach to disseminate their research.

Presentation

Two common ways of disseminating research information are poster presentations and oral paper presentations. In a **poster presentation**, the researcher visually presents information about a research study on a poster with graphics and text, answers questions about the study, and hands out papers detailing the research study. In an **oral paper presentation**, the researcher gives a formal talk about a research paper, often accompanied by visual aids, such as PowerPoint slides or flip charts.

Poster presentations and oral paper presentations occur at professional meetings, conferences, symposia, congresses, assemblies, and other events. These events are planned far in advance. Up to 12 months before an event, professional associations will issue a call for session proposals. (See figure 15.1.) In response to the call, researchers send brief descriptions of their proposed sessions. The meeting organizers and peer-review committees, as applicable, determine which proposals to accept based on the proposal's quality, the number of proposals received, and the relevance of the proposal's topic to the theme of the event.

Figure 15.1 Sample call for proposals

Call for Research Abstracts
Deadline for Abstracts: October 31, 20**
Abstracts for the Summer Symposium are being solicited.
Topics:
- Workforce initiatives

(Continued)

Figure 15.1 *(Continued)*

- Innovations in service delivery
- Organizational or administrative issues in healthcare enterprises
- Best practices or performance improvement
- E-health implementations

Content of the research abstract should include:

- Title of presentation
- Name(s) of author(s) with title, credentials, and organization
- Method
- Brief results

All applicants are invited to submit their abstracts for contributions to the symposium via the online submission form on the symposium Web site www.fictitious-URL.org/symposium20**. The submission deadline is October 31, 20**. Abstracts should be limited to 250 words. Questions should be e-mailed to Professor Qualef (qualefl@fictitious.edu).

Selection of abstracts will be made through a peer-reviewed process. The peer review committee will determine whether the mode of presentation will be oral presentation or poster. Applicants will be notified of acceptance or rejection and the mode of presentation by January 15, 20**. Accepted abstracts for poster presentations will be printed in the *Symposium Proceedings,* conditional upon payment of the registration fee.

Authors of accepted abstracts for oral presentations will be asked to submit the complete scholarly paper by February 15, 20**. Scholarly papers will be published in *Symposium Proceedings,* conditional upon payment of the registration fee.

Content for the scholarly paper should include all of the following, in the order listed:

1. Abstract
2. Title
3. Name(s) of author(s) with title, credentials, and organization
4. Literature review
5. Purpose or problem statement
6. Methods, including analytical technique
7. Results
8. Discussion
9. Conclusions and recommendations for future research

Authors of accepted abstracts for oral presentations will be asked to submit their PowerPoint presentations and handouts for their presentations by April 15, 20**. Presentations will be limited to 15 minutes, inclusive of questions.

All participants will receive a password that will allow online access to abstracts, *Symposium Proceedings,* and handouts by June 15, 20**, conditional upon payment of the registration fee.

Liz Qualef, PhD
Professor and Chair, Department of Health Informatics, Fictitious University
College of Related Professions City, ST 12345
e-mail: qualefl@fictitious.edu

Feedback and discussions with other researchers at poster and oral paper presentations provide valuable information on ways to improve or build on the research study. For example, a researcher who gives a presentation about a pilot study may receive from event attendees worthwhile suggestions, such as additional research questions or specific subpopulations to consider in the analyses. These suggestions often can be used to enhance the later full-scale study.

Abstracts and papers associated with poster and oral paper presentations may be published in the program or proceedings. *Abstracts* are brief summaries of the major parts of research studies, which include the literature review, purpose or problem statement, methods, results (also sometimes called *findings*), discussion, and conclusions and recommendations. Abstracts are used with poster presentations, oral paper presentations, and journal articles. **Papers** are written manuscripts that present research results related to the event's theme. They have been written with the goal of being accepted and being presented at the event. **Proceedings** are published collections of the papers, and often the abstracts, delivered at events.

Poster Presentation

Poster presentations communicate the results of research studies to attendees at events. Posters are displayed for multiple periods during the event in a designated area, such as a hall or a conference room, at the event's site.

When participating in a poster presentation, researchers must conform their posters to the event's poster guidelines, which state the size of the poster and other requirements and are distributed prior to the event by the meeting organizers. Institutional printing departments offer services that enhance posters. Commercial printing companies with staffs of commercial artists and graphic designers also print posters. These departments and companies have submission guidelines, such as requiring Microsoft Word documents or PowerPoint slides. Websites that offer the printing of posters may be a cost-effective option and may have templates that researchers can use to design their posters.

Typically, the posters contain the key information about research study as follows:

- Title of the study, names of the researchers, and their institutional affiliation(s)
- Background (of the study)
- Objectives
- Research design
- Results
- Conclusions
- Future plans

Effective posters are visually appealing, colorful, readable at a distance, and use charts, tables, pictures, and other graphics.

During the event, presenters have a session—a designated time—during which they are available to discuss their poster with attendees. During their session, presenters sit or stand near their posters. Typically, a presenter's session lasts two to five hours on one day. Attendees at the event read the posters and may ask the presenters questions about the study. Presenters have copies of their paper available for interested persons. Poster presentations are sometimes judged (juried). At judged poster presentations, judges mingle with the attendees, asking questions and inspecting and rating the research as depicted in the posters.

Oral Paper Presentation

Oral paper presentations occur during sessions of professional meetings, conferences, symposia, congresses, assemblies, or other events at the regional, state, national, and international levels. As described previously, researchers submit proposals in response to a call for papers, or they may be invited to present if their topic is particularly relevant. If accepted or invited, researchers receive a notice of their time slot.

Time slots, ranging in length from 15 minutes to 30 minutes, are on a certain day in the event's program. These slots include both the presentation of the oral paper and the question-and-answer period, during which attendees may ask questions or comment on the paper's contents. Presenters must pay attention to their allotted time as they prepare their presentation so that they stay within the time limits during the actual presentation. Event organizers attempt to strictly adhere to the program's schedule and may stop presenters who run too long. A presentation that is too short, although much less common than overly long talks, is also problematic because it, too, disrupts the schedule.

Presenters should remember their audience as they create and present their papers and accompanying slides. Presenters need to be sure to synthesize their results and state their take-home message. In the past 20 years, experts have found that presenters often run out of time before accomplishing these primary objectives (Edirisooriya 1996, 27; Wineberg 2004, 13–14; Reumann 2012, 7). In 1996, Edirisooriya published tips on how to improve oral paper presentations based on her research in which, over seven years, she attended 126 sessions and viewed 748 presenters (Edirisooriya 1996, 25). Her tips, validated by other experts over time, are still helpful to today's presenters. See table 15.1.

Table 15.1 Tips for content of oral paper presentations

Section	Include	Omit
Background	Brief update on status of the *current* body of knowledge with emphasis on gaps in the body of knowledge or the problem with a policy or method	Long discussions of the entire theory and all the related literature
Purpose or problem statement	Clear and explicit statement of purpose or problem Explicit linkage to the issue identified in the background	Disclaimers Involved qualifiers Claims of primacy
Method including analytic technique	Research design, time frame, method, sampling stratagem (if applicable), and major analytic technique	Justifications of research design, time frame, method, sampling stratagem (if applicable), and analytic techniques

(*Continued*)

Table 15.1 (*Continued*)

Section	Include	Omit
Results and discussion	Analyses that resulted in major findings Major findings explained in depth Interpretation of major findings	Trivia Unimportant findings Defense of theory Repetition of literature review
Conclusions and recommendations*	Relevance of findings Implications for field, policy, education, future research, or other consequence Recommendations for future research, including the presenter's own intended research	Statements, such as "I'm running out of time," or "Just one more point"

*This section is critical and should not be victim of poor planning or execution of other sections.
Source: Edirisooriya 1996, 28.

Presenters should be prepared to talk about their research to the audience. The following recommendations may help with that preparation:

- Know the background(s) of the audience, such as whether they are members of the general public or technical experts.
- Focus on the "take-home message" of the presentation, such as the study's actual findings or implications for practice.
- Keep the presentation simple.
- Allow one minute per slide.
- Use a logical flow that tells a story.
- Practice the presentation ahead of time. (Reumann 2012, 7)

Practice is important because it allows researchers to present their information rather than merely reading their notes or paper. Researchers should try to be animated and talk to the people in the room.

Journal Publication

Publication distributes the researchers' results to practitioners, decision makers, and other professionals so that they can use the researchers' information. Additionally, published research can be examined and critically analyzed by practitioners and other researchers.

An unpublished paper is known as a **manuscript**. An **article** is a manuscript or paper that has been published in a journal. Generally, the sections of a journal article are as follows:

- Introduction (including problem statement, literature review, and statement of hypothesis)
- Methods
- Results
- Discussion

As the chapters of this book moved through the steps of research, the documentation associated with each step was described. This documentation becomes the basis of these sections of the journal article. The sections may vary depending on the research method, the type of journal article, and specific requirements of the journal. Researchers now transform the documentation into an article manuscript by writing the abstract, assigning a title, and expanding and detailing the sections already written.

Abstract

It may seem counterintuitive that the abstract, the first section of a journal article, is written last. However, the abstract is written last because it encompasses the entire study, including the study's results. As stated previously, an abstract is a summary of the major parts of a research study.

Abstracts are important because they are used in bibliographic databases and electronic search engines to index and retrieve articles. Moreover, readers use the abstracts to decide whether articles contain the information that they need and whether they should read the full article. For example, chapter 8 describes how researchers use abstracts to filter articles for a systematic review or meta-analysis.

Abstracts generally have strict word limits, such as 150 to 500 words, depending upon the type of article. These word limits require authors to be brief and direct and to focus on the most important information in each part of their study.

An abstract generally summarizes the following information:

- Literature review
- Purpose or problem statement
- Method
- Results
- Discussion
- Conclusions and recommendations

Experts recommend that authors put the objective of the study at the abstract's beginning (Cals and Kotz 2013, 585). Then, authors should construct the abstract around key words from the major parts of the study.

Some journals have structured abstract formats that researchers must follow (see table 15.2 for examples). Not only do the formats vary by journal but the formats also may vary within journals by the type of article. Abstracts for research articles may have a different format than abstracts for commentary articles. Researchers read the journals' "Information for Authors" to determine exactly how they should structure their abstract.

Table 15.2 Structures and maximum word counts of abstracts for selected journals

Journal	Structure of Abstract	Maximum Word Count
Applied Clinical Informatics (2016)	❖ Background (optional) ❖ Objectives ❖ Methods ❖ Results ❖ Conclusions	300 words for the article type of research paper
BMC Medical Informatics and Decision Making (2016)	❖ Background ❖ Methods ❖ Results ❖ Conclusion	350 words for the article type of research article
Journal of Medical Internet Research (2016a)	❖ Introduction ❖ Objective ❖ Methods ❖ Results ❖ Conclusions	450 words for the article types of original paper, systematic review, and consensus paper
Journal of the American Medical Informatics Association (2016)	❖ Objective ❖ Materials and methods ❖ Results ❖ Discussion ❖ Conclusion	250 words for the article type of research and applications

Manuscript Title

A "title can be viewed as the shortest possible abstract" (Bordage et al. 2015, 57). Like the abstract, bibliographic databases and electronic search engines use titles to retrieve articles. Titles also need to appeal to readers' interests. An effective title indicates the way that the study was conducted and provides information about the study's results. Consider including the following items in the title (Cals and Kotz 2013, 585):

- *Type of article or study,* such as systematic review or randomized clinical trial
- *Population or setting,* such as pediatric patients with asthma or hospice
- *Implementation, system, or technique,* such as emergency department, diagnostic decision support system, or storyboarding
- *Independent variable(s) manipulated,* such as activity tracker alert
- *Dependent variable(s) measured or observed,* such as adherence to medication

- *Take-home message,* such as "Ready or not: HIM is changing—results of the new HIM competencies survey show skill gaps between education levels, students, and working professionals" (Sandefer and Karl 2015, 24)

Experts suggest strategies that can help researchers synthesize these items into a readable and clear title. For example, these experts recommend that an article's title be written using key terms and action verbs and including factors that make the study unique (Cals and Kotz 2013, 585). These words should be placed at the beginning of the title to catch the potential reader's attention. Titles should also be clear and specific. The title should portray the study's results accurately and without exaggeration (Bordage et al. 2015, 57). Journals sometimes have strict word limits on titles to which authors must adhere. Finally, though, even without word limits, titles need to concisely convey a message that attracts readers to retrieve the article.

Characteristics of Composition

The following paragraphs present general insights on expanding and detailing the article sections that were discussed in previous chapters. As authors begin to write their manuscripts, they also should review chapter 10 (research question, hypothesis, and literature review), chapter 11 (research design and method), and chapter 12 (analysis of data, results, and discussion). Table 15.3 serves as a final checklist for the composition and revision of a manuscript. Common pitfalls are also listed at the end of this section.

Table 15.3 Organization of research article manuscripts

Section	Contents
Title page	Concise and descriptive title, authors' names, authors' affiliations, grant information, disclaimer, corresponding author's mailing address, telephone number, fax number, and e-mail address
	Information about potential conflicts of interest and, when applicable, sources of funding
Abstract	Background, purpose, methods, results, conclusions *or* Context; objective; design, setting, and participants; interventions; main outcome measures; results, conclusions Word count within limit given in call for papers or journal instructions 3 to 10 key words using medical subject headings (MeSH)
Introduction	Background; pertinent literature review that provides rationale for research; brief statement of research plan; purpose, objectives, or research question
Methods	Protocol with detail for replication Design, setting, and participants Definition of variables Reference to established methods Sampling strategy Collection of data Statement about approval of institutional review board (IRB) or other oversight entity Analytic strategy
Results	Core findings Important results followed by less important results Neutral reporting
Discussion	Relationship between results and purpose, objectives, or research question Evidence of relationship Similarities to and differences from previous research New knowledge in terms of theoretical framework Limitations Conclusions as related to purpose, objectives, or research question Implications for future research Recommendations, if warranted Summary

(*Continued*)

Table 15.3 (*Continued*)

Section	Contents
Acknowledgments	Contributors whose level of involvement does not justify authorship
References	Citations per format in publisher's instructions
Tables	Consistent with narrative Expand abbreviations Units of measure Format per publisher's instructions
Figures	Consistent with narrative Expand abbreviations Units of measure Legend Format per publisher's instructions

Source: Forrestal 2016, p. 600.

Authors strive to be clear and explicit throughout the manuscript. The methods section fully details and explains the procedure or protocol. This section can be thought of as a "recipe" for the research, which other researchers should be able in a step-by-step manner.

As described in chapter 12, in the results section, authors are careful to neutrally report the results of their study. Structuring the results to match the order of the hypotheses gives the manuscript an organization and logic that readers can follow. In the results section, researchers do *not* interpret, explain, or compare their results.

It is in the discussion section that authors interpret, explain, and compare and contrast their results to those of other researchers, thus putting the results in context of the greater body of knowledge. Using the theory or model that framed the study to organize their discussion can be helpful. Authors clearly point out how the study filled a gap in the body of knowledge. They also include unexpected or contrary results because these results may become areas of future research. Researchers are cautious about making claims of primacy. A **claim of primacy** is when authors write that their study was "the first study ever" to do something. Instead of a claim of primacy, it is advisable to use qualifiers, such as "a comprehensive review of the literature did not reveal a similar study." Finally, the discussion section is the place to describe lessons learned or mistakes made, which can result in recommendations for future research.

Awareness of the common pitfalls that exist when writing papers, a list of which follows, can help authors avoid them:

- Interjecting subjective commentary and emotional hyperbole
- Duplicating information in narrative and graphic forms
- Creating confusing or inconsistent graphics
- Substituting verbosity, jargon, and inflated statements for clarity and accuracy

A good way to avoid these pitfalls is to allow sufficient time to write the results, to develop the research paper, and to revise the paper after taking a few days to gain perspective.

Selection of the Appropriate Journal

To select the appropriate journal to publish a manuscript, authors investigate various journals in their field of study. Authors can obtain lists of journals from their library's website or bibliographic databases. Authors may also consult with a librarian to obtain lists of journals related to various fields. Examples of a few journals related to health informatics journals and HIM are listed in table 15.2. Many other journals publish articles related to health informatics and HIM. Depending on the topic, appropriate journals may be identified in fields other than health informatics and HIM, such as allied health, bioethics, business, computer science, epidemiology, health policy, health services, healthcare management, information technology and systems, public health, and other fields. Authors may go to the journals' websites to check the journals' scopes and types of research articles and the journals' audiences. Additionally, when selecting a journal, authors match the purpose of their manuscript to the type of journal, such as practice-oriented or research-oriented.

Journals have defined missions and scopes. Editors only accept manuscripts within their journal's mission and scope. When writing and submitting a manuscript, authors try to match its content with the focus of the journal. For example, authors send manuscripts about research on the management of health information services, such as the effect of changes in coding guidelines on coding professionals' levels of stress, to journals in the field of HIM. If their results have an impact on reimbursement or health policy, the authors may consider submitting their manuscript to other journals with scopes that emphasize those topics.

Authors who match the design and method of their research to the types of designs and methods featured in the journal increase the likelihood that their manuscripts will be accepted for publication. Some journals include mostly experimental and quasi-experimental research; others include ethnographies, case studies, and personal histories.

Authors also strive to match their writing style and approach to the topic to the preferences of the journal's audience. The writing style in practice-oriented journals tends to be concise, with simple, direct sentences. On the other hand, the writing style for academic, scholarly journals has a more formal tone with longer, more complex sentences. If the intended audience includes a broad range of fields, authors write manuscripts that are of interest to all potential readers. Moreover, authors clearly state how their manuscript affects and benefits the journal's intended audience. For example, in the introduction to an article manuscript, this chapter's author explained how knowing about systematic reviews was important for healthcare managers and supervisors as follows (italics added):

> *Systematic reviews are the source of the evidence that supports evidence-based decision making. Therefore, understanding systematic reviews has become an essential skill for health care managers and supervisors.* This article provides an introduction to the technique by describing the types of systematic reviews and by overviewing the process of conducting them. (Forrestal 2014, 97)

Finally, authors consider their reasons for publishing. As stated earlier in the chapter, there are three common purposes for disseminating research: (1) building the body of knowledge, (2) advancing practice, and (3) advancing the researchers' careers. Authors may disseminate their research results for any of the three reasons or for a combination of the reasons. Authors who want to build the body of knowledge, advance their own careers, or both, publish in peer-reviewed journals (also called *research, refereed, academic,* and *professional journals*), and are covered later in this chapter.

Journals have varying levels of prestige. Authors who want to build the body of knowledge or advance their careers seek to publish in prestigious journals. Indirect measures of a journal's prestige are its status as refereed (peer reviewed) or non-refereed and its rejection rate. Another measure is the journal's **impact factor**, a ratio between citations and recently published citable items (Bensman 2012, 268). The impact factor is calculated by dividing the number of current-year citations to the source items published in that journal during the previous two years. For example, the *Journal of Medical Internet Research* is second in medical informatics journals by impact factor (*Journal of Medical Internet Research* 2016b).

Reporting and Submission Guidelines

To have their manuscripts considered for publication, authors are required to follow the journal's reporting guidelines and submission guidelines. Journals also have rules for the format of manuscripts. Paying attention to the details of the reporting and submission guidelines is important because some editors and peer reviewers may assume that sloppy writing and disregard for the journal's guidelines indicates a sloppy approach to research more generally.

IMRAD and Other Reporting Guidelines Editors and researchers have agreed upon reporting guidelines for the content of many types of scientific papers. Using these preexisting guidelines assists authors in producing quality manuscripts. One general guideline for scientific papers is **IMRAD**, which stands for *i*ntroduction, *m*ethods, *r*esults, *a*nd *d*iscussion (Cooper 2015, 67). However, there are many other reporting guidelines for health research, including the following:

- Consolidated Standards of Reporting Trials (CONSORT 2010) (Schulz et al. 2010)
- Consolidated Criteria for Reporting Qualitative Research (COREQ) (Tong et al. 2007)
- Preferred Reporting Items for Systematic Reviews and Meta-Analyses (PRISMA) (Moher et al. 2009)

The website of EQUATOR, which stands for *e*nhancing the *qua*lity and *t*ransparency *o*f health *r*esearch, lists many reporting guidelines and has links to specific websites (2016). These preexisting guidelines help authors include all key data and information in their manuscripts. Table 15.3 may also serve as a checklist for the composition and revision of the manuscript, and authors may want to check online recommendations for authors, such as those from the

International Committee of Medical Journal Editors (2016) or the Association of American Medical Colleges (Durning and Carline 2015).

Submission Guidelines **Submission guidelines** are explicit rules that authors are expected to follow if they want their manuscript published. Authors can find the explicit submission guidelines in journals or on the publishers' websites. Often, the submission guidelines refer authors to one of the four major style manuals listed in table 15.4 for detailed instructions about a wide range of issues related to grammar, spelling, word choice, how to use numbers and abbreviations, how to format citations, notes, and references, and many other topics of interest to authors. Selection of the style manual relates to the field of publication. For example, journals in education generally require American Psychological Association (APA) (2010) style whereas biomedical journals require American Medical Association (AMA) style (Iverson 2007) style. Journals in health informatics typically use AMA style, whereas journals in HIM require authors to use a modification of Chicago style (University of Chicago Press 2010). The variance in these style manuals isillustrated in table 15.4.

Table 15.4 Common style manuals and variations in their reference styles

Style Manual	Reference Style for Books	Reference Style for Journal Articles
American Psychological Association (APA). 2010. *Publication Manual of the American Psychological Association,* 6th ed. Washington, DC: APA. [Referred to as *APA style.*]	White, S. (2016). *A practical approach to analyzing healthcare data* (3rd ed.). Chicago, IL: American Health Information Management Association.	Kreiman, J. (2016). On peer review. *Journal of Speech, Language, and Hearing Research,* 59(3), 480–483.
Gibaldi, Joseph. 2016. *MLA Handbook for Writers of Research Papers,* 8th ed. New York: Modern Language Association of America. [Referred to as *MLA style.*]	White, Susan. *A Practical Approach to Analyzing Healthcare Data,* 3rd ed. Chicago, IL: American Health Information Management Association, 2016.	Kreiman, Jody. "On Peer Review." *Journal of Speech, Language, and Hearing Research,* vol. 59, no. 3, 2016, pp. 480–83.
Iverson, Cheryl. 2007. *American Medical Association Manual of Style: A Guide for Authors and Editors,* 10th ed. New York: Oxford University Press. [Referred to as *AMA Style.*]	White S. *A Practical Approach to Analyzing Healthcare Data.* 3rd ed. Chicago, IL: American Health Information Management Association; 2016.	Kreiman J. On peer review. *J Speech Lang Hear Res.* 2016;59(3):480–483.
University of Chicago Press. 2010. *Chicago Manual of Style,* 16th ed. Chicago: University of Chicago Press. [Referred to as *CMOS* or *Chicago style.*]	White, Susan. 2016. *A Practical Approach to Analyzing Healthcare Data,* 3rd ed. Chicago, IL: American Health Information Management Association.	Kreiman, Jody. 2016. "On Peer Review." *Journal of Speech, Language, and Hearing Research* 59(3):480–483.

In addition to directing authors to a style manual, the journal's submission guidelines include many requirements for the manuscript, such as the following:

- Information needed about the author and contact
- Length and representativeness of title
- Length of abstract in words
- Length of manuscript in maximum number of pages or number of words
- Fonts and font sizes for headings, paragraphs, lists, and so on
- Line spacing
- Justification of paragraphs
- Page margins
- Pagination
- Inclusive language (for example, non-sexist word choices)
- Blinding (names of authors on separate page)
- Format and design specifications of charts and tables

- Format of citations in text
- Format of references (a publisher's style may vary from the format shown in the recommended style manual)
- General organizational structure of manuscript
- Word processing software
- Electronic submission instructions

For instance, among the many formatting details that the editors of *Perspectives in Health Information Management (PHIM)* specify, are the following format requirements:

- Font: Times New Roman
- Font size: 12 points
- Text color: Black
- Spacing: Single spaced
- Margins: 1 inch and text in one column (AHIMA 2016a)

Submission guidelines indicate the journal's preferred organizational structure for the entire article, similar to the previously discussed structured abstracts. For instance, the editors of the *Journal of the American Medical Informatics Association* (2016) prefer that Research and Application manuscripts have sections to expand on each of the elements of the structured abstract (objective, materials and methods, results, discussion, and conclusion, see table 15.2), plus sections describing the study's background and the relevance of its results (JAMIA 2016). Often, the organizational structure varies by the type of article, such as research article versus case report. Moreover, many editors state that the organizational structure is flexible and that researchers should adapt the structure to suit their research. Most journals provide contact information with the guidelines should researchers have questions on formatting or style.

In addition to following the explicit submission guidelines, authors are also expected to adhere to journals' implicit rules when writing and formatting their manuscripts for submission. While these implicit rules are unwritten, they are important because editors and peer reviewers assume that researchers will naturally know and follow them. Different fields of research tend to have their own unique sets of implicit rules.

A journal's implicit rules reflect the culture of its audience. This culture is reflected in qualities of writing like the use of the first- or third-person voice, anthropomorphism, passive voice, and tone. For example, an audience of qualitative researchers may expect the use of the first person, whereas an audience of quantitative researchers may expect the use of the third person. Some readers and reviewers reject anthropomorphism as giving human traits to inanimate objects. Generally, audiences that reject first person and anthropomorphism also tend to prefer a detached, neutral tone. Spending time reading articles in a journal can provide insight into its implicit rules.

Peer Review

Peer review is a system in which journals' editors and peer reviewers work with authors to improve the quality of articles and advance scientific knowledge (Kreiman 2016, 483). Peer-reviewed journals have a publicized process of review and approval. Both print and electronic journals are peer reviewed. Information about whether a journal is peer reviewed and the peer-review process is found on the journal's website. Authors who want to advance practice may publish in peer-reviewed journals or in non-peer reviewed (popular or trade) publications. In peer review, experts critically examine the documentation of a study's design, method, and analytic techniques and they evaluate the researchers' interpretation of their data and the conclusions they reach. Functions of peer review include ensuring the research's relevance to the profession or field of study, its scientific validity, and the readability of the researchers' manuscripts. Peer review contributes to the growth of scientific knowledge.

Peer review has a long-established tradition in science. In 1731, the Royal Society of Edinburgh published the society's policy and objectives for its *Medical Essays and Observations*. The Royal Society of London is also credited with early adoption of peer review. In 1752, it established the Committee on Papers that reviewed all articles prior to publication in its *Philosophical Transactions* (Kronick 1990, 1321).

Peer reviewers judge the relevance of a research study to the field. As experts, they are aware of the field's body of knowledge and its current trends and crucial issues. Relevant studies are important to the field, such as adding critical new information to the field's knowledge or affecting many practitioners or sites of practice. For example, the manuscript review guidelines of the journal *Perspectives in Health Information Management* require that the manuscript's content be "valuable, important, and beneficial to readers" (2016b).

Peer review also attests to the study's rigor and face validity. As discussed in chapter 1, *rigor* refers to the procedures that researchers use to establish their studies' integrity. Peer reviewers check that, per the researchers' documentation, studies have been conducted appropriately using a suitable design, method, sampling stratagems, and analytic techniques. However, peer reviewers only check studies' face validity (discussed in chapter 11). They are generally unable to detect falsification or lies because they do not redo the researchers' data collection and analyses. Therefore, the reviewers only attest that, to the best of their knowledge based on the researchers' reporting, the studies' results are accurate, reliable, and valid. For example, using the manuscript review guidelines of *Perspectives in Health Information Management*, reviewers check 15 criteria related to how the research study was conducted, such as "the design of the research or investigation is sound" (2016b).

Finally, peer reviewers often improve the researchers' reporting of their studies' results. Peer reviewers attempt to follow the logic of the study as reported in the manuscript. Sometimes, the structure of the manuscript is illogical and the reviewers can neither understand nor evaluate what the researchers did in the study. Other times, the peer reviewers understand the overall activities of the study but believe that restructuring the manuscript would increase its readability. In these cases, peer reviewers make suggestions as to how manuscripts' logic or readability could be improved. Reviewers record their suggestions on a review form, and the feedback is relayed to the manuscripts' authors via the journals' editors. Again using the manuscript review guidelines of *Perspectives in Health Information Management* as an example, its reviewers check that the "manuscript is well organized and flows well" (2016b).

An expert who is an educator and researcher provided general types of questions for peer review:

1. Is the problem clearly stated? Are terms defined as needed? Has the problem been appropriately delimited?
2. Is the hypothesis stated (if applicable to the type of publication)? Does the hypothesis relate to the problem? Is the way the researcher intends to test the hypothesis clear?
3. To the best of the student's (reviewer's) knowledge, is the literature review thorough, complete, and pertinent? Is the literature review clear and organized? Is the reviewer convinced this problem is important? Does the literature review synthesize rather than merely summarize? Are all citations in the body of the article in the reference list? Is jargon kept to a minimum?
4. Does the study's design relate to the problem? Is the population clearly defined? Is the method of creating the sample clearly explained? Is bias reduced in sampling (if applicable)? Is the sample representative of the population (if applicable)?
5. Is the research instrument specified (if applicable)? Is the instrument related to the problem? Does the researcher state the instrument's reliability and validity?
6. Does the researcher explain the method clearly enough and with sufficient detail that another person could replicate the study? Are confidential data protected?
7. Does the researcher use the best mode to present the results? Do tables, figures, and graphs have clear titles? Do the numbers "add up?"
8. Do the conclusions relate to the findings? Does the researcher provide alternative explanations? Does the researcher relate the results back to the larger body of knowledge or theory? (Cohen 1991)

Readers of published articles as well as manuscripts can assess the quality of reporting by checking whether the authors used reporting guidelines (discussed earlier in the section) and whether the previous eight questions are answered in the article. Practitioners may also benefit from using these questions to evaluate research articles as they determine whether the results and conclusions are applicable to practice in their work setting.

Publication Bias

Editors, peer reviewers, authors, and some readers are aware of publication bias. *Publication bias*, also known as *reporting bias,* is the selective publication of studies based on the nature and the direction of the results (Sterne et al. 2011). Bias in the *nature* of results refers to the tendency of researchers to submit and journal editors to publish research results that are statistically significant rather than results that are nonsignificant. Bias in the *direction* of results refers to the preference for positive (conclusive) findings over inconclusive ones. As a result of publication bias, the overall effect of published research studies may be misleading because of the preponderance of favorable results. Registries of research studies, such as ClinicalTrials.Gov of the National Institutes of Health (NIH), are a means to reduce publication bias (NIH 2016). The registries contain the researchers' original proposed research design; thereby, any suppression or withholding of some results becomes detectable.

Response to a Journal's Feedback

Journal editors send the peer reviewers' decision and comments to the authors. The turnaround time between the submission of the manuscript and the receipt of the feedback is highly variable. Authors can make a rough estimate of the turnaround time by carefully reviewing the journal's published articles. Often, a footnote will state the dates of submission, revision, and acceptance. Online journals tend to have faster turnaround times than print journals.

Typically, decisions fit into the following five categories, although the third and fourth categories are sometimes merged:

- Accept
- Accept with minor revisions
- Accept with major revisions
- Reject, but request resubmission after major reworking
- Reject

All authors want to receive feedback stating, "Accept." Unfortunately, this response is rare. Peer reviewers and editors have a responsibility to improve the clarity and impact of the manuscript, and they diligently attempt to fulfill this responsibility. Therefore, reviewers usually make suggestions to authors on how to improve their manuscripts. Thus, authors can feel encouraged when they receive "accept with minor revisions" or "accept with major revisions." Authors are advised to turn the revision around quickly to maintain the timeliness of their topic.

Authors who receive feedback of "Reject, but resubmit" should consider the suggestion to resubmit. The editor and the peer reviewers found something of value in the manuscript, and they want to see that aspect developed. However, authors are cautioned to move expeditiously to return their revised manuscript. Editorial leadership and the direction of journals change over time, and this change could lead to a different, negative outcome.

In responding to the feedback, authors should focus on clearly and explicitly addressing each of the reviewers' comments. Creating a table that lists the reviewers' comments and the authors' actions is recommended for analyzing necessary changes. When authors disagree or cannot comply with the reviewers' comments, clarifying the passage or issue may be a viable strategy.

Peer review, by its very nature, is critical. Thus, authors will not receive much positive feedback. Therefore, authors should do the following:

- Accept feedback objectively because comments are not personal.
- Take feedback seriously, while understanding that some comments are not necessarily true or relevant; even if some feedback misses the mark, all comments deserve examination, analysis, and response.
- Persevere.

Authors will realize, though, much satisfaction and gratification when their manuscript becomes a journal article. The effort is well worth the result as they see their own contribution to the field's body of knowledge.

Checking Proofs Before Publication

Once a manuscript is accepted, authors can expect to receive galley (page) proofs that show how the article will look in print. Electronic galley proofs in PDF format are usually sent via e-mail or downloaded from a cloud-based program. Editors often include queries about wording, citations, and other issues requiring clarification. Authors must respond to every query. Authors also should inspect the galley proofs for the following:

- Grammatical errors
- Typographical errors
- Errors in their address, affiliation, or credentials
- Inaccuracies in editorial changes
- Distortions of facts through editorial changes
- Errors in tables or figures
- Inappropriate changes in the description or display of the instrument (survey, questionnaire, and so forth)

Journals expect a short turnaround time for feedback on proofs. Thus, authors should be prepared to review the pages quickly and carefully.

Alternative Dissemination Formats: White Paper and Research Project Website

The process of implementing research information in practice is slow (Glasgow et al. 2012, 1274.). Attention is now being given to ways of disseminating research findings beyond the traditional poster and oral paper presentations and journal publications. This section discusses two of those ways, white papers and research project websites.

White Paper

A **white paper** is a short document that seeks to inform or persuade readers (Willerton 2007, 191). Authors of white papers are often groups, such as a committee of a government agency, a taskforce of a professional association, a working group of a business or consulting firm, or a research team. Types of white papers are categorized based on their purpose, as follows:

- *Policy papers* and *position statement*s state or explain an organization's policy or position on a topic.
- *Research reports* and *technology papers* present research or data on a product, service, or topic.
- *Practice briefs* and *issues papers* describe a problem or issue and propose a solution.

The length of white papers typically ranges between 12 pages and 25 pages, with the research reports being the longest.

Generally, the organizational structure of white papers includes an abstract, a problem or issue statement, a review of the literature, a discussion section, a conclusion, references, and appendixes (such as graphs, tables, or case studies). White papers presenting research or data may also include a methods section and a section on research results and analysis. Policy papers or issue papers may also include potential responses to the problem or issue, such as a policy or a solution (Rotarius and Rotarius 2016, 183–184). A white paper may also have an executive summary that highlights the paper's recommendations or conclusions; the executive summary may be a separate document or included in the white paper's initial pages.

Research Project Website

Research project websites are used to make information about a research project accessible to practitioners, other researchers, policymakers, possible research participants, and other potentially interested persons or groups. The research project website may be a way to recruit subjects and keep the public and other researchers up-to-date on the progress of the research project.

An advantage of having a research project website is that the Internet is appealing to many users, such as youth and engaged patients. However, for other potential users of the website's information, such as the extremely elderly or the very poor, the Internet may be a barrier. To reach these users, another dissemination strategy should be planned and employed. Another advantage of the research project website is that it can be easily and inexpensively updated, unlike print documents.

The following are general recommendations for the development and maintenance of research project websites:

- Make the website visually appealing and easy to navigate.
- Organize the website by tabs, such as Home, Overview, Partners or Team, Research Method, Stories (Case Studies), Publications and Other Work Products, News and Events (press releases, newsletter, health fairs, or conferences), and Glossary.
- Update the website routinely, including such information as when the website was last reviewed and updated. (European Commission 2010, 1–2)

Some contracts with funding agencies require the researchers to build a research project website or create other research products (deliverables). In those instances, the researchers should follow the instructions from the funding agency for the content of the website. For example, the Agency for Healthcare Research and Quality (AHRQ) provides detailed guidelines for web publishing and communications (AHRQ 2016). These guidelines cover copyright, trademarks, web standards, creating press releases, social media policies, and many more topics. The US Department of Health and Human Services (HHS) provides an online searchable data of web standards and usability guidelines (HHS 2016).

Review Questions

1. Why is a manuscript title described as the shortest possible abstract?
2. What is the difference between the terms *manuscript* and *article*?
3. What is the term for a published compilation of research papers that were presented at a conference?
4. What advantages does presenting a pilot study at a poster presentation give a researcher?
5. Your abstract has been accepted for a poster presentation at a national symposium. Your friend's abstract has also been accepted. You both have been assigned to the same two-hour poster session, although the topics for your poster presentations are unrelated. At the last minute, your friend decides that he wants to attend another session that has oral presentations on a topic in which he has a particular interest. He asks whether you will "cover" his poster during your assigned time. He observes that "it would only be for two hours." Based on the chapter, what do you say to your friend and why?
6. Your abstract has been accepted for an oral presentation at your state's professional HIM meeting. The state's professional meeting has been organized into afternoon-long sessions. Each session has a theme; the theme of the session to which your oral presentation has been assigned is "Improving Practice." The topic of your paper is "Maintaining Integrity of the Enterprise Master Patient Index." The time limit for oral presentations in your session is 15 minutes. Who are members of your targeted audience and how will you frame your research results for them? According to the chapter, for an effective oral presentation, what are examples of content that you will include and of content that you will exclude?
7. What is peer review?
8. What are the parts of a manuscript and what do they include?
9. How is the quality of a journal evaluated?
10. What is a way to reduce publication bias in clinical trials?

Application Exercises

1. Compare (find similarities) and contrast (find differences) the instructions for authors of two journals, *Perspectives in Health Information Management* (PHIM 2016a) and the *Journal of the American Medical Informatics Association* (JAMIA 2016). You will be using the journals' home pages and their pages with instructions for authors.
   a. What areas of research are published in the journals (such as clinical, educational, and so forth)?
   b. What types (categories) of articles are published in the journals (such as systematic review, case study, and so forth)?
   c. In which word processing software do the publishers require the manuscript be submitted?
   d. According to JAMIA, what headings are contained in a structured abstract?
   e. What reference style do the journals require?
   f. What are the maximum word counts for articles in the journals?
2. Practice briefs are concise, research-based summaries of best practices and relevant federal statutes and regulations. Written by experts and routinely updated, practice briefs cover current issues. AHIMA disseminates practice briefs in the *Journal of the American Health Information Management Association* (*Journal of AHIMA*). The practice briefs are available in the *HIM Body of Knowledge*. On AHIMA's website, log into the HIM Body of Knowledge in MyAHIMA. Under the heading "Popular Resources" at the bottom of the web page, select the resource of "Practice Briefs."

   What are at least three topics that have recently been addressed in practice briefs?
3. A critique is a review or commentary that carefully analyzes and appraises works of literature or art. It is based on serious examination and reaches a sensible judgment. As a written evaluation, critique is a neutral term. The

purpose of critiquing an article is to build skills in assessing the quality of research and to hone critical reading skills. Your instructor will provide you with a rubric that is an expanded version of the questions in the section on Peer Review. Based on the rubric, critique an article assigned by your instructor or "Mining clinical text for signals of adverse drug-drug interactions" (Iyer et al. 2014).

References

Agency for Healthcare Research and Quality (AHRQ). 2016 (August). AHRQ Publishing and Communications Guidelines. http://www.ahrq.gov/research/publications/pubcomguide/index.html.

AHIMA. 2016a. Author's Style Guide. *Perspectives in Health Information Management (PHIM)*. http://perspectives.ahima.org/style-and-submission-guidelines.

AHIMA. 2016b. Manuscript Review Process. *Perspectives in Health Information Management (PHIM)*. http://perspectives.ahima.org/manuscript-review-process.

American Psychological Association (APA). 2010. *Publication Manual of the American Psychological Association,* 6th ed. Washington, DC: APA.

Applied Clinical Informatics. 2010 (August 16). Instructions for Authors. https://aci.schattauer.de/for-authors/instructions-to-authors.html.

Bartlett, R. 2013. Playing with meaning: Using cartoons to disseminate research findings. *Qualitative Research* 13(2): 214–227.

Bensman, S.J. 2012. The impact factor: Its place in Garfield's thought, in science evaluation, and in library collection management. *Scientometrics* 92(2):263–275.

BMC Medical Informatics and Decision Making. 2016. Instructions for Authors. http://old.biomedcentral.com/bmcmed-inform decismak/authors/instructions/researcharticle.

Bordage, G., W.C. McGaghie, and D.A. Cook. 2015. Title, Authors, and Abstract. Chapter 17 in *Review Criteria for Research Manuscripts,* 2nd ed. Edited by Durning, S.J. and J.D. Carline. Washington, DC: Association of American Medical Colleges. https://members.aamc.org/eweb/upload/Review%20Criteria%20For%20Research%20Manuscripts.pdf.

Cals, J.W.L. and D. Kotz. 2013. Effective writing and publishing scientific papers, part II: Title and abstract. *Journal of Clinical Epidemiology* 66(6):585.

Cleary, M., G. Walter, and G. Luscombe. 2007. Spreading the word: Disseminating research results to patients and carers. *Acta Neuropsychiatrica* 19(4):224–229.

Cohen, P.A. 1991. Criteria for evaluating research reports. Handout, educational research course. Augusta, GA: Medical College of Georgia.

Cooper, I.D. 2015. How to write an original research paper (and get it published). *Journal of the Medical Library Association* 103(2):67–68.

Durning, S.J. and J.D. Carline, eds. 2015. *Review Criteria for Research Manuscripts,* 2nd ed. Washington, DC: Association of American Medical Colleges. https://members.aamc.org/eweb/upload/Review%20Criteria%20For%20Research%20Manuscripts.pdf.

Edirisooriya, G. 1996 Research presentation in a democratic society: A voice from the audience. *Educational Researcher* 25(6):25–30.

EQUATOR Network: Enhancing the Quality and Transparency of Health Research. 2016. http://www.equator-network.org.

European Commission. 2010 (March). EU Project Websites—Best Practice Guidelines. http://www.eurosfaire.prd.fr/7pc/documents/1271333123_project_website_guidelines_en.pdf.

Forrestal, E.J. 2014. Foundation of evidence-based decision making for health care managers—part I: Systematic review. *Health Care Manager* 33(2):97–109.

Forrestal, E. 2016. Research methods. Chapter 19 in *Health Information Management: Concepts, Principles, and Practice,* 5th ed. Edited by Oachs, P.K. and A.L. Watters. Chicago: AHIMA Press.

Gibaldi, J. 2016. *MLA Handbook for Writers of Research Papers,* 8th ed. New York: Modern Language Association of America.

Glasgow, R.E., C. Vinson, D. Chambers, M.J. Khoury, R.M. Kaplan, and C. Hunter. 2012. National Institutes of Health approaches to dissemination and implementation science: Current and future directions. *American Journal of Public Health* 102(7):1274–1281.

International Committee of Medical Journal Editors. 2016. Manuscript Preparation. http://www.icmje.org/recommendations/browse/manuscript-preparation.

Iverson, C., ed. 2007. *American Medical Association Manual of Style: A Guide for Authors and Editors,* 10th ed. New York: Oxford University Press.

Journal of the American Medical Informatics Association (JAMIA). 2016. Instructions to Authors. http://jamia.oxfordjournals.org/for_authors/index.html.

Journal of Medical Internet Research (JMIR). 2016a. Instructions for Authors. https://www.jmir.org/content/author-instructions.

Journal of Medical Internet Research (JMIR). 2016b. Announcement: Impact Factor 2015 for Open Access Journals confirms JMIR as leading journal. http://www.jmir.org/announcement/view/133.

Kreiman, J. 2016. On peer review. *Journal of Speech, Language, and Hearing Research* 59(3):480–483.

Kronick, D.A. 1990. Peer review in the 18th-century scientific journalism. *Journal of the American Medical Association* 263(10):1321–1322.

Lafrenière, D., T. Hurlimann, V. Menuz, and B. Godard. 2014. Evaluation of a cartoon-based knowledge dissemination intervention on scientific and ethical challenges raised by nutrigenomics/nutrigenetics research. *Evaluation and Program Planning* 46:103–114.

Moher, D., A. Liberati, J. Tetzlaff, D.G. Altman, and the PRISMA Group. 2009. Preferred reporting items for systematic reviews and meta-analyses: The PRISMA statement. *PLoS Medicine/Public Library of Science* 6(7):e1000097.

National Institutes of Health (NIH). ClinicalTrials.Gov. https://clinicaltrials.gov.

Reumann, M. 2012. Preparing for conferences—basic presentation skills. *IEEE Pulse* 3(3):6–7, 12.

Rotarius, T. and V. Rotarius. 2016. Preparing a health care white paper: Providing structure to the writing process. *Health Care Manager* 35(2):180–185.

Sandefer, R. and E.S. Karl. 2015. Ready or not: HIM is changing—results of the new HIM competencies survey show skill gaps between education levels, students, and working professionals. *Journal of the American Health Information Management Association* 86(3):24–27.

Schulz, K.F., D.G. Altman, D. Moher, and the CONSORT Group. 2010. CONSORT 2010 statement: Updated guidelines for reporting parallel group randomized trials. *Annals of Internal Medicine* 152(11):726–732.

Sterne, J.A.C., M. Egger, and D. Moher; Cochrane Bias Methods Group. 2011. Addressing reporting biases. Chapter 10 in *Cochrane Handbook for Systematic Reviews of Interventions,* version 5.1.0. Edited by Higgins, J.P.T. and S. Green. The Cochrane Collaboration. http://handbook.cochrane.org.

Tong, A., K. Flemming, E. McInnes, S. Olive, and J. Craig. 2012. Enhancing transparency in reporting the synthesis of qualitative research: ENTREQ. *BMC Medical Research Methodology* 12(1):181. doi: 10.1186/1471-2288-12-181.

University of Chicago Press. 2010. *Chicago Manual of Style,* 16th ed. Chicago: University of Chicago Press.

US Department of Health and Human Services (HHS). 2016. HHS Web Standards and Usability Guidelines. http://webstandards.hhs.gov.

Willerton, R. 2007. Writing white papers in high-tech industries: Perspectives from the field. *Technical Communication* 54(2):187–200.

Wineberg, S. 2004. Must it be this way? Ten rules for keeping your audience awake during conferences. *Educational Researcher* 23(4):13–14.

Resources

Bailey, R.W., C. Barnum, J. Bosley, B. Chaparro, J. Dumas, M.Y. Ivory, B. John, H. Miller-Jacobs, S.J. Koyani, J.R. Lewis, S. Page, J. Ramey, J. Redish, J. Scholtz, S. Wigginton, C.A. Wolfson, L.E. Wood, and D. Zimmerman. 2006. *Research-Based Web Design and Usability Guidelines*. Washington, DC: Government Printing Office. https://www.usability.gov/sites/default/files/documents/guidelines_book.pdf.

Dolgin, E. 2009 (September 11). Publication bias continues despite clinical-trial registration. *Nature News*. http://www.nature.com/news/2009/090911/full/news.2009.902.html.

Goodhand, J.R., C.L. Giles, M. Wahed, P.M. Irving, L. Langmead and D.S. Rampton. 2011. Poster presentations at medical conferences: An effective way of disseminating research? *Clinical Medicine* 11(2):138–141.

Institute of Education Sciences. 2014 (June). Going Public Writing about Research in Everyday Language. http://ies.ed.gov/pubsearch/pubsinfo.asp?pubid=REL2014051.

Iyer, S.V., R. Harpaz, P. LePendu, A. Bauer-Mehren, and N.H. Shah. 2014. Mining clinical text for signals of adverse drug-drug interactions. *Journal of the American Medical Informatics Association* 21(2):353–362.

McCormack, L., S. Sheridan, M. Lewis, V. Boudewyns, C.L. Melvin, C. Kistler, L.J. Lux, K. Cullen, and K.N. Lohr. 2013. Communication and Dissemination Strategies to Facilitate the Use of Health-Related Evidence. Evidence Report/Technology Assessment no. 213. AHRQ publication no. 13(14)-E003-EF. Rockville, MD: Agency for Healthcare Research and Quality. https://www.ncbi.nlm.nih.gov/books/NBK179104.

Neta, G., R.E. Glasgow, C.R. Carpenter, J.M. Grimshaw, B.A. Rabin, M.E. Fernandez, and R.C. Brownson. 2015. A framework for enhancing the value of research for dissemination and implementation. *American Journal of Public Health* 105(1):49–57.

Plunkett, S.W. n.d. Tips on Poster Presentations at Professional Conference. California State University Northridge. https://www.csun.edu/plunk/documents/poster_presentation.pdf.

Rosenthal, R. 1979. The "file drawer problem" and tolerance for null results. *Psychological Bulletin* 86(3):638–641.

Stelzner, M.A. 2007. *Writing White Papers: How to Capture Readers and Keep Them Engaged*. Poway, CA: WhitePaperSource Publishing.

Strunk, W. and E.B. White. 1999. *The Elements of Style*, 4th ed. Boston: Allyn and Bacon.

US Department of Health and Human Services (HHS). 2016 (August 19). Digital Communications. http://www.hhs.gov/web/index.html.

Web of Science. 2016. Essays and White Papers. http://wokinfo.com/essays.

Wilson, P.M., M. Petticrew, M.W. Calnan, and I. Nazareth. 2010. Disseminating research findings: What should researchers do? A systematic scoping review of conceptual frameworks. *Implementation Science* 5(91)1–16.

Wolf, L.A. 2015. Getting the word out: Dissemination of research results. *Journal of Emergency Nursing* 41(5):451–452.

World Health Organization. 2014 (March). Implementing Research Toolkit: Workbook. http://www.who.int/tdr/publications/year/2014/ir-toolkit-manual/en.

Young Adult Library Services Association. 2007. Proposed Guidelines for White Papers. http://www.ala.org/yalsa/sites/ala.org.yalsa/files/content/workingwithyalsa/board/boarddoc/midwinter/pdf07/13WhitePaperGuidelin.pdf.

Glossary

2 × 2 table: A table containing two variables (e.g. system prediction of sepsis and actual health outcome of sepsis) with each variable having two values (e.g. sepsis and no sepsis)

Absolute risk (AR): The probability of an occurrence of an event in an entire population of subjects (experimental group and control group)

Absolute risk reduction (ARR): The arithmetic difference between the event rate of two groups

Abstract: A succinct description of the proposed work that can be read separately from the application

Advisory committee: A group of subject matter experts (SMEs) with experience in survey design as well as the topic of study

Agent: The cause, for example, of a disease

Alpha level (α): *See* **Significance level**

Alternative hypothesis: States that there is a difference or an association between the independent and dependent variables

Analytic study: Determines whether there is a relationship between the independent variable and the dependent variable; in epidemiology, this determines a relationship between the exposure or risk factor (independent variable) and the disease or health outcome (dependent variable)

Annotated bibliography: A list of citations, each with a paragraph that summarizes the issues that the citation addressed, its main contentions or claims, and its methodological soundness

Annual review: Entire journals or books on recently published research articles on a topic

Applied research: Answers the questions "What?" "How?" "When?" or "For Whom?" Most health informatics and HIM researchers who conduct applied research focus on the implementation of theories and models into practice. Applied research, particularly clinical applied research, is often done in healthcare settings, such as at the bedside or in the clinic.

Approach: Methodology for carrying out research

Area under the curve (AUC): The performance of the predictive algorithm or other detection technology

Article: A manuscript or paper that has been published in a journal

Artifact: Object that humans make that serves a purpose and has meaning

Association rule mining: A data-mining technique that analyzes identifying attributes that frequently occur together in a data set; also called dependency modeling

Attrition: The withdrawal of subjects from the study

Autonomy: In the research context, refers to the ability of research participants to understand what their participation in a research study involves and to give their informed consent

Bar chart: Visual presentation of data that shows comparisons between and among variables and illustrates major characteristics in the distribution of data

Basic research: Answers the question "Why?" and focuses on the development of theories and their refinement. Basic research is sometimes called *bench science* because it often occurs in laboratories. In health informatics and HIM, basic research comprises the development and evaluation of new methods and theories for the acquisition, storage, maintenance, retrieval, and use of information.

Belmont Report: The ethical and regulatory foundation for biomedical and behavioral research on human subjects in the United States
Beneficence: Doing good for others
Beta (B): Designates the probability of making a type II error because power is 1.0 – B
Bibliographic databases: Collection of publication data about published literature such as journals, magazines, newspaper articles, books, book chapters, and other information sources
Bioethics committees: Provide guidance on ethical issues related to patient care
Biographical sketch: Component of a grant application that typically includes the name and title of each key personnel, along with that person's educational background, relevant publications, roles in research, and professional experience (including employment history)
Biomedical research: The broad area of science that looks for ways to prevent and treat diseases that cause illness and death in people and in animals
Bivariate: Designation for statistical tests that involve two variables
Box-and-whisker plots: Display variation in a data set and summarize its key features; also called box plots
Budget: Money allowed for a research project. It can be specific or broad-based, depending on the requirements of the grant application
Caring: An ethical principal that focuses on the importance of relationships and on the connections between oneself and others
Case–control study design: Studies with cases and controls to investigate whether exposure to a factor or phenomenon is associated with an outcome
Cases: Individuals who have the disease under study
Case study: An in-depth investigation of one or more examples of a phenomenon, such as a trend, occurrence, or incident
Categorical data: Data that can be grouped, such as by race or age group
Categorical items: Require the respondent to select the appropriate category or grouping
Causal-comparative research: Involves a variable from the past or phenomenon that has already occurred; also called quasi-experimental or ex post facto (retrospective) research
Causal relationship: Demonstrates cause and effect, such that one variable *causes* the change in another variable
Census survey: Examines an entire population
Centers for Scientific Review (CSR): Part of the NIH peer review process that provides referral officers to review applications, assign applications to integrated review groups, and receive reviews and scores
Chronic disease model: Demonstrates that a mix of factors may increase risk for a chronic disease, and that the presence of multiple factors over a long period of time may also increase risk of chronic disease
Civil monetary penalties: Fines imposed by the Office for Civil Rights (OCR) for failure to take satisfactory action to resolve a HIPAA violation
Claim: Means interpretation in qualitative research
Claim of primacy: Occurs when authors write that their study was "the first study ever" to do something
Clinical trial: Designed to test new approaches to the diagnosis, treatment, or prevention of specific diseases
Closed-ended (structured) questions: Require the participant to choose a particular response, similar to a multiple-choice exam; also known as *quantitative questions*
Clustering: Groups data objects within the database that are similar to each other and are dissimilar to data objects in other groups; also called segmentation
Cluster sampling: Method that separates the total population into "clusters" (smaller groups), such as neighborhoods within a city, and then randomly samples the clusters
Cochrane Collaboration tool: Assesses risk of bias in a study's design by evaluating sequence generation, allocation concealment, blinding, incomplete outcome data, and selective outcome reporting
Code of ethics: Incorporates ethical principles to express a profession's core values and promote ethical behavior of the profession's members
Cohen's kappa (κ) coefficient: A value that states whether the levels of agreement seen among reviews by different abstractors are real or due to chance
Cohort study: An analytic study design that follows two groups of study participants—one with exposure to an independent variable and one without the exposure—forward in time to determine whether and when they develop the disease or outcome variable under study

Common Rule: Subpart A of the Federal Policy for the Protection of Human Subjects that offers a basic set of protections for all human subjects of research conducted or supported by HHS; *See also* **Federal Policy for the Protection of Human Subjects**
Community trial: Like a clinical trial except that a community trial takes place in a community and researchers therefore have less control over the intervention than they would have with the clinical trial (which is usually conducted in a controlled environment such as a clinic rather than the participant's community or home environment); *See also* **Clinical trials**
Comparison group: A group that is used when a different intervention is used as a comparison for the intervention being investigated
Comparative effectiveness research (CER): Research that generates and synthesizes comparative evidence about the benefits and harms of alternative methods to prevent, diagnose, treat, and monitor a clinical condition, or to improve the delivery of care
Complex adaptive system (CAS): An entity with many diverse and autonomous components or parts that are interrelated and interdependent with many interconnections
Conclusion validity: The extent to which observations, patterns, and inferences are reasonable
Concurrent validity: The instrument's ability to discriminate between groups it should differentiate
Confidence interval (CI): A range of values for a sample's characteristic, such as the mean, within which it is estimated that the population's characteristic lies
Confidence level: The probability that the CI includes the population's value
Confidentiality form: A document signed and dated by a proposal reviewer that states that the reviewer will keep all information in the proposal application confidential
Conflict of interest form: Asks the reviewer to inform the program officer of any conflicts of interest based on the area of focus for the grant application
Confounding (extraneous, secondary) variable: An unknown variable that could be creating an apparent difference or association identified in a correlational study
Constant comparative method: Analyzes data by coding categorization and comparison; *See also* **Grounded theory**
Constructs: Abstractions of theoretical, non-observable concepts
Construct validity: Agreement between a theoretical concept and the survey instrument. Can be separated into two parts: *convergent validity* (agreement among ratings collected independently on issues that should be agreed on theoretically) and *discriminate validity* (disagreement on issues measured that should be disagreed on theoretically); The degree to which an instrument measures the constructs that it claims to measure
Content analysis: The process of examining all textual data collected and detecting the number of recurrent words or phrases to determine emerging themes and factors reflective of the culture or institution examined
Content validity: The survey instrument captures the information the researchers intended to measure
Content validity index (CVI): A numerical representation of the SMEs' aggregate level of agreement for the entire instrument
Content validity ratio (CVR): The ratio of the number of items that the SMEs scored as essential and the total number of SMEs, adjusted for 50 percent agreement (Lawshe's assumption)
Context: The specific conditions of the situation, including time, space, emotional attitude, social situation, and culture
Contingency table: Visually presents information on two or more variables
Continuous data: Represent values or observations that have an infinite number of points along a continuum
Control group: Comprises those who do not receive the study's intervention
Convenience sample: Obtained by selecting units from the population based on easy availability or accessibility; they are not random, so the results are not generalizable
Convergent validity: The degree of correlation between the instrument and other instruments designed to measure similar constructs, or the degree of correlation among items measuring the same construct
Correlational research: Detects the existence, direction, and strength (or degree) of associations among characteristics
Cost-benefit analysis (CBA): Weighs the inputs (cost) to the outcome (benefit) of a program, showing strengths and weaknesses from an institutional or societal perspective
Cost-effectiveness analysis (CEA): Compares the costs to the outcomes of various courses of action
Cost-sharing: *See* **Matching requirements**

Coverage error: Occurs when elements of the population are missing from the sampling frame, creating a systematic (nonrandom) discrepancy between the target population and the sampling frame
Criterion-related validity: Measurement of the accuracy of the intended survey instrument through comparison to another method that has been shown to be valid
Cronbach's alpha: A measure of internal consistency and determines whether all the variables within the instrument are measuring the same concept
Cross-industry process for data mining (CRISP-DM): Breaks the process of data mining into six distinct phases that apply to any project: business understanding, data understanding, data preparation, modeling, evaluation, and deployment
Crossover design: Uses two groups of participants as both the experimental and control group
Cross-sectional: Time frame that collects or reviews the data at one point in time
Cross-sectional (prevalence) study: Explores a disease by determining the prevalence in a community or geographic area at a particular point in time
Curvilinear associations: Common nonlinear associations named for their shapes, such as *s*-curves, *j*-curves, and *u*-curves
Database: An organized collection of data typically represented by multiple tables that are connected by keys
Data cleaning: The process of detecting, diagnosing, and editing faulty data; also called data cleansing and data scrubbing
Data dictionary: A descriptive list of names (also called representations or displays), definitions, and attributes of data elements to be collected in an information system or database
Data mining: The semiautomated and automated processes for exploring large databases and detecting relevant patterns and relationships (knowledge) in the data contained in those databases
Data science: The application of methods related to extracting value from existing data to solve problems, including analyzing existing data sets to identify patterns
Data set: A file of related data, which are typically organized in rows and columns
Data visualization: The use of graphics to examine data
Decision tree: A machine-learning technique used to predict categorical or numerical variables by creating rules from training data that result in the best performance of the model
Declaration of Helsinki: An international statement of ethical principles for biomedical research involving humans
Deductive reasoning: Involves drawing conclusions based on generalizations, rules, or principles. Deductive reason is "top down," meaning that deductive reasoning goes from the general to the specific.
Dependent samples: Matched or paired samples or repeated measures
Dependent variable: The hypothesized change, is measured *before* and *after* the intervention
Descriptive analytics: Summarize data into meaningful charts and reports
Descriptive research: Determines and reports on the current status of topics and subjects; descriptive research studies seek to accurately capture or portray dimensions or characteristics of people, organizations, situations, technology, or other phenomena
Descriptive statistics: Describe "what is" by classifying, organizing, and summarizing numerical data about a particular group of observations
Diagnostic trials: Conducted to find better tests, procedures, or screenings to detect a disease or condition
Direct observation: Researchers are present in the environment they are observing so they can personally conduct the observation
Discrete data: Separate and distinct values or observations that can be measured across a set of fixed values
Discriminant (divergent) validity: The degree to which the instrument does *not* positively correlate to instruments measuring dissimilar constructs or the degree to which items measuring dissimilar constructs are uncorrelated
Dissemination: The planned, strategic distribution of information to a targeted audience
Distributed computing: Spreads data and analytics tasks equally across many computers to speed processing time
Effect size: Index that quantifies the degree to which a study's results should be considered important or unimportant
Elicitation: A technique of data collection that evokes, brings out, or draws out knowledge, ideas, perceptions, beliefs, memories, needs, and other, often hidden, phenomena
Eligibility criteria: Specify the types of facilities eligible to apply for funding
Empiricism: The theory that true knowledge is based on observations and direct experiences that can be perceived through the physical senses, such as eyesight or hearing; one component of scientific inquiry

Environment: The physical surroundings of the host and agent as well as environmental influences such as disasters (tornado, flood, hurricane, war), crowding, neighborhood density, housing, and workplace conditions
Epidemiologists: Scientists who study changes in the incidence and prevalence of diseases over time, variations in the incidence of diseases among communities, and whether individuals with a disease have characteristics or risk factors that distinguish them from individuals without the disease
Epidemiology: Scientific field that examines the patterns of disease occurrence in human populations and the factors that influence these patterns in relation to time, place, and persons.
Error rate: The number of observations the model incorrectly predicts divided by the actual number of observations
Ethics: The norms for conduct that distinguish between acceptable and unacceptable behavior
Ethnography: The exhaustive examination of a culture by collecting data and making observations while being in the field (a naturalistic setting)
Evaluation methods: Used to measure program activities and determine value of the program, to undertake quality improvement, and to contribute to generalizable scientific knowledge
Evaluation research: The systematic application of criteria to assess the value of objects
Exclusion criteria: The criteria used to remove articles from the study
Exempt from review: A category of review for research projects that do not collect identifiable information and do not pose a risk to subjects
Expedited review: A category of review for minor changes in previously approved research during the period (of one year or less) for which approval is authorized, and research projects that involve no more than minimal risk for subjects and are in one of the authorized categories
Experimental procedures: How the intervention or treatment is applied in the study
Experimental research: A research design in which researchers follow a strict procedure to randomly assign subjects to groups, manipulate the subjects' experience, and finally measure any resulting physical, behavioral, or other changes in the subjects.
Experimental (study) group: Comprises the research subjects who receive the study's intervention
Exploratory data analysis (EDA): Involves getting a basic understanding of a dataset through numerous variable summaries and visual plots
External validity: The extent to which a research study's findings can be generalized to the broader population, people, or groups.
Face page: Introductory material on a grant proposal, similar to a title page
Face validity: Confirmation at the surface level ("face value") that the survey seems to measure what it set out to measure.
Factor analysis: A statistical technique in which a large number of variables are summarized and reduced to a smaller number based on similar relationships among those variables
Federal Policy for the Protection of Human Subjects: Set of federal regulations created by the HHS and FDA that protect the rights, welfare, and well-being of subjects involved in research and gives the Office for Human Research Protections (OHRP) oversight of compliance with the federal regulations; *See also* **Office for Human Research Protections (OHRP)**
Federal-wide assurance of compliance (FWA): A formal, written, and binding commitment in which an institution promises to comply with applicable regulations governing research with human subjects and stipulates the procedures through which compliance will be achieved, "regardless of whether the research is subject to federal regulation" (45 CFR 46.103(b)(1))
Fidelity: Keeping promises and honoring contracts and agreements
Field notes: The documentation the ethnographic researcher maintains
Five rights of clinical decision support: States that optimal design and implementation of clinical decision support will be achieved if the system provides (1) the right information (2) to the right person, (3) in the right format, (4) through the right channel, and (5) at the right time in the workflow
Fixed-effects model: Calculates a pooled effect estimate by assuming all the variations among studies are caused by chance
Focused interview: Uses open-ended questions to solicit the interviewee's opinions about a specific topic
Focus group: A group of subjects, who are often experts in an area of study, who discuss a specific topic in a focused interview with a moderator

Forecasting: Predicting outcomes at a date in the future
Forest plot: A graphical display of estimated results from multiple studies on the same topic, the amount of variation, and the overall estimate of the effect
Formative evaluation: Measures or assesses improvement in delivery methods with regard to technology used; quality of implementation of a new process or technology; information about the organizational placement of a given process; type of personnel involved in a program; or other important factors such as the procedures, source, and type of inputs
Frequency distribution: The frequency with which values of a variable occur in a sample or population
Full review: A category of review for research projects that represent more than minimal risk for the subjects and, therefore, are presented to a quorum of IRB members, who may discuss the proposal at length
Funding opportunity announcement (FOA): *See* **Request for application (RFA)**
Funnel plot: A scatter plot of the intervention effect estimated from individual studies against some measure of each study's size or precision
Gelsinger case: The first publicly reported case of a death in a gene therapy clinical trial.
General interview guide: An outline or checklist used to guide interviews rather than standardized questions; the interviewer can choose which areas to cover and may not cover all of them
Generalizability: Means capable of being applied to other similar situations and people.
Geospatial analysis: Uses geographical maps to illustrate differences in data across variables
GRADE (Grading of Recommendations, Assessment, Development and Evaluation) system: Used to judge the quality of evidence in healthcare literature and evidence-based research
Grant: In healthcare research, receipt of a financial assistance award for peer-reviewed research that extends health and decreases illness and disability
Grantee: Recipient of grant money
Grey literature: The body of publications that is available in print, electronically, or both, but is not published in easily accessible publications, such as journals
Grounded theory: Analyzes data and generates theories through coding, categorization, and comparison; uses both quantitative and qualitative findings and enables researchers to develop a theory substantiated by data; *See also* **Constant comparative method**
Group case study: Resembles the individual case study except the interviews or observations are performed on a group of individuals instead of just one individual.
Hand search: Visiting the websites of journals and performing keyword search there
Health informatics research: The investigation of the process, application, and impact of computer science, information systems, and communication technologies to health services
Health information management (HIM) research: Involves investigations into the practice of acquiring, analyzing, storing, disclosing, retaining, and protecting information vital to the delivery, provision, and management of health services. HIM research has a narrower scope than health informatics research
Health Information National Trends Survey (HINTS): A population-based survey that could be used to track trends in the use of communication technologies, such as the Internet, as a source of cancer information
Health Information Technology for Economic and Clinical Health (HITECH) Act: Legislation created to promote the adoption and meaningful use of health information technology and provide for additional privacy and security requirements that will develop and support electronic health information, facilitate information exchange, and strengthen monetary penalties
Health Research Extension Act: Mandated the secretary of HHS to issue a regulation requiring institutions receiving research awards to establish an administrative process to review reports of scientific misconduct and report to the federal government their investigations into the misconduct
Health services research: Multidisciplinary research that studies how social factors, financing systems, organizational structures and processes, health technologies, and personal behaviors affect access to healthcare, its quality and cost, and overall health and well-being
Health technology assessment (HTA): Evaluation of the usefulness (utility) of a health technology in relation to cost, efficacy, utilization, and other factors in terms of its impact on social, ethical, and legal systems
Heterogeneity: Means variation or diversity
Histogram: Shows major characteristics in the distribution of data and summarizes data about variables whose values are numerical and measured on an interval or ratio scale (continuous data)

Historical-prospective study: Study groups are identified from data about characteristics in existing data sources and the groups are followed over time, usually from the time the data were first collected to the present or into the future, to examine their outcomes
Historical research: Examines historical materials to explain, interpret, and provide a factual account of events
History: The events happening in the course of the experiment
Holmesburg Prison studies: Unjust experiments conducted with prisoners as subjects at Holmesburg Prison in Philadelphia, PA, from the early 1950s through the mid-1970s
Honesty: In the context of a research study, a complete, truthful accounting for all parts of the research study
Host: The person who has the disease under study
Human Genome Project (HGP): An international, collaborative research program whose goal was the complete mapping and understanding of all the genes of human beings, prioritized the ethical implications of its investigations
Human radiation experiments: A series of unethical experiments sponsored by the several federal agencies and conducted by researchers affiliated with government agencies, universities, hospitals and other research institutions between 1944 and 1974
Hypothesis: A statement of the researchers' predictions on the outcome of the study
Impact evaluation: Assesses the overall effects of the program or software implementation in terms of the larger organization, community, or system
Impact factor: A ratio between citations and recently published citable items
Implementation evaluation: Used to examine the fidelity of the actual program delivery as compared to the planned delivery
Implementation science: A discipline that studies how and why implementation of evidence in clinical practice succeeds or fails
Imputation: The substitution of values for the missing values
IMRAD: A general guideline for scientific papers that stands for *i*ntroduction, *m*ethods, *r*esults, *a*nd *d*iscussion
Incidence cases: Patients newly diagnosed with a disease
Incidence rate: The rate at which new cases of a disease or health characteristic occur
Inclusion criteria: The criteria used to keep articles in the study
Independent samples: Samples that have no effect on one another and are not correlated
Independent variable: Manipulatable factor or action that the researchers are proposing will cause the hypothesized change
Indirect costs: Cover such items as office space, use of library resources, electricity, and so forth; also called facilities and administration costs
Indirect observation: Researchers use audio or video recording so that the environment is not changed in any way from the norm
Individual case study: The researcher collects as much relevant information as they can on an individual as he or she progresses through a certain disease, procedure, treatment, cultural, or health information system change
Inductive reasoning: Involves drawing conclusions based on a limited number of observations; inductive reasoning is "bottom up," meaning that it goes from the specific to the general
Infectious disease model: Demonstrates how infectious disease is influenced by three factors: the agent, the host and the environment
Inferential statistics: Allow investigators to detect differences or associations between groups and to generalize those findings from the sample to the entire population of interest
Informal conversational interviews: Which are loosely structured and may flow like a conversation between the person being interviewed and the researcher
Informed consent: Signifies that the subject was given a complete and understandable explanation of the experiment and its risks and based his or her decision to participate or not to participate on that information, without being coerced or unduly influenced
Innovation: 1. Having unique and original qualities; 2. An idea or proposal that challenges existing clinical practice and uses novel concepts, approaches, and technologies
Institutional case study: Is used to observe a healthcare institution or facility to determine how it conducts a process, system, or procedure. Individual case studies may be included within the institutional case study, but the focus is on the institution-wide system, process, or procedure

Institutional ethics committees: *See* bioethics committees
Institutional review board (IRB): Which is the institutional body that provides review, oversight, guidance, and approval for research projects carried out by employees serving as researchers, regardless of the location of the research (such as a university or private research agency) and which is responsible for protecting the rights and welfare of the human subjects involved in the research
Instrument: A standardized, uniform way to collect data
Instrumentation: How a particular survey, interview, procedure or intervention may be performed; may affect internal validity
Intention-to-treat (ITT) analysis: Defined as the principle in which subjects of a randomized controlled trial (RCT) are analyzed within the group to which they were originally allocated with no regard to noncompliance or deviations from the protocol
Interaction of factors: A combination of the factors affecting validity, may also bias the final results
Internal consistency reliability: The homogeneity of an instrument's items
Internal validity: An attribute of a research study design that contributes to the accuracy of its findings and can be threatened by factors or influences outside the study, such as confounding variables.
Interquartile range (IQR): Range within which the middle 50 percent of values fall. Interquartile ranges can be calculated for ordinal and metric data
Interrater reliability: Means that different persons completing the instrument or test have reasonably similar results
Interval data: Represent values or observations that occur on an evenly distributed scale that does not begin with a true zero
Interval scale: Measure in which the intervals between adjacent scale values are equal with respect to the attributes being measured; does not have a meaningful absolute zero
Intervention: *See* **Independent variable**
Intrarater reliability: Means that the same person completing the instrument or test at different times will have reasonably similar results
Investigators: Personnel who carry out the research
Jewish Chronic Disease Hospital study: An experiment conducted in 1963 in which live cancer cells were injected into 22 weak and chronically ill patients
Justice: In research, means individuals are treated fairly during enrollment and when they participate in a study
Key personnel: All staff, professional and non-professional
***k*-means clustering:** An algorithm for partitioning a data set into multiple groups (clusters) and systematically analyzing the data to identify observations that are similar based on multiple characteristics
Knowledge discovery in databases (KDD): Algorithmic means by which patterns are extracted and enumerated from data
Kurtosis: A measure of the heaviness of both tails of a frequency distribution
Letter of intent: Describes the focus and goal of the research project and enables the granting agency to determine whether a full application is of interest
Likelihood ratio (LR): One number into which sensitivity and specificity can be merged
Likert scale: Allows respondents to record their level of agreement or disagreement along a range of five categories
Line graph: Displays trends for one variable over time
Logic model: A graphic representation of the logic of how things work
Logistic regression: Aims to predict a categorical target, which is a dependent variable that is qualitative and falls into groups
Longitudinal: Time frame collects data from participants in at least three or more *waves* (phases) to compare changes in health, satisfaction, effectiveness, perceptions, and other variables of interest
Manuscript: An unpublished paper
Matching requirements: Any costs of the specific research project that are not going to be funded by the granting agency and therefore can be shared or matched with the entity submitting the grant, who in turn can seek these funds through their own entity or other funding agencies
Maturation: The natural changes of research subjects that occur during the length of time that they are in the study
Mean: Average calculated by adding up all the values and dividing by the number of values. Calculating the mean is only appropriate for metric data

Measures of central tendency: The clustering of the majority of a data set's values around its middle value
Measures of dispersion: The distribution of observations away from the central value
Median: Middle value when all the values are placed in numeric order
Meta-analysis: The statistical arm within the systematic review; it combines both quantitative and qualitative research studies to arrive at a statistically sound conclusion
Meta-regression: A regression analysis of the data from multiple studies. Meta-regression is typically used when the number of selected studies is large (> 10)
Metric data: Interval and ratio data
Midtests: Observations that are administered at the midpoint of a study
Mixed-methods research: Combines (mixes) quantitative and qualitative theoretical perspectives, methods, sampling strategies, data collection techniques, data sets, analytic procedures, representational modes, or any combination of these aspects of research ; also known as mixed research
Mode: Value that occurs most frequently
Model: An idealized representation that abstracts and simplifies a real-world situation so the situation can be studied, analyzed, or both
Modeling: The process of using existing data to construct an explanation of how they were created
Mortality: *See* **Attrition**
Multinomial logistic regression: Analysis method used if the target variable has more than two levels,
Multiple linear regression: Analysis method used when multiple predictors are used to predict the outcome.
Multiple logistic regression: Term for a regression method if the target variable is binary
Multivariate: Correlational tests involve multiple dependent (outcome) variables
Multivariate analysis: Shows the relationship between multiple independent variables and a dependent variable
National Center for Health Statistics (NCHS): A part of the CDC and provides data and statistics to identify and address health issues within the United States, use survey research to compile useful statistics
National Health Interview Survey (NHIS): A study from the NCHS that describes the health status of individuals and their families
National Institutes of Health (NIH): The primary federal agency that provides grant funding to researchers so that they are able to conduct clinical research
National Library of Medicine (NLM): The world's largest medical library and a branch of the National Institutes of Health
National Research Act: Provides a framework for the protection of human subjects in biomedical and behavioral research
Naturalistic observation: Researchers record observations that are unprompted and unaffected by the investigators' actions.
Needs assessment: Determines organizational goals and gaps between the actual state and the desired state. It also identifies the parties that need resources and what kinds of resources are needed
Negative (inverse) linear relationship (association): Exists when the scores of the variables proportionately move in *opposite (inverse)* directions
Negative predictive value (NPV): The probability that a person does *not* have a characteristic when the measure is *negative*
Newcastle-Ottawa Scale (NOS): An assessment tool designed for evaluating the quality of nonrandomized studies, can be used to assess the quality of case-control and cohort studies.
Nominal data: Values or observations that can be named or labeled
Nominal scales: Scales that simply name, label, or categorize the response and assign a numerical value to the response for purposes of easier data analysis.
Nonmaleficence: Ethical principle that means doing no harm
Nonparametric: Tests that generally make no assumptions about the distribution of the population's parameters
Nonparametric data: Discrete data, nominal data, and ordinal data
Nonparticipant observation: Researchers act as neutral observers who neither intentionally interact with nor affect the actions of the participants being observed
Nonrandom (nonprobability) sampling: Does not use statistical methods of probability to select samples, and all members of the target population do *not* have an equal and independent chance of being selected for the research study

Nonrandom selection: The selection of subjects that is not random; it is also known as nonprobability sampling because each subject's probability of being selected is unknown and could be either equal or unequal; generally associated with the qualitative approach
Normal (bell) curve: Symmetrical distribution of data that underlies many statistical tests
Normal distribution: When the frequencies of a variable's values are graphed, they form a bell-shaped curve
Null hypothesis: States that there is no difference or there is no association between the independent variable and the dependent variable
Null hypothesis significance testing (NHST): Method used to determine the likelihood that the research study's findings are *not* the result of random chance or a biased sample
Number needed to treat (NNT): The number of people who need to receive the intervention for one person to benefit from the intervention
Numerical items: Request that the respondent enter a number
Nuremberg Code: Set of 10 ethical principles that guide human experimentation
Observational research: Exploratory research that identifies factors, contexts, and experiences through observations in natural settings
Odds ratio (OR): The chance of an event occurring in one group compared to the chance of it occurring in another group
Office for Civil Rights (OCR): The agency within the HHS that enforces federal civil rights laws and HIPAA of 1996
Office for Human Research Protections (OHRP): Government body that oversees compliance with the Federal Policy for the Protection of Human Subjects. *See also* **Federal Policy for the Protection of Human Subjects**
Office of Research Integrity (ORI): The agency in the HHS that monitors compliance with the Health Research Extension Act. The ORI is charged with promoting research integrity and preventing research misconduct
One group pretest-posttest method: Similar to the one-shot case study except that the pretest is used before the intervention
One-shot case study: A simple design in which an intervention is provided to one group and they are followed forward in time after intervention to assess the outcome (posttest).
One-tailed hypothesis: The researcher predicts the direction of the results as being more or less (greater or smaller, higher or lower)
Open-ended (unstructured) questions: Do not have a specific choice of answers, and the participant can provide their oral or written responses in their own words, similar to an essay exam; also known as qualitative questions
Operational definition: Term from the literature (the body of published studies and authoritative books) that is measurable and capable of generating data
Operationalize: To formulate a problem statement using operational definitions obtained during the literature review
Oral paper presentation: The researcher gives a formal talk about a research paper, often accompanied by visual aids, such as PowerPoint slides or flip charts
Ordinal data: Represent values or observations that can be ranked (ordered)
Ordinal scale: Used when the answer to a question or value can be rank-ordered
Outcome evaluation: Assesses whether the specifically defined target outcomes were demonstrated
Panel of reviewers: Experts in a scientific area who evaluate grant applications
Papers: Written manuscripts that present research results related to the event's theme
Parametric data: Continuous data, interval data, and ratio data
Parametric test: A type of statistical procedure, such as the *t*-test or ANOVA, that is based on the assumption that a variable is normally distributed in a population
Parsimony: In the context of research, means that explanations of phenomena should include the fewest assumptions, conditions, and extraneous complications
Participant observation: Researchers participate in the observed actions, activities, processes, or other situations
Peer review: A system in which journals' editors and peer reviewers work with authors to improve the quality of articles and advance scientific knowledge
Peer-reviewed research: Research that is examined and evaluated by experts in the same or a related research field or scientific area
Phase I clinical trials: Usually test a new drug or treatment in a small group of people (20 to 100) for the first time to evaluate its safety, determine a safe dosage, and identify any side effects

Phase II clinical trials: Study the intervention in a larger group of people (100 to 300)
Phase III clinical trials: Study it in even larger groups of people (300 to 3,000) to confirm its effectiveness, monitor side effects, compare other treatments, and collect data to affirm that the drug or treatment can be used safely
Phase IV clinical trials: Carried out after a drug or device has been approved by the FDA; these postmarket safety monitoring studies collect additional information after the drug has been marketed, such as the drug's risks, benefits, and optimal use
PICO(TS): An acronym that stands for the elements of a well-developed, manageable research question, patent, intervention, comparison, outcome, timing, and setting
PICOS: Stands for *participants, interventions, comparisons, outcome(s),* and *study design setting*; may also be seen as PICO (no S) or as PICOT with T standing for *time*
Pie chart: Visually shows the proportions (percentages) of a variable in each value, relationships among the values, and the whole
Pilot test: A trial run on a small scale that enhances the likelihood of a study's successful completion because it provides an opportunity to work out the details of the research plan, on the survey questionnaire
Policy and Procedure Order 129: Contained directives concerning research and investigations involving human subjects in institutions receiving PHS grant money
Positive (direct) linear relationship (association): Exists when the scores for variables proportionately move in the *same* direction
Positive predictive value (PPV): The probability that a person has the characteristic when the measure is positive
Positivism: Proposes that knowledge should be based on universal laws, objectivity, and observed facts
Poster presentation: Session in which the researcher visually presents information about a research study on a poster with graphics and text, answers questions about the study, and hands out papers detailing the research study
Posttest-only control group method: Similar to the pretest-posttest control group method except that the posttest-only method does not use a pretest
Precision: The degree of certainty
Predictive analytics: Provide forecasts for the future based on analysis of past performance as demonstrated in historical data
Predictive modeling: The use of models to forecast from existing data whether an event will occur
Preferred Reporting Items for Systematic Review and Meta-Analysis Protocols (PRISMA-P): 17 items that are considered essential, minimum components to include in systematic reviews and meta-analyses
Prescriptive analytics: Technique used to identify the best alternatives to minimize or maximize some objective
Pretest-posttest control group method: A classic experimental design in which participants are randomly assigned to either the intervention (experimental) or nonintervention (control) group with measurements taken before and after intervention or observation
Prevalence rate: The proportion of people in a population who have a particular disease or health characteristic at a specific point in time or over a period of time
Prevalence study: A study that examines existing diseases to generate new hypotheses rather than to prove existing hypotheses; does not answer questions regarding causation; *See* **Cross-sectional study**
Prevarication bias: Respondents may exaggerate or lie in their answers to the questions, especially when answering questions related to salary or other sensitive matters
Prevention trials: Aim to prevent disease in a person who has never had the disease or to prevent it from advancing or recurring
Primary analysis: The analysis of original research data by the researchers who collected the data for a specific study
Primary data: The data researchers collect to answer their own specific research question
Primary source: Firsthand source, including original documents, artifacts (objects, such as computers or paper records), and oral histories (first-person, spoken accounts)
Principal investigator (PI): The leader of the research project for which the grant proposal is being written
Privacy Rule: Element of HIPAA that establishes minimum standards to protect the privacy of health information that identifies individuals who are living or deceased
Problem statement: A single sentence with an action verb, such as *explore* or *compare,* that specifically and succinctly states what the researcher will be doing to investigate the problem or question
Proceedings: Are published collections of the papers, and often the abstracts, delivered at events

Process evaluation: Used to determine how well the project was carried out
Program officer: Person who leads a specific RFA, RFP, or FOA and is the primary person who will address any questions that investigators may have while developing the proposal
Proportion: A type of ratio in which the numerator's quantity is included in the denominator
Proposal reviewer: An individual with an extensive background or experience in a research area who reviews the grant proposals and provides comments
Prospective: Study design time frame that follows subjects into the future to examine relationships between variables and later occurrences
PROSPERO: An international prospective register of systematic reviews
Protocol: A step-by-step plan on how the trial will be conducted; *See also* **Research protocol**
Publication bias: Results when researchers or scientific journal editors treat studies that demonstrate positive results differently from studies that demonstrate negative results
Purpose statement: A declarative sentence that summarizes the specific topic and goals of the research study
Purposive sampling: Method in which qualitative researchers use their expertise to select both representative units and unrepresentative units of the population
***P* value:** A statistical summary of the compatibility between the observed data and what would be predicted or expected if all the assumptions, such as normal distribution, used to compute the *P* value were correct
Qualitative approach: Involves investigations to describe, interpret, and understand processes, events, and relationships as perceived by individuals or groups
Qualitative data analysis: A systematic process of working with data to create coherent descriptions and explanations of phenomena
Quality appraisal: The assessment of the quality of selected studies
Quality-of-life (QOL) trials: Explore methods used to improve comfort and the QOL for individuals, such as people with a chronic disease or disability
Quantitative approach: Explains phenomena by making predictions, collecting and analyzing evidence, testing alternative theories, and choosing the best theory
Quantitative data analysis: Examines, probes, and transforms large amounts of numerical data into understandable information through the application of descriptive statistics and inferential statistics
Quasi-experimental research: Searches for *plausible* causal factors or indicates that a causal relationship *could* exist. They often do not use randomization.
Quota sampling: Subjects are selected to ensure proportionate representation of various strata present in the population
Random-effects: Model calculates the effect estimate by assuming there are other sources of variation among included studies
Randomization: The random allocation of subjects to the comparison groups
Randomized controlled trial (RCT): Study in which subjects are randomly selected and randomly assigned to an experimental group or a control group
Random sampling: Which is the unbiased selection of subjects from the population of interest
Range: Difference between greatest and smallest value
Rater reliability: Consistency in the scoring of tests by one or more raters, indicating the extent to which subjectivity has been eliminated
Ratio data: Represent values or observations that occur on an evenly distributed scale that begins at a true zero
Ratios: Comparison of two values
Ratio scale: Continuous data have both equal intervals and an absolute zero (0) point that is clearly defined and meaningful
Recall bias: Respondents may not remember correctly so their answers will be inaccurate
Receiver operating characteristic (ROC) curves: Plot sensitivity versus specificity at different thresholds and graphically show a measure's ability to predict an outcome
Relative risk (RR): A measure of the strength of an association between the exposure (independent variable) and the disease or outcome (dependent variable)
Relative risk reduction (RRR): The percentage that an intervention reduces risk in the experimental group compared to the control group
Reliability: The extent to which a procedure or an instrument yields similar results over repeated trials, over time, across similar groups, within individuals, and across raters

Request for application (RFA): The project announcement that describes the project and encourages researchers to apply; may list additional criteria specific to the announcement
Request for proposal (RFP): *See* **Request for application (RFA)**
Research: A systematic process of inquiry aimed at discovering or creating new knowledge about a topic; confirming or evaluating existing knowledge; or revising outdated knowledge
Research design: A plan to achieve the researchers' purpose: answering a question, solving a problem, or generating new information
Research frame: The overarching structure of a research project
Research method: A set of specific procedures used to gather and analyze data
Research methodology: The study and analysis of research methods and theories
Research misconduct: Act that includes falsifying data, fabricating data and results, and plagiarizing
Research project website: Used to make information about a research project accessible to practitioners, other researchers, policymakers, possible research participants, and other potentially interested persons or groups
Research protocol: Defines the detailed steps the research team should follow to conduct the research; *See also* **Protocol**
Research question: An explicit statement of the question a research team wants to answer in a research project
Respect for persons: Recognition of the personal dignity and autonomy of individuals and special protection of those persons with diminished autonomy
Response bias: When there is a systematic difference, such as computer-savviness or age, between the responders (participants) and nonresponders (nonparticipants)
Response rate: The percentage of subjects answering the survey
Retrospective: Research time frame that looks back in time on that which has already occurred
Rich data: Thick descriptions and layers of extensive details from multiple sources
Rigor: For quantitative researchers, rigor is the "strict application of the scientific method to ensure unbiased and well-controlled experimental design, methodology, analysis, interpretation and report of results … and includes transparency in reporting full experimental details so that others may reproduce and extend the findings" (NIH/AHRQ 2015). For qualitative researchers, rigor is the trustworthiness of the interpretation of the study's findings
Risk of bias: The chance that a systematic error or deviation from the truth exists in results or inferences
Robust: Characteristic of parametric tests that are relatively unaffected by deviations from the assumptions and are still able to produce accurate, unbiased results
Sample size: The number of subjects needed in a study to represent the population
Sample size calculation: Refers to the quantitative and qualitative procedures used to estimate the appropriate sample size
Sample survey: Collects data from representative members of the population
Sampling: The process of selecting the units to represent the target population
Sampling error: A difference between the population and sample due to pure chance
Sampling frame: The list of subjects from which the sample is drawn
Sanctity: Ethical principle meaning that humans are valued and have rights just because they exist
Saturation: A point of closure when there is repetition and convergence of information and no new themes, ideas, or concepts are emerging
Scale: A form of categorical item that uses progressive categories, such as size, amount, importance, rank, or agreement
Scatter graph: Plot or diagram that shows the association between two variables
Scientific inquiry: Use of diverse ways to systematically gather data about phenomena, critically analyze the data, propose explanations based on their evidence, and develop understanding and knowledge
Scientific review group (SRG): Entity that assesses the proposal's scientific and technical merit
Scientific review officer (SRO): Reviews the application for completeness and content, and assigns the most appropriate proposal reviewer
Screening process: The process of selecting (filtering) articles according to predetermined inclusion and exclusion criteria
Screening trials: Examine the best method to detect diseases or health conditions
Secondary analysis: Any research in which researchers use data for purposes not defined nor predicted in the original study's design

Secondary data: Data that were originally collected for another specific purpose
Secondary source: In historical research, sources created by people uninvolved with the event; generally, secondary sources aggregate, summarize, critique, analyze, or manipulate the primary sources, and, as such, they are derived from primary sources
Security Rule: Portion of HIPAA that protects the security of electronically stored PHI that is created, received, used, or maintained by a covered entity
Seed money: Funding, often from an internal source or a foundation, that enables an investigator to begin research in a new area of interest
Selection bias: The ability of some participants to choose to answer the survey questionnaire or be part of the survey research study
Semantic differential scales: Allow respondents to rate products, healthcare organizations, or other services using adjectives that are polar opposites on the ends of a continuum
Semistructured interview: Follows a guide but allows additional questions that seem appropriate or that are triggered by the participants' comments
Semistructured questions: Begin with structured questions and then follow with open-ended questions to clarify
Sensitivity: The ability of a measure to detect a characteristic (such as disease) when the characteristic exists
Sensitivity analysis: Analytic technique to test whether a study's results change if assumptions, statistical techniques, inputs, or other elements of a research plan are varied
Sensitivity rate: A measure of validity; percentage of all true cases correctly labeled where TP/(TP + FN)
Significance: Importance of the research area
Significance level: A pre-established threshold that determines whether the null hypothesis is rejected
Simple linear regression: Aims to predict an outcome (dependent variable) based upon a single predictor (independent variable)
Simple random sampling: Which gives every member of the population under study an equal chance of being selected
Simulation observation: Researchers stage events rather than allowing them to occur naturally
Skewness: The nonsymmetrical slant or tilt of the distribution. It occurs when values are overly represented in one of the tails of the distribution
Snowball sampling: Initial contacts (units) suggest additional contacts who also could be informative; also called *chain* or *nominated sampling*
Sociotechnical system: The interaction of HIT functions and processes, such as information governance, EHRs, computer-assisted coding, clinical decision support, and computerized patient order entry
Solomon four-group method: Similar to the pretest-posttest design but includes two intervention or experimental groups and two control groups; pretests are used for one of the intervention groups and one of the control groups and posttests are used for all groups.
Specific aims: Component of a grant application that consists of the research objectives and goals for the project
Specificity: The ability of a measure to detect the absence of a characteristic (again, such as disease) when the characteristic is absent
Specificity rate: A measure of validity; percentage of all true non-cases correctly labeled where TN/(TN + FP)
Stakeholders: In evaluation projects and evaluation research, the recipients of the product, service, technology, or process being evaluated as well as participants in the evaluation.
Standard deviation: Average distance from the mean that each value lies
Standardized open-ended interviews: Researchers develop a set of questions ahead of time and then follow the wording and order of questions closely when conducting the interview.
Static group comparison method: When two groups are examined, one with the intervention and one without, and then a posttest is given to assess the result of the intervention
Statistical analysis plan (SAP): A document that contains technical and detailed descriptions of the statistical analyses that will be performed on a research study's variables and other data
Statistical conclusion validity: The extent to which the statistical conclusions about the relationships in the data are reasonable
Statistical regression: Can affect the internal validity of a study when extreme values (outliers) unduly affect the calculation of the mean

Statistics: The science of collecting, classifying, displaying, analyzing, and interpreting numerical data, to benefit from and make sense of the numerical data that surround them
Stem-and-leaf diagrams: Summarize data while maintaining all the individual data points
Stratified random sampling: Separate the population by certain characteristics, such as physician specialties, nursing units, or diagnosis-related groups (DRGs), and then choose the random sample.
Streamlining: Not discussing proposals that fall in the lower half of the scoring at the meeting to discuss proposals, but critiquing and returning them to the applicants for resubmission
Structured questions: *See* **Closed-ended (structured) questions**
Subgroup analysis: Evaluation of data representing subsets of participants or subsets of studies
Subject matter experts (SMEs): Authorities in the instrument's domain, topic, or field
Submission guidelines: Explicit rules that authors are expected to follow if they want their manuscript published
Summative evaluation: Occurs at or near the end of the project or research and is undertaken to assess effectiveness of the program.
Supervised learning: A model built on a training database when the values or other attributes of the independent variables are *known* and the target is *known*. During the model's training phase, the algorithms learn the relationship (dependency) and, then, during subsequent deployment in other databases, can predict the target
Survey: Systematically collects data about a population (entire group) to determine its current status regarding certain factors
Survey research: Collects research data by asking questions, with the responses being collected via the mail, through websites, mobile apps, or by telephone, fax, e-mail or text message
Survival analysis: Also called life table analysis, examines survival of study subjects over time and compares whether the intervention group survived longer than the control group
Systematic random sampling: Draw the sample from a list of items such as diagnoses, ICD-10-CM codes, or discharges and select every *nth* case
Systematic review: Uses a predetermined plan to search, evaluate, and synthesize the results on a topic area
System Usability Scale (SUS): A 10-item questionnaire that measures usability of products and services based on the respondents' Likert-scale responses indicating their level of agreement with the questions; these scores are then converted to numbers
Target population: The set of individuals (or objects) of interest to the researchers and the focus of their research study
Tearoom Trade study: A research project to examine the sexual behavior of men in public restrooms conducted by Laud Humphreys in St. Louis, MO, in the late 1960s, a time when engaging in homosexual sex was illegal
Testing: The effect created when participants are exposed in the pretest to questions that may be on the posttest
Test-retest reliability: Determines whether the survey instrument is consistent over time or when given multiple times
Theoretical sampling: Subjects are selected as topics emerge to ensure representation of those topics and to build theory.
Theory: The systematic organization of knowledge that explains or predicts phenomena, such as behavior or events
Theory of change: A statement that explains how activities will produce a series of results
Time-series tests: Observations that may be conducted at intervals throughout the study period
Translational research: Two aspects: applying discoveries generated during basic research to the development of research studies with human subjects, and enhancing the sector's adoption of best practices and cost-effective strategies to prevent, diagnosis, and treat health conditions
Treatment trials: Test experimental treatments, new combinations of medicines, and various types of surgery, radiation therapy, or chemotherapy
Trend analysis: Involves collecting data over time to determine changes, trends, or patterns in the data
Triangulation: The use of multiple sources or perspectives to investigate the same phenomenon.
Tuskegee Study of Untreated Syphilis in the Negro Male: Also known as the US Public Health Service Syphilis Study, was conducted by the US Public Health Service (PHS) between 1932 and 1972 in rural counties around Tuskegee, AL
Two-tailed hypothesis: The researcher makes no prediction about the direction of the results
Type I error: Occurs when the researcher erroneously rejects the null hypothesis when it is true; in actuality, there is no difference or relationship
Type II error: Occurs when the researcher erroneously fails to reject the null hypothesis when it is false
Unit of analysis: The group, object, or phenomenon for which the researchers have collected data to analyze

Unit of analysis error: A mismatch between the unit of randomization and the data (measurements or observations) that are used for statistical tests

Univariate: Characteristic of descriptive statistics meaning they analyze one variable. Researchers begin with descriptive statistics to verify the accuracy of the data entry

Univariate association: The relationship between a variable and a dependent variable

Unstructured questions: *See* **Open-ended (unstructured) questions**

Unsupervised learning: Type of modeling that is exploratory in that there is no dependent variable of interest (target) and the algorithm searches through the database to discover potentially significant relationships or patterns among fields in the database

Usability testing: Evaluation that assesses whether a product or service achieves its intended goals effectively, efficiently, and satisfactorily for representative users in a typical setting

User-centered design: Founded on an "explicit understanding of users, tasks, and environments; is driven and refined by user-centered evaluation; and addresses the whole user experience" (HHS 2017a)

Utility: Ethical principle that involves considering the usefulness of an act, which is evaluated by its effects, including its benefits and costs

Validity: As it relates to instruments, means the extent to which the instrument measures what it is intended to measure

Variables: Characteristics that are measured and may take on different values

Vioxx case: Involves a pharmaceutical company that violated the principle of honesty by marketing a drug while knowingly suppressing information about its serious adverse side-effects

Vulnerable population: Those people who "are likely to be vulnerable to coercion or undue influence, such as children, prisoners, pregnant women, mentally disabled persons, or economically or educationally disadvantaged persons" (45 CFR 46.111(b))

Warrant: Justification in qualitative research

Web-based surveys: Surveys that are administered to participants via a website

White paper: A short document that seeks to inform or persuade readers

Willowbrook hepatitis studies: A series of experiments on institutionalized children with severe intellectual disabilities at Willowbrook State School

Index

2×2 table, 173

absolute risk (AR), 252
absolute risk reduction (ARR), 252–253
abstract, 206, 280, 317, 319–320
accuracy, 22
administrative safeguards, 305
adverse events, 302
advisory committee, 38
Affordable Care Act, 90
Agency for Healthcare Research and Quality (AHRQ), 214, 274, 328
agent, 102, 113
AHIMA Foundation, 276
alpha level (α), 244
American Health Information Management Association (AHIMA), 13, 276
American Hospital Association (AHA), 89, 214
American Hospital Association (AHA) guide, 47
American Medical Association (AMA), 324
American Medical Informatics Association (AMIA), 13
American Psychological Association (APA), 324
American Recovery and Reinvestment Act (ARRA) of 2009, 306
analogy, 105
analysis of covariance (ANCOVA), 182, 254
analysis of variance (ANOVA), 181, 221, 253–254
  one-way ANOVA, 181
  one-way repeated measures ANOVA, 181, 254
  two-way ANOVA, 181, 254
analysis, evaluation, and synthesis of information sources, 207
analytic study, 90
  case-control study design, 90
  cohort study design, 93
  historical-prospective study, 95
annotated bibliography, 194
annual review, 200
appendixes, 282
application for grant proposal, 278–282
  content, 279–282
  entity funding priorities, 278–279
  geographic area, 279
  intervention requirements, 279
  project objectives, 278
  target population, 279
  timelines, 278
applied research, 8
approach, 276
approvals, 229
  of oversight committees, 234
area under the curve (AUC), 136, 250
article, 319
artifacts, 16
association rule mining, 136
attrition, 81
audience, 43
autonomy, 292–293
AVDR, 76

basic research, 8
Belmont Report, 298–299, 303
beneficence, 293, 296, 298
Beta (B), 245
bias
  meta-bias, 146
  nonresponse bias, 36
  prevarication bias, 36, 44
  publication bias, 153, 326
  recall bias, 36, 91
  reporting bias, 26
  response bias, 233

risk of, 153–154,
selection bias, 48, 81,
sources of, 24
subjective bias, 23
bioethics committees, 307
biographical sketch, 280
biological plausibility, 104
biomedical research, 290
biostatistics, 163
bivariate, 178
blinding in research, 23–24
body mass index (BMI), 145
breast cancer research, 95–98, 98–99
budget, 280
business understanding, 127

CAQDAS (computer-aided qualitative data analysis software), 262
caring, 293–294
case-control study design, 90–93
examples, 92–93
steps in, 90–91
case deletion, 247
case study, 17, 56
group case study, 57
individual case study, 57
institutional case study, 57
cases, 90
categorical data, 166
categorical items in instruments, 224–225
causal-comparative research, 25
causal relationship, 16
causation, 185
epidemiological models of, 102
census survey, 46, 228
Centers for Disease Control and Prevention (CDC), 36, 62
Centers for Medicare and Medicaid Services (CMC), 15
Centers for Scientific Review (CSR), 284
Chicago Manual Style, 324
chi-square test, 179
chronic disease model, 102–103
civil monetary penalties, 304
claim of primacy, 262
classification, 134
clinical decision making in nursing scale (CDMNS), 79
clinical trial, 99–102
in health informatics, 101
phases of, 101
prevention trials, 101
protocols, 100
quality-of-life (QOL) trials, 101
treatment trials, 100
types of, 100–101
closed-ended questions, 39, 224
clustering, 135
cluster sampling, 46, 231
Cochrane collaboration tool, 153
codes of ethics, 296–297. *See also* international protection of human research subjects
for health informatics and HIM professionals, 296
Cohen's kappa (κ) coefficient, 92, 221
coherence, 104
cohort study design, 90, 93–95
collection and recording of information sources, 206
medical subject headings (MeSH), 206
Common Rule, 299–304
community trial, 99
in health informatics, 101
protocols, 100
comparative content analysis (CCA), 154
comparative effectiveness research (CER), 20
comparators, 147
comparison group, 72
complex adaptive system (CAS), 113–114
coevolution, 113
diverse agents, 113
emergence, 113
nonlinear interdependencies, 113
self-organization, 113
comprehension, 304
computer-assisted coding (CAC), users' resistance to, 103
Computerized Pediatric Infection Surveillance System (COMPISS), 79
computerized provider order entry (CPOE) system, 58, 274
conclusion validity, 261–262
concurrent validity, 220
confidence interval (CI), 251
confidence levels, 251
confidential responses, 44
confidentiality form, 285
conflict of interest form, 285
confounding (extraneous, secondary) variable, 16
Consolidated Criteria for Reporting Qualitative Research (COREQ), 323
Consolidated Standards of Reporting Trials (CONSORT 2010), 323
constant comparative method, 65, 260
construct validity, 42
constructs, 219–220
content analysis, 55, 65, 261
AHIMA computer-assisted coding (CAC) fraud and abuse study, 65

constant comparative method of, 65, 67–68
software for, 68
content validity, 42
content validity index (CVI), 218
content validity ratio (CVR), 217
context, 9, 112
contingency table, 173–174, 180
continuous data, 41, 155–156, 166, 182, 221, 254
control arm, 23. *See also* control group
control group, 23, 72, 74
convenience sample, 46
convenience sampling, 231
convergent validity, 219
correlation, 178, 185
correlational research, 14–16
cost-benefit analysis (CBA), 111
cost-effectiveness analysis (CEA), 111
covariables, 14
covariates, 14
coverage error, 230
criterion validity, 220. *See also* criteron-related validity
criterion variables, 14
criterion-related validity, 35, 220
Cronbach's alpha, 37, 43
cross-industry process for data mining (CRISP-DM), 126, 133, 136
crossover design, 73
cross-product ratio, 250
cross-sectional study, 86–89
cross-sectional time frame, 26
curvilinear associations, 167

data
access, 229–230
assembling and storing, 234–235
cleaning, 247
dictionary, 127
dredging, 257
individual or aggregate, 229–230
location of, 230
mining, 229–230, 254–256
preparation of, 245–247
primary, 255
public-domain or proprietary, 230
rich, 16, 228
scrubbing, 247
secondary, 255
set, 124
sources, 229
understanding, 127
visualization, 133
database, 124
data collection, 215–216
procedures, 234–235
qualitative plan, 216
quantitative plan, 215–216
techniques and tools of, 227–230
data science, 124–126
descriptive analytics, 126
predictive analytics, 126
prescriptive analytics, 126
decision support systems (DSS), 228–229
decision tree, 134
Declaration of Helsinki, 297
deductive reasoning, 10
dependency modeling, 136
dependent sample, 170
dependent variables, 23, 24
deployment, 137
descriptive analytics, 126
descriptive research, 13–14
descriptive statistics, 171, 247–253
absolute risk reduction (ARR), 252
analysis of variance (ANOVA), 253
box-and-whisker plots, 176
confidence interval (CI), 251
negative predictive value (NPV), 249
odds ratio (OR), 251–252
positive predictive value (PPV), 249
purposes of, 171
receiver operating characteristic (ROC) curves, 249–250
relative risk reduction (RRR), 252–253
relative risk (RR) ratios, 252–253
sensitivity, specificity, and predictive values, 247–249
stem-and-leaf diagrams, 176
development of a research question, 193
FINER, 193
process of, 194
quantitative process, 194
qualitative process, 194
sources of questions, 194
diagnostic trials, 101
direct observation, 55
disclosure, 304
discrete data, 166
discriminant (divergent) validity, 220
dissemination of information, 315
formats for, 316–327
distributed computing, 130

distribution of survey, 45–46
distribution-free tests, 170
dose-response relationship, 104
dual-eligible beneficiaries, 242

effect sizes, 253
electronic health record (EHR), 25, 57, 74, 130, 143, 217, 274, 286
  example of sample size, 46–48
  physician-patient encounters and, 65
elicitation, 228–229
eligibility criteria, 277
e-mail survey, 45
empiricism, 9
entity relationship diagram (ERD), 128
environment, 102
epidemiological models of causation, 102
  chronic disease model, 102
  infectious disease model, 102
  uses, 103
epidemiological study designs, 87
  analytic, 90
  descriptive, 87
  experimental, 99
epidemiologists, 85
epidemiology, 85–86
  effectiveness in eradicating disease, 86–87
  epidemiological study designs, 87–102
  health informatics and, 86–87
EQUATOR, 323
error rate, 136
ethical climate for research, 307
Ethical, Legal, Social Implications (ELSI) program, 292
ethics in research, 290. *See also* international protection of human research subjects
  approaches to, 290–292
  autonomy, 292–293
  beneficence, 293
  caring, 293–294
  codes of, 296–297
  fidelity, 294
  honesty, 294–295
  importance of, 290
  informed consent, 292–293
  justice, 295–296
  local-level ethical research guidelines and procedures, 306–307
  nonmaleficence, 296
  principles in biomedical research, 292–296
  sanctity, 296
  utility, 296
ethnography, 18–19, 63
evaluation data collection, 117
evaluation methods, 109
evaluation plan, 110
  evaluation data collection and activities, 117–118
  evaluation questions, 117
  theory of change, 116
evaluation research, 20–23, 112
  evaluation projects *vs*, 111–112
  evaluation resources in health informatics, 119
  examples of, 118–119
  identifying a theoretic framework, 112–113
  identifying scientific gaps, 112
  scientific gaps, 112
  theoretic framework, 112
evidence-based medications, 110
evidence for causality rules, 104
exempt from review, 300
expedited review, 301
experimental (study) group, 23
experimental procedures, 81
experimental research, 16, 23–25, 71–72
experimental research study design, 72, 75, 99–102
  control group, 74
  clinical and community trial protocols, 100
  clinical and community trial applications in health informatics, 101
  crossover design, 73
  observation, 73
  pretests and posttests, 73–74
  randomization, 72–73
  summary, 75
  treatments or interventions, 74
experimental study design types, 74–77
  posttest-only control group method, 75
  pretest-posttest control group method, 75
  Solomon four-group method, 76
  experimental (study) group, 23
explanatory studies. *See* descriptive research
exploratory data analysis (EDA), 130
ex post facto research, 25
external validity, 72, 79–82, 214–215
  factors affecting, 81

face page, 279
face validity, 42
factor analysis, 43
factors in selecting a statistical test, 167
  purpose of the research, 169
  type of variable, 169
  number of variables, 169

nature of the target population, 169
number, size, and independence of groups, 170
false negatives (FN), 248
feasibility, 22
federal laws and regulations
American Recovery and Reinvestment Act (ARRA), 306
Belmont Report, 298–299
Ethical, Social, Legal Implications (ELSI) program, 292
Federal Food, Drug, and Cosmetic Act, 299
Genetic Information Nondiscrimination Act (GINA), 292
Health Information Technology for Economic and Clinical Health (HITECH) Act, 304–306
Health Insurance Portability and Accountability Act (HIPAA) of 1996, 229–230, 298, 304–306
Health Research Extension Act of 1985, 306
National Research Act of 1974, 298
Policy and Procedure Order 129, 298
support and training for researchers, 306
Federal Policy for the Protection of Human Subjects ("Common Rule"), 299–304
federal-wide assurance of compliance (FWA), 299
fidelity, 294
field notes, 63
FINER, 193
Fisher exact test, 180
fishing, 257
five rights of clinical decision support, 114
fixed-effects model, 155
focused interviews, 54, 58–62, 228
focus groups, 58
general interview guide, 58
informal conversational interview, 58
standardized open-ended interview, 58
forecasting, 135
forest plot, 155
formative evaluation, 111
implementation evaluation, 111
needs assessment, 111
process evaluation, 111
framing of questions, 43
frequency distribution, 171
bar chart, histogram, and other graphical displays, 174
nonnormal distributions, 172
normal distribution, 171
tables, 172
frequency measures, 177
ratios, 177
proportions, 177
full review, 301
full-information likelihood (FIML), 247
funding entity, 286
funding opportunity announcements (FOAs), 274
funnel plot, 153

Gelsinger case, 294
general interview guide, 54
general interview guide interviews, 58, 61
generalizability, 9
Genetic Information Nondiscrimination Act (GINA) of, 2008, 292
geospatial analysis, 130
Glass's delta (D), 253
goal-based and impact evaluation, 118
GRADE (Grading of Recommendations, Assessment, Development, and Evaluation) system, 153
grant, 273, 306
application criteria, 276–277
budgets, 278
federal funding, 276
format and submit documents, 277–278
minimum requirements for applications, 278–282
preparing to write, 274
review criteria, 282–283
revising proposals, 287
sections of, 279
seed money, 275
sources of, 275–276
state or local, 276
submission procedures, 278
writing a proposal, 276–282
grantee, 274
granting agency
key individuals in, 283–284
review process, 284–287
grant proposal review process, 284–287
confidentiality form, 285
conflict of interest form, 285
funding entity's decision, 286
panel assessment and ranking, 286
proposal reviewers, role of, 284–285
reasons for rejection of grant, 287
scoring and commenting on proposals, 285
graphical displays, 174
bar chart, 175
box-and-whisker plots, 176
histogram, 176
line graphs, 176
pie charts, 176
scatter graphs, 176
stem-and-leaf diagrams, 176

grey literature, 148, 154, 203, 205
grounded theory, 67, 259–260
  general interview guide, 54
  general interview guide interviews, 58, 61

hand search, 148
Health Belief Model (HBM), 113
health informatics, 216, 290
health informatics research
  clinical and community trial applications in, 101
  correlational research, 14–16
  defined, 4
  descriptive research, 13–14
  evaluation research, 20–23
  examples of hypothetical historical research investigations, 13
  experimental research, 23–25
  historical research, 12–13
  observational research, 16–19
  purposes of, 4–5
  quasi-experimental studies, 26
  reasons for using observational research, 19
  theories and models used in, 5–6
health information exchange (HIE), 73
health information exchange (HIE) systems, 135
health information management (HIM), 110, 216, 290, 315–316
  assessment of health information technology (HIT) workforce, 223
  elicitation techniques, use of, 229
  instruments used in, 227
  use of scale in, 226
health information management (HIM) research
  correlational research, 14–16
  defined, 4
  descriptive research, 13–14
  evaluation research, 20–23
  examples of hypothetical historical research investigations, 13
  experimental research, 23–25
  historical research, 12–13
  observational research, 16–19
  purposes of, 4–5
  quasi-experimental studies, 26
  reasons for using observational research, 19
  theories and models used in, 5–6
Health Information National Trends Survey (HINTS), 37
health information technology (HIT), 110, 143, 274
Health Information Technology for Economic and Clinical Health (HITECH) Act of 2009, 14, 22, 230, 304–306
Health Information Technology Research Center (HITRC), 22
Health Insurance Portability and Accountability Act (HIPAA) of 1996, 62, 74, 229–230, 298, 304–306
Health Research and Educational Trust (HRET), 214
Health Research Extension Act of 1985, 306
Health Resources and Services Administration (HRSA), 276
health services research, 20
health technology assessment (HTA), 20
healthcare leaders, 4
healthcare-acquired infections (HAIs), 124
Healthcare Information and Management Systems Society (HIMSS), 47
heterogeneity, 232, 257
historical-prospective study design, 90, 95–98
historical research, 12–13
Holmesburg Prison Studies, 295–296
homogeneity of variance, 170
honesty, 294–295
host, 102
human genome project (HGP), 290, 292
human immunodeficiency virus (HIV), 78
human radiation experiments, 293
human subjects committees, 234
hunting, 257
hypothesis, 197
  alternative hypothesis, 198
  null hypothesis, 198
  qualitative hypotheses, 197
  quantitative hypotheses, 197
  one-tailed hypothesis, 198
  two-tailed hypothesis, 198

impact evaluation, 111, 118–119
impact factor, 323
implementation science, 112
imputation, 247
IMRAD, 323
incentives, 44
incidence cases, 92
incidence rate, 93
independent one-sample *t*-test, 179
independent sample, 170
independent variables, 23, 24
independent-measures *t*-test 179
indirect costs, 283
indirect observation, 55
individual case study, 54, 57
individual or aggregate data, 229–230
inductive reasoning, 9–10

infectious disease model, 102
inferential statistics, 178, 253–257
  other tests and terms, 184
  paired *t*-test, 254
  parametric tests, 253
influential data mining methods, 256
informal conversation, 54
informal conversational interviews, 58
informed consent, 292–293, 302–304
innovation, 282
institutional assurance of compliance, 299
institutional case study, 54, 57–58
institutional ethics committees, 307
institutional review board (IRB), 44, 111, 300–302
instrumentation, 80
instruments, 216–227
  attributes of items in, 223–227
  categorical items in, 224–225
  factors in selecting, 222–227
  feasible logistics, 227
  in public domain, 227
  numerical items in, 224
  operational definitions, 222–223
  proprietary, 227
  purchasing, 227
  reliability of, 220–222
  satisfactory ratings for validity and reliability, 223
  scales, 225–226
  sources of, 216
  standardized categories in, 226
  structured, unstructured, and semistructured types of questions, 224
  style and format of, 223
  theoretical underpinning, 222
  used in health informatics and HIM, 227
  validity of, 216–220
intention-to-treat (ITT) analysis, 246
interaction of factors, 81
internal consistency reliability, 222
internal validity, 72, 79–82, 214–215
  attrition, 81
  history, 80
  instrumentation, 80
  maturation, 80
  nonrandom selection, 80
  statistical regression, 80
  testing, 80
International Classification of Diseases, Ninth Revision, Clinical Modification (ICD-9-CM), 62
International Classification of Diseases, 10th Revision, Clinical Modification (ICD-10-CM), 62, 90, 275, 281
International Classification of Diseases, 10th Revision, Procedure Classification System (ICD-10-PCS), 275, 281
international protection of human research subjects, 297. *See also* codes of ethics
  Declaration of Helsinki, 297
  Nuremburg Code, 297
interrater reliability, 220
interval data, 165
interval scale, 41
intervention, 71
intervention arm, 23. *See also* experimental group
interview survey, 228
intraclass correlation coefficient, 221
intrarater reliability, 220–221
introductory materials, 279–280
investigators, 274

Jewish Chronic Disease Hospital study, 290, 296
journal publication
  abstract, 319–320
  bias in, 326
  characteristics of composition, 321–322
  impact factor, 323
  manuscript title, 320–321
  reporting and submission guidelines, 323–325
  response to a journal's feedback, 327
  sections, 319
  selection of appropriate journal, 322–323
justice, 295–296

Kefauver-Harris Amendments (Public Law 87-781) to the Federal Food, Drug, and Cosmetic Act, 299
key personnel, 280
k-means clustering, 135
knowledge discovery in databases (KDD), 133
kurtosis, 172

letter of intent, 277
likelihood ratio (LR), 248–249
Likert scale, 226
limited data set (LDS), 127
linearity, 166
literature review, 142, 200
  development of, 208
  equitable coverage, 209
  organizational structure, 208
  pertinence, 209
  process of, 202
  progression, 208
  purposes of, 201

rapid reviews, 200
scoping systematic reviews, 200
style, 209
transparency, 208
logic model, 116
logistic regression, 134
longitudinal time frame, 26
long-term care facility (LTCF), 40

mail survey, 45
Mann-Whitney U Test, 179
manuscript, 319
market basket analysis, 136
matching requirements or cost-sharing rules, 278
maturation, 80
maximum likelihood estimation (MLE), 247
measures of central tendency, 177
mean, 177
median, 178
mode, 178
measures of dispersion, 178
interquartile range, 178
normality of distribution, 178
range, 178
standard deviation, 178
measures of effect, 250
medical record, 14
Medicare beneficiaries, 242
meta-analysis, 142
meta-regression, 155
metric data, 166
midtests, 74
missing at random (MAR), 247
missing completely at random (MCAR), 246
missing not at random (MNAR), 247
misuse of statistics, 184
confusing correlation with causation, 185
invalid statistics for ordinal data, 185
lying with statistics, 185
unit of analysis error, 185
mixed-methods research, 9
model, 7
modeling, 133
classification, 134
clustering, 135
decision tree, 134
regression, 134
monitoring of research trends, 275
mortality, 81
multinomial logistic regression, 134
multiple linear regression, 134
multiple logistic regression, 134
multiple regression, 183
multivariate, 183
multivariate analysis, 97–98
multivariate ANOVA (MANOVA), 254

National Center for Health Statistics (NCHS), 36
National Health Interview Survey (NHIS), 37
National Institute of Aging (NIA), 276
National Institute on Disability, Independent Living, and Rehabilitation Research (NIDILRR), 276
National Institutes of Health (NIH), 276
National Library of Medicine (NLM), 276
National Research Act of 1974, 298
National Survey of Family Growth (NSFG), 36
naturalistic approach, 9
naturalistic observation, 17, 55
negative (inverse) linear relationship (association), 15
negative likelihood ratio, 249
negative predictive value (NPV), 249
Newcastle-Ottawa scale (NOS), 153
nominal data, 165
nominal scale, 40
nonmaleficence, 296
nonparametric data, 166
nonparametric test, 170, 253
nonparticipant observation, 17, 55
direct observation, 55
indirect observation, 55
nonprobability sampling, 80
nonrandom (nonprobability) sampling, 231
nonrandom selection, 80–81
nonresponse bias, 36
normal (bell) curve, 171
NoSQL, 130
null hypothesis significance testing (NHST), 244–245
number needed to treat (NNT), 253
numerical data, 166
numerical items, 224
in instruments, 224
Nuremburg Code, 297
Nurses' Health Study, 26

observational research, 16–19, 53
observations, 228
observations in experimental research, 73–74
odds ratio (OR), 91, 251–252
Office for Civil Rights (OCR), 304
Office for Human Research Protections (OHRP), 299–300
Office of Research Integrity (ORI), 306
one-group pretest-posttest method, 77–79

one-shot case study, 77–78
one-way ANOVA, 181
one-way repeated measures ANOVA, 181, 254
open-ended (unstructured) questions, 39, 224
operational definition, 197
operationalize, 197
oral paper presentation, 316, 318–319
ordinal data, 165
ordinal scale, 40
outcome evaluation, 111, 119
outcomes research, 20
outcome variables. *See* criterion variables

P value, 97–98, 244–245, 251
paired *t*-Test, 180
panel of reviewers, 286
Papanicolaou (Pap) test, 248
papers, 317
parametric data, 166
parametric test, 170
parsimony, 6
participant observation, 17–18, 62
Pearson product-moment correlation coefficient, 182
peer review, 325–326
peer-reviewed journals, 323
peer-reviewed research, 275
permissions, 229
personal health record (PHR), 72, 134, 260
Perspectives in Health Information Management (PHIM), 325–326
p-hacking, 257
phases of clinical trials, 101
phone survey, 45
physical safeguards, 306
PICO(TS), 195–197
PICOS, 146
pilot studies, 234
pilot test, 37
pilot test survey, 42
Policy and Procedure Order 129, 298
population health, 214
  importance of research, 214
positive (direct) linear relationship (association), 15
positive likelihood ratio, 249
positivism, 9
poster presentation, 316–318
posttest-only control group method, 75, 76–77
posttests, 73–74, 76
power, 245, 257
precision, 251
predictive analytics, 126
predictive modeling, 133
predictor variables (predictors), 14
Preferred Reporting Items for Systematic Reviews and Meta-Analyses (PRISMA), 323
Preferred Reporting Items for Systematic Review and Meta-Analysis Protocols (PRISMA-P), 145
presentation
  oral paper, 316, 318–319
  poster, 316–318
  tabular and graphical displays, 263
presentation of results
  interpretation of results, 264
  narrative, 263–264
  results and discussion, 263–264
pretest-posttest control group method, 74–76
pretests, 73–74, 76
prevalence rate, 87
prevalence study. *See* cross-sectional study
prevarication bias, 36
prevention trials, 101
primary analysis, 255
primary care providers (PCPs), 114
primary data, 255
primary sources, 12
principal investigator (PI), 276, 286
Privacy Rule, 304–305
probability, 164
problem statement, 196
problem-solving inventory (PSI), 79
proceedings, 317
process evaluation, 111, 118
product information form, 59–60
program officer, 283–284
Promoting Action on Research Implementation in Health Services, (PARIHS) framework, 112
proposal reviewers, 284–285
proprietary instruments, 227
propriety, 22
prospective time frame, 26
PROSPERO, 146
protected health information (PHI), 305
protocol, 100
Public Health Institute (PHI), 214
publication bias, 153, 326
public-domain or proprietary data, 230
purpose statement, 199
purposive sampling, 231

qualitative analysis, 154
qualitative analytic software programs, 262
qualitative approach to research, 8–9

qualitative data, 166
qualitative data analysis, 214–215, 258–262
  conclusion validity, 261–262
  content analysis, 261
  grounded theory, 259–260
qualitative questions. *See* open-ended (unstructured) questions
quality appraisal, 152
quality-of-life (QOL) trials, 101
quantitative analysis, 154
quantitative analytic software programs, 258
quantitative approach to research, 8–9
quantitative data, 166
quantitative data analysis, 214–215
  addressing missing values, 246–247
  intention-to-treat (ITT) analysis, 246
  null hypothesis significance testing (NHST), 244–245
  power, 245
  preparation of data, 245–247
  significance level, 244–245
  statistical analysis plan (SAP), 243–244
  statistical significance *vs* practical significance, 244
  type I error and type II error, 245
  unit of analysis, 246
quantitative questions. *See* closed-ended (structured) questions
quasi-experimental research, 25–26, 72
quasi-experimental study design types, 77
  one-group pretest-posttest method, 77–79
  one-shot case study, 77–78
  static group comparison, 77, 79
  summary of, 78
Questionnaire for User Interaction Satisfaction (QUIS), 227
questionnaire surveys, 228
questions
  closed-ended (structured), 39
  evaluation, 117
  framing of, 43
  open-ended (unstructured), 39, 59, 61
  standardized open-ended, 59, 61
quota sampling, 231

random number generator, 231
random sampling, 23, 165, 231
random-effects model, 155
randomization, 23, 72
randomized controlled trial (RCT), 24–25, 142, 246
rater reliability, 220–221
ratio data, 165
ratio scale, 41, 176
reasoning, 9–10
recall bias, 36
receiver operator characteristic (ROC), 136
  receiver operating characteristic (ROC) curves, 249–250
refinement of the research question, 192
Regional Extension Center (REC) program, 22
regression, 134–135
relative difference, 253
relative odds, 250
relative risk (RR), 91, 93–94
  relative risk (RR) ratios, 252–253
relative risk reduction (RRR), 252–253
reliability, 43
reliability of instruments, 220–222, 257
  Cohen's kappa (κ) coefficient, 221
  internal consistency reliability, 222
  interrater reliability, 220
  intraclass correlation coefficient, 221
  intrarater reliability, 220–221
  rater reliability, 220–221
  test-retest reliability, 221–222
requests for applications (RFAs), 274, 277
requests for proposals (RFPs), 274
research, 4
research design, 10–26
  correlational research, 14–16
  descriptive research, 13–14
  evaluation research, 20–23
  experimental research, 23–25
  historical research, 12–13
  observational research, 16–19
  quasi-experimental research, 25–26
  time frame in, 26
research design and method
  factors in selecting, 215
  internal validity and external validity, 214–215
  purpose of selecting, 214
  regulators, 234
  selection of instruments, 216–227
research frame, 5
  theories and models, 5–8
research method, 8
research methodology, 8
research misconduct, 306
research plan, 280–281
research project websites, 328
research protocol, 145
research question, 144
respect for persons, 298
response bias, 233–234
response rate, 48, 233–234
retrospective time frame, 26
rich data, 16, 228

rigor, 10
risk of bias, 153
risk reduction statistics, 252
robust, 170

sample, 4, 230
sampling
  data, 230–231
  error, 231
  frame for, 231
  nonrandom (nonprobability), 231
  random, 231
sample size, 46, 230–233
  calculation, 46
sample call for proposals, 316
sanctity, 296
saturation, 228
scales, 225–226
  Likert, 226
  points in, 225
  semantic differential, 226
scientific inquiry, 9
  reasoning, 9–10
  rigor, 10
scientific review group (SRG), 284
scientific review officer (SRO), 284
screening process, 149
screening trials, 101
search and retrieval of information sources, 204
  bibliographic database, 204
  digital collections, 204
secondary analysis, 255
secondary data, 255
secondary sources, 12
Security Rule, 305
seed money, 275
selection bias, 48, 81
semantic differential scales, 226
semistructured interview, 118
semistructured questions, 224
sensitivity, 247–249
sensitivity analysis, 155, 254
sensitivity rates, 89
significance, 276
simple linear regression, 134
simple random sampling, 46, 231
  cluster sampling, 46, 231
  stratified random sampling, 46, 231
  systematic random sampling, 46
simple regression, 183
simulation observation, 17, 56
Sittig's and Singh's sociotechnical model, 7–8
skewness, 172
snooping, 257
snowball sampling, 231
sociotechnical system, 113
Software Usability Measurement Inventory (SUMI), 227
Solomon four-group method, 74, 76
sources of information, 202
  credibility of sources, 203
  grey literature, 203
  primary sources, 203
  secondary sources, 203
Spearman rank order correlation, 182, 254
specific aims, 100
specificity rates, 89
specificity, 247–249
stakeholders, 111
standardized categories, 226
standardized open-ended interview, 54, 58–61
standardized open-ended questions, 59, 61
static group comparison method, 77
statistical analysis, 49, 101
statistical analysis plan (SAP), 243–244
  data elements in, 243–244
  purpose of, 243
  statistical tests and criteria for significance, 243
statistical conclusion validity, 257–258
statistical regression, 80
statistical significance testing (SST), 244
statistical significance *vs* practical significance, 244
statistics, 163
stratified random sampling, 46, 231
streamlining, 284
strength of the association, 104
structured query language (SQL), 130
structured questions, 224. *See* closed-ended questions
subgroup analysis, 155
subject matter experts (SMEs), 38, 216–218
submission guidelines in journals, 324–325
summative evaluation, 110–111
  impact evaluation, 111
  supervised learning, 255
survey creation, 37–44
  audience, 43
  building a new questionnaire, 37–39
  confidential responses, 44
  framing of questions, 43
  incentives to survey participants, 44
  measurement scales, 40–41
  pilot survey, 42
  types of questions, 39
  using exisiting surveys, 37
  validity and reliability testing of, 42–43

survey questionnaire, 36, 45
survey research, 35–36
  by e-mail, mail, fax, and phone, 45
  census survey, 46
  exclusion criteria, 39
  group-administered surveys, 45
  inclusion criteria, 39
  limitations, bias, and error, 44
  medium and distribution of surveys, 44–46
  response rate, 48
  sample and sample size, 46–48
  statistical analysis of survey data, 49–50
  web-based survey, 44
surveys, 228
survival analysis, 101
systematic random sampling, 46
System Usability Scale (SUS), 115, 227
systematic review, 142
  exclusion criteria, 146
  final report, 157
  inclusion criteria, 146
  performing searches, 147
  quality appraisal and data analysis, 152
  research question, 144
  reviewing and extracting data, 151
  selecting articles, 149
  systematic review protocol, 145
  terms of the project, 146
  validity systematic sampling, 231
systematic sampling, 231

tabular and graphical displays, 263
target population, 165, 230, 279
team-based learning (TBL), 61
Tearoom Trade study, 292
technical safeguards, 306
technology acceptance model (TAM), 7
temporality, 104
testing, 80–81
testing of research instruments, 234
test-retest reliability, 43, 221–222
test-retest reliability coefficient, 43
theoretical sampling, 231
theory, 6
theory of change, 116
threats, 215
time-series tests, 74
training of investigators, 234
translational research, 8
traumatic brain injury (TBI), 79
treatments (intervention), 23, 24
treatment trials, 100
trend analysis, 135
triangulation, 17
true negative rate, 248
true positive rate, 248
true positives (TP), 248
t-test, 254
Tuskegee Study of Untreated Syphilis in the Negro Male, 290–292
two-way ANOVA, 254
type I error, 245, 248
type II error, 245, 248

unanticipated problems, 302
understanding, 303
unit of analysis, 246
univariate, 171
univariate association, 96
unstructured questions, 224. *See* open-ended questions
unsupervised learning, 255
usability testing, 21
user-centered design, 114
utility, 22, 296

validity
  concerns affecting, 81–82
  internal and external, 79–82
  for survey research, 42–43
validity of instruments, 216–220
  concurrent validity, 220
  construct validity, 219–220
  content validity, 217–219
  convergent validity, 219
  criterion validity, 220
  discriminant (divergent) validity, 220
  face validity, 216–217
variables, 14
  dependent, 23–24
  independent, 23–24
vendor interview form, 60
venous thromboembolism (VTE) research, 93
Vioxx case, 294–295
voluntariness, 303–304
vulnerable populations, 290, 299

warrant, 262
web-based surveys, 44–45
white paper, 328
Wilcoxon Signed-Rank Test, 180
Willowbrook hepatitis studies, 294